MOLECULAR PHARMACEUTICS AND NANO DRUG DELIVERY

MOLECULAR PHARMACEUTICS AND NANO DRUG DELIVERY

Fundamentals and Challenges

Edited by

UMESH GUPTA

Nanopolymeric Drug Delivery Lab, Department of Pharmacy, School of Chemical Sciences and Pharmacy, Central University of Rajasthan, Ajmer, Rajasthan, India

AMIT K. GOYAL

Department of Pharmacy, School of Chemical Sciences and Pharmacy, Central University of Rajasthan, Ajmer, Rajasthan, India

ELSEVIER

ACADEMIC PRESS

An imprint of Elsevier

Academic Press is an imprint of Elsevier
125 London Wall, London EC2Y 5AS, United Kingdom
525 B Street, Suite 1650, San Diego, CA 92101, United States
50 Hampshire Street, 5th Floor, Cambridge, MA 02139, United States
The Boulevard, Langford Lane, Kidlington, Oxford OX5 1GB, United Kingdom

ISBN: 978-0-323-91924-1

For Information on all Academic Press publications
visit our website at https://www.elsevier.com/books-and-journals

Publisher: Mica H. Haley
Acquisitions Editor: Andre G. Wolff
Editorial Project Manager: Gonzalez Pat
Production Project Manager: Jayadivya Saiprasad
Cover Designer: Rogers Mark

Typeset by MPS Limited, Chennai, India

Contents

List of contributors

Tuanny Leite Almeida Department of Biochemistry and Tissue Biology, Institute of Biology, University of Campinas (UNICAMP), Campinas, SP, Brazil

Sumel Ashique Department of Pharmaceutics, Pandaveswar School of Pharmacy, Pandaveswar, West Bengal, India

Sanya Batheja Nanopolymeric Drug Delivery Lab, Department of Pharmacy, School of Chemical Sciences and Pharmacy, Central University of Rajasthan, Ajmer, Rajasthan, India

Viviane Lucia Beraldo-de-Araújo Faculty of Pharmaceutical Sciences, University of Campinas (UNICAMP), Campinas, SP, Brazil

Prativa Biswasroy School of Pharmaceutical Science, Sikhsa "O" Anusandhan University, Bhubaneswar, Odisha, India

Akash Chaurasiya Translational Pharmaceutics Research Laboratory, Department of Pharmacy, Birla Institute of Technology and Science, Pilani, Hyderabad, Telangana, India

Juliana Souza Ribeiro Costa Faculty of Pharmaceutical Sciences, University of Campinas (UNICAMP), Campinas, SP, Brazil

Mariana Rodrigues Da Silva Department of Biochemistry and Tissue Biology, Institute of Biology, University of Campinas (UNICAMP), Campinas, SP, Brazil

Marcelo Bispo de Jesus Department of Biochemistry and Tissue Biology, Institute of Biology, University of Campinas (UNICAMP), Campinas, SP, Brazil

Laura de Oliveira-Nascimento Faculty of Pharmaceutical Sciences, University of Campinas (UNICAMP), Campinas, SP, Brazil

Sonu Gandhi DBT-National Institute of Animal Biotechnology (DBT-NIAB), Hyderabad, Telangana, India

Fernanda Garcia-Fossa Department of Biochemistry and Tissue Biology, Institute of Biology, University of Campinas (UNICAMP), Campinas, SP, Brazil

Ashish Garg Department of Pharmaceutics, Guru Ramdas Khalsa Institute of Science and Technology (Pharmacy), Jabalpur, Madhya Pradesh, India

Goutam Ghosh School of Pharmaceutical Science, Sikhsa "O" Anusandhan University, Bhubaneswar, Odisha, India

Amit K. Goyal Department of Pharmacy, School of Chemical Sciences and Pharmacy, Central University of Rajasthan, Ajmer, Rajasthan, India

Ujjwal Gupta Department of Pharmaceutics, National Institute of Pharmaceutical Education and Research, Raebareli, Uttar Pradesh, India

Umesh Gupta Nanopolymeric Drug Delivery Lab, Department of Pharmacy, School of Chemical Sciences and Pharmacy, Central University of Rajasthan, Ajmer, Rajasthan, India

Prathap Madeswara Guptha Amity Institute of Pharmacy, Amity University Madhya Pradesh (AUMP), Gwalior, Madhya Pradesh, India

Shaifali Gurjar Neuropsychopharmacology Division, Department of Pharmacy, Birla Institute of Technology and Science-Pilani Campus, Rajasthan, India

Jitu Haldar School of Pharmaceutical Science, Sikhsa "O" Anusandhan University, Bhubaneswar, Odisha, India

Afzal Hussain Department of Pharmaceutics, College of Pharmacy, King Saud University, Riyadh, Saudi Arabia

Keerti Jain Drug Delivery and Nanomedicine Research Laboratory, Department of Pharmaceutics, National Institute of Pharmaceutical Education and Research (NIPER)—Raebareli, Lucknow, Uttar Pradesh, India

Amin Janghorbani Department of Biotechnology, Faculty of New Sciences and Technologies, Semnan University, Semnan, Iran

Jovita Kanoujia Amity Institute of Pharmacy, Amity University Madhya Pradesh (AUMP), Gwalior, Madhya Pradesh, India

Biswakanth Kar School of Pharmaceutical Science, Sikhsa "O" Anusandhan University, Bhubaneswar, Odisha, India

Aadil Sk Khatik Nanopolymeric Drug Delivery Lab, Department of Pharmacy, School of Chemical Sciences and Pharmacy, Central University of Rajasthan, Ajmer, Rajasthan, India

Ameya Kothekar Neuropsychopharmacology Division, Department of Pharmacy, Birla Institute of Technology and Science-Pilani Campus, Rajasthan, India

Pramod Kumar Pulmonary Aerosol Delivery Group, Institute of Lung Health and Immunity (LHI), Helmholtz Zentrum, München, Bayern, Germany

Priyanka Kumari Department of Pharmacy, School of Chemical Sciences and Pharmacy, Central University of Rajasthan, Ajmer, Rajasthan, India

Satish Kurdhane Nanopolymeric Drug Delivery Lab, Department of Pharmacy, School of Chemical Sciences and Pharmacy, Central University of Rajasthan, Ajmer, Rajasthan, India

S. Mohana Lakshmi Amity Institute of Pharmacy, Amity University Madhya Pradesh (AUMP), Gwalior, Madhya Pradesh, India

Sabyasachi Maiti Department of Pharmacy, Indira Gandhi National Tribal University, Amarkantak, Madhya Pradesh, India

Akanksha Malaiya Nanomedicine and Bioengineering Research Laboratory, Department of Pharmacy, Indira Gandhi National Tribal University, Amarkantak, Madhya Pradesh, India

Farhan Mazahir Department of Pharmaceutics, National Institute of Pharmaceutical Education and Research, Raebareli, Uttar Pradesh, India

Elisabetta Mazzotta Department of Pharmacy, Health and Nutritional Sciences, University of Calabria, Rende, Italy

Ansit Mishra Neuropsychopharmacology Division, Department of Pharmacy, Birla Institute of Technology and Science-Pilani Campus, Rajasthan, India

Neeraj Mishra Amity Institute of Pharmacy, Amity University Madhya Pradesh (AUMP), Gwalior, Madhya Pradesh, India

Thaís Moraes-Lacerda Department of Biochemistry and Tissue Biology, Institute of Biology, University of Campinas (UNICAMP), Campinas, SP, Brazil

Rita Muzzalupo Department of Pharmacy, Health and Nutritional Sciences, University of Calabria, Rende, Italy

Priyamvada Nair Neuropsychopharmacology Division, Department of Pharmacy, Birla Institute of Technology and Science-Pilani Campus, Rajasthan, India

Gautami Nirbhavane Drug Delivery and Nanomedicine Research Laboratory, Department of Pharmaceutics, National Institute of Pharmaceutical Education and Research (NIPER)—Raebareli, Lucknow, Uttar Pradesh, India

Laura de Oliveira-Nascimento Faculty of Pharmaceutical Sciences, University of Campinas (UNICAMP), Campinas, SP, Brazil

Rishi Paliwal Nanomedicine and Bioengineering Research Laboratory, Department of Pharmacy, Indira Gandhi National Tribal University, Amarkantak, Madhya Pradesh, India

Shivani Rai Paliwal Department of Pharmacy, Guru Ghasidas Vishwavidhyalaya (A Central University), Bilaspur, Chhattisgarh, India

Kanan Panchal Translational Pharmaceutics Research Laboratory, Department of Pharmacy, Birla Institute of Technology and Science, Pilani, Hyderabad, Telangana, India

Anchal Pathak Drug Delivery and Nanomedicine Research Laboratory, Department of Pharmaceutics, National Institute of Pharmaceutical Education and Research (NIPER)—Raebareli, Lucknow, Uttar Pradesh, India

Gajanan Paul Department of Pharmaceutics, National Institute of Pharmaceutical Education and Research, Raebareli, Uttar Pradesh, India

Rafaella Mascarelli Pereira Department of Biochemistry and Tissue Biology, Institute of Biology, University of Campinas (UNICAMP), Campinas, SP, Brazil

Deepak Pradhan School of Pharmaceutical Science, Sikhsa "O" Anusandhan University, Bhubaneswar, Odisha, India

Drishya Prakashan DBT-National Institute of Animal Biotechnology (DBT-NIAB), Hyderabad, Telangana, India

Vineet Kumar Rai School of Pharmaceutical Science, Sikhsa "O" Anusandhan University, Bhubaneswar, Odisha, India

Tushar Kanti Rajwar School of Pharmaceutical Science, Sikhsa "O" Anusandhan University, Bhubaneswar, Odisha, India

Goutam Rath School of Pharmaceutical Science, Sikhsa "O" Anusandhan University, Bhubaneswar, Odisha, India

Martina Romeo Department of Pharmacy, Health and Nutritional Sciences, University of Calabria, Rende, Italy

Garima Sahu Department of Pharmacy, School of Chemical Sciences and Pharmacy, Central University of Rajasthan, Ajmer, Rajasthan, India

Hinal Shah Department of Pharmaceutics, National Institute of Pharmaceutical Education and Research, Raebareli, Uttar Pradesh, India

Deepshikha Shahdeo DBT-National Institute of Animal Biotechnology (DBT-NIAB), Hyderabad, Telangana, India

Sonali Singh Translational Pharmaceutics Research Laboratory, Department of Pharmacy, Birla Institute of Technology and Science, Pilani, Hyderabad, Telangana, India

Victória Soares Soeiro Faculty of Pharmaceutical Sciences, University of Campinas (UNICAMP), Campinas, SP, Brazil

Rajesh Sukhija Neuropsychopharmacology Division, Department of Pharmacy, Birla Institute of Technology and Science-Pilani Campus, Rajasthan, India

Kunjbihari Sulakhiya Neuro Pharmacology Research Laboratory, Department of Pharmacy, Indira Gandhi National Tribal University, Amarkantak, Madhya Pradesh, India

Teeja Suthar Drug Delivery and Nanomedicine Research Laboratory, Department of Pharmaceutics, National Institute of Pharmaceutical Education and Research (NIPER)—Raebareli, Lucknow, Uttar Pradesh, India

Rajeev Taliyan Neuropsychopharmacology Division, Department of Pharmacy, Birla Institute of Technology and Science-Pilani Campus, Rajasthan, India

Marcelo Van Vliet Lima Faculty of Pharmaceutical Sciences, University of Campinas (UNICAMP), Campinas, SP, Brazil

A.K. Yadav Department of Pharmaceutics, National Institute of Pharmaceutical Education and Research, Raebareli, Uttar Pradesh, India

Fatemeh Yazdian Department of Life Science Engineering, Faculty of New Sciences and Technologies, University of Tehran, Tehran, Iran

Preface

Molecular pharmaceutics deals with the science of dosage forms and formulation design. It is the major area of pharmaceutical sciences, which focuses and emphasizes on the technological aspects of how a new chemical entity is converted into a suitable dosage form and subsequent formulation. Traditionally, the tablets, capsules, syrup, solutions, and ointments were the most popular dosage forms for delivering drugs to patients for different ailments. However, in the last few decades, the introduction of novel dosage forms has completely shifted the traditional paradigm of drug delivery technologies. The so-called "novel drug delivery systems" are numerous, and each has different approaches with respect to their production, characterization, and evaluation. Some of these are at the laboratory levels, while some of these have successfully made their way into the market. A proper understanding of these dosage forms as well as their critical attributes such as toxicity and regulatory requirements are some of the aspects which researchers should know before starting to work on these carriers. Individual literature is available at discrete levels for each of these novel drug carriers such as liposomes, nanoparticles, niosomes, phytosomes, dendrimers, quantum dots, and carbon nanotubes. This book is an attempt to provide fundamental information to readers, from a beginner to an established scientist, on the key challenges of these carriers at the molecular level. This book satisfies the need for availability of literature in a single platform with the detailed knowledge to understand the crucial aspects such as regulatory, clinical, toxicological, and formulation requirement of these carriers. This book will help the readers to design and develop novel drug delivery systems and devices for the treatment of different disorders by taking advantage of recent advances in nanomedical technologies.

This book is a fair attempt to address the basic aspects of molecular pharmaceutics as well as nano drug delivery through different chapters. This book comprises 14 chapters: Protein and Enzyme-Based Formulations; Vaccine and Sera; Aptamers and Antisense Oligonucleotide-Based Delivery; Monoclonal Antibodies: Recent Development in Drug Delivery; Hormonal Delivery Systems; Vesicular Drug Delivery Systems: a Novel Approach in Current Nanotherapies; Polymeric Micelles in Drug Delivery and Targeting; Physicochemical Characterization of Drug Delivery Systems Based on Nanomaterials; Inorganic and Metal-based Nanoparticles; Dendrimers: Promises and Challenges in Drug Delivery; Development of the Different Advanced Diagnostic Platform for Detection of Infectious Diseases; Fundamentals of a Targeted Drug Delivery System; Toxicological and Regulatory Aspects of Nanomaterials: Recent Updates; and Gene Therapy: Advocacies, Perspectives, and Ethical Provocations.

Umesh Gupta
Amit K. Goyal

CHAPTER

1

Protein and enzyme-based nanoformulations

Biswakanth Kar, Deepak Pradhan, Prativa Biswasroy, Jitu Haldar, Tushar Kanti Rajwar, Vineet Kumar Rai, Goutam Ghosh and Goutam Rath

School of Pharmaceutical Science, Sikhsa "O" Anusandhan University, Bhubaneswar, Odisha, India

1.1 Introduction

In several biological processes, such as catalysis, transport, gene expression control, immunity-related activities, and so forth, proteins and enzymes are essential. Additionally, they play a role in various clinical disorders, including "cancer, diabetes, and hypertension" [1]. Proteins are desirable therapeutic agents for treating many diseases due to their wide variety of functions and their involvement in diseases. "The first commercially available recombinant therapeutic protein was human insulin, which was approved by the US Food and Drug Administration (FDA) in 1982" [2]. Since then, it has replaced other treatments as the primary option for those with type I and types II diabetes. There are currently more than 100 authorized peptide-based medications on the market [3]. The market for protein and peptide pharmaceuticals is expanding significantly more quickly than for small molecule pharmaceuticals. "Notably, since the approval of Muromonab-CD3 in 1986, monoclonal antibodies (mAbs) have represented a promising area of protein therapy research." One of the most exciting developments in cancer immunotherapy is the recent clinical validation of immune checkpoint mAbs that target the programmed death-1 (PD-1) receptor, such as Nivolumab and Pembrolizumab [4]. Compared to small-molecule drugs, these therapies have several benefits, including high potency, activity, reduced unspecific binding, decreased toxicity, minimal drug–drug interactions, and biological and chemical diversity. However, proteins' physicochemical characteristics make their application as medications challenging. First, oral administration of proteins and peptides

Molecular Pharmaceutics and Nano Drug Delivery
DOI: https://doi.org/10.1016/B978-0-323-91924-1.00011-3

is unsuitable due to their instability in the gastrointestinal tract. Its usefulness is constrained by physical and chemical degradation, a short in vivo circulation half-life and biodistribution, and the lack of an effective, secure, and targeted administration mechanism. Their ability to penetrate cell membranes and be cleared by mononuclear phagocytes of the reticuloendothelial system, as well as the possibility of an immunogenic reaction, solubility problems, high molecular weight, and structural complexity, all reduce the effectiveness of their treatments. Therefore, to achieve high therapeutic efficacy, it is necessary to establish appropriate delivery platforms for proteins and enzymes [5]. Over the past few decades, significant research has been conducted to develop protein and peptide delivery systems that get around the issues outlined above. Numerous methods have been used to achieve this goal, including mucoadhesive polymers, enzyme inhibitors, absorption enhancers, nanoparticle carriers, and chemically altering protein or peptide structures. Among these, nanocarrier systems demonstrated a tremendous application for the delivery of proteins. Particularly, nanoparticles with sizes typically between 10 and 30 nm, including liposomes, micelles, polymer nanoparticles, and inorganic nanomaterials, have significant benefits as drug carriers [6]. Generally, nanoparticles aggregate to reduce surface energy. After being systemically delivered, these aggregates and the surface properties of the particles, such as charge and hydrophobicity, can lead to opsonization in the blood, which increases the visibility of nanoparticles to biological defense systems like the mononuclear phagocyte system and exposes them to removal from circulation by defense cells, significantly reducing their effectiveness [7]. For example, "Wu et al., in 2014, prepared LGA–polycation nanoparticles for encapsulation and delivery of protein bioactive for sustained release of proteins while maintaining protein bioactivity. They reported that nanoconjugate systems effectively interact with proteins with high protein loading (20–40 wt.%)" [8]. The nanotherapeutic approach enhanced the circulation half-life, biodistribution, and targeted delivery of intracellular-acting protein. Kim and a coworker developed a nano composed of lipid and apolipoprotein for targeted delivery to the lung cancer cell. The resulting nanocomposite with a particle size of 20–30 nm showed 64%–75% loading efficiency and exhibited significant apoptosis in H460 cells [9]. Numerous nanomedicines for protein delivery have already received clinical approval, and many more are undergoing clinical trials. For example, the FDA approved pegaptanib in 2004 [10], an RNA oligonucleotide aptamer that specifically binds to the angiogenic vascular endothelial growth factor protein. After a year, the FDA approved Abraxane1, an albumin-bound nanoparticle formulation of paclitaxel that boosts albumin delivery to tumor cells by encouraging receptor-mediated trans-cytosis. This chapter provides a brief overview of the nanocarrier systems for the transport of proteins and enzymes and emphasizes the benefits of their use in enhancing functionality. We also go over the numerous difficulties with protein delivery.

1.2 Challenges associated with protein and enzymes delivery

Proteins and peptides are the preferred drugs for treating a variety of disorders due to their powerful and efficient actions. Protein delivery research priorities include creating appropriate target-specific protein carriers and stabilizing proteins in delivery devices.

Due to its fragility, complexity, higher molecular weight, protein denaturation, and changing spatial properties, the distribution of proteinaceous drugs has presented significant challenges for pharmaceutical and biomedical research. The success of developing carrier systems hinges on their capacity to preserve protein activity and structure during the development process, throughout delivery to the targeted region, and during long-term storage [11]. Improved protein stability is required for the delivery of therapeutic proteins. Despite significant advancements in the mass production of therapeutic proteins, it is still difficult to deliver these medications to the body in a way that is both practical and efficient. The challenges that proteins and peptides face by different routes of administration are summarized in Table 1.1. Although the oral route for the delivery of therapeutic peptide and protein therapeutics has been studied for decades, additional routes, including the nasal, pulmonary, ophthalmic, buccal, and transdermal routes, are also being investigated today [12].

Additionally, an intriguing membrane that limits the majority of hydrophilic molecules is the blood–brain barrier. Endothelial cells that surround the brain capillaries provide this barrier, which is supported by numerous cells such as pericytes, astrocytes, and microglial cells. This barrier's function is to protect the brain from harmful substances, germs, and toxins, while maintaining the brain's homeostasis [13]. For this purpose, the cerebral endothelium is outfitted with very tight junctions that significantly restrict the movement of water and polar solutes across the membrane, as well as highly effective efflux systems made up primarily of organic anion transporters and transporters from the

TABLE 1.1 Challenges that proteins and peptides face by different routes of administration.

Route of administration	Challenge offered by the route of administration
Ocular	• Tear turnover • Low patient compliance • Corneal irritation possible • Chance of degradation by protease enzyme • Extensive protein binding
Oral	• Extreme pH condition • Restricted absorption of the larger molecules • Epithelial cell barrier-based protease degradation • Kidney filters small molecules and rapidly leaves them in urine • Insoluble molecules may cause aggregation in the kidneys • Larger molecules are metabolized extensively by the liver proteolytic enzymes
Nasal	• Epithelial cell barrier-based protease degradation • Prone to alveolar macrophages • Limits on the higher dose of the protein • Extremely rapid rate of absorption
Buccal	• Lack of drug retention for a long duration • Oxidases, reductases, cyclooxygenases, and peptidases metabolize the protein drugs
Subcutaneous	• Nearly 80% of the dose is lost • Protease and macrophage degradation • Limited surface is for absorption • Depot injections may get precipitated at the injection site
Intravenous	• The immune system produces immunogenicity

ATP binding cassette (ABC transporters) (OAT). The LRP1, transferrin, insulin, and amino acid receptors or transporters are a few examples of transporters that are used to move necessary substances across the blood–brain barrier. Some substrates can also be transported into the brain by OAT. However, the majority of therapeutic medicines, particularly macromolecules, cannot enter the brain through the bloodstream, the aforementioned transporter systems virtually always reject lipophilic compounds, and tight junctions prevent the transport of hydrophilic chemicals [14]. As per "Galliani et al., in 2018, the systemic administration of proteins and large molecules suffers from degradation majorly, poor biodistribution, and inability to cross most biological barriers that severely affect the efficacy of protein and enzyme replacement therapies for many diseases, in particular for those involving the central nervous system" [15].

1.3 Nanocarrier system for protein and enzyme delivery

The use of proteins as therapeutics has increased in the healthcare industry to treat several disease conditions because it helps to create potentially specialized medicines. Instability, short half-life, and immunogenicity frequently limit their safety and effectiveness. Nanocarriers have the potential to improve protein delivery as therapeutics. The nanotherapeutic approach can overcome these limitations by increasing the systemic circulation half-life of protein, by protecting proteins from premature degradation, denaturation, and release. Additionally, nanotechnology helps targeted delivery of proteins with controlled or sustained release [16].

1.3.1 Polymeric nanocarrier system

Protein–polymer conjugates have been shown to have a unique combination of characteristics from both materials (i.e., the protein and the polymer), which can be individually modified to produce acceptable effects as a treatment strategy. Several works have been done for protein delivery through a nanotherapeutic approach. For example, Rebekah et al. prepared a magnetic nanoparticle-decorated graphene oxide-chitosan composite as an efficient nanocarrier for bovine serum albumin (BSA) delivery and studied its activity and stability performance. The result showed enhanced drug loading and better release profile compared to the free drug. Also, the nanocomposite protects the protein from enzymatic degradation [17]. Protein transportation through nanocarriers has been used in different disease conditions. "Zhang and colleagues developed a zwitterionic chitosan-based nanocarrier for the pulmonary delivery of therapeutic proteins for treating pulmonary lungs. The ionic gelation method was used to load the antifibrosis therapeutic protein (msFGFR2c), into a zwitterionic nanocomplex. Results showed after orotracheal administration, the nanocombination can inhibit the transforming growth factor beta 1-induced α-smooth muscle actin expression, responsible for fibroblasts, while the naked protein showed poor efficacy" [18]. In another study, Xie and group developed a customized nanocarrier for interleukin 10 plasmid (pIL-10) delivery. The novel carrier improved muscle repair outcomes and biocompatibility in several acute muscle damage mouse models.

The novel carrier had the potential for safe nuclear acid delivery in vivo to treat numerous muscle disorders [19]. Nanocarrier systems also help to deliver protein biomolecules through the oral route. Lee and coworkers developed a "zonula occludins toxin-derived peptide and chitosan-functionalized pluronic-based nanocarrier for enhanced transepithelial transport of insulin orally, both in vitro and in vivo." For effective oral delivery of insulin, the protein must be shielded from gastric and enzymatic destruction, allowed to persist on the intestinal surface for an extended period to improve protein absorption, and successfully penetrated through the tight epithelial junction. Only chitosan functionalization can boost the mucoadhesive property of the nanocarriers in the small intestine, but it is unable to go beyond the small intestine wall's absorption barrier. Contrarily, dual functionalization with chitosan and peptide permitted extended small intestine residence as well as efficient junction penetration. As a result, the synergistic effect of the dual targeting of nanocarrier showed the largest reduction in blood sugar level after 12 hours of oral administration [20].

1.3.2 Lipidic nanocarrier system

"Fatty acids, fatty alcohols, phospholipids, long and medium-chain monoglycerides, diglycerides, and triglycerides are among the natural, semisynthetic, or synthetic lipids utilized to create lipid-based nanoparticles." Dietary fats or oils are used to make the majority of lipid excipients. Because of their biocompatibility, biodegradability, low toxicity, and ability to pass through a variety of biological barriers (including digestive fluids, mucus layer, and intestinal epithelium), lipid nanoparticles are thought to be a promising protein delivery technique [21].

Csiszar and coworkers developed fusogenic liposomes for intracellular protein delivery ranging in size from 2.3 to 240 kDa (R-phycoerythrin). In general, interactions between proteins or peptides and liposomal components like lipids, surfactants, polymers, or inorganic compounds have a significant impact on how well they are encapsulated and how quickly they are released. These elements, which are connected on the liposomal surface, may improve the stability of nanocarriers, regulate the drug release period, and encourage protein distribution at the desired location [22].

It has been discovered that programmable cell death is dysregulated in a number of diseases, and the ability of cells to evade it is a defining characteristic of cancer. The mitochondrion is a strong candidate for anticancer treatment in this case. The essential outer mitochondrial membrane (OMM) component voltage-dependent anion channel (VDAC) regulates connections and communication between mitochondria and other cell compartments. Liguori and coworkers described an optimized cell-free production of a pivotal protein (VDAC), directly into liposomes for integration with biomimetic membrane systems. A supported lipid bilayer membrane that enables electrical evaluations of the ionic conductance of integrated membrane proteins was combined with a cell-free expression method to construct a functioning VDAC. The main benefit is in the analysis of the pure VDAC protein's properties to identify particular impacts to support, examine, and comprehend the various membrane pathways that VDAC affects in the cell. Additionally, because membrane proteins are a main target for therapeutic drugs, we can increase the number of transporters, channels, and exchanger proteins created by cell-free methodologies so they can be integrated into the connected membrane for the creation of biomimetic tools like biosensors or diagnostic tools [23].

There has been a lot of interest in the targeted intracellular delivery of medicines to boost biological activity during the past few decades. There are many different kinds of biomaterials, and it is well known that employing them to treat serious diseases has advanced significantly. Protein-based therapeutic materials are widely used for the treatment of a variety of illnesses like cancer, diabetes, and inflammatory diseases in the medical industry. By altering liposomes by adding hydrophobic polyampholytes within, Matsumura et al. created a novel protein delivery carrier. The adsorption and internalization of protein-incorporated polyampholyte liposomes were improved after freezing compared to that seen in unfrozen complexes, according to flow cytometry and microscopic examination. Studies on inhibition showed that polyampholyte-modified and unmodified liposomes have different internalization mechanisms. Additionally, polyampholyte-modified liposomes demonstrated high efficiency in promoting endosomal escape to improve protein transport to the cytoplasm with minimal damage [24].

Another type of lipidic nanocarrier is solid lipid nanoparticles (SLNs), which have been considered as a promising technology for delivering genes and proteins due to their exceptional biodegradability and biocompatibility, ability to perform a specific function through the appropriate chemical modification, and speedy uptake by cells [25].

Oral administration of insulin as a noninvasive treatment for diabetes mellitus is currently impractical because of its high molecular weight and lack of lipophilicity, as well as its quick enzymatic deterioration in the stomach, slight decrease and metabolism by enzymes in the intestinal lumen, and poor permeability throughout the intestinal epithelium. Oral insulin, however, has an advantage over endogenous insulin, in that it is transported to the liver, which is where it works most effectively via portal circulation. Zahang and group "designed and characterized SLNs of insulin, modified with stearic acid−octaarginine (SA-R8), to improve the stability and bioavailability for oral administration. According to the result, SLNs and SA-R8 were able to partially shield insulin from proteolysis in an in vitro enzyme degradation experiment." The prepared SLNs boosted Caco-2 cell internalization up to 18.44 times the normal insulin solution. In vivo tests on diabetic rats revealed a significant hypoglycemic impact compared to controls with prepared SLNs. These findings showed that SA-R8-modified SLNs facilitate the absorption of insulin orally [26].

The challenge of enhancing protein therapeutic bioavailability persists despite the recent focus on oral protein delivery. The gastrointestinal enzymatic barrier and the absorption barrier, which are composed of mucus layer and intestinal epithelial cells, must be broken down in addition to the negative physicochemical effects of drugs. The salmon calcitonin-loaded SLNs are synthesized and characterized by Huang and colleagues using the affinity peptides "CSKSSDYQC (CSK) and CPP IRQRRRR (IRQ) for goblet cells." Studies conducted in vitro and in vivo revealed that the modified SLNs with peptides altered the internal accumulation of protein therapeutics on Caco-2/HT29-MTX co-cultured cells and penetration in excised rat duodenal mucosa. The protein can also be changed with functional ligands to improve the therapy of diseases, in addition to altering the lipids surface to improve the targeted protein delivery [27].

1.3.3 Inorganic nanocarrier systems

Proteins are biomacromolecules with therapeutic value, but due to large size and shape, protein molecules cannot penetrate the cell membrane. Inorganic nanoparticles have the potential to overcome the barriers associated with delivery of proteins and protein-based drugs to different cells [28]. Inorganic nanoparticles like metal nanoparticles, silica nanoparticles, graphene oxides, silica nanoparticles, magnetic nanoparticles, and so forth are used for delivery of protein molecules and protein-based drugs [29]. Recently, aquasomes have emerged as an efficient drug delivery system for proteins and peptides. Aquasomes are self-assembled nanostructures consisting of a spherical hydroxyapatite inner membrane and carbohydrate at the outer membrane, which absorb proteins and penetrate the cellular barriers [30]. Damera et al. showed that aquasomes are used as the intracellular delivery system for BSA along with hydrophobic drugs warfarin (War), Ibuprofen (Ibu), and Coumarin (C153). Experimental findings showed that ~30% of BSA released from the aquasomes after 120 hours in a sustained release manner. Also, it has been found that aquasomes-encapsulated BSA and hydrophobic drugs showed improved biocompatibility and low hemolytic activity [31]. Similarly, Omar et al. found that biodegradable Magnetic silica @Iron oxide nanovectors have potency to deliver large proteins (diameter above 15 nm). It has been found that prepared magnetic hybrid nanovectors are potential candidates to deliver large proteins (~534 kDa, HD~20 nm) inside the cancerous cells. Also, it has been reported that large-scale cavities of prepared nanovectors provide electrostatic immobilization to large proteins up to 23 wt.% [32]. Among various nanoparticles, quantum dots (QDs) have shown distinct benefits in bioimaging, biosensing, and drug delivery compared to any other nanoparticles due to their particular photostability and photochemical features, QDs, among other metallic nanoparticles. Dynamic processes, temperature, and QDs' size are the key determinants of their photochemical characteristics. Zhao and coworkers prepared a pH-activated charge-convertible QD as a novel nanocarrier for targeted protein delivery and cancer cell imaging. According to experimental findings, the complex provided legible real-time imaging for lung cancer cells and demonstrated improved internalization and quick endo/lysosomal escape. Additionally, the complex killed cancer cells more efficiently than the control groups did due to its pH-triggered charge-convertible ability [33] (Table 1.2).

TABLE 1.2 List of various nanoformulations based on therapeutic proteins and peptides.

Sl. No.	Proteins/enzymes	Nanoformulation	Outcomes	References
1	Interleukin 10 (IL10), erythropoietin, insulin, and human growth hormone.	Two-stage polymeric thermosponge nanoparticles incorporated with poly (D, L-lactide) as core material and Pluronic F127 as the outer polymer.	• It has been found that thermosponge nanoparticles induce the half-life of IL-10 and insulin up to 5.9-fold and 1.6-fold, respectively. • Also, it has been reported that thermosponge nanoparticles increased the in vivo efficacy of the protein molecules without affecting their biological activity.	[34]

(Continued)

TABLE 1.2 (Continued)

Sl. No.	Proteins/enzymes	Nanoformulation	Outcomes	References
2	Insulin	Ethyl palmitate and hydroxypropyl methyl cellulose acetate succinate lipid polymeric nanoparticles.	• Lipid polymeric nanoparticles incorporated with insulin have 80% increased efficiency as compared to the standard. • In vitro release assays showed 9% and 14% of insulin release at pH 1.2 and at pH 6.8 for 6 h in simulated gastrointestinal conditions.	[35]
3	Insulin	Alginate/dextran sulfate coated with a dual layer of chitosan and albumin.	• 70% of insulin is retained inside the nanoparticles in a simulated gastric environment. • Also, it has been reported that the prepared nanoparticles increased the interactions and permeability of insulin in intestinal cells.	[36]
4	BSA	Aquasomes	• BSA incorporated with hydrophobic drug coumarin (C153) released ~30% in 120 h, while those incorporated with warfarin and ibuprofen showed a release rate of ~80% in 50 h. • It has been reported that the aquasomes are a biocompatible delivery system for proteins and hydrophobic drugs.	[37]
5	Monoclonal antibody (mAb) 2C-5	Immunoliposomes	• It has been reported that prepared liposomes have 170–220 nm size (−13 to −20 mV) of zeta potential and (<0.2) polydispersity indices. • The prepared liposomes showed drug encapsulation efficiency ~150 μg/mL and ~210 μg/mL for salinomycin and paclitaxel respectively in a ratio of 1:1.	[38]
6	Programmed death-ligand 1 (PD-L1) monoclonal antibody	Polyethylene glycol-poly (ε-caprolactone) nanoparticles	• It has been found that docetaxel-loaded polyethylene glycol-poly (ε-caprolactone) nanoparticles induce the mortality rate of tumor cell up to 65% and also induce cell apoptosis. • The author has found that polyethylene glycol-poly (ε-caprolactone) nanoparticles with monoclonal antibody have less side effects and increased synergistic effects against cancer cells.	[39]
7	Concanavalin A.	Cisplatin complexed gelatin (CG) nanoparticles	• The author investigated that CG nanoparticles incorporated with concanavalin A, that is, CCG nanoparticles at low concentration 1 μg/mL and 5 μg/mL increased the early apoptosis up to 21.3% and late apoptosis up to 60.6%. • Also, it has been found that at high concentration 10 μg/mL prepared nanoparticles showed late apoptosis up to 91.8%.	[40]

(Continued)

TABLE 1.2 (Continued)

Sl. No.	Proteins/enzymes	Nanoformulation	Outcomes	References
			• It has been concluded that the prepared nanoparticles are highly biocompatible, coherent in mannose receptor-mediated cellular uptake, thus effective in treatment of lung cancer.	
8	Ovalbumin	Dextran sulfate and ε-poly-lysine nanogel.	• It has been found that prepared nanogel eliminates 43% ovalbumin within 72 h, with enhanced immune response.	[41]
9	Insulin	Solid lipid nanoparticles.	• Experimental investigation showed that bipolymeric encapsulation of insulin improved the chemical stability and entrapment efficiency of insulin by 2.5-fold. • The author also found that the encapsulation of insulin by the bipolymeric nanoparticles avoids degradation of insulin inside a gastrointestinal environment.	[42]
10	Cytokines (interleukin-10) IL-10	Pluronic-based nanocarriers (NCs)	• It has been found that intravenous administration of encapsulated IL-10 has more efficacy as compared to the free IL-10. • The result indicated that NC-encapsulated IL10 showed more therapeutic activity both in vivo and in vitro.	[43]
11	Interleukin-10	Poly lactic acid–polyethylene glycol nanoparticles	• Experimental investigation showed that encapsulated IL-10 has prolonged release up to 60 days with an encapsulation efficiency of ~77%.	[44]
12	Urokinase	Cyclic arginyl-glycyl-aspartic acid (cRGD) liposomes	• It has been found that 60% of urokinase is released within 5 h from the cRGD liposomes. • The author has concluded that urokinase encapsulated within cRGD liposomes is effective in treatment of thrombolysis as compared to free urokinase.	[45]
13	Insulin	Poly (anhydride) thiamine conjugated zein nanoparticles	• It has been found that the prepared nanoparticles release insulin up to 4 h after administration in serum and have 5.2% of relative bioavailability as compared to standard formulation of insulin.	[46]

1.4 Conclusion

There are numerous uses for nanoparticles in both industry and medicine. They can be utilized as medicines or as carriers of therapeutic compounds depending on their physical and chemical characteristics. Protein delivery through the use of nanocarriers might lessen undesired restrictions and lower the dosage of drug required to produce the desired therapeutic effect. In order to prevent the medicine from degrading, extend its time in the body, and lessen its toxic effects, protein pharmaceuticals and other therapeutic compounds are combined to form nanoparticle conjugates. Such a conjugation facilitates targeted delivery of the medicine to the cells, tissues, and organs where it is needed. Numerous nanoparticles are available, depending on how and where a targeted protein needs to be administered to humans. The administration and efficacy of therapeutic proteins could be enhanced by the use of nanoparticles as the protein delivery method. Nanoparticles can cross biological barriers like the blood–brain barrier and perform cellular functions as a result of their small size. Through accumulating in target tissues, nanoparticles enhance the efficiency and effectiveness of medications, lowering the required dose and minimizing adverse effects. Although protein therapies have also demonstrated remarkable potential for nanotechnology-based techniques, the clinical development of protein delivery systems using nanoparticles is still in its early phases, and there are still a number of obstacles to overcome. To retain the protein cargo characteristics and prevent batch-to-batch variability, drug encapsulation must first be carefully managed.

References

[1] Bruno BJ, Miller GD, Lim CS. Basics and recent advances in peptide and protein drug delivery Ther Deliv [Internet] 2013;4(11):1443–67. Nov [cited 2022 Oct 29]. Available from: https://www.future-science.com/doi/10.4155/tde.13.104.

[2] Mark Terry. First recombinant insulin marks 36th year of DNA technology [Internet] 2018;. Available from: https://www.biospace.com/article/first-recombinant-insulin-marks-36th-year-of-dna-technology/#:~:text=It's%20been%2036%20years%20since,using%20recombinant%20insulin%20DNA%20technology.

[3] Dimitrov DS. Therapeutic proteins In: Voynov V, Caravella JA, editors. Therapeutic proteins [Internet]. Totowa, NJ: Humana Press; 2012;1–26. [cited 2022 Oct 29]. Available from: http://link.springer.com/10.1007/978-1-61779-921-1_1.

[4] Jiang Y, Chen M, Nie H, Yuan Y. PD-1 and PD-L1 in cancer immunotherapy: clinical implications and future considerations Hum Vac Immunother [Internet] 2019;15(5):1111–22. May 4 [cited 2022 Oct 29]. Available from: https://www.tandfonline.com/doi/full/10.1080/21645515.2019.1571892.

[5] Varanko A, Saha S, Chilkoti A. Recent trends in protein and peptide-based biomaterials for advanced drug delivery Adv Drug Deliv Rev [Internet] 2020;156:133–87. [cited 2022 Oct 29]. Available from: https://linkinghub.elsevier.com/retrieve/pii/S0169409X20301198.

[6] Zhu Q, Chen Z, Paul PK, Lu Y, Wu W, Qi J. Oral delivery of proteins and peptides: Challenges, status quo and future perspectives Acta Pharm Sin B [Internet] 2021;11(8):2416–48. Aug [cited 2022 Oct 29]. Available from: https://linkinghub.elsevier.com/retrieve/pii/S2211383521001167.

[7] Gustafson HH, Holt-Casper D, Grainger DW, Ghandehari H. Nanoparticle uptake: the phagocyte problem Nano Today [Internet] 2015;10(4):487–510. Aug [cited 2022 Oct 29]. Available from: https://linkinghub.elsevier.com/retrieve/pii/S1748013215000766.

[8] Wu J, Kamaly N, Shi J, Zhao L, Xiao Z, Hollett G, et al. Development of multinuclear polymeric nanoparticles as robust protein nanocarriers Angew Chem Int Ed [Internet] 2014;53(34):8975–9. Aug 18 [cited 2022 Oct 29]. Available from: https://onlinelibrary.wiley.com/doi/10.1002/anie.201404766.

[9] Kim SK, Foote MB, Huang L. The targeted intracellular delivery of cytochrome C protein to tumors using lipid-apolipoprotein nanoparticles Biomater [Internet] 2012;33(15):3959–66. May [cited 2022 Oct 29]. Available from: https://linkinghub.elsevier.com/retrieve/pii/S0142961212001755.

[10] Stapleton M. Pegaptanib sodium. In: xPharm: the comprehensive pharmacology reference [Internet] 2010;1–8. Elsevier. [cited 2022 Oct 29]. Available from: https://linkinghub.elsevier.com/retrieve/pii/B9780080552323640826.

[11] Zaman R, Islam RA, Ibnat N, Othman I, Zaini A, Lee CY, et al. Current strategies in extending half-lives of therapeutic proteins J Contr Rel [Internet] 2019;301:176–89. May [cited 2022 Oct 29]. Available from: https://linkinghub.elsevier.com/retrieve/pii/S0168365919300914.

[12] Jain A, Jain A, Gulbake A, Shilpi S, Hurkat P, Jain SK. Peptide and protein delivery using new drug delivery systems Crit Rev Ther Drug Carr Syst [Internet] 2013;30(4):293–329. [cited 2022 Oct 29]. Available from: http://www.dl.begellhouse.com/journals/3667c4ae6e8fd136,38d647663ccd959a,6cf9a7241b969ee3.html.

[13] Gürsoy-Özdemir Y., Tas Y.C. Anatomy and physiology of the blood–brain barrier. In: Nanotechnology methods for neurological diseases and brain tumors [Internet] 2017;3–13. Elsevier. [cited 2022 Oct 29]. Available from: https://linkinghub.elsevier.com/retrieve/pii/B9780128037966000010.

[14] Tosi G, Duskey JT, Kreuter J. Nanoparticles as carriers for drug delivery of macromolecules across the blood-brain barrier Exp Opin Drug Deliv [Internet] 2020;17(1):23–32. Jan 2 [cited 2022 Oct 29]. Available from: https://www.tandfonline.com/doi/full/10.1080/17425247.2020.1698544.

[15] Galliani M, Santi M, Del Grosso A, Cecchettini A, Santorelli FM, Hofmann SL, et al. Cross-linked enzyme aggregates as versatile tool for enzyme delivery: application to polymeric nanoparticles Bioconjugate Chem [Internet] 2018;29(7):2225–31. Jul 18 [cited 2022 Oct 29]. Available from: https://pubs.acs.org/doi/10.1021/acs.bioconjchem.8b00206.

[16] Moncalvo F, Martinez Espinoza MI, Cellesi F. Nanosized delivery systems for therapeutic proteins: clinically validated technologies and advanced development strategies Front Bioeng Biotechnol [Internet] 2020;8:89. Feb 14 [cited 2022 Oct 29]. Available from: https://www.frontiersin.org/article/10.3389/fbioe.2020.00089/full.

[17] Rebekah A, Sivaselvam S, Viswanathan C, Prabhu D, Gautam R, Ponpandian N. Magnetic nanoparticle-decorated graphene oxide-chitosan composite as an efficient nanocarrier for protein delivery Colloids Surf A: Physicochem Eng Asp [Internet] 2021;610:125913. Feb [cited 2022 Oct 29]. Available from: https://linkinghub.elsevier.com/retrieve/pii/S0927775720315065.

[18] Zhang G, Mo S, Fang B, Zeng R, Wang J, Tu M, et al. Pulmonary delivery of therapeutic proteins based on zwitterionic chitosan-based nanocarriers for treatment on bleomycin-induced pulmonary fibrosis Int J Biol Macromol [Internet] 2019;133:58–133:66. Jul [cited 2022 Oct 29]. Available from: https://linkinghub.elsevier.com/retrieve/pii/S0141813019307822.

[19] Xie X, Jiang J, Liu X, Cao Y, Li J, Xia T, et al. Interleukin-10 plasmid delivery by polymeric nanocarrier shows efficient and safe tissue repair in acute muscle damage models in mice Nano Today [Internet] 2022;46:101544. Oct [cited 2022 Oct 29]. Available from: https://linkinghub.elsevier.com/retrieve/pii/S1748013222001724.

[20] Lee JH, Sahu A, Choi WI, Lee JY, Tae G. ZOT-derived peptide and chitosan functionalized nanocarrier for oral delivery of protein drug Biomater [Internet] 2016;103:160–9. Oct [cited 2022 Oct 29]. Available from: https://linkinghub.elsevier.com/retrieve/pii/S0142961216303192.

[21] Martins S, Sarmento B, Ferreira DC, Souto EB. Lipid-based colloidal carriers for peptide and protein delivery–liposomes versus lipid nanoparticles. Int J Nanomed 2007;2(4):595–607.

[22] Kube S, Hersch N, Naumovska E, Gensch T, Hendriks J, Franzen A, et al. Fusogenic liposomes as nanocarriers for the delivery of intracellular proteins Langmuir [Internet] 2017;33(4):1051–9. Jan 31 [cited 2022 Oct 29]. Available from: https://pubs.acs.org/doi/10.1021/acs.langmuir.6b04304.

[23] Liguori L, Stidder B, Alcaraz JP, Lenormand JL, Cinquin P, Martin DK. Cell-free production of VDAC directly into liposomes for integration with biomimetic membrane systems Prep Biochem Biotechnol [Internet] 2016;46(6):546–51. Aug 17 [cited 2022 Oct 29]. Available from: https://www.tandfonline.com/doi/full/10.1080/10826068.2015.1068800.

[24] Ahmed S, Fujita S, Matsumura K. Enhanced protein internalization and efficient endosomal escape using polyampholyte-modified liposomes and freeze concentration Nanoscale [Internet] 2016;8(35):15888–901. [cited 2022 Oct 29]. Available from: http://xlink.rsc.org/?DOI = C6NR03940E.

[25] Almeida A, Souto E. Solid lipid nanoparticles as a drug delivery system for peptides and proteins. Adv Drug Deliv Rev [Internet] 2007;59(6):478–90. Jul 10 [cited 2022 Oct 29]. Available from: https://linkinghub.elsevier.com/retrieve/pii/S0169409X07000439.

[26] Lv Hui-Xia H, Zhang ZH, Zhang Ylong, Wang X, Xu XR, Zhou JP, et al. Solid lipid nanoparticles modified with stearic acid–octaarginine for oral administration of insulin IJN [Internet] 2012;3333. Jul [cited 2022 Oct 29]. Available from: http://www.dovepress.com/solid-lipid-nanoparticles-modified-with-stearic-acidndashoctaarginine-peer-reviewed-article-IJN.

[27] Fan T, Chen C, Guo H, Xu J, Zhang J, Zhu X, et al. Design and evaluation of solid lipid nanoparticles modified with peptide ligand for oral delivery of protein drugs Eur J Pharm Biopharm [Internet] 2014;88(2):518–28. Oct [cited 2022 Oct 29]. Available from: https://linkinghub.elsevier.com/retrieve/pii/S0939641114002033.

[28] Luther DC, Huang R, Jeon T, Zhang X, Lee YW, Nagaraj H, et al. Delivery of drugs, proteins, and nucleic acids using inorganic nanoparticles Adv Drug Deliv Rev [Internet] 2020;156:188–213. [cited 2022 Oct 22]. Available from: https://linkinghub.elsevier.com/retrieve/pii/S0169409X20300661.

[29] Shi Z, Zhou Y, Fan T, Lin Y, Zhang H, Mei L. Inorganic nano-carriers based smart drug delivery systems for tumor therapy Smart Mater Med [Internet] 2020;1:32–47. [cited 2022 Oct 22]. Available from: https://linkinghub.elsevier.com/retrieve/pii/S2590183420300065.

[30] Asfour MH. Advanced trends in protein and peptide drug delivery: a special emphasis on aquasomes and microneedles techniques Drug Deliv Transl Res [Internet] 2021;11(1):1–23. Feb [cited 2022 Oct 22]. Available from: https://link.springer.com/10.1007/s13346-020-00746-z.

[31] Damera DP, Kaja S, Janardhanam LSL, Alim S, Venuganti VVK, Nag A. Synthesis, detailed characterization, and dual drug delivery application of BSA loaded aquasomes ACS Appl Bio Mater [Internet] 2019;2(10):4471–84. Oct 21 [cited 2022 Oct 22]. Available from: https://pubs.acs.org/doi/10.1021/acsabm.9b00635.

[32] Omar H, Croissant JG, Alamoudi K, Alsaiari S, Alradwan I, Majrashi MA, et al. Biodegradable magnetic silica@iron oxide nanovectors with ultra-large mesopores for high protein loading, magnetothermal release, and delivery J Contr Rel [Internet] 2017;259:187–94. Aug [cited 2022 Oct 22]. Available from: https://linkinghub.elsevier.com/retrieve/pii/S0168365916312251.

[33] Zhao T, Fu Y, Jang MS, Sun XS, Wu T, Lee JH, et al. A pH-activated charge convertible quantum dot as a novel nanocarrier for targeted protein delivery and real-time cancer cell imaging Mater Sci Eng: C [Internet] 2021;118:111449. Jan [cited 2022 Oct 29]. Available from: https://linkinghub.elsevier.com/retrieve/pii/S0928493120333671.

[34] Choi WI, Kamaly N, Riol-Blanco L, Lee IH, Wu J, Swami A, et al. A solvent-free thermosponge nanoparticle platform for efficient delivery of labile proteins Nano Lett [Internet] 2014;14(11):6449–55. Nov 12 [cited 2022 Oct 18]. Available from: https://pubs.acs.org/doi/10.1021/nl502994y.

[35] Sgorla D, Lechanteur A, Almeida A, Sousa F, Melo E, Bunhak É, et al. Development and characterization of lipid-polymeric nanoparticles for oral insulin delivery Expert Opin Drug Deliv [Internet] 2018;15(3):213–22. Mar 4 [cited 2022 Oct 18]. Available from: https://www.tandfonline.com/doi/full/10.1080/17425247.2018.1420050.

[36] Lopes M, Shrestha N, Correia A, Shahbazi MA, Sarmento B, Hirvonen J, et al. Dual chitosan/albumin-coated alginate/dextran sulfate nanoparticles for enhanced oral delivery of insulin J Contr Rel [Internet] 2016;232:29–41. Jun [cited 2022 Oct 18]. Available from: https://linkinghub.elsevier.com/retrieve/pii/S0168365916301997.

[37] Damera DP, Kaja S, Janardhanam LSL, Alim S, Venuganti VVK, Nag A. Synthesis, detailed characterization, and dual drug delivery application of BSA loaded aquasomes ACS Appl Bio Mater [Internet] 2019;2(10):4471–84. Oct 21 [cited 2022 Oct 18]. Available from: https://pubs.acs.org/doi/10.1021/acsabm.9b00635.

[38] Narayanaswamy R, Torchilin VP. Targeted delivery of combination therapeutics using monoclonal antibody 2C5-modified immunoliposomes for cancer therapy Pharm Res [Internet] 2021;38(3):429–50. Mar [cited 2022 Oct 18]. Available from: http://link.springer.com/10.1007/s11095-021-02986-1.

[39] Xu S, Cui F, Huang D, Zhang D, Zhu A, Sun X, et al. PD-L1 monoclonal antibody-conjugated nanoparticles enhance drug delivery level and chemotherapy efficacy in gastric cancer cells IJN [Internet] 2018;Volume 14:17–32. Dec [cited 2022 Oct 18]. Available from: https://www.dovepress.com/pd-l1-monoclonal-antibody-conjugated-nanoparticles-enhance-drug-delive-peer-reviewed-article-IJN.

[40] Vaghasiya K, Ray E, Singh R, Jadhav K, Sharma A, Khan R, et al. Efficient, enzyme responsive and tumor receptor targeting gelatin nanoparticles decorated with concanavalin-A for site-specific and controlled drug delivery for cancer therapy Mater Sci Eng: C [Internet] 2021;123:112027. Apr [cited 2022 Oct 18]. Available from: https://linkinghub.elsevier.com/retrieve/pii/S0928493121001661.

[41] Bonaccorso A, Carbone C, Tomasello B, Italiani P, Musumeci T, Puglisi G, et al. Optimization of dextran sulfate/poly-l-lysine based nanogels polyelectrolyte complex for intranasal ovalbumin delivery J Drug Deliv Sci Technol [Internet] 2021;65:102678. Oct [cited 2022 Oct 19]. Available from: https://linkinghub.elsevier.com/retrieve/pii/S1773224721003580.

[42] Boushra M, Tous S, Fetih G, Xue HY, Wong HL. Development of bi-polymer lipid hybrid nanocarrier (BLN) to improve the entrapment and stability of insulin for efficient oral delivery J Drug Deliv Sci Technol [Internet] 2019;49:632–41. Feb [cited 2022 Oct 19]. Available from: https://linkinghub.elsevier.com/retrieve/pii/S1773224718307809.

[43] Kim M, Sahu A, Hwang Y, Kim GB, Nam GH, Kim IS, et al. Targeted delivery of anti-inflammatory cytokine by nanocarrier reduces atherosclerosis in Apo E − /- mice Biomater [Internet] 2020;226:119550. Jan [cited 2022 Oct 19]. Available from: https://linkinghub.elsevier.com/retrieve/pii/S0142961219306490.
[44] Duncan SA, Dixit S, Sahu R, Martin D, Baganizi DR, Nyairo E, et al. Prolonged release and functionality of interleukin-10 encapsulated within PLA-PEG nanoparticles Nanomaterials [Internet] 2019;9(8):1074. Jul 26 [cited 2022 Oct 20]. Available from: https://www.mdpi.com/2079-4991/9/8/1074.
[45] Zhang N, Li C, Zhou D, Ding C, Jin Y, Tian Q, et al. Cyclic RGD functionalized liposomes encapsulating urokinase for thrombolysis Acta Biomater [Internet] 2018;70:227–36. Apr [cited 2022 Oct 20]. Available from: https://linkinghub.elsevier.com/retrieve/pii/S1742706118300497.
[46] Inchaurraga L, Martínez-López AL, Martin-Arbella N, Irache JM. Zein-based nanoparticles for the oral delivery of insulin Drug Deliv Transl Res [Internet] 2020;10(6):1601–11. Dec [cited 2022 Oct 20]. Available from: https://link.springer.com/10.1007/s13346-020-00796-3.

CHAPTER

2

Vaccines and sera

Garima Sahu, Priyanka Kumari and Amit K. Goyal

Department of Pharmacy, School of Chemical Sciences and Pharmacy, Central University of Rajasthan, Ajmer, Rajasthan, India

2.1 Introduction

Vaccines and sera are biological products that work by boosting the body's immune defenses against foreign agents (mostly infecting organisms or their toxins). Vaccines confer active immunity; they function as antigens that stimulate the recipient's own production of specific antibodies. Antisera and immunoglobulins confer passive immunity; antibodies (produced by another person or animal who has been actively immunized) that are already present are transferred.

2.1.1 Vaccines

Vaccines are fundamentally purified preparations that trigger the immune system by producing antibodies that can offer long-term protection in the future against being exposed to a particular microbe; therefore, this is medical wonder for human health. These are biological preparations that increase resistance to specific diseases. The majority of vaccines contain an agent that closely resembles a microbe that causes disease and is usually prepared using the microbe's toxins, attenuated/weakened or killed, or surface proteins of the microorganism. The immune system is stimulated by this agent to identify the foreign agent, eliminate it, and "remember" it so that the immune system can more easily identify and eliminate these pathogens, which are easily encountered in the coming decades. In historical public health, vaccination is a major turning point. Since millions of people were once killed by these pathogenic diseases, this is the most successful medical intervention that has ever been created [1]. Vaccines used in national immunization programs are thought to be secure and efficient when properly administered. However, there are some risks associated with vaccinations, and occasionally, there may be some unfavorable reactions. Vaccine risk does exist. However, some adverse events may occur on occasion during vaccination.

Molecular Pharmaceutics and Nano Drug Delivery
DOI: https://doi.org/10.1016/B978-0-323-91924-1.00009-5

Currently, immunization prevents between 3.5 and 5 million deaths annually from the diseases like as influenza, pertussis, diphtheria, tetanus, and measles [2]. Between the 17th and 20th centuries, French, British, and German scientists made significant contributions to vaccine evolutions. In order to immunize millions of people, Spain was the first country to put in place a general public health vaccination program by bringing smallpox vaccines from Europe to the Americas [3].

2.1.2 Revolution of vaccines development

Numerous lessons can be learned from history while tackling infectious diseases. It is also obvious that our ongoing global collaboration is necessary to effectively combat COVID-19 and other potential pandemics because "no one is safe until everyone is safe."

2.1.2.1 18th century

Several significant events occurred in the 18th century, beginning with the introduction of variolation from Turkey and China to England and America and ending with Edward Jenner's development of vaccination in the latter half of the century. After the pursuit of Lady Mary Wortley Montague, an English aristocrat who had experienced a case of smallpox firsthand, variolation was brought to England by 1715. In Turkey in 1718, she was forced to perform the variolation procedure on her 5-year-old son by Charles Maitland, the physician for the consulate. Lady Montague became a strong supporter of the procedure and put a lot of effort into promoting it as a means of preventing the spread of smallpox. Every level of society was affected by smallpox. Europe experienced 400,000 smallpox deaths per year in the 18th century, and one-third of those who survived went blind [4]. Based on this, an English physician by the name of Edward Jenner (1748–1823) set out to discover a treatment for the crippling illness known as smallpox, which rendered the entire world defenseless. In the latter half of the 18th century, he discovered vaccination as a safer method of immunizing than variolation. He was renowned throughout the world for his ground-breaking work in vaccine development and the eventual eradication of smallpox. He was recognized for introducing the modern idea of vaccination.

An English farmer by the name of Benjamin Jesty personally oversaw the vaccination of his wife and children using fresh material from a cowpox lesion in one of his cows during that time of the smallpox pandemic. He employed this strategy because he had cowpox and believed that made him immune to smallpox. He never published his findings, even though his wife and kids showed no clinical signs after being exposed to smallpox. Smallpox epidemics continued to occur throughout this time [5]. In contrast, Jenner's 1798 recommendation of cowpox vaccination appeared to be less harmful and equally effective. It gave humans adequate protection through a type of cross-immunity, albeit probably less robust than that brought on by the smallpox vaccination [6].

Bishop Marius of Avenches coined the term "variola," Latin word "varius," which means "stained," or "varus," which means "mark on the skin." Around the end of the 15th century, the term "small pockes" (pocke meaning "sac") was first used in England to distinguish the condition from syphilis, which was then known as the "great pockes" [7].

2.1.2.2 19th century

Despite Jenner's historic achievement, no new vaccines were introduced until the following century due to a lack of adequate information and fundamental understanding of microbes and microbiology. The development of immunization science led to the rise of scientists like Paul Ehrlich, Robert Koch, and Louis Pasteur, and the end of the 19th century heralded the start of a new era in vaccine research [8].

In late 19th century, Pasteur earned the title "father of vaccines" after creating the first laboratory vaccine and was also the first person to lodge the "Germ Theory" of the disease in addition to the development of principles of vaccination [9]. In the years 1879 and 1880, Pasteur invented the term "vacciner" to describe his capacity to offer total body immunity through vaccination by inoculating an attenuated virulence. This was the first vaccine developed by a human in a lab [8]. The 4th quarter of the 19th century was a time of great awakening where the practical science of vaccination emerged. Through World War I, it continued for more than 40 years. The leading figures in the early era were Koch, Pasteur, Ehrlich, and von Behring. It was a time when research on bacteria, medical applications, and empirical immunologic discoveries involving primarily antibodies commanded the majority of attention [10]. Robert Koch was hailed as the father of pure culture technology in Berlin, where he also received praise for discovering the cholera and tubercle bacilli. The discovery of clinical hypersensitivity by Koch was comparable to Metchnikof's discovery of phagocytic cells in terms of innate immunity, where Koch hypothesized a strict definition to identifying specified etiologies for disease. Emil von Behring, the first recipient of the Nobel Prize for developing passive immunotherapy, used Roux and Yersin's ability to induce the soluble toxins of diphtheria and tetanus bacilli which might be detoxified for the aim of immunization. This was to dominate therapeutic medicine for many years to come in the fight against infectious diseases [11].

Military objectives sparked intense motivation in the creation of vaccines between 1930 and 1950, particularly during World War II. Additionally, from that point on, foundations and government organizations, like the WHO and research institutions, significantly increased their support. At this time, vaccines for influenza, polio, and Japanese encephalitis B were developed. Because of the scientific developments made in vaccine screening and industrial production, the second half of the 20th century is known as the "golden age of vaccine science." During this time, new vaccine generations were developed. During this time, which began in the 1960s, vaccines against mumps, rubella, and measles, as well as those against chickenpox and inactivated Japanese encephalitis, were created [12].

After World War II, vaccination campaigns were widely used as a tool to improve public health. The worldwide vaccination campaign and the availability of vaccines led to a significant drop in related mortality and the eradication of smallpox and polio [13]. The process of producing vaccines in large quantities has involved the use of cultivation methods under controlled circumstances. Following this time, in the 1980s, proteins and capsular polysaccharide were combined to create the conjugated vaccine. The issue of a dysregulated immune response to carbohydrate antigens was resolved by the use of conjugated vaccines with carrier proteins. Recombinant vaccines were created as a result of advancements in genetic engineering. With regard to a class of pathogens like hepatitis B, these vaccines improved the efficiency of the immune response and the secure application of antigens for immunogenicity. With the advent of DNA vaccines in the 1990s, the evolution of vaccines eventually entered a daring and unexpected final phase. A cytotoxic lymphocyte response against the influenza antigen is induced when a plasmid containing the influenza virus gene is injected into muscle, according to research. Wolf stated at the time that an immune response results from intramuscular DNA injection [14].

COVID-19, the newly discovered human coronavirus illness since the 1918 flu pandemic, has been designated as the fifth pandemic. COVID-19 spread quickly after it was discovered in China, Wuhan. Phylogenetic analysis was used by the International Committee on Taxonomy of Viruses to give the coronavirus that causes SARS the name SARS-CoV-2 (short for SARS-CoV-2). With unprecedented speed, efficient COVID-19 vaccines were produced and distributed by using cutting-edge messenger RNA (mRNA) technology. The first doses of the COVID-19 vaccine are given out in December 2020, just 1 year after the first case of the disease was discovered [15]. The evolution of vaccine from centuries is mentioned in Fig. 2.1.

2.2 Vaccine types and generations

Vaccines are typically divided into four types, as mentioned in Fig. 2.2.

2.2.1 Live attenuated vaccines

In order to prevent serious illness in people with healthy immune systems, live attenuated vaccines contain a variant of the live virus that has been weakened. There are various processes for producing live attenuated vaccines. The most popular techniques involve repeatedly exposing animal or cell cultures to the disease-causing virus (typically chick embryos). Viruses are frequently attenuated by permitting them to continue for several generations in cells where they would not normally grow. With each passage, the virus' ability to replicate in human cells decreases, but it becomes more adept at doing so in new cells. The virus can eventually be used in a vaccine because it has lost some of its ability to survive in human cells. This method selects mutants that are better suited to growth in unusual culture conditions than in natural hosts. As a result, attenuated viruses do not have the capacity to reproduce to the extent that they would in the wild, but they still cause an immune reaction that can serve as protection against subsequent infection [16]. Some of the vaccines are as follows:

The varicella, measles, mumps, and rubella vaccines were developed by Albert Sabin, and the oral polio vaccine was also produced by in vitro cell culture passage selection clones. The poliovirus that is used in the Sabin vaccine is weakened by the growth of monkey kidney epithelial cells. A strain of rubella virus used in the measles vaccine multiplies first in duck embryo cells and then in human cell lines [17]. A technique was developed in the late 1930s to produce yellow fever vaccine and live attenuated influenza vaccine in embryonated hen's egg. Live attenuated vaccines were found to be the best one in training the immune system to combat particular viruses. Only a single vaccination had the ability to eliminate the need for ongoing boosters [18].

Attenuated vaccines have the potential to revert to a virulent form and spread disease, which is their main drawback. Immune systems compromised due to human immunodeficiency virus

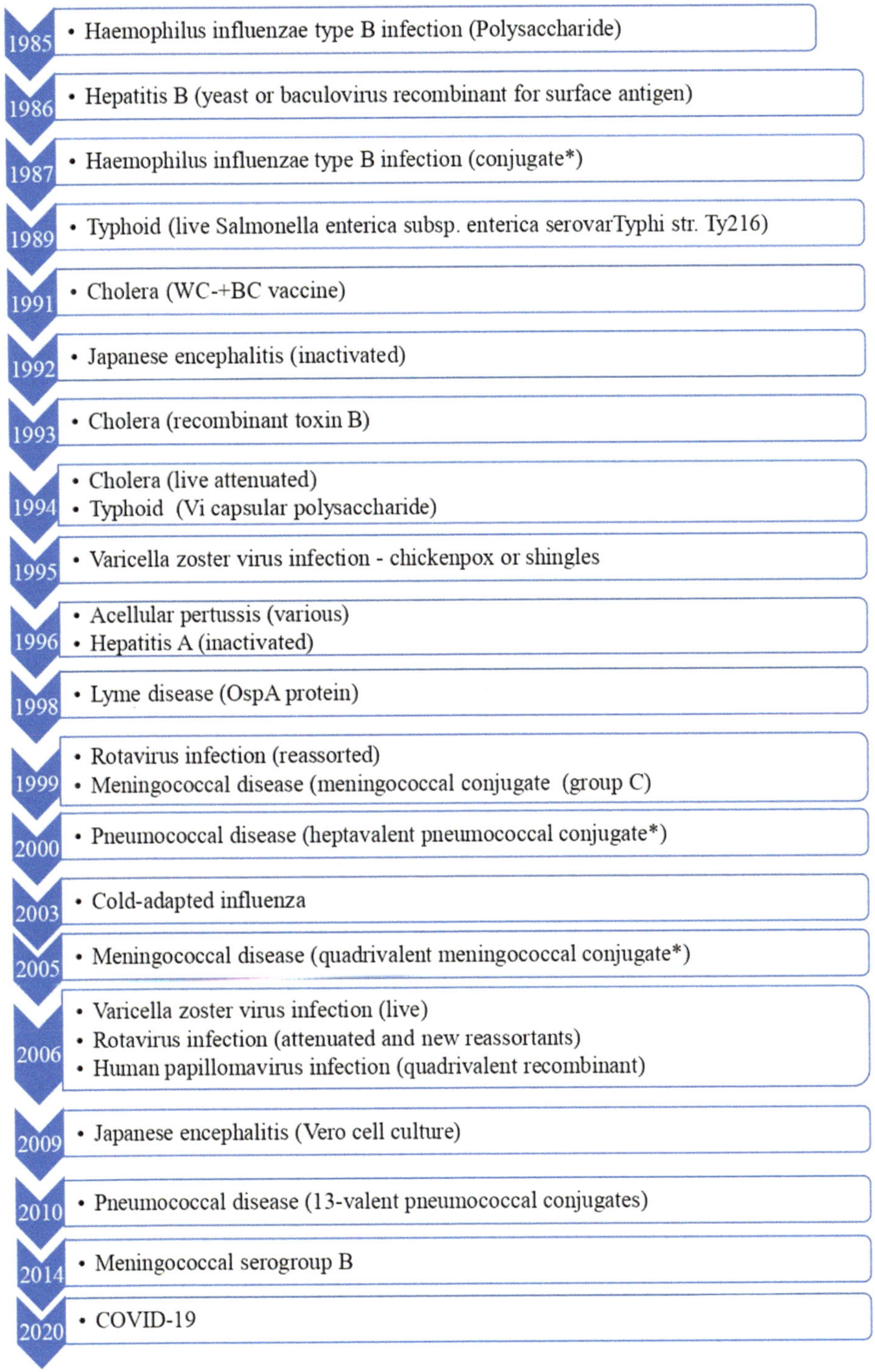

FIGURE 2.1 Revolution of vaccines development.

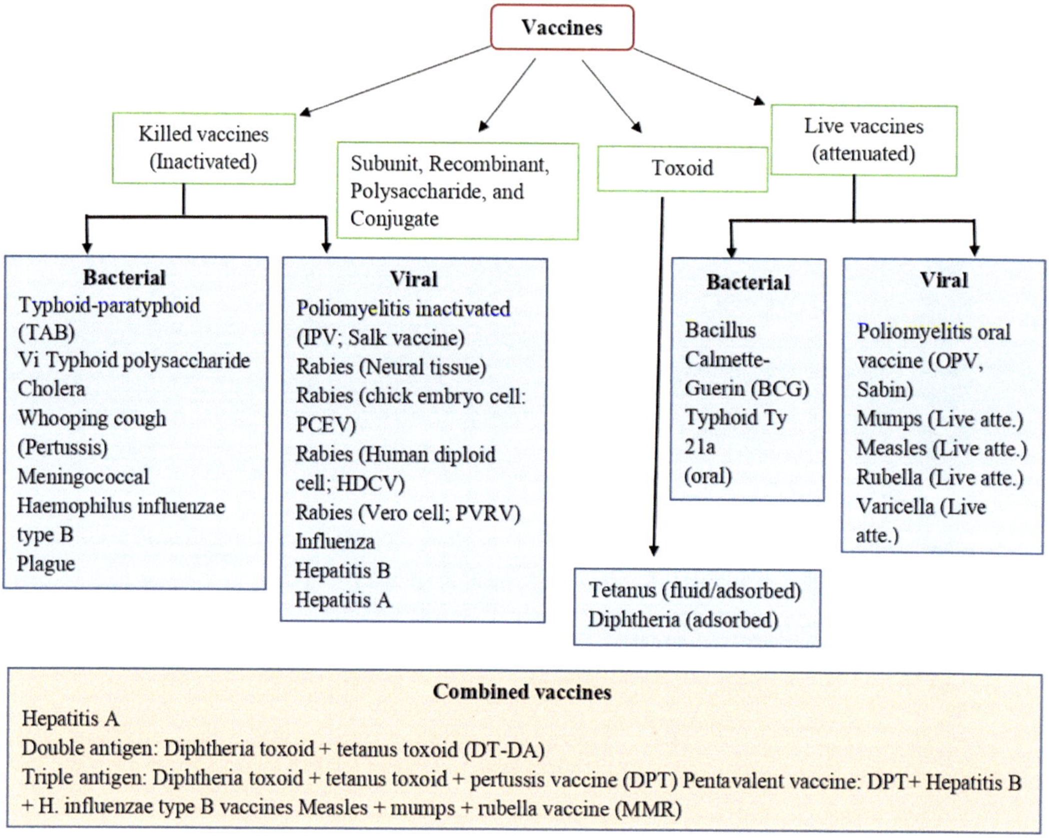

FIGURE 2.2 Types of vaccines.

(HIV), cancer, or any other immune system-depressive diseases cannot receive these vaccines. Currently, researchers are working to weaken specific bacteria by removing crucial genes in order to produce vaccines [19].

2.2.2 Subunit vaccine

Subunit vaccines were created by combining pathogen components, or antigens, that stimulated the immune system and elicited appropriate immune responses. Because subunit vaccines cannot replicate in the host, there is no risk of pathogenicity. Instead, they take advantage of the possibility of using only a portion of the infectious microorganism to elicit a protective immune response. An important benefit in terms of safety considerations and side effect minimization is the normal ability to define the composition of a subunit vaccine. Subunit vaccines frequently required multiple doses and the addition of adjuvants to induce a strong immune response. Based on peptides, proteins, or polysaccharides that have been shown to contain protective epitopes, these vaccines may be developed [20].

2.2.3 Recombinant vaccine

Recombinant DNA technology is used to create recombinant vaccines. Using rDNA technology, DNA from two or more sources can be combined. The Flublok brand of vaccines for influenza, human papillomavirus (HPV), and hepatitis B were made by inserting a segment of the relevant viral gene into the gene of a yeast cell or virus. When the modified yeast cell or virus multiplies, it secretes only pure forms of the hepatitis B surface antigen, the HPV capsid protein, or influenza hemagglutinin. The outer membrane vesicles and proteins used in serogroup B meningococcal vaccines were produced through recombinant technology [21]. The controlled production of protein-subunit vaccines in heterologous hosts is made possible by recombinant DNA technology. Such tactics have a number of benefits, including the use of safe and economical production systems. Additionally, recombinant approaches provide the option of delivering protein subunits via live delivery systems, such as bacteria or viruses or even antigen-encoding genes, or so-called nucleic acid vaccines [22]. Recombinant vaccines for hepatitis B are those that have been authorized for use in people. It contains the recombinant DNA-produced hepatitis B surface antigen (HBsAg), which is made by the yeast Saccharomyces cerevisiae [23]. The vaccine against the HPV is another one created through genetic engineering. There are two HPV vaccines on the market: Gardasil, marketed by Merck and protecting against HPV types 6, 11, 16, and 18, and Cervix (protects for age group 16–18 only and GlaxoSmithKline markets the vaccine) [24].

2.2.4 Polysaccharide vaccine

Polysaccharides are typically the most prevalent antigens found on the exterior of bacterial cells. Vaccines against human diseases are created using bacteria-derived lipopolysaccharides and capsule polysaccharides [25]. Typically, the immune response to a pure polysaccharide vaccine does not require a T cell. This indicates that these vaccines have the ability to stimulate B cells without the aid of T-helper cells. It is likely due to the immaturity of the immune system that T-cell-independent antigens, such as polysaccharide vaccines, do not consistently elicit an immune response in children under the age of 2. In populations where a polysaccharide vaccine is ineffective or only offers transient protection, it is possible to prevent bacterial infections by coupling the polysaccharide antigen to a protein. Millions of people around the world have been helped by polysaccharide vaccines to prolong their lives since the late 20th century. Nevertheless, pure polysaccharide vaccines have a number of drawbacks. Specifically, children under 2 suffer from hyporesponsiveness and poor immunogenicity [26].

2.2.5 Conjugate vaccines

In fact, conjugate subunit vaccines such as those for pneumococcal and *Haemophilus influenzae* type B were developed by chemically joining a polysaccharide from the surface of bacteria to a protein molecule known as "conjugation." A polysaccharide antigen can produce long-lasting protective immunity when it can be conjugated to a protein molecule. Conjugate vaccines were made of combining two different components, similar to how recombinant vaccines are made. Fragments from the bacterial coats were used to prepare the conjugate vaccine. The carrier protein that serves as a vaccine is chemically connected to these coatings. In order to elicit a stronger co-immune response, conjugate vaccines are used. Like recombinant vaccines, conjugate vaccines are created by combining two unique components. The conjugate vaccine was made using pieces of the bacterial coats.

The carrier protein that serves as a vaccine is chemically connected to these coatings. In general, the presented "fragments" of the bacteria do not themselves produce a strong immune response, whereas the carrier protein produces a strong immune response. Conjugate vaccines are used to produce a more potent co-immune response. Examples of conjugated vaccines are hepatitis B, part of the DTaP combined vaccine (whooping cough), meningococcal disease, *H. influenzae* type B (Hib) disease, pneumococcal disease, HPV, and shingles [27].

2.2.6 Inactivated vaccines

Inactivating the pathogen using heat or chemicals had been the common method of producing vaccines. The pathogen is kept "intact" so that the immune system can still detect it even though its ability to reproduce is destroyed. During inactivation, it was crucial to preserve the epitope structure on the epitope antigen. Because extensive denaturation of the protein occurs during heat inactivation, it was generally unsatisfactory because any epitope that depends on higher levels of protein structure may change significantly. Successful chemical inactivation techniques were used like formaldehyde or formalin. Formaldehyde inactivation was used to create the Salk polio vaccine. A microbe that has been destroyed or rendered inactive cannot change back into a more virulent, disease-causing form because it was unable to reproduce in any way (as discussed above with live attenuated vaccines). In most cases, attenuated vaccines only need one dose to produce lifelong immunity. In contrast, inactivated vaccines frequently need booster shots to produce long-lasting immunity and typically offer a shorter window of protection than live vaccines. Glenny and Hopkins used formalin treatment in 1923 to lessen the diphtheria toxin's toxicity. Some of the examples of inactivated vaccines are hepatitis A, polio (shot only), flu (shot only), and rabies [28].

Vaccines are also categorized in generation based on the process of evolution. Each generation has unique traits and a different range of protection, as mentioned in Table 2.1.

2.2.7 Toxoid vaccines

Inactivated toxins produced by bacteria were used to create toxoid vaccines. Heat, chemicals, or other techniques were used to deactivate these protein-based toxins. Tetanus and diphtheria are two examples of bacteria that produce toxins that lead to illness. The immune system's capacity to identify and get rid of these toxins offers defense against the illness. A toxoid vaccine produces an antitoxoid antibody that can bind to toxins and counteract their effects. Toxoid vaccines, like some other types of vaccines, may require booster shots to obtain ongoing protection against diseases because they typically do not have immunity duration comparable to attenuated viral vaccines. Depending on the risk factors associated with each patient, revaccination (a booster) may be necessary more than once in a single year. The examples of toxoid vaccines were tetanus and diphtheria [30].

TABLE 2.1 Vaccine generations [29].

First generation		Second generation		Third generation
Live attenuated vaccines	**Inactivated vaccines**	**Subunit vaccines**	**Recombinant vaccines**	**DNA vaccines**
Influenza	Influenza	Hepatitis B	Hepatitis B	HIV
Hepatitis A	Hepatitis B	Pertussis	HSV	Cancer
MMR	Cholera	Diphtheria	Rotavirus	Ebola
OPV	IPV	Haemophilus influenzae	Anthrax	Malaria
Chickenpox	Rabies			Influenza
Yellow fever	Pertussis			Hepatitis

2.3 Immunization

Immunization can be acquired either passively or actively, depending upon the situation. These methods may come from both natural and man-made sources. Natural sources include enviroment, people, and animal, whereas medical methodologies include artificial sources. An unimmunized person receives preformed antibodies through passive immunization. The presence of these preformed antibodies would then cause this person to temporarily develop a resistance to a specific organism or toxin. Then, the person will no longer be immune to this microorganism or toxin after these preformed antibodies that had been destroyed.

Both natural and artificial processes can result in passive immunization. Excellent examples of natural passive immunization are the transmission of maternal antibodies to the fetus through the placenta and the transmission of these maternal antibodies to the infant through colostrum and milk. The administration of combined human immunoglobulin and antivenin were an excellent example of artificial passive immunization. These gamma globulins and antivenins offer momentary immunity to a specific disease or venom. The body of the individual is probably still in the early stages of forming its own active immune response, which occurs concurrently with the effects of this transient immunity from the preformed antibodies [31].

Passive immunization, which typically entails the administration of a globulin product, results in transient immunity for a particular exposure through the direct transfer of an antibody. It offers those who had been exposed to a specific antigen momentary protection. An individual who was bitten by a rabid animal, for instance, can be protected from contracting rabies by receiving an injection of Ig against the virus [32]. When a person who had never received an immunization was exposed to a pathogenic agent, active immunization takes place. The process of this person's immune system developing immunity to this agent then starts. Active immunization typically results in long-term immunity compared to passive immunization because it stimulates the individual's immune system. Both natural and artificial active immunization were possible. Influenza exposure was a prime illustration of a natural active immunization. The process of the body building long-term immunity to the influenza virus then starts. Although they do not cause active disease, these immunizations mimic the stimulation required for immune development [31].

2.4 Immunology of vaccines

The investigation of the body's infection-fighting mechanisms is renowned as immunology. Edward Jenner's successful vaccination against smallpox in 1796 marks the beginning of immunology as an experimental science. Smallpox was the first and only human disease that had been eradicated, and vaccination's widespread adoption had contributed to humanity's greatest successes in disease prevention. The influence of immunology had expanded throughout the 20th century beyond infection protection. The study and treatment of many human diseases had been benefited greatly from our expanding the understanding of the immune system, which had several impacts on the number of different biomedical disciplines. It is still evident that the immune system's main function is infection resistance [33].

2.4.1 Immune system

The two main immune system subsystems are the innate (or general) resistance system and the adaptive system. To deliver a successful immune response, the innate system and the adaptive system constantly interact with one another. The humoral immune system is a component of the acquired or adaptive immune system that focuses on vaccinology. The humoral and cell-mediated immune systems make up the adaptive immune system, which had a high level of specificity and memory. The term "humoral immune system" describes immune reactions involving antibodies produced by B cells. Cell-mediated immunity, on the other hand, refers to T cell responses without the use of antibodies. Using serum that contains antibodies, humoral immunity can be passed from one person to another [34]. An adaptive immune response occurs when the pathogen manages to avoid the innate immune response, which detects and quickly eliminates organisms by defense mechanisms that were not antigen-specific and do not require prolonged induction. The dendritic cell (DC), also known as the Langerhans cell in the skin, is the most significant of the various antigen-presenting cells because it is designed specifically for the capture of antigens, subsequent processing, and presentation at the cell surface for T cell receptor recognition. However, B-cell receptors have the potential to directly identify foreign antigens. Plasma cells are produced when immunoglobulin (Ig) receptors on B cells recognize foreign antigen epitopes. Subclasses of antibodies were subsequently secreted by plasma cells (IgG, IgA, IgM, and IgE). These antibodies work to stop or restrict the spread of infection and were involved in the lysis of infected cells via complement-mediated lysis or antibody-dependent cellular cytotoxicity [35,36]. After being exposed to an antigen again, the immune system can respond quickly due to immunological memory or the anamnestic nature of the immune system. One of the tenets of vaccination is this characteristic, which is crucial to the immune system's operation [37].

2.4.2 General immune response mechanism

IgG, IgM, and IgA class antibodies are produced as a result of immunization and natural infection. IgM antibody typically manifests during an acute infection within the first few days of the onset of symptoms and peaks between 7 and 10 days later. IgM gradually drops to undetectable levels over the course of the following few months as the infection is treated. IgM antibodies are therefore indicative of a recent or ongoing infection, though there are some exceptions to this rule. Serum IgG antibodies typically appear concurrently with IgM antibodies in a natural infection or shortly after immunization. After that, IgG concentration quickly rises. IgG antibodies typically last for years at low levels that can be found using sensitive enough tests and the right tests. A booster response happens after reinfection or revaccination. The primary systemic or mucosal component of the IgA antibody response depends on the route of immunization or infection. Parenterally administered vaccines or infections with microorganisms that replicate in and spread to internal organs and the systemic circulation result in a systemic IgA antibody response. Compared to the IgM and IgG antibody responses, the serum IgA antibody response is less consistent in terms of level, onset, and duration.

2.4.2.1 *Activation of immunity*

Specific antigen-presenting cells, which are essentially DCs, must be recruited into the reaction in order to activate antigen-specific B and T cell responses. DCs in their infancy patrol the entire body. Mature DCs play a crucial role in the induction of vaccine responses due to their exceptional ability to activate T cells by sending them "danger signals" that are both antigen-specific and costimulatory. Thus, delivering adequate danger signals via vaccine antigens and/or adjuvants is the first requirement to elicit vaccine response, to start an inflammatory response that is mediated by innate immune system cells. A set of receptors on DCs, monocytes, and neutrophils are directed against evolutionarily conserved pathogen patterns that are not present in self-antigens and are therefore quickly recognized as "danger." When they come into contact with a pathogen, these host cells detect the potential danger through these receptors, among which Toll-like receptors play a crucial role. They make pro-inflammatory cytokines and chemokines and modulate the expression of the molecules on their surface [38]. Due to these granulocytes, monocytes, and natural killer cells are drawn to the area and extravasate there. This creates an inflammatory microenvironment in which immature DCs are activated and monocytes differentiate into macrophages. DCs remain immature in the absence of warning signs of danger. T cells differentiate into regulatory CD^{4+} T cells, which uphold immune tolerance, rather than immune effectors when they encounter nave T cells.

2.4.2.1.1 Immune response of live vaccine

Live viral vaccines effectively activate the innate immune system, most likely through pathogen-associated signals (such as viral RNA), which enables pattern recognition receptors to recognize the vaccines. Viral particles are injected, and they quickly spread throughout the vascular network and reach their intended tissues. This pattern, which includes the initial mucosal replication stage for vaccines given orally or nasally, is strikingly similar to what happens after a natural infection. DCs are thus activated at multiple sites after the administration of a live viral vaccine and its spread, migrate toward the corresponding draining lymph nodes, and start multiple foci of T and B cell activation [39].

2.4.2.1.2 Immune response of nonlive vaccine

All nonlive vaccines, whether they contain glycoconjugates, polysaccharides, proteins, or inactivated microorganisms, may still have pathogen recognition patterns that can trigger innate defenses. However, vaccine-induced activation is still more confined in time and space when microbial replication is not present. In essence, innate responses are triggered at the injection site by nonlive vaccines [40].

2.5 Side effects and safety of vaccines

One of the most significant advancements in public health over the past century is the development of vaccines which resulted in notable decreases in the morbidity and mortality caused by numerous infectious diseases. The effectiveness and safety of vaccines are both necessary for vaccination programs to be successful. As diseases that can be prevented by vaccines become less common, the public knows less about them and pays more attention to how safe vaccines are. Low vaccination rates and a resurgence of diseases that can be prevented by vaccines can result from widespread worries about the possibility of adverse events. Before vaccines are approved, their safety is thoroughly tested in clinical trials. However, the main focus of clinical trials is efficacy; they frequently have insufficient sample sizes and follow-up times to detect rare adverse events or those with delayed onset.

Additionally, only healthy volunteers are typically allowed to participate in prelicensure trials, and trial protocols specifically exclude certain vulnerable subpopulations, like expectant mothers, for whom a vaccine may be recommended. Monitoring vaccines is therefore necessary to identify rare adverse reactions, those that may develop years after vaccination, and those that may affect particular subpopulations [41,42].

2.5.1 Adverse event following immunization detection: to strengthen vaccine safety monitoring in all countries

A "vaccine adverse event," also renowned as an "adverse event following immunization" (AEFI), is a detrimental health activity or health issue that tends to happen during or after the administration of a vaccine. Adverse reactions are sudden, unanticipated events that could be brought on by a vaccine or could just be coincidences unrelated to immunization. In addition to elements of infectious agents, vaccines frequently include additional ingredient [43]. These include egg protein, thimerosal, aluminum salts, gelatin, and leftover antibiotics. Recent data suggest that these components may be crucial in the adverse reactions to vaccinations. Several vaccines have been linked to a variety of adverse reactions based only on anecdotal or weak evidence. Due to the fact that vaccines are foreign substances, they may cause some local inflammation, a systemic reaction, or even anaphylaxis. Phase I–III trial characteristics such as structure, animal testing, and limited human testing may not adequately predict rare adverse outcomes due to idiosyncratic reactions. As an illustration, rare hypotonic or hyporesponsive episodes may occur after receiving the whole-cell pertussis vaccine. A small percentage of newborn infants who receive the hepatitis B vaccine may experience a febrile reaction that necessitates an unnecessary medical examination and, in some cases, presumptive antibiotic therapy. A week after receiving the first dose of the rhesus rotavirus vaccine in infants, there seems to be an increased risk of developing intussusception. Since 1999, the Global Advisory Committee for Vaccine Safety (GACVS) has examined the evidence on various vaccine components (like aluminum adjuvants used in several and thiomersal in multidose nonlive vaccines) as well as any associations between vaccination and general categories of unfavorable health outcomes, such as autism, immune system overload, a potential link between vaccines and autoimmune syndromes, and possibly increased mortality among vaccine recipients [44].

The Vaccine Adverse Event Reporting System (VAERS), a joint project of the US Food and Drug Administration (FDA) and the Centers for Disease Control and Prevention, tracks adverse events that may be related to vaccinations (CDC). Its main job is to look for early warning signs and come up with theories about potential new vaccine side effects or variations in the frequency of already known ones. A passive surveillance system called VAERS depends on medical professionals and others to voluntarily report cases of illness following vaccination. All adverse events of which manufacturers become aware must be reported. VAERS is a passive reporting system, which means it depends on people to send the CDC and FDA reports of their experiences. It is particularly helpful for identifying unusual or unexpected patterns of adverse event reporting that might indicate a potential safety issue with a vaccine. It is not intended to determine whether a vaccine caused a health problem. In this manner, VAERS can offer the CDC and FDA valuable information, and more research and analysis are required to fully assess a potential safety concern [45]. On November 1, 1990, VAERS took the place of the FDA's Spontaneous Reporting System for the private sector and manufacturer reporting as well as the CDC's Monitoring System for Adverse Events Following Immunization (MSAEFI) for public sector reporting. Maintaining the database was primarily done so that it can act as an early warning or signaling system for adverse events that were not found during premarket testing. Each report was coded before being added to the VAERS database. From November 1990 to January 16, 2007, the FDA's Coding Symbols for a Thesaurus of Adverse Reaction Terms (COSTART) was used to code the adverse events detailed in each report. The VAERS coding system was changed to a universally accepted international coding system on January 17, 2007. The Medical Dictionary for Regulatory Activities was the name of this system (MedDRA). With an estimated 1.9 billion vaccinations administered during the decade beginning in 1991, VAERS received 128,717 reports of adverse events, translating to a rate of 11.4 cases per 100,000 vaccinations [46]. Fever (25.8%), injection-site hypersensitivity (15.8%), rash (11%), injection-site edema (10.8%), and vasodilation (10.8%) were the most frequently reported side effects. 14.2% of the reports were for serious adverse events, which were defined as death, serious illness, hospitalization, or permanent disability; however, in most cases (2% of cases), death could not be directly linked to the vaccine. Several vaccines with side effects are mentioned in Table 2.2 [47].

According to VAERS data, the most frequent side effects include pain at the fever, injection site, neck pain, headache, nausea, drowsiness, vomiting, dizziness, diarrhea, decreased alcohol tolerance, enlarged lymph nodes, cough, excessive sweating, dyspnea, fainting, thirst, stuffy nose, loss of appetite, insomnia, sore throat, irritability, photosensitivity, stupor, numbness in the extremities, eye pain, and malaise. Each year, a different

TABLE 2.2 Several vaccines with their adverse effects.

Name of vaccine	Adverse events/side effects
Hepatitis B vaccine	Multiple sclerosis, allergic reactions, diabetes, rheumatoid arthritis, lymphoblastic leukemia, and chronic fatigue syndrome
Influenza	Allergic reactions, fever, myalgia, and malaise Chronic obstructive pulmonary disease
Measles, mumps, and rubella	Allergic reactions, acute arthritis, thrombocytopenia, anaphylaxis, febrile seizures, and autism
Diphtheria, tetanus, and pertussis	Fever, irritability, and drowsiness Anorexia, pain, tenderness, edema, erythema, and extensive limb swelling
Polio	Meningitis, allergic reactions, allergic reaction, headache, anaphylactic shock, convulsion, high fever causing seizure (febrile seizure), arthralgia, hypersensitivity reaction, mass, joint pain, and injection-site rash
Haemophilus influenzae type b	Allergic reactions, edema, injection-site erythema, fever, and warmth
Varicella	Allergic reactions, soreness, redness, or swelling at the site of the injection, fever, rash, fussiness, headache, seizures, and meningitis
Rotavirus	Allergic reactions, irritability, mild, temporary diarrhea or vomiting, fussiness, decreased appetite, low-grade fever
Coronavirus	Allergic reactions, myocarditis and pericarditis, anaphylaxis, headache, thrombosis with thrombocytopenia, and Guillain–Barré syndrome
BCG	Fever, bladder irritability, arthritis/arthralgia, bladder contracture, cytopenias, cystitis, respiratory failure, disseminated intravascular coagulation, epididymitis, hepatitis, miliary tuberculosis, pneumonitis, loss of bladder capacity, polyarthritis, pyelonephritis, and prostatitis.

number of VAERS reports are submitted [48]. Over 48,000 reports were received by VAERS in 2019 (Center of Disease Control and Prevention). Due to VAERS' potential coverage of the entire US population, it may be possible to study extremely rare occurrences like anaphylaxis, following the administration of the mumps, measles, and rubella (MMR) vaccine or poliomyelitis and the administration of a live oral poliovirus vaccine. Nevertheless, VAERS has significant limitations. Reports to VAERS represent temporal, but not always causal, relationships between vaccination and negative events, and it is only occasionally possible to actually establish causality [49]. In addition, VAERS attracted more attention after the 2019 coronavirus disease (COVID-19). The majority of COVID-19 vaccines were authorized for use under emergency use authorizations, which mandate that medical professionals document certain AEFIs, including death, in VAERS [50].

Over the period of 1990 to 2021, there were 228 vaccines reported in 1,396,280 domestic and 346,210 nondomestic reports. The highest reporting rate for both domestic and nondomestic reports was in 2021 (48.52% and 70.33%), and notable changes in AEFIs patterns were also noted in 1991, 1998, 2000, 2006, 2009, 2011, and 2017. The following AEFIs were recorded: lethal threats (1.42% and 4.38%), hospitalizations (5.84% and 27.78%), hospitalizations (13.37% and 2.27%), and deaths (1.00% and 4.08%) (1.4% and 7.96%). With the exception of 2021, when headaches were the most frequently reported symptom, pyrexia has dominated the past 31 years. The top three reported vaccines for COVID-19 were manufactured by Moderna, Pfizer-Biontech, and Janssen. The most common adverse events (AEFIs) were headache, pyrexia, and fatigue [51].

The WHO established the GACVS in 1999 to provide impartial, fact-based guidance on vaccine safety issues that might have global implications. This was carried out in response to several vaccine safety issues that have drawn considerable attention over the past few decades. The GACVS carefully examined these issues in its early years. In 1990, 1479 million vaccine doses were administered globally. Numerous serious diseases were successfully managed, thanks to vaccinations. However, vaccine administration also carries a risk of adverse reactions. Given that vaccinations are given to healthy individuals, frequently children, there is a strong obligation to ensure a favorable benefit-to-risk ratio. For vaccinations that are required or advised by national health services, this obligation is especially strong. The evaluation of vaccine safety will become more difficult as more vaccines and vaccine combinations are used. The prevalence of serious infectious diseases has significantly decreased as a result of advancements in modern medicine. The most significant factor in this advancement has been vaccination, and vaccines may also become more and more crucial in preventing the spread of viruses and bacteria that are resistant to antibiotics and other treatments. The public must continue to have faith in vaccine efficacy and vaccine safety in order for global vaccination programs to maintain their progress [52].

2.6 Vaccine preparation

Depending on the type of vaccine and the pathogen it is designed to fight, different techniques are used in the preparation of vaccines. The standard procedures for the vaccine preparation are mentioned in Fig. 2.3.

The vaccines are made up of several fundamental steps that combine to form the finished products are approved. The production of the immune response-inducing antigen is the first step. In this step, either the pathogen itself is produced (for later inactivation or isolation of a subunit) or a recombinant protein derived from the pathogen is produced. In cells, which can either be primary cells like chicken fibroblasts (used in, e.g., the yellow fever vaccine) or continuous cell lines like MRC-5, viruses are grown (e.g., hepatitis A vaccine). In bioreactors, bacterial pathogens are raised on a medium designed to maximize antigen yield while preserving its integrity. Recombinant proteins can be produced in cell culture, yeast, or bacteria. The cell lines and seed cultures for bacteria and viruses that are used in the production of viruses are carefully regulated, preserved, characterized, and frequently guarded. The creation of a "master cell bank" is the first stage of manufacturing. This is a set of cell vials that serve as the raw material for all upcoming production. Performance and the absence of any adversative agents are two of its many distinguishing characteristics. Working cell banks, which serve as the standard starting culture for production lots, are created from this bank. The vaccine's final product is directly related to its raw materials, and altering these materials can be as challenging as starting a new product development process from scratch. The antigen must then be separated from the substrate and the majority of the environment that served as its growth environment [53]. The vaccines are made up of several fundamental steps that combine to form the finished products that are approved. The production of the

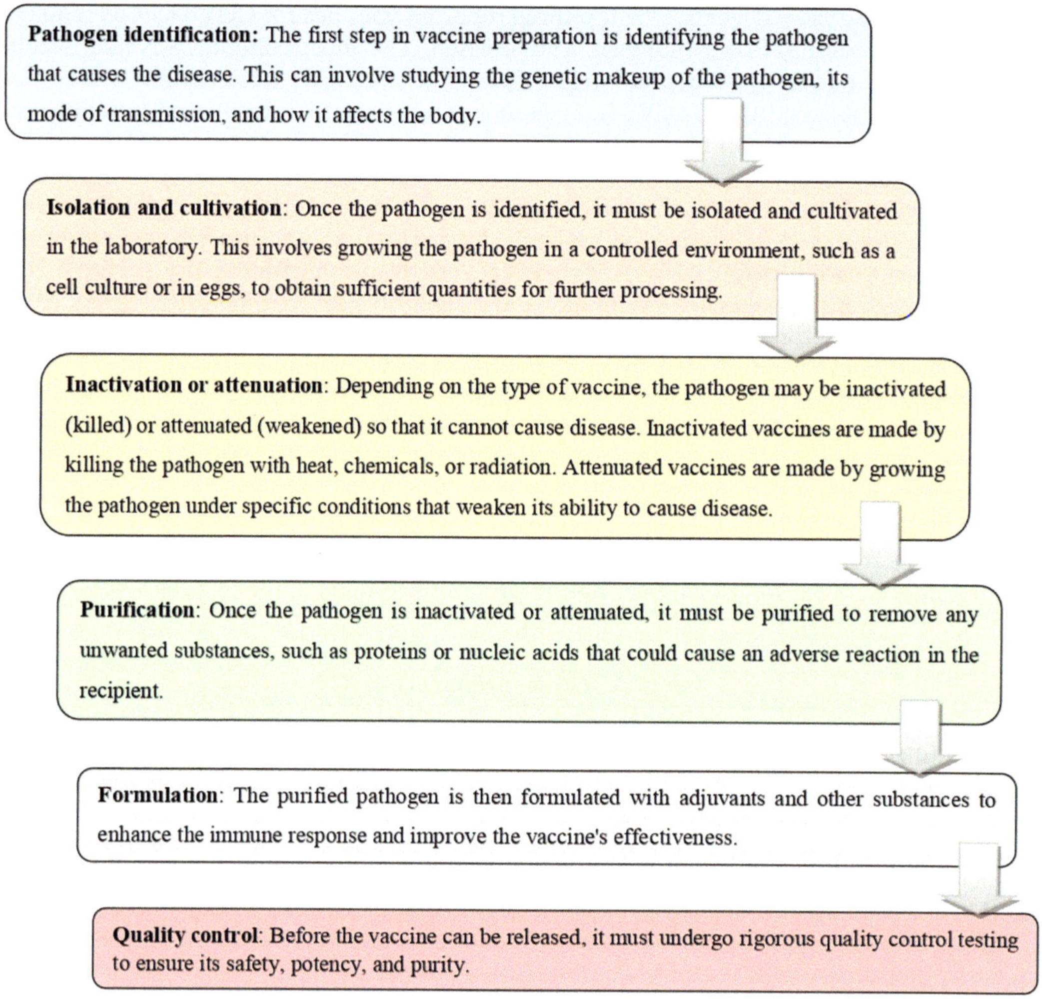

FIGURE 2.3 Steps for the preparation of vaccines.

immune response-inducing antigen is the first step. In this step, either the pathogen itself is produced (for later inactivation or isolation of a subunit) or a recombinant protein derived from the pathogen is produced. In cells, which can either be primary cells like chicken fibroblasts (used in, e.g., the yellow fever vaccine) or continuous cell lines like MRC-5, viruses are grown (e.g., hepatitis A vaccine). In bioreactors, bacterial pathogens are raised on a medium designed to maximize antigen yield, while preserving its integrity. Recombinant proteins can be produced in cell culture, yeast, or bacteria. The viral and bacterial seed cultures and the cell lines used for viral production are carefully controlled, stored, characterized, and, often, protected. The creation of a "master cell bank" is the first stage of manufacturing. This is a set of cell vials that serve as the raw material for all upcoming production. Performance and the absence of any adversative agents are two of its many distinguishing characteristics. Working cell banks, which serve as the standard starting culture for production lots, are created from this bank. The vaccine's final product is directly related to its raw materials, and altering these materials can be as challenging as starting a new product development process from scratch. The antigen must then be separated from the substrate and the majority of the environment that served as its growth environment. The removal of free viruses, cell-secreted proteins, or cells containing the antigen from the used medium are examples of this. The antigen is then purified in the following step. This step may involve numerous unit operations of column chromatography and ultrafiltration for vaccines made of recombinant proteins. An isolated virus may be inactivated for a viral vaccine without any additional purification. The vaccine's formulation aims to maximize stability while delivering it in a way that facilitates effective distribution and the preferred clinical delivery of the drug. The vaccine formulation may include an adjuvant to boost the immune response, stabilizers to extend shelf life, and/or preservatives to enable the delivery of multidose vials. The formulation entails combining and evenly mixing each of the parts that make up the finished vaccine in a single vessel. Employees wear specialized protective clothing to prevent exposure to adversative agents, while working in a highly controlled environment. During operations, critical surfaces and the environment are monitored for control. At this stage, the product is typically subjected to quality control (QC) testing for safety, potency, purity, sterility, and other factors. The potency of vaccines is designed to last past the maximum dose that has been shown to be effective in human clinical trials [54].

2.6.1 Examples of vaccine preparations

2.6.1.1 Measles vaccine

The measles virus was discovered in 1954 and belongs to the family Paramyxoviridae's genus *Morbillivirus*. The strains used in current vaccines are Edmonston, Moraten, or Schwarz. The MMR vaccine was introduced to the market in the 1970s, but these vaccines have been available since the 1960s. In more than 90% of recipients, the final vaccine, a live attenuated viral vaccine, results in immunity. The production of one measles vaccine begins with a set of pathogen-free embryonated chicken eggs that are incubated for a number of days. To get chick embryo fibroblasts ready for cell culture, the embryos are collected and trypsinized. All procedures are carried out by skilled workers in strict aseptic conditions. Hanks media and fetal calf serum are used to grow cell cultures in roller bottles for optimum cell growth. The viral working seed is further transmitted to chick embryo fibroblast cells, which are then incubated for a number of days to produce the viral culture. The cells are mechanically lysed to release the virus at the conclusion of the viral culture. The virus is filtered and centrifuged to remove impurities before being frozen for storage. The vaccine is prepared alone or in combination with the mumps and rubella vaccines and lyophilized to produce a stable product following the release of all QC tests. Just before use, the vaccine is reconstituted [55].

2.6.1.2 Diphtheria vaccine

A purified form of the inactivated diphtheria toxin is known as diphtheria toxoid. Although antibodies might not stop the spread or acquisition of the organism, they are very effective at producing disease-preventing antibodies. The first diphtheria vaccine was created in the early 1800s and became widely used in the United States in 1914 (Vitek and Wharton, 2008). It was discovered that the vaccine, which contained both a toxin and an antitoxin, successfully prevented diphtheria in 85% of cases. In particular, *Corynebacterium diphtheriae* is grown in a liquid medium that is advantageous to toxin production. The strain of *C. diphtheriae* is known to produce large amounts of toxin, such as the Park Williams 8 strain. The appropriate incubation, centrifugation, and filtration aid in sterilization. After potency testing, the filtrate is incubated with formalin to cause the toxin to turn into a toxoid. To achieve the required dosage, the product is then further purified and concentrated. It is adsorbed onto an aluminum salt, typically aluminum phosphate, or hydroxide. The proper tests for potency and sterility are performed after each step [56].

2.6.1.3 *Tetanus vaccine*

The toxigenic strains of *Clostridium tetani* are rendered inactive in order to create the tetanus toxoid. The pathogenic properties of the toxic strains are eliminated by formaldehyde treatment after they have been purified and grown in liquid media. Tetanus toxoid is combined with calcium or aluminum salts after being purified and sterilized. Then, typically, a vaccination form containing this toxoid antigen, diphtheria, and pertussis antigens is used. Using *C. tetani* seeds that have been approved, tetanus protein is produced in bioreactors. Continuous-flow centrifugation and diafiltration are used to separate the crude toxin from the culture supernatant. After that, fractional ammonium sulfate precipitation and ultrafiltration are used to purify the crude toxin. The resulting purified toxin is concentrated by ultrafiltration, detoxified with formaldehyde, and stored between 2°C and 8°C for further processing [57].

2.6.1.4 *Influenza vaccine*

The influenza virus vaccine is a sterile suspension made from influenza viruses propagated in chicken embryos and is intended for intramuscular administration. Two influenza A virus strains (H1N1 and H3N2) and one influenza B virus are typically included in the influenza vaccine. A new strain of the influenza B virus was discovered, and in 2012, the first vaccine with four antigens was granted a license. Hemagglutinin and neuraminidase subtypes are used to distinguish between the two type A viruses. The primary immunizing antigens and major surface proteins of the influenza A virus are the glycoproteins hemagglutinin and neuraminidase. In a ratio of roughly 4:1, these proteins are inserted as spike-line projections into the viral envelopes [58].

2.6.1.5 *Hepatitis vaccine*

The "S" gene, which codes for HBsAg, was inserted into an expression vector that could control the synthesis of a significant amount of HBsAg in Saccharomyces cerevisiae in order to create this vaccine. It has been proven that the HBsAg particles produced by and purified from yeast cells are identical to those produced from the plasma of a chronic hepatitis B carrier [59].

2.6.1.6 *Haemophilus influenzae type B*

Type B *H. influenzae* Capsular polysaccharide from *H. influenzae* type B (Hib) and a carrier protein, such as tetanus protein from *C. tetani* (purified tetanus toxoid), CRM protein from

C. diphtheriae, or the outer membrane protein complex of Neisseria meningitis, are produced separately to create the conjugate. Utilizing Hib-approved seeds, the capsular polysaccharide is produced in industrial bioreactors. Using a cationic detergent, a crude intermediate is extracted from the fermentation supernatant. Continuous-flow centrifugation is used to collect the resulting material. The disrupted paste is then redissolved in buffer, where the polysaccharide is then selectively separated from it by raising the ionic strength. After that, phenol extraction, ultrafiltration, and ethanol precipitation are used to further clean the polysaccharide. The finished product is precipitated with alcohol, vacuum-dried, and stored for further processing at −35°C. Hib capsular polysaccharide activation and conjugation to tetanus protein via a spacer constitute the two steps that make up the preparation of the conjugate. The native polysaccharide is chemically fragmented to a target molecular weight as part of activation, and adipic acid dihydrazide is covalently linked. By using 1-ethyl-3-(3-dimethylaminopropyl)carbodiimide to condense, the activated polysaccharide is then covalently joined to the purified tetanus protein. To obtain high-molecular-weight conjugate molecules free of chemical residues, free proteins, and free polysaccharides, the conjugated material must be purified. After being diluted in the proper buffer, the conjugate bulk is then poured into unit-dose and/or multidose vials and lyophilized [60].

2.6.1.7 *BCG vaccine*

A Mycobacterium tuberculosis (TB) strain referred as the bacillus of Calmette and Guérin was used to make this suspension of living cells. Instead of using human strain, bovine (cattle) strain was found to be safer for men. It was raised on a medium containing ox bile cultures in which it had been used to break up cell clumps that had shown reduction in the the virulence of the organisms. After 13 years of subculture on this medium, it was stable and deemed safe to administer to people [61].

2.6.1.8 *Smallpox vaccine*

The vaccination induces protection against the smallpox virus in 95% or more of recipients and is a live, unattenuated preparation of the vaccinia virus. On the chorioallantoic membrane of a fertile hen's egg, viruses are grown to make vaccines. The products of tissue culture techniques using calf embryo skin or chick embryo cells appear to be immunologically equivalent to vaccines from other sources. The 3-day incubation period is followed by the aseptic removal of the shell and separation of the thickened and infected chorioallantoic membrane into saline. The material is frozen and ground, while it is still frozen to remove any viruses. A similar diluent to that used for vaccine made from free-living animals is used to dilute the suspension [62].

2.6.1.9 *Rabies vaccine*

The rabies vaccine is an inactivated virus vaccine made in either purified chick embryo cell culture or human diploid cell culture. Preexposure prophylaxis for people who are likely to be exposed to rabies (such as veterinarians, forest rangers, and travelers who may be at high risk based on countries and activities) and after exposure to animals that are known or suspected to be rabid are the two situations in which rabies vaccination is advised [63].

2.7 Vaccines evaluation and standardization

2.7.1 Evaluation of vaccines

There are a number of things that make it hard for regulators to check the quality of vaccines to make sure they are safe and effective.

1. Biological sources used to create vaccines, such as eggs, mammalian cells, fetal bovine serum, and others, carry a risk of contamination due to their complexity and diversity.
2. Common purification and decontamination techniques, such as those used for pure chemical compounds or less complex biologics (like recombinant proteins), are often ineffective for many vaccines.
2. A bioassay, such as a challenge test on animals, a virus titration using cell culture, and so forth, is frequently used to evaluate the efficacy of a vaccine. However, reproducibility and reliability are problems with bioassays.

These issues could all be resolved by carrying out the following actions: Identifying the components of the vaccine that trigger the protective immune response will allow for the development of new quality control methods for vaccines. Strong manufacturing procedures and stringent control of the source materials will be used as part of the evaluation [64].

Vaccines must pass a stringent process of clinical trials before they can be used to ensure their safety, efficacy, and high quality. The following steps are typically involved in the evaluation process:

1. Preclinical research: A vaccine undergoes numerous tests in the lab and on animals to determine its safety and efficacy before being tested on humans.
2. Phase I: The vaccine is tested on a small number of healthy volunteers during Phase I clinical trials to determine its safety and determine the best dose.
2. Phase II involves testing the vaccine on a larger population to learn more about its safety and efficacy.
4. Phase III: The vaccine is examined in Phase III clinical trials on a sizable population to determine its efficacy and safety as well as how well it prevents disease.
5. Regulatory acceptance: Following the completion of the clinical trials, the vaccine manufacturer submits an application for approval to regulatory organizations like the FDA or European Medicines Agency (EMA).
6. Post-marketing surveillance: Following a vaccine's approval and use, it is continuously monitored to ensure its safety and efficacy as well as to look for any potential side effects.

Vaccines are assessed according to these procedures as well as their cost-effectiveness, usability, and acceptance by the general public. Overall, evaluating a vaccine is a difficult, multistep process that involves a lot of parties, including those responsible for creating the vaccine, those in charge of its regulation, medical professionals, and members of the general public [65].

2.7.2 Standardization of vaccines

By measuring and comparing a vaccine's physical, chemical, and biological characteristics to a reference standard, standardization determines a vaccine's quality, efficacy, and safety. To ensure that every batch of the vaccine is of the same quality and meets the requirements for how well it functions and how safe it is, this is done. The WHO and national regulatory organizations have established rules and guidelines for the standardization of vaccines. The creation and application of reference standards are covered in great detail in these rules. Additionally, they demonstrate how to measure potency, purity, and other crucial elements. The reference standard for standardizing vaccines is typically a very pure and well-known preparation of the vaccine antigen or its active ingredient. Typically, a recognized laboratory or organization, like the WHO International Laboratory for Biological Standards, produces this reference standard. The capacity of the vaccine to elicit a specific immune response serves as a measure of its efficacy. Examining the number of antibodies produced in response to the vaccine is typically how this is done. Analyzing the vaccine for contaminants or impurities, such as bacterial endotoxins or leftover chemicals from the manufacturing process, reveals its purity. To ensure that vaccines are both effective and safe for use in humans, it is crucial to standardize them. Additionally, it assists in ensuring that each batch of vaccines has the same level of quality and efficacy [66].

2.8 Regulatory consideration of vaccines

Almost every stage of creating, manufacturing, and obtaining approval to sell a vaccine involves regulatory issues. From the time they are created and tested on humans to the time they are manufactured and given to the general public, vaccines are subject to regulations. A manufacturer of biological products must first obtain a license under Section 351 of the Public Health Service Act (P.L. 78–410) in order to export or import the product (vaccine) into the United States. Manufacturers must follow an approved process, use an approved facility, and employ an approved staff in order to obtain a license. The Center for Biologics Evaluation and Research (CBER) at the US FDA develops and upholds standards and requirements for vaccine licensure in the country (FDA) [67]. Since being classified as "vaccines, sera, toxins, antitoxins, and analogous products" in the 1919 US regulations, biologic products have been handled differently compared to chemical medications. Regulators understood that these substances are challenging to characterize and frequently contaminated and that ensuring standard parameters like potency, consistency, and safety presents unique challenges. Because they require biological testing systems, regulators have frequently labeled biological products as such. However, other nations' regulatory frameworks are identical to those in the United States. Since each nation has historically adhered to its own set of standards, some specifics vary from one nation to the next. However, just as the creation and application of medicines and biologics have become more universal, so too has their regulation. Prophylactic (e.g., against measles, polio, HPV, etc.) or therapeutic (e.g., against HIV or other chronic infectious diseases) vaccines must be produced in accordance with stringent standards set by national regulatory authorities (NRAs), like the US FDA [68]. Although the NRAs have the legal authority to ensure that products are safe, effective, and of high quality, vaccine manufacturers have the primary legal responsibility for ensuring these factors. Additionally, NRAs are in charge of overseeing and approving clinical trials, licensing applications, lot releases, and product performance evaluations over the course of a product's lifecycle. Although they are not legally binding, the FDA also publishes guidance documents that give sponsors and manufacturers access to the FDA's most recent thoughts on a range of scientific and regulatory issues [69]. Fig. 2.4 enlists the general phases of a vaccine's development cycle. Initial actions are primarily exploratory in nature. The exploratory stage, which frequently lasts 2–4 years, involves fundamental laboratory research.

Scientists from academia, government, and business conduct research to find natural or artificial antigens that may be used to treat or prevent disease. These antigens may take the form of viruses, bacteria, or viruses that have been weakened, bacterial toxins that have been weakened, or other compounds derived from pathogens that cause infectious diseases. The objective of research and development at this point is to find and create a marketable product that complies with all applicable regulatory requirements set forth by the NRA of record while being safe and immunogenic [70].

Purity and preclinical safety, which are necessary before a vaccine can be used in humans, are the first regulatory requirements that must be considered. Both must be proven before clinical trials can start. The candidate vaccine needs to be thoroughly described, and its purity needs to be proven. All vaccines must pass the general safety and sterility tests mandated by the FDA. By injecting some vaccines into rabbits, it is possible to check if they contain any components that could result in fever. After it is established that the limulus amoebocyte lysate assay for endotoxins is effective with the product, it can be used in place of the pyrogen test with FDA approval [69].

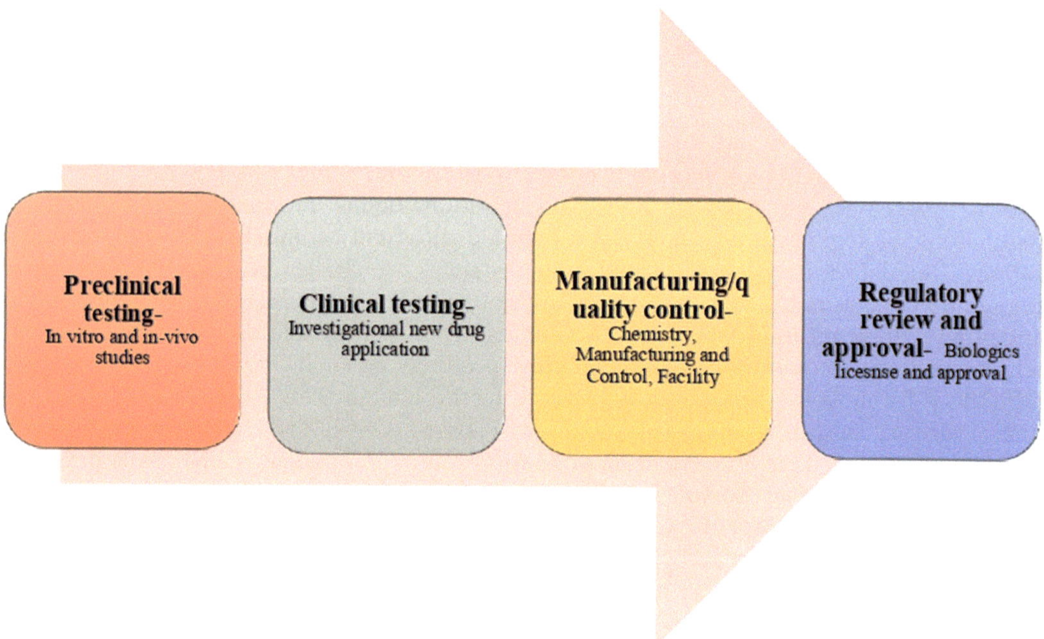

FIGURE 2.4 Development stages of new vaccines.

Exploratory phase: If the vaccine shows promise in this stage, it advances to preclinical or animal testing. Although the basic research and discovery phase is not subject to regulatory oversight, the regulatory process has an impact on each stage of product development, starting with the preclinical stage. There are obstacles to be overcome once product development enters the regulated environment. Before a vaccine is tested on humans, it goes through a preclinical stage of development and testing. Preclinical study considerations are assessed for each individual product, and specifications may change depending on the type of vaccine, the manufacturing process, and the mechanism of action.

Preclinical stage: Preclinical toxicity study requirements are determined by taking into account the potential advantages and disadvantages of the vaccine, the target population, available clinical data from the use of related products, the product characteristics, and the availability of animal models. The FDA might ask for more preclinical studies as product development advances. To determine how safe and effective the candidate vaccine is at immunizing people, preclinical studies are conducted on tissue or cell cultures, animals, and tissue cultures. These investigations may also shed light on the cellular reactions anticipated in people. The results of these studies may also point to a safe starting dose for the following stage of research and a secure way to administer the vaccine. The candidate vaccine may undergo preclinical modifications based on the clinical data in an effort to improve the vaccine's efficacy and safety. Important information regarding the effects of the investigational product on the target organs and whether or not the toxic effects can be reversed can be found in preclinical safety studies. Compliance with good laboratory practices should be followed when conducting toxicity studies. In order for the FDA to decide that the vaccine is reasonably safe to move forward with a clinical investigation, adequate preclinical data must be provided in the submission of an IND to the FDA [71].

Clinical development: The sequential phases of clinical evaluation begin after the FDA have reviewed and accepted the preclinical data package. The clinical testing stage, also known as the investigational new drug (IND) stage, is made up of several phases where the investigational product is tested on humans under precisely controlled conditions.

Phase I studies are designed to examine a vaccine's safety and tolerability as well as to gather preliminary evidence regarding how well it immunizes individuals.

Phase II studies, which typically include several hundred participants, assess the vaccine's immunogenicity and offer rough estimates of the prevalence of common adverse events. A common goal of phase II studies is to gather information for phase III study design.

Vaccine efficacy trials in *phase III* are carried out on a sizable subject population. Phase II clinical development also includes dose ranging studies. The phase III trial offers the vital evidence of the vaccine's efficacy and safety required to assess the vaccine's benefit-risk relationship and support licensure.

After the vaccine is given the go-ahead, *Phase IV* of clinical testing is carried out. Its main objective is to offer extra safety information for sporadic events. Evaluation of breakthrough infections may also be done through phase IV trials.

Clinical studies primarily need to demonstrate safety, immunogenicity, and efficacy in order to obtain a vaccine's license. Immunogenicity might be sufficient in some circumstances. Effectiveness is best proven in randomized, double-blind, tightly controlled studies [72].

Method to produce vaccines: The method used to create a vaccine depends on the type of antigen used to create it. Depending on the particular type of antigen that makes up the vaccine, there are various manufacturing processes for vaccines. Before an IND is filed, many steps in developing a vaccine, like fermentation and cell culture, purification, formulation, analytical testing, and characterizing the vaccine, can be done at the same time.

The four interconnected areas of process development are (1) process, analytical, formulation, and development; (2) production and testing of preclinical supplies; (3) production and testing of clinical supplies (prepared in accordance with cGMP regulations); and (4) production and testing of the final product for marketing authorization. Manufacturers continue to test the bulk, intermediate, and finished vaccine products even after receiving a license. They are typically required to submit the results and to adhere to all product and process specifications. Before CBER approved the release of the lot and administration of the vaccine, key test results and product samples were evaluated. The final product may be subjected to tests for sterility, identity, purity, and potency to evaluate immunogenicity and/or antigen content, as well as additional tests mandated by the NRAs to ensure vaccine safety and quality, depending on the vaccine's composition and manufacturing process. To guarantee safety and consistency in production, it is essential to establish analytical testing procedures for vaccines and all intermediates. Establishing the identity, quality, purity, and potency of a vaccine requires the use of appropriate analytical test methods. In accordance with Title 21 CFR 211.194(a), test procedures used to determine whether pharmaceutical products, including vaccines, adhere to established specifications must be accurate and reliable. Even though it is not required to have analytical methods qualified for testing process development demonstration run materials or scale-up engineering run materials, during the early stages of the vaccine development and manufacturing program, all test methods must at least be qualified for any good manufacturing practices (GMP) lot material [73].

2.9 Licensed vaccines

Licensed vaccines are vaccines that have undergone rigorous testing and regulatory processes to demonstrate their safety and efficacy in preventing specific diseases. These vaccines have been approved by regulatory authorities such as the US FDA and the EMA and are considered safe and effective for use in humans. Some of the licensed vaccines are mention in Table 2.3 [75].

2.10 Sera

A significant portion of the antibodies present in the plasma of an immune person or animal are found in the serum that separates when blood is withheld and allowed to clot. Antitoxic, antibacterial, or antiviral serums are those that contain antitoxic, antibacterial, or antiviral antibodies. However, antitoxic sera are more frequently referred to as antitoxins. However, there are some diseases, like measles and German measles, that cannot be reproduced in animals, and for these, human serum or products derived from it are used. The majority of antisera are obtained from animals in which active immunity has been artificially stimulated. The study of proteins, primarily antibodies, found in blood and

TABLE 2.3 Licensed vaccines [74].

Name of disease	Source (microorganism)	Year of vaccine availability	Strain bacterial/viral	Parts used	Doses	Route of administration	Vaccine strategy/type
Cholera	*Vibrio cholerae*	1896	Bacterial	Cholerae O1and O139 serogroup	2–3 dose Of 1.5 mL	Oral	Killed/inactivated whole organisms
Anthrax	*Bacillus anthracis*	1881 1960 2008	Bacterial	toxins	0.5 mL	Intramuscular	Live vaccine
Diphtheria	*Corynebacterium diphtheriae*	1923	Bacterial	Toxin	0.5 mL	Hep-B–Transcutaneous	Toxoid
Adenovirus	*Adenovirus*	2011	Viral	Viral vector	0.5 mL	Intramuscular	Live vaccine
Hepatitis A (HepA)	*Hepatitis A virus (HAV)*	1995	Viral	HM17 and CR326F	0.5 ml (≤18 yrs) 1.0 mL (≥19 yrs)	Intramuscular	Inactivated and live attenuated vaccines
Hepatitis B (HepB)	*Hepatitis B virus*	1986	Viral	HepB surface antigen *HBsAg*	0.5 mL (≥19 yrs) 1.0 mL (≥20 yrs)	Intramuscular	HepA-killed HepB-recominant protein
Influenza	*Influenza virus*	1938	Viral	Viral Strain	0.5 mL inactivated	Intramuscular	Inactivated vaccine
Influenza	*Influenza virus*	2003 1970	Viral	Viral strain and HA and NA antigens	0.2 mL Live (0.1 mL each nostril)	Intranasal	Killed subunit and Live
HPV	*HPV*	2009	Viral	VLP capsid protein	0.5 mL	Intramuscular	Killed/ inactivated/ recombinant
Japanese encephalitis	*Japanese encephalitis*	1944	Viral	Nakayama strain	0.5 mL	Subcutaneous	Extract and subunits
Measles	*Paramyxoviridae*	1963	Viral	Edmonston–Enders strain	0.5 mL	Subcutaneous	Live attenuated
Mumps	*Paramyxovirus*	1948	Viral	Jeryl–Lynn strain	0.5 mL	Intramuscular or Subcutaneous	Live attenuated
Plague	*Yersinia pestis*	1897	Bacteria	Antigen F1 and V	3 doses of 1.0, 0.2, 0.2 mL (≤ 11 yrs) 1.0,0.04,0.08 mL (≥ 11)	Intramuscular	Killed/inactivated whole organisms

(Continued)

TABLE 2.3 (Continued)

Name of disease	Source (microorganism)	Year of vaccine availability	Strain bacterial/viral	Parts used	Doses	Route of administration	Vaccine strategy/type
Poliomyelitis OPV	*Poliovirus*	1955	Viral	Viral capsid and RNA	2 drops	Oral	Sabin-live attenuated Salk-killed
Poliomyelitis IPV	*Poliovirus*	1955	Viral	Viral capsid and RNA	0.5 mL	Intramuscular or Subcutaneous	Live weakened or inactivated
Pneumococcal PCV PPSV	*Streptococcus pneumoniae*	1977 2002-	Bacteria	Capsular polysaccharide antigen	0.5 mL	Intramuscular or Subcutaneous	PS/protein conjugated capsular polysaccharides
Meningococcal	*Neisseria meingitidis*	1974 2002	Bacteria	Capsular polysaccharide antigen	0.5 mL	Intramuscular	PS-protein/ Recombinant
Rotavirus RV	*Neisseria meningitidis*	2005	Viral	G1, G2, G3, G4, and P	5 drops (1.0 mL) (2.0 mL)	Oral	VLPs
Rubella	*Rubella virus*	1969	Viral	Wister RA 27/3 strain	0.5 mL	Subcutaneous	Live attenuated
Smallpox	*Vaccinia variola*	1798	Viral	Lister strain	0.5 mL (> 18 yrs) 0.1 mL (< 18 yrs)	Subcutaneous	Live organisms
Tetanus	*Clostridium tetani*	1927	Bacterial	Exotoxin	0.5 mL	Intramuscular	Toxoid
Tuberculosis	*Mycobacterium tuberculosis*	1921	Bacterial	*Bacillus Calmette-Guérin*	0.05 mL to Infants 0.1 mL to Children	Intradermal	Live organisms
Typhoid	*Salmonella typhi*	1896 1989 1995	Bacterial	Vi polysaccharide or Ty 21	0.5 mL	Intramuscular	PS/Killed/inactivated whole organisms
Varicella (VAR)	*Varicella zoster*	1995	Viral	Oka VZV	0.5 mL	Intramuscular	Live attenuated
Yellow fever	*Yellow fever virus (Arbovirus)*	1935	Viral	17 D strain	0.5 mL	Intramuscular or Subcutaneous	Live attenuated

Zoster (Zos)	*Varicella zoster*	2006	Viral	VZV glycoprotein E	0.5 mL	Intramuscular	Live attenuated
Tick-borne Encephalitis	*Tick-borne Encephalitis virus*	2021	Viral	Purified whole virions and recombinant E protein	0.5 mL	Intramuscular	Killed/Inactivated whole organism
Diphtheria and tetanus toxoids and pertussis	Combined strains	1949	Bacterial	Combined cell	0.5 mL	Intramuscular	Inactivated
MR	Paramyxoviridae and Rubella	2006	Viral	Combined cell	0.5 mL	Subcutaneous	Live attenuated
DTaP-IFV/Hib	Combined strains	2008	Bacterial and viral	Combined cell	0.5 mL	Intramuscular	Inactivated
DTaP-IPV	Combined strains	2008	Bacterial and viral	Combined cell	0.5 mL	Intramuscular	Inactivated
DTaP-IPV-Hib-HepB	Combined strains	2018	Bacterial and viral	Combined cell	0.5 mL	Intramuscular	Inactivated
MMR vaccine	Combined strains	1963	Viral	Combined cell	0.5 mL	Subcutaneous	Live attenuated
HepA-HepB	Combined strains	1981	Viral	Combined cell	1.0 mL $\leq$ 18 yrs	Intramuscular	Inactivated
Typhoid-Paratyphoid A and B (TAB) Vaccine	Combined strains	1983 and 1989	Bacterial	Combined cell	1 capsule 0.50 mL	Oral Intramuscular	Live, attenuated Inactivated
MMRV	Combined strains	2005	Viral	Combined cell	0.5 mL	Subcutaneous	Live, attenuated

other secretions like saliva is known as serology [76]. Following the discovery that administering immune sera could be used to prevent or treat specific infections in experimental animals, passive antibody therapies were first applied in the 1890s. With the exception of some viral diseases like measles, animal sera were frequently used because it was impractical to obtain enough human convalescent sera for therapeutic purposes. The type of infection affected the serum's efficacy. For the treatment of pneumococcal pneumonia, highly effective sera were available, but serum therapy for TB had varying degrees of success [77]. Even though serum therapy worked well in the clinic, using heterologous sera was very dangerous. There was a high risk of both immediate and delayed allergic reactions.

2.11 Revolutions in serum therapy

Emil von Behring won the first Nobel Prize in medicine and physiology in 1901 "for his work on serum therapy and especially for its use against diphtheria, which opened a new path in medical science and gave doctors a powerful tool to fight disease and death" [78]. The revolutionary changes are mentioned in Table 2.4.

Infections in humans were first treated with antibody-based (serum) therapies in the 1890s. Several bacterial infections were treated with serum therapy in the early 20th century, including those brought on by *Neisseria meningitidis, C. diphtheriae, H. influenzae, Streptococcus pneumoniae, C. tetani*, and *group A streptococcus*. Serum therapy for lobar pneumonia had become the norm by the 1930s. Large-scale controlled trials revealed that giving patients type-specific serum reduced their risk of dying from pneumococcal pneumonia by about 50% [79].

TABLE 2.4 Revolutionary changes of sera.

Years	Revolutions
Early 1890s	Discovery of specific antibodies from the protection of bacteria and toxins
1890s to early 1930s	Serum therapy is used to treat diseases that spread from person to person.
1935	Introduction of sulfonamide antimicrobial therapy
1935 to late 1940s	Removal of serum therapy from practice
1940s	Introduction of beta-lactam antibiotics
1960–90	Invention of particular immune globulins
1975	The emergence of monoclonal antibodies using hybridoma technology
1980s	mAb to CD3 introduced into clinical practice
1990s	Sepsis treatment failure with mAb
1998	Respiratory syncytial virus diseases are approved for the use of Palivizuman.
2004	In order to treat noninfectious diseases, more than 12 mAbs have received authorization

However, serum therapy for bacterial infections was quickly dropped after the discovery of antimicrobial chemotherapy in the middle of the 1930s. Over serum therapy, antimicrobial chemotherapy had several significant advantages, including greater efficacy and lower toxicity.

Serum therapy had immediate side effects like fevers, chills, and allergic reactions. "Serum sickness," a syndrome with rash, proteinuria, and arthralgia, was a delayed toxic effect of serum therapy. This happened in 10% to 50% of patients who got heterologous serum. It was usually triggered by immune complexes. Despite the fact that serum therapy was effective, it was frequently accompanied by side effects, ranging from immediate hypersensitivity reactions to serum sickness, a type of antigen–antibody complex disease. Inadequate dosage, postponed treatment, mislabeled serum, and complicated or mixed infections can all cause serum therapy to fail (i.e., empyema). Due to the high costs of animal husbandry, antibody purification, refrigeration, and standardization through mouse protection tests, producing therapeutic sera was very expensive [80].

The idea of combining serum therapy and antimicrobial chemotherapy was enthusiastically discussed when it was first introduced. However, many studies showed that combined therapy had a lot more side effects than antimicrobial chemotherapy alone, without being any more effective. Serum therapy was abandoned at the beginning of the 20th century due to its toxicity and unfavorable side effects (i.e., serum sickness). It has only been within the last 40–50 years that serum therapy, also known as antibody therapy, has become a significant form of treatment for many chronic inflammatory and infectious diseases. Since then, monoclonal antibodies (mAbs), transgenic antibodies, recombinant mAbs (such as antibody fragments), and most recently the development of recombinant polyclonal antibodies have all contributed to the rapid development of antibody therapy. Immunoglobulins have been used for a very long period to avoid and treat autoimmune and infectious diseases like the newborn hemolytic anemia and rabies virus. Immunoglobulins can be obtained from normal or hyperimmunoglobulin donors, and in some cases, animals [81].

Kohler and Milstein created a method for creating mouse mAbs in 1975; they were able to consistently produce pure, specialized, and reproducible antibodies. In a variety of clinical settings, including cancer and autoimmune diseases, mAbs have proven to be effective therapeutic agents due to their purity and specificity. One type of immortal hybridoma cell continuously and infinitely produces large amounts of mAbs (a hybrid cell between spleen cells usually of murine origin and myeloma cells). mAbs are less expensive and simpler to make than immunoglobulins derived from human or animal plasma, and they are also safe. However, there are some restrictions related to the use of murine mAbs in therapy. These entail the requirement for repeated and higher doses of the antibody, especially in chronic diseases, which enhances the risk of side effects; their short serum half-life; weak immune response recruitment; the development of human anti-mouse antibodies; the possibility of a fatal allergic reaction; and the loss of efficacy and function after small epitopic changes, which mostly happens with highly mutagenic viruses and often leads to drug resistance. The majority of therapeutic antibodies that are currently on the market are humanized mAbs, which are 85%–90% human, are less immunogenic, and have reduced or completely stopped.

Instead of the live animal or human donors needed for serum therapy, modern technology makes it possible to produce mAbs relatively easily and effectively using only tissue culture or microbial expression systems. Therefore, the potential toxicity of human and humanized mAbs is lower than serum therapy and comparable to that of antibiotics, particularly heterologous preparations. In addition, mAbs treat diseases more effectively and with fewer side effects than conventional therapies because they have a higher level of specificity and affinity for their targets. As a result, the pharmaceutical industry has increased its production and application of mAbs [82].

The current focus of research is on creating novel approaches to enhance and improve the specificities and modes of action of the existing mAbs as well as to create risk-free and affordable expression systems. Recently, there has been research into a method for producing recombinant polyclonal antibodies.

As of 30 June 2022, there were 162 approved and marketed antibody therapies, which were used to treat a variety of illnesses, including cancer, immune-related disease, infectious disease, and hematological disease. Golimumab, Cetrolizumab, Eculizumab, Ranibizumab, Panitumumab, Natalizumb, Nimotuzumab, Bevacizumab, Omalizumab, Cetuximab, Daclizumab, and others are examples of therapeutic antibodies that are currently approved [83].

2.12 General method of preparation of sera

2.12.1 Antibacterial sera

Passive immunity against diseases brought on by endotoxin-producing bacteria is provided by this kind of serum. In the past, chemotherapy took the place of the antisera used to treat a number of these illnesses, including typhoid, meningitis, and pneumonia.

They are prepared similarly to antitoxins, with the following key distinctions:

1. The organism is injected into the horse either as a dead or living suspension.
2. The intravenous route is used because reactions frequently occur after the intramuscular injection of large numbers of bacterial cells.
2. There are different ways to clean up the sera because antibacterial antibodies are linked to the gamma-globin fraction.

As a result, in order to produce antitoxins that are pure, various techniques must be used, including precipitation, ultrafiltration, and ion exchange chromatography. These techniques aid in the concentration of the antitoxin for therapeutic use and the removal of unwanted impurities [84].

2.12.2 Antiviral sera

Antiviral antibodies are thought to behave differently than other types of antibodies. Because viruses are intracellular parasites and antibodies cannot penetrate cells, virus inactivation must occur in body fluids or on surfaces where invasion is taking place. The mode of attack appears to involve the virus blocking sites used in adsorption on host cells prior to penetration. Human serum is the primary source of antiviral antibodies used in passive immunization (see Human Normal Immunoglobulin Injection). This is due to the horse's immunity to several major diseases against which protection may be needed, such as German measles, measles, and poliomyelitis. Moreover, the official rabies antiserum is prepared in horses [85].

2.13 Evaluation of sera

Evaluation of sera is a key step in making sure they work well in diagnostic and therapeutic applications. Sera can be evaluated based on their purity, potency, specificity, and stability. Several methods are used to evaluate these characteristics of sera, including gel electrophoresis, immunodiffusion, enzyme-linked immunosorbent assay (ELISA), and Western blotting.

1. Gel electrophoresis is a method used to separate proteins based on their size and charge. It is often used to check the purity of sera by identifying for viruses, bacteria, and other unwanted substances that might be there.
2. Immunodiffusion is a technique that visualizes the presence of specific antigens or antibodies in a sample by using antigen–antibody reactions. It is frequently used to assess sera specificity by determining their ability to recognize and bind to a specific antigen.
2. ELISA is a popular method for the quantitative detection of antigens or antibodies in a sample. Testing the concentration of particular antibodies in a serum sample is a common way to evaluate its efficacy.
4. Western blotting is a method for detecting specific proteins within a sample. It is frequently used to evaluate the purity and specificity of serum by detecting the presence of particular proteins or antibodies.

In addition to these techniques, stability testing is an essential component of the evaluation of sera. Stability testing involves exposing sera to a variety of environmental conditions, such as temperature and humidity, in order to evaluate their ability to maintain their activity over time. This type of testing is essential for ensuring that sera remain effective and safe to use throughout their shelf life, which is crucial for patient safety and regulatory compliance. In addition, it assists manufacturers in determining the proper storage conditions and expiration dates for their products.

Sera are typically evaluated in accordance with guidelines established by organizations such as the WHO and the International Organization for Standardization (ISO). These guidelines offer suggestions for evaluating sera and establishing international standards for their use [86].

2.14 Standardization of sera

The process of establishing a set of quantitative measures for the potency and quality of sera used in diagnostic and therapeutic applications is referred to as sera standardization. The goal of standardization is to ensure that different batches of sera produced by different manufacturers have the same composition and activity and can be compared and used interchangeably.

The establishment of international reference standards or units of measurement for the activity of specific sera components, such as antibodies or antigens, is typically involved in the standardization of sera. These reference standards are used to calibrate assays used to measure the activity of serum components and to assign potency values to different batches of sera.

One of the major organizations in charge of standardizing sera is the WHO. The WHO creates and disseminates international reference standards for a variety of sera components, including antibodies, antigens, and cytokines, through its International Biological. The development of global reference standards for sera components enables producers to calibrate their assays against these norms and guarantee that their goods comply with global norms. This in turn makes it easier to use sera products in clinical and research settings and to compare the outcomes of various assays and laboratories [87].

2.15 Regulatory consideration of sera

Regulations and guidelines that control the production, testing, and use of sera in diagnostic and therapeutic applications are known as regulatory considerations for sera. The goal of these rules and suggestions is to make sure that sera products work, are safe, and are of good quality. Under Title 21 of the Code of Federal Regulations (CFR), the US FDA controls the production, testing, and distribution of serum products. As biological products, sera products must follow rules called GMP and get FDA approval before they can be sold.

In accordance with the European Pharmacopoeia (EP) and European Union Directives, the EMA also controls the production and use of sera products in the European Union (EU). The EU Directives establish guidelines for their production, testing, and distribution. The European Parliament (EPr) establishes standards for the quality, purity, potency, and safety of serum products.

The following additional regulatory factors for sera products are as follows:

1. Adverse event reporting: Companies that make or sell sera products have to tell regulatory agencies about any bad things that happen because of their products.
2. According to labeling regulations, sera products must include the necessary information on their packaging, such as the product's name, intended use, recommended storage conditions, and any potential risks or adverse effects.
2. Traceability: In order to be found in the event of a recall or other issue, regulatory authorities may require manufacturers and distributors of sera products to keep records of where their products came from and how they were sold.

Norms applied internationally:

The rules and regulations established by international organizations like the WHO and the International Conference on Harmonization may also apply to sera products [88].

2.16 Marketed products of vaccines and sera

These are just a few examples of marketed serum products mentioned in Table 2.5. There are many other types of sera, each with their own specific applications and indications.

TABLE 2.5 Marketed products of vaccines and sera [89,90].

Generic name of vaccine/sera	Abbreviation	Marketed products/trade name
Vaccines		
Adenovirus vaccine	AdVs	Adenovirus Type 4 and Type7
Anthrax vaccine	AVA	BioThrax
Cholera vaccine	Oral cholera vaccine	Dukoral, Shancol, Euvichol, Vaxchora
Diphtheria and tetanus vaccine	DT/Td,	Generic, Tenivac (Td)
Diphtheria, tetanus, and whooping cough vaccine	DTwP/DTaP	Daptacel, Infanrix (DTaP) Adacel (Tdap)
Diptheria, tetanus, and pertussis-polio vaccine	DTaP-IPV	Kinrix, Quadracel
Diptheria, tetanus, and pertussis-Hepatitis B-polio vaccine	DTaP-HepB-IPV	Pediarix
Diptheria, tetanus, and pertussis-*Haemophilus influenzae* type-b-polio vaccine	DTaP-IPV/Hib	Pentacel
Diptheria, tetanus, and pertussis-polio *H. influenzae* type b-hepatitis B vaccine	DTaP-IPV-Hib-HepB	Vaxelis
Dengue vaccine	DenV	Dengvaxia
Hepatitis A vaccine	HepA	Havrix, Vaqta
Hepatitis B vaccine	HepB	Engerix-B, Recombivax HB, Heplisav-B
Hepatitis A-B vaccine	HepA-HepB	Twinrix
H. influenzae type b vaccine	Hib (PRP-T) Hib (PRP-OMP) Hib (PRP-T)	ActHIB, PedvaxHIB, Hiberix
HPV vaccine	9vHPV	Gardasil9
Influenza vaccine	IIV LAIV	Afluria, Fluad, Flublok, Flucelvax, FluLaval, Fluarix, Fluzone FluMist
Japanese Encephalitis vaccine	JE	Ixiaro
Measles Mumps vaccine Meningococcal vaccine	MMR MMRV MenACWY MenB	M-M-R II ProQuad Menactra, Menveo MenQuadfi, Bexsero, Trumenba
Pneumococcal vaccine	PCV13 PCV15 PCV20 PPSV23	Prevnar13 Vaxneuvance Prevnar20 Pneumovax 23
Polio vaccine	IPV DTaP-IPV DTaP-HepB-IPV	Ipol Kinrix, Quadracel Pediarix

(*Continued*)

TABLE 2.5 (Continued)

Generic name of vaccine/sera	Abbreviation	Marketed products/trade name
	DTaP-IPV/Hib DTaP-IPV-Hib-HepB	Pentacel Vaxelis
Rabies vaccine	Rabies	ImovaxRabies, RabAvert
Rotavirus vaccine	RV1 RV5	Rotarix RotaTeq
Rubella vaccine	MMR MMRV	M-M-R II ProQuad
Herpes Zoster (Shingles) vaccine	RZV	Shingrix
Smallpox vaccine	Vaccinia	ACAM2000
Tetanus vaccine	DTaP DT Td	Daptacel, Infanrix Generic Tenivac
Typhoid fever vaccine	Typhoid-oral Typhoid polysaccharide	Vivotif Typhim Vi
Varicella vaccine	VAR	Varivax
Yellow fever vaccine	YF	YF-Vax
Sera		
Anthrax vaccine	Anthrax immune globulin intravenous	ANTHRACIL
Botulism	Botulism antitoxin bivalent (Equine) types A and B (BIG-IV) Botulism antitoxin heptavalent (A, B, C, D, E, F, and G)	BabyBIG BAT
Black widow spider bite	Antivenin (*Latrodectus mactans*)	Black widow spider antivenin
Cytomegalovirus disease	Cytomegalovirus immune globulin	CytoGam
Coronavirus	COVID-19	Casirivimab and Imdevimab Sotrovimab
Hepatitis A	Hepatitis A immunoglobulin (HepA-Ig)	GamaSTAN GamaSTAN S/D
Hepatitis B	Hepatitis B immunoglobulin (HepB–Ig)	Bayhep B HepaGam B HyperHEP B Nabi-HB Nabi-HB NovaPlus
Human Rabies immunoglobulin	Human rabies immunoglobulin	Imogam Rabies—HT Kedrab Hyperrab
Tetanus	TET	Hyper-TET S/D, Tetglob
Scorpian Venomation	Centruroides (Scorpion) Immune F(ab')2 (Equine) Injection	Anascorp
Vaccinia	Vaccinia immune globulin	VIGIV VARIZIG

(*Continued*)

TABLE 2.5 (Continued)

Generic name of vaccine/sera	Abbreviation	Marketed products/trade name
		CNJ-016
Viper Venomation	Crotalidae Immune F(ab')2 (Equine)	ANAVIP
Eastern coral snake	Antivenin (*Micrurus fulvius*)	North American coral snake antivenin
Crotalid envenomation	Crotalidae Polyvalent Immune Fab	CROFAB

2.17 Challenges to vaccine and sera success

One of the biggest problems with public health is the emergence of new pathogens that are easier to spread, kill more people, or can get around the immune system. The development of vaccines for diseases like HIV, TB, and malaria that evade the immune system has not been particularly successful and remains a difficult task. Certain pathogens' genomic variability and capacity for rapid mutation present difficulties for vaccine development and pose a risk of evasion, which would reduce the efficacy of existing vaccines. New infectious diseases with high death rates or rates of spread pose a serious threat to public health as well as the local and global economies, as the Ebola outbreak and COVID-19 pandemic have demonstrated. Monitoring, pandemic preparedness programs, cooperation between the government and non-government organizations, national policies, and current technologies and platforms for vaccine production and distribution are just a few of the many variables that affect how quickly one can respond to such threats. Although immediate response tactics like social isolation, quarantine, and lockdown effectively stop the spread of an emerging pathogen, they are difficult to maintain over the long term from a practical standpoint. By limiting disease transmission, preventing the clinical manifestation of infection in a short amount of time, and establishing herd immunity, rapid rollout of mass vaccination programs lowers treatment costs and prevents overloading the healthcare system [91].

Important prerequisites for vaccine production include an understanding of the immune elements that stimulate the production of antibodies against infection and an understanding of the metrics to be used to assess the vaccine's effectiveness. This kind of information is mostly gathered from patients who have recovered from an infection on their own or from animal models that respond to infection in a similar way to how humans get sick. Every time one of these elements is absent, the development of vaccination is made more difficult and serious safety concerns are raised. For instance, the lack of validated animal models to facilitate vaccine candidates against COVID-19 and the absence of fundamental aspects of virus biology and immunity are the main obstacles in the development of the COVID-19 vaccine.

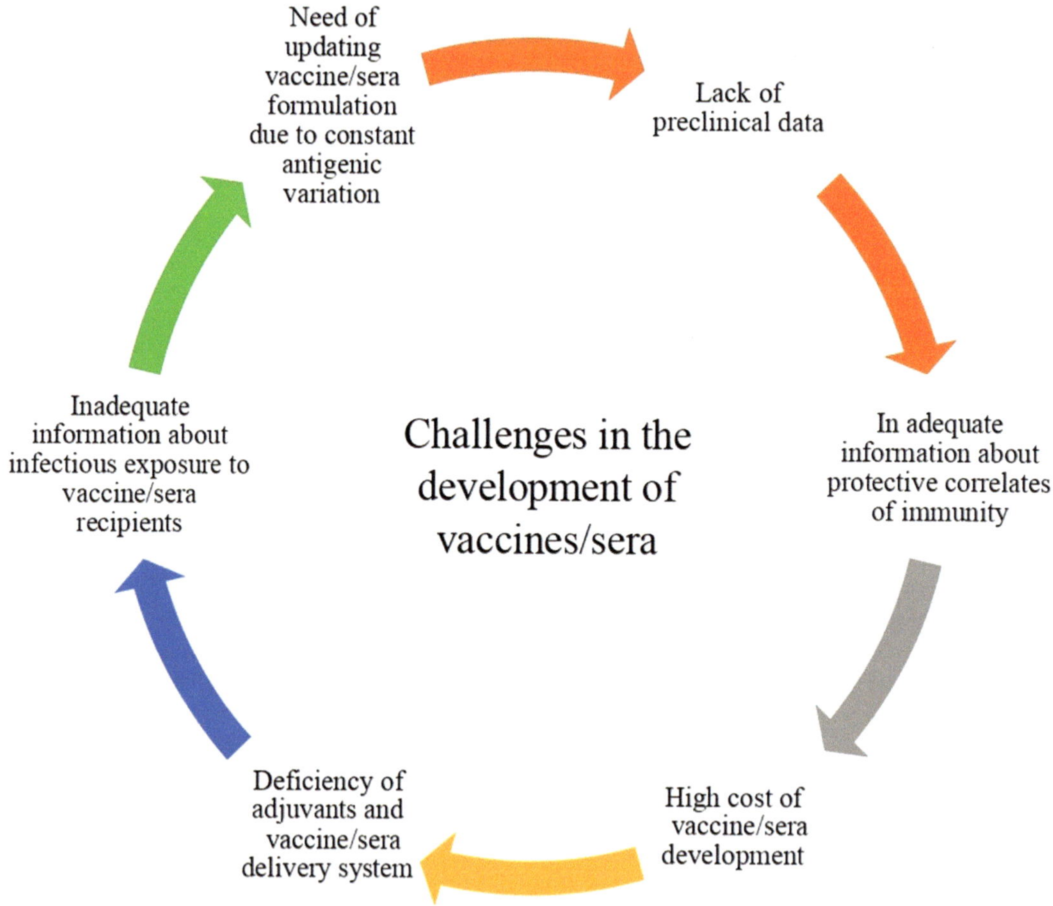

FIGURE 2.5 Challenges of vaccines and sera.

The current state of antigen selection techniques has changed as a result of the advancement of bioinformatics and high throughput screening. These methods allow researchers to find novel and recently discovered pathogens. Despite these more recent technologies, the antigenic diversity of pathogens, the delay in the availability of adjuvants, and delivery methods limit the market impact of genomic approaches [92]. Additionally, due to the high costs and several other challenges mentioned in Fig. 2.5 associated with vaccine research, potentially beneficial products are shelved too soon.

2.18 New approaches for vaccines and sera

Traditional vaccinations have been very effective, but there are still many infectious diseases for which there are insufficiently effective vaccines. Human pathogens like the TB, HIV, respiratory syncytial virus, herpes simplex virus, Epstein–Barr virus, and cytomegalovirus, are yet to have vaccines developed against them. New vaccine technologies have been developed because existing platforms for traditional vaccines have limitations [93]. In the 1970s, the development of rDNA technology marked the beginning of a new era in vaccine development. With the aid of the new technology, single proteins or proteins that make up virus-like particles (VLP) could be produced and potentially modified to create an improved vaccine. Additionally, it made it possible for modified vectors to be created to carry antigens from various pathogens and the use of RNA or DNA encoding antigens as vaccines. In the interim, key antigens have been identified and some aspects of the immune responses they elicit have been elucidated by structural biology and systems biology. Vaccines that are rationally designed to protect against a specific pathogen should have well-defined active ingredients and excipients. These vaccines consist of antigens, delivery systems, and adjuvants that frequently elicit predictable immune responses against specific epitopes. These new technologies can fill unmet medical needs, such as those for novel pathogens for which rapid development is essential or vaccines involving difficult-to-manufacture antigens. Two mRNA vaccines and two adenovirus vectored vaccines are among the four most advanced programs being tested in Phase 3 trials in the United States for the ongoing COVID-19 pandemic [94].

However, due to limited information, this is not always possible. The development of vaccines is still typically a time-consuming and expensive empiric process, and there are no generally accepted methods and tools for rationally designing vaccines [95]. The development of new vaccine candidates, as well as vaccine candidates undergoing active clinical trial phases 1–3, will all be covered in the following sections, followed by a brief overview of the most frequently used technologies. Finally, the discussion of the new generation vaccines that have received FDA and EMA approval will take place [96].

2.18.1 Nucleic acid

2.18.1.1 mRNA vaccine

In recent years, mRNA vaccines have drawn a lot of attention due to their potential to speed up vaccine development, improve safety and efficacy, and combat diseases that have previously been impossible to prevent using conventional methods. The risk of toxicity and long-term side effects is reduced by the fact that mRNA is nonintegrative, noninfectious, and quickly degraded by normal cellular processes after injection. In extensive Phase 3 clinical trials, the safety and high efficacy of two mRNA-based SARS-CoV-2 vaccines (Moderna mRNA-1273 and Pfizer/BioNTech BNT162b2 lipid nanoparticles) were established in both adult and elderly subjects. These are the first licensed mRNA vaccines, and if they are well received and used, it will be possible to develop new mRNA vaccines that target other infectious diseases.

The initial clinical trials for the H10 and H7 influenza hemagglutinin mRNA LNP vaccines took place in 2015 and 2016. With doses of modified uridine mRNA of 25 and 100 mg, respectively, phase I clinical data demonstrated 100% seroconversion with a side effect profile comparable to other approved vaccines [97].

2.18.1.2 DNA vaccine

Inactivated viruses, live attenuated viruses, VLP, subunit proteins, virally vectored recombinant organisms, and even closely related mRNA vaccines have all been successfully replaced by DNA vaccines as a viable and compelling alternative. Since DNA vaccines are stable at room temperature, they do not require the cold chain transportation and ultralow temperature storage required for mRNA vaccines. Since the simplified DNA sequences lack the ability to transform into a virulent form of the virus and there is no evidence of integration into host DNA as a safety concern, DNA vaccines have a safer clinical profile than live attenuated vaccines. Clinical trials for prophylactic DNA vaccines against hantaviruses, alphaviruses, the HIV, influenza, the Zika virus, West Nile File (WNV), the Ebola virus, and the severe acute respiratory syndrome coronavirus 2 have recently been conducted (SARS-CoV-2) [98]. When Zydus Lifesciences received approval from the Drug Controller General of India for the coronavirus disease 2019 (COVID-19) vaccine, ZyCoV-D, using the PharmaJet Tropis intradermal needle-free injection system, the first DNA vaccine for administration to humans was licensed in 2021 [99].

2.18.2 Viral vectors

Viral vectors that mimic a live infection by expressing antigens in situ after vaccination include those based on adenoviruses or pox viruses (de Cassan and Draper, 2013). This facilitates the induction of cytotoxic T lymphocytes and other potent T-cell responses. Because they can target both the infected cells (rather than the pathogen itself) and epitopes that are consistent across strains, these types of responses are advantageous for intracellular pathogens that change a lot. One of the most cutting-edge methods relies on a prime-boost vaccination using two different viral vectors (chicken pox and vaccinia virus, respectively) that express prostate cancer antigen and three different co-stimulatory molecules (B7−1, LFA-3, and ICAM1) [100].

2.18.3 Recombinant viral vector

Recombinant viral vector platforms make use of the viral vector's natural capacity to deliver the desired antigen's genetic material into the cell, where it is subsequently expressed as a foreign protein and recognized as such by the immune system. Compared to nonviral techniques like liposome nanoparticles or naked plasmid DNA, this method is frequently more efficient. Another design for this technology is where a "ready-made" antigen is carried on the viral vector's particle and presented as the vaccine's own protein to the immune system. Recombinant viral vectors have a number of important advantages over competing technologies. Adenoviruses, lentiviruses, nonsegmented negative-stranded RNA viruses (like Sendai virus, measles virus, and vesicular stomatitis virus), poxviruses, herpes viruses, and baculoviruses have all been considered as viral vectors for new vaccines [101].

2.18.4 Virus-like particles

Multiprotein nanostructures called VLP can assemble by themselves. They are made from viral structural proteins and mostly look like how viruses form on their own. Depending on the desired properties of the protein, VLP-forming proteins can be produced in any expression host system (e.g., *E. coli*, *S. cerevisiae*, baculovirus expression systems, mammalian cell lines). VLPs are highly effective at promoting the activation of the CD^{8+} immune response and B cell immunity. Due to its simplicity, stability, uniformity, and effectiveness in inducing humoral and cellular immunity, and safety, VLP-based vaccine development is a field that is expanding quickly [102].

2.18.5 Tuberculosis vaccine

Mycobacterium TB (*M. tuberculosis*), which causes TB, is still a threat to global public health. TB, an ageing illness, will continue to be the leading cause of human death from a single pathogen in 2021. However, it is claimed that BCG's protection only lasts for 10 to 15 years and varies greatly, ranging from 0% to 80%. Although it is well tolerated, it can spread in immunocompromised people, particularly HIV-infected people, and cause a condition known as BCGosis. As a result, BCG is not advised for newborns who have been exposed to HIV in many nations. Therefore, the urgent and difficult task of finding a new, efficient TB vaccine for governments and scientists is to eradicate TB. Some vectored vaccines are currently being developed as prime boost strategies, which may include a variety of viral vectors and/or M. TB antigen combinations, in addition to BCG boosters. There are currently two candidates in separate phase I trials based on the adenovirus-borne mycobacterial antigen 85A: Prime-boost Ad5-Ag85A and ChA-dOx185A-MVA85A. The whole-cell freeze-dried Mtb vaccine AEC/BC02 was created by Anhui Zhifei Longcom, China, and is administered intramuscularly six times. The Phase I trial was nonrandomized, open-label, and placebo-controlled. The Russian company Gamaleya Research Institute of Epidemiology and Microbiology's subunit recombinant vaccine GAMTBVac, which contains the mycobacterial antigens 85A and ESAT-CFP10, demonstrated safety and underwent dose selection in phase I. M72/AS01, a different strategy based on an adjuvanted recombinant protein antigen, was immunogenic and well tolerated in a phase I trial, and phase II trials are currently evaluating it [103,104].

2.18.6 Cancer vaccine

Infectious disease vaccines have been available for many years. Contrarily, only a small number of cancer vaccines have been authorized for use in humans. These include therapeutic vaccines used as immunotherapy agents to treat cancers as well as preventative vaccines against infectious agents linked to cancer. Heterogeneity within and between cancer types, the selection of vaccine delivery platforms, and the screening and identification of appropriate tumor-specific antigens are challenges in the development of cancer vaccines. The FDA approved ipilimumab for the treatment of metastatic or incurable melanoma in 2011. The phase III double-blind study, which showed an overall response rate of 10.9% with 60% of patients maintaining the response for at least 2 years, served as the foundation for the approval. Seven deaths were attributed to immune-related toxicity, which was observed in 60% of the patients. Despite the fact that this was a fantastic advancement, the low response rate though durable and the high rate of immune-related toxicity (20% grade III and IV) made it necessary to develop safer and more potent immunotherapy medications [105]. Patients with metastatic melanoma still receive the anti-CTLA-4 mAb therapy in addition to other immunotherapy medications. In some studies, melanoma, Hodgkin's lymphoma, non-small-cell lung cancer, and other human cancers have been treated with mAbs that target PD-1/PD-L1 interactions. Examples include the treatment of advanced melanoma (December 22, 2014), metastatic renal cell carcinoma (November 23, 2015), Hodgkin's lymphoma (May 17, 2016), and metastatic urothelial carcinoma (February 2, 2017) with Nivolumab, a PD-1 mAb. Another PD-1 mAb, pembrolizumab, has received FDA approval for the treatment of advanced melanoma (September 4, 2014), advanced non-small-cell lung cancer (October 2, 2015), head and neck squamous cell carcinoma (August 5, 2016), classical Hodgkin's lymphoma (March 15, 2017), and advanced renal cell carcinoma (August 11, 2021).

The goal of developing cancer vaccines is to trigger an immune response against tumor antigens. Only a few cancer vaccines have been given the go-ahead for use in humans despite years of research and development. Other vaccines are being tested in various stages of clinical trials (described below). The antigens used, the tumor microenvironment, the immune landscape of the tumor, and the various vaccine formulations all play a role in how well these cancer vaccines work. The objectives of nucleic acid vaccines for pathogens and nucleic acid vaccines for cancers are very different from one another. Similar to vaccines used to prevent disease, therapeutic nucleic acid vaccines are used to treat cancer by instructing the immune system to recognize and eliminate tumors. This is accomplished by focusing on antigens that cancer cells frequently express [106]. These antigens include elements that promote growth or ones that are specific to cancer cells as a result of somatic mutations (neoantigens).

2.18.6.1 *Neoantigen vaccines*

These vaccines are made to target particular mutations in the tumor cells of a patient. By examining the genetic profile of a patient's tumor, researchers can identify mutations that can be targeted by a vaccine. Early-stage clinical trials have demonstrated the potential of this strategy [107].

2.18.6.2 *RNA-based vaccines*

An innovative method that uses a patient's own cells to produce cancer antigens is the RNA vaccine. The injected RNA molecules are absorbed by immune cells, which then use them to produce the antigens in the patient's body [108].

2.18.6.3 *Peptide-based vaccines*

Peptides, or small fragments of protein from cancer cells, are used in these vaccines to stimulate an immune response. Peptide-based vaccines can be made relatively quickly and affordably, and they are less complex than other kinds of cancer vaccines [109].

2.18.6.4 *Dendritic cell–based vaccines*

Immune cells called DCs display antigens to other immune cells. DCs may be used to trigger the immune system to attack cancer cells, according to researchers. This procedure involves removing DCs from the patient's blood, exposing them to cancer antigens in a lab, and then reintroducing them into the patient's body. Sipuleucel-T (Provenge), for instance, has prostate cancer approval [110].

In a randomized Phase 2 clinical trial, a personalized mRNA cancer vaccine created by Moderna and Merck Co. demonstrated promising outcomes [111].

2.18.7 HIV vaccine

HIV is still a major threat to health around the world. In 2021, between 33.9 million and 43.8 million people became infected with HIV. Antiretroviral therapy is being implemented globally, and there is a growing arsenal of nonvaccine HIV prevention tools, but, as is covered elsewhere in this special issue, an efficient vaccine will likely be required to put an end to the epidemic. The HIV vaccine field has been able to create a number of vaccine platforms, thanks to cutting-edge clinical studies. The only evidence that an HIV vaccine can shield people from contracting the disease is still the RV144 Thai trial. To improve the elicitation of immune correlates derived from RV144, prime-boost strategies, combination mosaic antigens, novel viral vectors, antigens intended to elicit broadly neutralizing antibodies, new nucleic acid platforms, and potent adjuvants are currently used in vaccine development. "Engineered Fc receptor ligands target HIV-1 env immunogens to B cells" by Matteo Bianchi outlines a novel method for designing an HIV vaccine that involves engineering Fc receptor ligands to target env immunogens to B cells [112].

2.18.8 Malaria vaccines

Malaria is a dangerous disease that can cause death. It is caused by parasites that are transmitted through the bites of female Anopheles mosquitoes that are infected. It can be avoided and treated. The estimated number of malaria cases and deaths worldwide in 2021 is 247 million cases and 619,000 deaths, respectively.

There are no vaccines that are widely used. At the moment, bed nets treated with pyrethroid insecticide and indoor residual insecticide spraying are the best vector control methods for prevention. Additionally, there are antimicrobials for chemoprophylaxis. There are no vaccines that are widely used. RTS,S/AS01 is the only vaccine that has shown some level of malaria protection (MosquirixTM by GlaxoSmithKline). The main circumsporozoite protein (PfCSP), which coats the surface of the infecting sporozoite, is the target of this vaccine's immune responses. In order to achieve this, RTS,S was created as VLP with two parts: 18 copies of the central repeat and the C-terminal domain of PfCSP fused to extra HBsAg on the hepatitis B virus surface. In the preliminary analysis of a significant phase 3 study carried out in southern Africa, the vaccine's efficacy against clinical malaria in infants aged 5 to 17 months was estimated to be 50%. Diverse whole sporozoite vaccine (WSV) strategies have shown high levels of protection against homologous CHMI in preclinical animal models and humans; current studies seek to define efficacy in populations with high rates of malaria as well as the breadth and duration of protection. WSV relies on the administration of live-attenuated sporozoites, which stop developing at different stages before the fulminant blood-stage infection, or live sporozoites, which enter the blood but are destroyed by medications. The timing of the arrest has significant effects on the breadth and potency of the immune response, according to preclinical research in rodents. When transmitted to humans by mosquito bites, radiation-attenuated sporozoites, the first WSV to be studied in both rodents and humans, arrest at various points early in the liver-stage development. These sporozoites were the first to be shown to confer protection in humans.

Recently, subunits against pregnancy-associated malaria using VAR2CSA and a chemically attenuated whole-parasite blood-stage vaccine have been created. These vaccines may replicate some aspects of natural acquired immunity.

The upcoming years look to be an exciting time that should inspire hope that a highly effective vaccine may be within reach when combined with ongoing progress in terms of vaccine biomanufacture, human vaccine delivery platforms, and efficacy assessment by long-term and heterologous CHMI controlled human malaria infection [113].

2.18.9 Dengue vaccines

The viral disease dengue, which is spread by mosquitoes, can result in life-threatening conditions like dengue hemorrhagic fever and dengue fever. Currently, there is no known cure for dengue, and mosquito control is the main method of prevention. Additionally, vaccines are being created to guard against dengue infection. Here are a few fresh ideas for developing a dengue vaccine [114].

Research on dengue vaccines has been ongoing for a while, with a focus on making the available vaccine candidates safer, more efficient, and more cost-effective. Here are a few current instances of innovative studies in the creation of dengue vaccines:

2.18.9.1 Nanoparticle-based vaccines

To increase the efficacy and safety of dengue vaccines, researchers are investigating the use of nanoparticle-based vaccines. As an illustration, a recent study developed a tetravalent dengue vaccine using VLP. The VLP resembled the dengue virus in shape, but they lacked any of the virus' genetic material. It was less likely that someone would react negatively as a result of this [115].

2.18.9.2 Tetravalent dengue vaccine

Dengvaxia, the first dengue vaccine, was a tetravalent vaccine that protected against all four dengue virus serotypes. However, it was not very effective and raised safety issues, particularly for those who had never had dengue before. New tetravalent dengue vaccines are being developed by researchers, such as the TAK-003 vaccine, which uses a live attenuated virus and has demonstrated promising outcomes in clinical trials [116].

2.18.9.3 Nonstructural protein targets

The majority of dengue vaccine candidates go after the structural proteins of the virus, which can change quickly and result in vaccine failure. Nonstructural proteins are more conserved than structural proteins and may offer broader protection against dengue. Researchers are investigating the use of vaccines that target these proteins [117].

2.18.9.4 Vaccines with additives

To boost the immune response, certain substances are added to vaccines. Toll-like receptor agonists are one of the new adjuvants being studied by researchers to improve the efficacy of dengue vaccines [118].

2.18.9.5 RNA-based vaccines

A more recent strategy that has shown promise in combating other viral diseases like COVID-19 is the use of RNA-based vaccines. Researchers are investigating the possibility of treating dengue with RNA vaccines. Early preclinical research has produced encouraging findings [119].

2.19 Conclusion

Immunization is essential for protecting from diseases. Vaccine technologies like nucleic acid, inactivation, attenuation, subunits, viral vectors, and viral particle-based techniques are used to make a safer and an effective vaccines. Despite the fact that there are many limitations, ongoing efforts have been made to develop highly effective and competent vaccines for many human and animal-related diseases due to their unlimited potential. This article focuses on the historical perspective and development of the vaccine because it is a critical area of research where human life is saved from various potential diseases. However, there are still significant knowledge gaps and problems that need to be resolved. The development of effective vaccines against serious diseases has been hindered by insufficient knowledge of immune mechanisms and a lack of strategies to deal with antigenic variability. Additionally, social barriers prevent everyone from receiving a safe and effective vaccine. The combination of current information, continuous development, and a rising understanding of human immunology can provide methods to successfully address developing future global outbreaks.

References

[1] Rappuoli R, Pizza M, Del Giudice G, De Gregorio E. Vaccines, new opportunities for a new society. Proc Natl Acad Sci U S A 2014;111:12288–93. Available from: https://doi.org/10.1073/pnas.1402981111.

[2] World Health Organisation Vaccines and Immunization. Available from: https://www.who.int/health-topics/vaccines-and-immunization#tab = tab.

[3] Kayser V, Ramzan I. Vaccines and vaccination: history and emerging issues. Hum Vaccin Immunother 2021;17:5255–68. Available from: https://doi.org/10.1080/21645515.2021.1977057.

[4] Barquet N, Domingo P. Smallpox: the triumph over the most terrible of the ministers of death. Ann Intern Med 1997;127:635–42. Available from: https://doi.org/10.7326/0003-4819-127-8_Part_1-199710150-00010.

[5] Riedel S. Edward Jenner and the history of smallpox and vaccination. Bayl Univ Med Cent Proc 2005;18:21–5. Available from: https://doi.org/10.1080/08998280.2005.11928028.

[6] Lombard M, Pastoret P-P, Moulin AM. A brief history of vaccines and vaccination. Rev Sci Tech l'OIE 2007;26:29–48. Available from: https://doi.org/10.20506/rst.26.1.1724.

[7] Moore J. The history of the small pox. 1815. https://books.google.co.in/books?hl = en&lr = &id = 3kUSAAAAYAAJ&oi = fnd&pg = PA1&dq = The + History + of + the + Small + Pox + by + Moore, + J.C. + The + year + 1815%3B + Longman, + Hurst, + Rees, + Orme, + and + Brown&ots = vGxGqt2Go_&sig = h0x1Q8XoONPhRhpyOTCRo_9rOIw&redir_esc = y#v = onepage&q&f = false.

[8] Plotkin S. History of vaccine development. Springer Science & Business Media; 2011.

[9] Dubé E, Laberge C, Guay M, Bramadat P, Roy R, Bettinger J. Vaccine hesitancyAn overview. Hum Vaccin Immunother 2013;9:1763–73. Available from: https://doi.org/10.4161/hv.24657.

[10] Wever PC, van Bergen L. Prevention of tetanus during the first world war. Med Humanit 2012;38:78–82. Available from: https://doi.org/10.1136/medhum-2011-010157.

[11] Hilleman MR. Vaccines in historic evolution and perspective: a narrative of vaccine discoveries. Vaccine. 1999;1436–47.
[12] Ehreth J. The global value of vaccination. Vaccine 2003;21:596–600. Available from: https://doi.org/10.1016/S0264-410X(03)00377-3.
[13] Hoyt K. Vaccine innovation: lessons from world war II. J Public Health Policy 2006;27:38–57. Available from: https://doi.org/10.1057/palgrave.jphp.3200064.
[14] Rappuoli R. Bridging the knowledge gaps in vaccine design. Nat Biotechnol 2007;25:1361–6. Available from: https://doi.org/10.1038/nbt1207-1361.
[15] Liu Y-C, Kuo R-L, Shih S-R. COVID-19: the first documented coronavirus pandemic in history. Biomed J 2020;43:328–33. Available from: https://doi.org/10.1016/j.bj.2020.04.007.
[16] KATZ SL. Studies on an attenuated measles-virus vaccine. Am J Dis Child 1960;100:942. Available from: https://doi.org/10.1001/archpedi.1960.04020040944023.
[17] Hilleman MR, Buynak EB, Weibel RE, Stokes J. Live, attenuated mumps-virus vaccine. N Engl J Med 1968;278:227–32. Available from: https://doi.org/10.1056/NEJM196802012780501.
[18] Minor PD. Live attenuated vaccines: historical successes and current challenges. Virology 2015;479–480:379–92. Available from: https://doi.org/10.1016/j.virol.2015.03.032.
[19] Kumar V. Vaccines: the history and future. BoD-Books; 2019.
[20] Moyle PM, Toth I. Modern subunit vaccines: development, components, and research opportunities. ChemMedChem 2013;8:360–76. Available from: https://doi.org/10.1002/cmdc.201200487.
[21] Dai X, Xiong Y, Li N, Jian C. Vaccine types. Vaccines – history and future. IntechOpen; 2019. Available from: https://doi.org/10.5772/intechopen.84626.
[22] Hansson M, Nygren P-Å, Ståhl S. Design and production of recombinant subunit vaccines. Biotechnol Appl Biochem 2000;32:95. Available from: https://doi.org/10.1042/BA20000034.
[23] Adkins JC, Wagstaff AJ. Recombinant hepatitis B vaccine*. BioDrugs 1998;10:137–58. Available from: https://doi.org/10.2165/00063030-199810020-00005.
[24] Markowitz LE, Tsu V, Deeks SL, Cubie H, Wang SA, Vicari AS, et al. Human papillomavirus vaccine introduction–the first five years. Vaccine 2012;30:F139–48. Available from: https://doi.org/10.1016/j.vaccine.2012.05.039.
[25] Santana VF, Balbin YV, Calderón JC, Icart LP, Verez-Bencomo V. Polysaccharide-based vaccines. Glycoscience. Berlin, Heidelberg: Springer Berlin Heidelberg; 2008. p. 2699–723. Available from: https://doi.org/10.1007/978-3-540-30429-6_69.
[26] Wilder-Smith A. Meningococcal vaccines: a neglected topic in travel medicine? Exp Rev Vac 2009;8:1343–50. Available from: https://doi.org/10.1586/erv.09.102.
[27] Perera SR, Sokaribo AS, White AP. Polysaccharide vaccines: a perspective on non-typhoidal salmonella. Polysaccharides 2021;2:691–714. Available from: https://doi.org/10.3390/polysaccharides2030042.
[28] Glenny B, Hopkins AT. Diphtheria toxoid as an immunising agent. Br J Exp Pathol 1923;4:283.
[29] Tahamtan A, Charostad J, Hoseini Shokouh SJ, Barati M. An overview of history, evolution, and manufacturing of various generations of vaccines. J Arch Mil Med Press 2017;. Available from: https://doi.org/10.5812/jamm.12315.
[30] Atkinson W. Epidemiology and prevention of vaccine-preventable diseases. 9th ed. 2006. https://books.google.co.in/books?hl = en&lr = &id = h9BQG90D9e4C&oi = fnd&pg = PR1&dq = Hall + E, + Wodi + AP, + Hamborsky + J, + Morelli + V, + Schillie + S. + Epidemiology + and + prevention + of + vaccine-preventable + diseases. + Centers + for + Disease + Control + and + Prevention. + Public + Health + Foundat.
[31] Clem A. Fundamentals of vaccine immunology. J Glob Infect Dis 2011;3:73. Available from: https://doi.org/10.4103/0974-777X.77299.
[32] Bartlett BL, Pellicane AJ, Tyring SK. Vaccine immunology. Dermatol Ther 2009;22:104–9. Available from: https://doi.org/10.1111/j.1529-8019.2009.01223.x.
[33] Abbas AK, Janeway CA. Immunology. Cell 2000;100:129–38. Available from: https://doi.org/10.1016/S0092-8674(00)81689-X.
[34] Casadevall A, Dadachova E, Pirofski L. Passive antibody therapy for infectious diseases. Nat Rev Microbiol 2004;2:695–703. Available from: https://doi.org/10.1038/nrmicro974.
[35] Delves PJ, Roitt IM. The immune system. N Engl J Med 2000;343:37–49. Available from: https://doi.org/10.1056/NEJM200007063430107.

[36] Giese M, editor. Molecular vaccines. Vienna, Vienna: Springer; 2013. Available from: https://doi.org/10.1007/978-3-7091-1419-3.

[37] Nauta J. Basic concepts of vaccine immunology. Stat. Clin. Vaccine Trials. Berlin, Heidelberg: Springer Berlin Heidelberg; 2011. p. 1–12. Available from: https://doi.org/10.1007/978-3-642-14691-6_1.

[38] Hoebe K, Janssen E, Beutler B. The interface between innate and adaptive immunity. Nat Immunol 2004;5:971–4. Available from: https://doi.org/10.1038/ni1004-971.

[39] L.S. Leo. Oberdan; Anthony, Cunningham; Peter, Vaccine immunology; 2011.

[40] C.-A. Siegrist. Vaccine immunology; 2008.

[41] Chen RT, Glasser JW, Rhodes PH, Davis RL, Barlow WE, Thompson RS, et al.the Vaccine Safety Datalink Team Vaccine safety datalink project: a new tool for improving vaccine safety monitoring in the United States. Pediatrics 1997;99:765–73. Available from: https://doi.org/10.1542/peds.99.6.765.

[42] McNeil MM, Gee J, Weintraub ES, Belongia EA, Lee GM, Glanz JM, et al. The vaccine safety datalink: successes and challenges monitoring vaccine safety. Vaccine 2014;32:5390–8. Available from: https://doi.org/10.1016/j.vaccine.2014.07.073.

[43] Varricchio F, Iskander J, Destefano F, Ball R, Pless R, Braun MM, et al. Understanding vaccine safety information from the vaccine adverse event reporting system. Pediatr Infect Dis J 2004;23:287–94.

[44] Day MJ. Vaccine side effects: fact and fiction. Vet Microbiol 2006;117:51–8. Available from: https://doi.org/10.1016/j.vetmic.2006.04.017.

[45] Iskander JK, Miller ER, Chen RT. The role of the vaccine adverse event reporting system (VAERS) in monitoring vaccine safety. Pediatr Ann 2004;33:599–606. Available from: https://doi.org/10.3928/0090-4481-20040901-11.

[46] Shimabukuro TT, Nguyen M, Martin D, DeStefano F. Safety monitoring in the vaccine adverse event reporting system (VAERS). Vaccine 2015;33:4398–405. Available from: https://doi.org/10.1016/j.vaccine.2015.07.035.

[47] Song BJ, Katial RK. Update on side effects from common vaccines. Curr Allergy Asthma Rep 2004;4:447–53. Available from: https://doi.org/10.1007/s11882-004-0010-8.

[48] Meissner HC. Understanding vaccine safety and the roles of the FDA and the CDC. N Engl J Med 2022;386:1638–45. Available from: https://doi.org/10.1056/NEJMra2200583.

[49] Hibbs BF, Moro PL, Lewis P, Miller ER, Shimabukuro TT. Vaccination errors reported to the vaccine adverse event reporting system, (VAERS) United States, 2000–2013. Vaccine 2015;33:3171–8. Available from: https://doi.org/10.1016/j.vaccine.2015.05.006.

[50] Cai C, Peng Y, Shen E, Huang Q, Chen Y, Liu P, et al. A comprehensive analysis of the efficacy and safety of COVID-19 vaccines. Mol Ther 2021;29:2794–805. Available from: https://doi.org/10.1016/j.ymthe.2021.08.001.

[51] Almadani OA, Alshammari TM. Vaccine adverse event reporting system (VAERS): evaluation of 31 years of reports and pandemics' impact. Saudi Pharm J 2022;30:1725–35. Available from: https://doi.org/10.1016/j.jsps.2022.10.001.

[52] Conklin L, Hviid A, Orenstein WA, Pollard AJ, Wharton M, Zuber P. Vaccine safety issues at the turn of the 21st century. BMJ Glob Heal 2021;6:e004898. Available from: https://doi.org/10.1136/bmjgh-2020-004898.

[53] Soler E, Houdebine L-M. Preparation of recombinant vaccines. Biotechnol Annu Rev 2007;65–94. Available from: https://doi.org/10.1016/S1387-2656(07)13004-0.

[54] Chiodini J. Safe storage and handling of vaccines. Nurs Stand 2014;28:45–52. Available from: https://doi.org/10.7748/ns2014.02.28.25.45.e8486.

[55] Gomez PL, Robinson JM, Rogalewicz JA. Vaccine manufacturing. Vaccines. Elsevier; 2013. p. 44–57. Available from: https://doi.org/10.1016/B978-1-4557-0090-5.00019-7.

[56] Bagriacik EU. Biotechnological approaches in maintenance of a healthy immune system for protection against diseases. Nanotechnol Appl Health Environ Sci in:2021;291–8. Available from: https://doi.org/10.1007/978-3-030-64410-9_15.

[57] Blencowe H, Lawn J, Vandelaer J, Roper M, Cousens S. Tetanus toxoid immunization to reduce mortality from neonatal tetanus. Int J Epidemiol 2010;39:i102–9. Available from: https://doi.org/10.1093/ije/dyq027.

[58] Stanley WM. The preparation and properties of influenza virus vaccines concentrated and purified by differential centrifugation. J Exp Med 1945;81:193–218. Available from: https://doi.org/10.1084/jem.81.2.193.

[59] Qureshi H. editor. Hepatitis B infection in Eastern Mediterranean Region: challenges and the way forward; 2013.

[60] Schneerson R, Barrera O, Sutton A, Robbins JB. Preparation, characterization, and immunogenicity of *Haemophilus influenzae* type b polysaccharide-protein conjugates. J Exp Med 1980;152:361–76. Available from: https://doi.org/10.1084/jem.152.2.361.

[61] Bedwell J, Kairo SK, Behr MA, Bygraves JA. Identification of substrains of BCG vaccine using multiplex PCR. Vaccine 2001;19:2146–51. Available from: https://doi.org/10.1016/S0264-410X(00)00369-8.

[62] Parrino J, Graham B. Smallpox vaccines: past, present, and future. J Allergy Clin Immunol 2006;118:1320–6. Available from: https://doi.org/10.1016/j.jaci.2006.09.037.

[63] Frazattigallina N, Mouraofuches R, Paoli R, Silva M, Miyaki C, Valentini E, et al. Vero-cell rabies vaccine produced using serum-free medium. Vaccine 2004;23:511–17. Available from: https://doi.org/10.1016/j.vaccine.2004.06.014.

[64] Page M, Wilkinson DE, Mattiuzzo G, Efstathiou S, Minor P. Developing biological standards for vaccine evaluation. Fut Virol 2017;12:431–7. Available from: https://doi.org/10.2217/fvl-2017-0003.

[65] Beutels P, Van Doorslaer E, Van Damme P, Hall J. Methodological issues and new developments in the economic evaluation of vaccines. Expert Rev Vac 2003;2:649–60. Available from: https://doi.org/10.1586/14760584.2.5.649.

[66] Trivedi B, Valerio C, Slater JE. Endotoxin content of standardized allergen vaccines. J Allergy Clin Immunol 2003;111:777–83. Available from: https://doi.org/10.1067/mai.2003.1338.

[67] Plitnick LM. Global regulatory guidelines for vaccines. Nonclinical Dev. Nov. Biol. Biosimilars, Vaccines Spec. Biol. Elsevier; 2013. p. 225–41. Available from: https://doi.org/10.1016/B978-0-12-394810-6.00009-5.

[68] Baylor NW. The regulatory evaluation of vaccines for human use in:Vaccine Des 2016;773–87. Available from: https://doi.org/10.1007/978-1-4939-3389-1_51.

[69] Powell MF, Newman MJ, editors. Vaccine design. Boston, MA: Springer US; 1995. Available from: https://doi.org/10.1007/978-1-4615-1823-5.

[70] Stern PL. Key steps in vaccine development. Ann Allergy, Asthma Immunol 2020;125:17–27. Available from: https://doi.org/10.1016/j.anai.2020.01.025.

[71] Schalk JAC, Mooi FR, Berbers GAM, van Aerts LAGJM, Ovelgönne H, Kimman TG. Preclinical and clinical safety studies on DNA vaccines. Hum Vaccin 2006;2:45–53. Available from: https://doi.org/10.4161/hv.2.2.2620.

[72] Thomas S, editor. Vaccine design. New York, NY: Springer New York; 2016. Available from: https://doi.org/10.1007/978-1-4939-3389-1.

[73] Conner J, Wuchterl D, Lopez M, Minshall B, Prusti R, Boclair D, et al. The Biomanufacturing of biotechnology products. Biotechnol. Entrep. Elsevier; 2014. p. 351–85. Available from: https://doi.org/10.1016/B978-0-12-404730-3.00026-9.

[74] Del Giudice G, Rappuoli R, Didierlaurent AM. Correlates of adjuvanticity: a review on adjuvants in licensed vaccines. Semin Immunol 2018;39:14–21. Available from: https://doi.org/10.1016/j.smim.2018.05.001.

[75] Pickering LK, Meissner HC, Orenstein WA, Cohn AC. Principles of vaccine licensure, approval, and recommendations for use. Mayo Clin Proc 2020;95:600–8. Available from: https://doi.org/10.1016/j.mayocp.2019.11.002.

[76] Wine Y, Horton AP, Ippolito GC, Georgiou G. Serology in the 21st century: the molecular-level analysis of the serum antibody repertoire. Curr Opin Immunol 2015;35:89–97. Available from: https://doi.org/10.1016/j.coi.2015.06.009.

[77] Glatman-Freedman A, Casadevall A. Serum therapy for tuberculosis revisited: reappraisal of the role of antibody-mediated immunity against Mycobacterium tuberculosis. Clin Microbiol Rev 1998;11:514–32. Available from: https://doi.org/10.1128/CMR.11.3.514.

[78] Winau F, Winau R. Emil von Behring and serum therapy. Microbes Infect 2002;4:185–8. Available from: https://doi.org/10.1016/S1286-4579(01)01526-X.

[79] Casadevall A, Scharff MD. Return to the past: the case for antibody-based therapies in infectious diseases. Clin Infect Dis 1995;21:150–61. Available from: https://doi.org/10.1093/clinids/21.1.150.

[80] Saylor C, Dadachova E, Casadevall A. Monoclonal antibody-based therapies for microbial diseases. Vaccine 2009;27:G38–46. Available from: https://doi.org/10.1016/j.vaccine.2009.09.105.

[81] Koudstaal W, UytdeHaag FG, Friesen RH, Goudsmit J. Human monoclonal antibodies for prophylaxis and treatment of influenza. Influ. Vaccines Futur. Basel: Springer Basel; 2011. p. 383–98. Available from: https://doi.org/10.1007/978-3-0346-0279-2_17.

[82] Rasmussen SK, Rasmussen LK, Weilguny D, Tolstrup AB. Manufacture of recombinant polyclonal antibodies. Biotechnol Lett 2007;29:845–52. Available from: https://doi.org/10.1007/s10529-007-9331-8.
[83] Lyu X, Zhao Q, Hui J, Wang T, Lin M, Wang K, et al. The global landscape of approved antibody therapies. Antib Ther 2022;5:233–57. Available from: https://doi.org/10.1093/abt/tbac021.
[84] Romanov VA, Kulibin AI, Zaĭtseva IP. [Antibacterial antibodies in human immunoglobulins and sera: past and present]. Zhurnal Mikrobiol Epidemiol i Immunobiol 2010;40–3. Available from: http://www.ncbi.nlm.nih.gov/pubmed/21061576.
[85] Herd S, Macwilliam K. Preparation of antiviral sera for immunofluorescence on infected tissue culture. J Clin Pathol 1971;24:304–7. Available from: https://doi.org/10.1136/jcp.24.4.304.
[86] Hubby B, Talarico T, Maughan M, Reap EA, Berglund P, Kamrud KI, et al. Development and preclinical evaluation of an alphavirus replicon vaccine for influenza. Vaccine 2007;25:8180–9. Available from: https://doi.org/10.1016/j.vaccine.2007.09.038.
[87] Pinheiro de Oliveira TF, Fonseca AA, Camargos MF, de Oliveira AM, Pinto Cottorello AC, Souza Ados R, et al. Detection of contaminants in cell cultures, sera and trypsin. Biologicals 2013;41:407–14. Available from: https://doi.org/10.1016/j.biologicals.2013.08.005.
[88] Vannice KS, Wilder-Smith A, Barrett ADT, Carrijo K, Cavaleri M, de Silva A, et al. Clinical development and regulatory points for consideration for second-generation live attenuated dengue vaccines. Vaccine 2018;36:3411–17. Available from: https://doi.org/10.1016/j.vaccine.2018.02.062.
[89] Charles RC, Ryan ET. Cholera in the 21st century. Curr Opin Infect Dis 2011;24:472–7. Available from: https://doi.org/10.1097/QCO.0b013e32834a88af.
[90] Centers for Disease. Control and Prevention, Markted vaccines. 2022Available from: https://www.cdc.gov/vaccines/terms/usvaccines.html.
[91] Ghattas M, Dwivedi G, Lavertu M, Alameh M-G. Vaccine technologies and platforms for infectious diseases: current progress, challenges, and opportunities. Vaccines 2021;9:1490. Available from: https://doi.org/10.3390/vaccines9121490.
[92] Oyston P, Robinson K. The current challenges for vaccine development. J Med Microbiol 2012;61:889–94. Available from: https://doi.org/10.1099/jmm.0.039180-0.
[93] Bansal S, Prakash A, Medhi B. New generation vaccine: novel approaches of vaccine design and delivery and current challenges of vaccine development. Indian J Pharmacol 2022;54:241. Available from: https://doi.org/10.4103/ijp.ijp_555_22.
[94] Gebre MS, Brito LA, Tostanoski LH, Edwards DK, Carfi A, Barouch DH. Novel approaches for vaccine development. Cell 2021;184:1589–603. Available from: https://doi.org/10.1016/j.cell.2021.02.030.
[95] Rueckert C, Guzmán CA. Vaccines: from empirical development to rational design. PLoS Pathog 2012;8:e1003001. Available from: https://doi.org/10.1371/journal.ppat.1003001.
[96] Matić Z, Šantak M. Current view on novel vaccine technologies to combat human infectious diseases. Appl Microbiol Biotechnol 2022;106:25–56. Available from: https://doi.org/10.1007/s00253-021-11713-0.
[97] Feldman RA, Fuhr R, Smolenov I, (Mick) Ribeiro A, Panther L, Watson M, et al. mRNA vaccines against H10N8 and H7N9 influenza viruses of pandemic potential are immunogenic and well tolerated in healthy adults in phase 1 randomized clinical trials. Vaccine 2019;37:3326–34. Available from: https://doi.org/10.1016/j.vaccine.2019.04.074.
[98] Gaudinski MR, Houser KV, Morabito KM, Hu Z, Yamshchikov G, Rothwell RS, et al. Safety, tolerability, and immunogenicity of two Zika virus DNA vaccine candidates in healthy adults: randomised, open-label, phase 1 clinical trials. Lancet 2018;391:552–62. Available from: https://doi.org/10.1016/S0140-6736(17)33105-7.
[99] Ledesma-Feliciano C, Chapman R, Hooper JW, Elma K, Zehrung D, Brennan MB, et al. Improved DNA vaccine delivery with needle-free injection systems. Vaccines 2023;11:280. Available from: https://doi.org/10.3390/vaccines11020280.
[100] Kantoff PW, Higano CS, Shore ND, Berger ER, Small EJ, Penson DF, et al. Sipuleucel-T immunotherapy for castration-resistant prostate cancer. N Engl J Med 2010;363:411–22. Available from: https://doi.org/10.1056/NEJMoa1001294.
[101] Schöne D, Hrycak CP, Windmann S, Lapuente D, Dittmer U, Tenbusch M, et al. Immunodominance of adenovirus-derived CD8 + T cell epitopes interferes with the induction of transgene-specific immunity in adenovirus-based immunization. J Virol 2017;91. Available from: https://doi.org/10.1128/JVI.01184-17.

[102] Mohsen MO, Gomes AC, Cabral-Miranda G, Krueger CC, Leoratti FM, Stein JV, et al. Delivering adjuvants and antigens in separate nanoparticles eliminates the need of physical linkage for effective vaccination. J Control Rel 2017;251:92–100. Available from: https://doi.org/10.1016/j.jconrel.2017.02.031.
[103] Ottenhoff THM, Kaufmann SHE. Vaccines against tuberculosis: where are we and where do we need to go? PLoS Pathog 2012;8:e1002607. Available from: https://doi.org/10.1371/journal.ppat.1002607.
[104] Jeyanathan M, Fritz DK, Afkhami S, Aguirre E, Howie KJ, Zganiacz A, et al. Aerosol delivery, but not intramuscular injection, of adenovirus-vectored tuberculosis vaccine induces respiratory mucosal immunity in humans. JCI Insight 2022;7:1–20. Available from: https://doi.org/10.1172/jci.insight.155655.
[105] Hodi FS, O'Day SJ, McDermott DF, Weber RW, Sosman JA, Haanen JB, et al. Improved survival with ipilimumab in patients with metastatic melanoma. N Engl J Med 2010;363:711–23. Available from: https://doi.org/10.1056/NEJMoa1003466.
[106] Pardi N, Hogan MJ, Porter FW, Weissman D. mRNA vaccines—a new era in vaccinology. Nat Rev Drug Discov 2018;17:261–79. Available from: https://doi.org/10.1038/nrd.2017.243.
[107] Peng M, Mo Y, Wang Y, Wu P, Zhang Y, Xiong F, et al. Neoantigen vaccine: an emerging tumor immunotherapy. Mol Cancer 2019;18:128. Available from: https://doi.org/10.1186/s12943-019-1055-6.
[108] Faghfuri E, Pourfarzi F, Faghfouri AH, Abdoli Shadbad M, Hajiasgharzadeh K, Baradaran B. Recent developments of RNA-based vaccines in cancer immunotherapy. Exp Opin Biol Ther 2021;21:201–18. Available from: https://doi.org/10.1080/14712598.2020.1815704.
[109] Zhang L, Huang Y, Lindstrom AR, Lin T-Y, Lam KS, Li Y. Peptide-based materials for cancer immunotherapy. Theranostics 2019;9:7807–25. Available from: https://doi.org/10.7150/thno.37194.
[110] Matsuo K, Yoshie O, Kitahata K, Kamei M, Hara Y, Nakayama T. Recent progress in dendritic cell-based cancer immunotherapy. Cancers (Basel) 2021;13:2495. Available from: https://doi.org/10.3390/cancers13102495.
[111] Miao L, Zhang Y, Huang L. mRNA vaccine for cancer immunotherapy. Mol Cancer 2021;20:41. Available from: https://doi.org/10.1186/s12943-021-01335-5.
[112] Hsu DC, O'Connell RJ. Progress in HIV vaccine development. Hum Vaccin Immunother 2017;13:1018–30. Available from: https://doi.org/10.1080/21645515.2016.1276138.
[113] Duffy PE, Patrick Gorres J. Malaria vaccines since 2000: progress, priorities, products. NPJ Vac 2020;5:48. Available from: https://doi.org/10.1038/s41541-020-0196-3.
[114] Deng S-Q, Yang X, Wei Y, Chen J-T, Wang X-J, Peng H-J. A review on dengue vaccine development. Vaccines 2020;8:63. Available from: https://doi.org/10.3390/vaccines8010063.
[115] Quach QH, Ang SK, Chu J-HJ, Kah JCY. Size-dependent neutralizing activity of gold nanoparticle-based subunit vaccine against dengue virus. Acta Biomater 2018;78:224–35. Available from: https://doi.org/10.1016/j.actbio.2018.08.011.
[116] Biswal S, Reynales H, Saez-Llorens X, Lopez P, Borja-Tabora C, Kosalaraksa P, et al. Efficacy of a tetravalent dengue vaccine in healthy children and adolescents. N Engl J Med 2019;381:2009–19. Available from: https://doi.org/10.1056/NEJMoa1903869.
[117] Chen H-R, Lai Y-C, Yeh T-M. Dengue virus non-structural protein 1: a pathogenic factor, therapeutic target, and vaccine candidate. J Biomed Sci 2018;25:58. Available from: https://doi.org/10.1186/s12929-018-0462-0.
[118] España G, Yao Y, Anderson KB, Fitzpatrick MC, Smith DL, Morrison AC, et al. Model-based assessment of public health impact and cost-effectiveness of dengue vaccination following screening for prior exposure. PLoS Negl Trop Dis 2019;13:e0007482. Available from: https://doi.org/10.1371/journal.pntd.0007482.
[119] Idris F, Ting DHR, Alonso S. An update on dengue vaccine development, challenges, and future perspectives. Expert Opin Drug Discov 2021;16:47–58. Available from: https://doi.org/10.1080/17460441.2020.1811675.

CHAPTER

3

Aptamers and antisense oligonucleotide-based delivery

Fatemeh Yazdian[1] and Amin Janghorbani[2]

[1]Department of Life Science Engineering, Faculty of New Sciences and Technologies, University of Tehran, Tehran, Iran [2]Department of Biotechnology, Faculty of New Sciences and Technologies, Semnan University, Semnan, Iran

3.1 What is the aptamer?

Aptamers are single-stranded DNA or RNA oligonucleotides (often 20–80 bases in length with ~6–30 kDa molecular weight). They are made for a specific and variety of targets ranging from small ions to an entire organism, such as ATP, proteins, peptides, amino acids, viruses, whole cells, receptors, antibiotics, small chemicals, antigens, or even metal ions compared to the antibodies and enzymes. One of their most important features is having high affinity and specificity [1–5].

Since aptamers have competitive advantages over protein antibodies, their clinical application is remarkably higher than antibodies. Like the antibody–antigen reactions, the target-specific binding happens through a structural recognition process, so aptamers are often called "chemical antibodies" [6–8]. So, aptamers can be substituted for antibodies in therapeutic applications [9–11]. They are physically smaller than intact antibodies (150 kDa) or antibody-derived Fab fragments (50 kDa). In addition, storing and transporting aptamers are easier than antibody-based products.

On the other hand, aptamers have no immune system-modulating functionality carried out by the Fc region of biological antibodies. Furthermore, as small-sized oligonucleotides, aptamers are nearly nonimmunogenic and nontoxic compared to protein antibodies [12,13]. Also, they generally show weaker binding and dissociation constants (Kd) in the low micromolar range to the high nanomolar. In contrast, antibodies display picomolar and even femtomolar binding. Oligonucleotides are natural substrates of nuclease enzymes, so aptamers generally have short in vivo half-lives, in the order of minutes.

Molecular Pharmaceutics and Nano Drug Delivery
DOI: https://doi.org/10.1016/B978-0-323-91924-1.00012-5

To partially solve this problem, a fluoro, amino, or O-methyl group at the 20 positions of the sugar moiety and capping the 30 ends of the oligonucleotide are used [14,15].

In recent decades, aptamers have been applied in many therapeutics and drug delivery systems that include innovative delivery mechanisms and carry various types of drug cargos. In comparison, some limitations affect the successful translation of all aspects of aptamer research and slow down the realization of promising aptamer applications as therapeutics at the clinical level. The main constraints are susceptibility to degradation by nucleases, low thermal stability, fast renal clearance, and limited functional group diversity. It seems that the key to solving the problem lies in the chemistry of aptamers [16]. The synthesis of aptamers is not dependent on biological systems; so that they can be modified with chemical methods. Aptamers' stabilization against nuclease degradation can be obtained by chemical modification using various approaches. In addition, introducing chemical modifications into nucleic acid libraries raises the interaction abilities of aptamers and, thereby, their target spectrum [17]. Aptamer's modification may improve their chemical diversity and expand their applications in diagnostics, therapeutics, and nanotechnology compared to aptamers composed entirely of natural DNA or RNA nucleotides [18].

Chemical modifications of aptamers can disturb the 3D structure of the aptamer that adversely affects aptamer function [19]. Aptamers are easily modified by incorporating different functional parts. In addition, storage, regeneration, and reuse of aptamer-based analytical reagents are simple [20]. Also, since molecules smaller than 30 kDa are rapidly cleared from the body through renal filtration, the relatively small size of aptamers is another problem [19]. However, covalently attaching polyethylene glycol or other bulky molecules to the aptamer can be a helpful approach to solve this problem [21]. One of the highly desirable aptamer features is discrimination between closely related proteins or other molecules. So, this feature can be used in aptamer-based diagnostics or therapeutics [22–25]. Aptamers have ability to bind different targets and their conformation will change upon binding to them [26].

Aptamers are chemically and thermally stable and, compared to antibodies, are rapidly and reproducibly synthesized at a low cost. For example, the fluorophore-labeled CD4 aptamer, as a flow cytometric probe in multicolored cell-phenotyping, is about 0.002 dollars per assay, while the cost per assay of CD4 antibody was 2 dollars [27]. Since 2 decades ago, with the onset of aptamer technology, many advances have been made in different biomedical fields. As chemical antibodies, aptamers are a beneficial alternative or supplement for protein antibodies in disease diagnostics and therapeutics [11]. In addition, they can be used for targeting tumor biomarkers, cancer cell detection, tumor tissue IHC staining, and in vivo tumor imaging [28].

3.2 Aptamer design

Designing aptamers with a high binding affinity to a target molecule is based on empirical in vitro approaches and computational methods. In this section, both groups of aptamer designing methods called systematic evolution of ligands by exponential enrichment (SELEX) and in silico SELEX are reviewed.

3.2.1 Systematic evolution of ligands by exponential enrichment

SELEX is a chemical process for making aptamers in the laboratory. It requires a series of repetitive selection and amplification steps after exposure to the target cell type or ligand [11,29,30]. It is an experimental method based on the assumption that many candidate sequences may contain nucleotide strands with the ability of binding to any target molecule [31]. Since aptamer selection by SELEX has many rounds of selection and enrichment processes, it needs much time and effort and has a low-efficiency rate and results. Among several SELEX methodologies, there are two main steps to design and optimize aptamers. In the first step, many polynucleotides with possible binding affinity toward a target are screened using the SELEX method and then chosen. Shortening, modification, and stabilization of aptamers with high affinity will be in the second step. This process is helpful for both DNA and RNA aptamers design [32].

3.2.2 In silico systematic evolution of ligands by exponential enrichment

SELEX is an iterative process initiated with a random pool of 10^{14} to 10^{15} aptamers and continued with selecting and amplifying aptamer sequences with a higher binding affinity to the targets. This process consists of several rounds of incubation, binding, washing, target-bound elution, and amplification, which can last for a few days to several months [33]. This situation makes this process complex, expensive, and time-consuming. In addition, the success rates of aptamer candidates are not high enough, and only a limited number of selected aptamer candidates from the next-generation sequencing data could be synthesized [34].

Since the computational methods are relatively rapid, cost-effective, repeatable, and without the need for any particular sources, they can help decrease various costs of the SELEX process and deal with its challenges to improve its performance [35]. So, several studies have recently paid attention to computational predictive methods in aptamer characteristics [36–40]. These computational methods benefit from scalability, repeatability, and consistency, which lead to efficiency and promote the identification and characterization of these ligands. The computational method can be categorized into two main groups; structure-based and machine learning (ML)-based techniques. In this section, these methods will be explained briefly.

Structure-based methods:

In these methods, aptamers' predicted structures' information using different computational methods is applied to select aptamers with high affinity. This process can be summarized as follows (Fig. 3.1) [32]:

- Prediction of the secondary structure of aptamers using their sequences
- Optimization of the tertiary structure based on the secondary structure
- Investigation of aptamer target interaction using rigid or flexible docking
- Selection of complexes based on binding energy
- Stability assessment of aptamer–target complex through molecular dynamic simulations

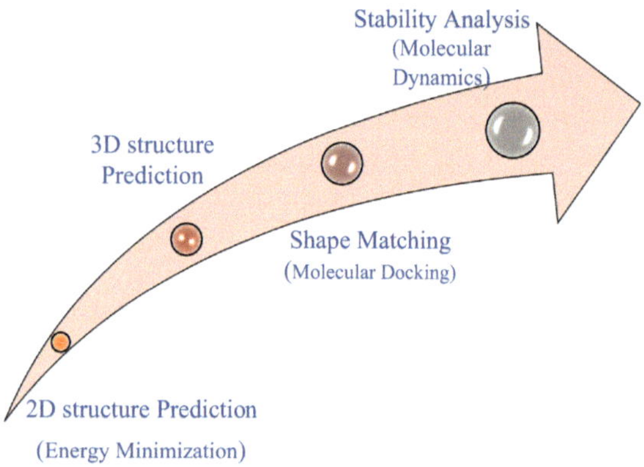

FIGURE 3.1 Different stages of structure-based aptamer selection.

The secondary structure of aptamers that provide abstract information from their 3D structure plays a critical role in the binding affinity of aptamers. They can be determined based on their sequences and using different online computational algorithms such as RNAfold, Mfold, RNAstructure, Vfold2D, and Centroidfold. These algorithms worked based on sequence alignment and free energy minimization to determine the secondary structure. The unique 3D structure of aptamers makes them suitable for recognizing their target and provides helpful information about their interaction with its target [41]. So, the 3D structure of aptamer and its target, as a biological complex, plays a significant role in their biological functionality such that predicting the aptamer 3D structure is critical. Different online web servers provide an aptamer 3D structure prediction based on the fragment method and energy-based methods [34].

After 3D construction of the aptamers, molecular docking is applied to identify and evaluate binding sites in the aptamer and target. Different molecular docking tools such as ZDOCK, MDockPP, AutoDock, AutoDock Vina, and DOCK showed good potential in the aptamer design procedure. The final step is applying molecular dynamic simulation for stability assessment of the target–aptamer complex and binding energy estimation.

3.2.3 Machine learning-based methods

The structure-based techniques are very time-consuming and inefficient in evaluating a high number of aptamer sequences. Also, they depend on the availability of homologous sequences and structural analogs in the reference library of software [42,43]. In recent years, several studies have used ML methods to predict the interaction of different aptamers and targets [33,37,40,44–47]. This process can be summarized into the following steps and will be explained in this section.

- Dataset preparation
- Feature extraction
- Features selection
- Training ML models using training sets
- Evaluation of the trained models using the testing set

3.2.3.1 *Data preparation*

Interaction prediction of aptamers and targets can be considered as a two-class classification task. Each supervised ML algorithm for a classification task needs a dataset consisting of both positive and negative classes. The positive class is the group of aptamers that bind to the target, and the negative one is the group of aptamers that do not bind to the target. These datasets can be created from public aptamer–target interaction databases such as the Aptamer database, Riboapt DB, Aptamer Base, and Aptagen [43].

3.2.3.2 *Feature extraction*

Feature extraction is analyzing the input data to reduce the dimensionality of data and extract valuable and useful information related to the classification task. In the ML-based aptamer design, these features should be independent, informative, nonredundant, and relative characteristics of aptamers and targets. The procedure can be considered as encoding the aptamers and targets to a numerical feature vector [48]. These features can be categorized as follows:

3.2.3.2.1 Sequence-based features

These features provide us with information about the pattern of aptamer sequences and targets. These features can be as simple as the statistical features of nucleotides and amino acids in an aptamer sequence, such as k-mer frequency, frequency of each nucleotide acid, and their statistics such as average, minimum, and maximum [36,48].

Also, correlation-based features, reflecting sequence-order information, such as dinucleotide auto-covariance, dinucleotide cross-covariance, trinucleotide auto-covariance, and trinucleotide cross-covariance for aptamers and pseudo-K-tuple nucleotide composition, amino acid composition, dipeptide composition, tripeptide composition, and pseudoamino acid composition for targets such as proteins, can be considered as the sequence-based features [33]. In some studies, aptamer sequences are transformed to numeric values based on their physicochemical characteristics. Then, mathematical transformations such as fast Fourier transform or discrete cosine transform are applied to targets to extract frequency domain features [36].

3.2.3.2.2 Structure-based features

These features provide information about the functionality of amino acids and nucleotides at the molecular level. Biochemical contacts, salt bridges, hydrogen bonds, and conformational information such as frequency and statistical features of the normalized length of protein secondary structure are the main structure-based features for protein as targets [43,48]. Moreover, bend, twist, shift, rise, roll, twist, slide, and tilt are the structural features of aptamers that determine their affinity and interaction with targets.

3.2.3.2.3 Energy-based features

These features have information about molecular and environmental energies that can be applied to predict aptamer–target interaction and binding affinity [43]. Electrostatic charges, side-chain intramolecular energies, side-chain intermolecular energies, van der

Waals potential, hydrogen-bonding potential, environment intermolecular energies, and interface propensity are some examples of energy-based features.

3.2.3.3 *Feature selection*

On the one hand, extracting individual groups of features leads to a limited representation of targets and aptamers characteristics and adversely affects the performance of a classifier. On the other hand, extraction of different features leads to a high dimensional feature vector that makes the classification model overfitted. So, selecting an optimum and informative subset of features is essential for improving ML model generalization. Several methods such as statistical methods like t-test or analysis of variance [48] and heuristics methods such as genetic algorithm or incremental feature selection [36] and gradient-based decision tree [49] are the examples of feature selection algorithms applied in some studies.

3.2.3.3.1 Prediction models of aptamer–target interaction

ML models are used to predict the interaction of aptamers and targets according to the input feature vectors. ML models such as support vector machine [49], decision tree [33], random forest [35,36], naive Bayes, and logistic regression [42] were used for this purpose. A training dataset consisting of both samples from positive and negative classes is required for training models, and a testing dataset is essential to evaluate the generalization of the trained model. It is common to select 80% of the whole dataset as the training dataset and 20% as the testing dataset. The number of positive cases in a database is often much lower than negative ones, making the classification task unbalanced. So, some methods such as weighting to the minority class and SMOTE applied to prevent classifiers from biasing to the majority class [33,42].

3.2.3.4 *Model evaluation*

Evaluating prediction models of aptamer–target interaction is based on the model's performance in classifying the testing dataset. These performances are based on some quantitative metrics as follows [Eq. (3.1)]:

3.2.3.4.1 Accuracy: fraction of correctly classified samples

$$\frac{\mathrm{TP} + \mathrm{FN}}{\mathrm{TP} + \mathrm{TN} + \mathrm{FP} + \mathrm{FN}} \tag{3.1}$$

in which TP is True Positive, FN is False Negative, FP is False Positive, and FN is False Negative

3.2.3.4.2 Sensitivity

The fraction of samples that the model correctly classified as negative classes to all the negative samples is given in Eq. (3.2)

$$\frac{\mathrm{TN}}{\mathrm{FN} + \mathrm{TN}} \tag{3.2}$$

3.2.3.4.3 Specificity

The fraction of samples that the model correctly classified as positive classes to all the positive samples is given in Eq. (3.3)

$$\frac{TP}{FP + TP} \tag{3.3}$$

3.3 Drug delivery by aptamers

In many cases, aptamers are better and more effective than antibodies in finding new biomarkers, in vitro and in vivo diagnosis, targeted therapy, and controlled drug release [11]. Conjugation of determined ligands like aptamers or antibodies developed against a specific molecule on the target cell leads to the drug targeting [50]. Aptamers can detect cancerous cells with quick penetration into tissues without any immunogenicity [51]. It is easy to identify between two different cancerous cells or between cancerous and normal cells by using aptamers [52]. For example, in breast cancer MUC-1, a glycoprotein in the cells' membrane, is underglycosylated and highly overexpressed. 5TR1 aptamer can attach to this glycoprotein specifically and get inside the cell via endocytosis [53].

During tumor treatment, aptamers have low molecular weights and can make a hole in tissue barriers and quickly enter tumor cells. So, tumor-to-blood and tumor-to-normal tissue ratios will be improved, which is so practical [54,55]. Another therapeutic application of aptamers is in in vivo diagnostics during fast blood clearance. This process has various side effects, such as aptamer's rapid renal filtration and short circulating half-lives [56,57].

3.4 Binding to different molecules

Aptamers are a class of DNA or RNA with unique 3D conformations and have the ability to bind with target molecules specifically. Aptamers can be relatively easily screened, designed with program, reproduced, and chemically modified for various biomedical applications, like targeted therapy. Chemical modification improves enzymatic degradation resistance or pharmacological behaviors, ensuring chemical integration and bioavailability under physiological conditions. Aptamer–nanocarrier conjugations have been extensively investigated for targeted drug delivery, based on nanoplatforms like liposomes, DNA/RNA nanostructures, and silicon nanomaterials [58].

3.4.1 Aptamers and liposomes

One of the most prevalent drug nanocarriers is the liposome. It has valuable protective hollow sections to be confident of the in vivo integrity and half-life of nucleic acid therapeutics. If not protected, they are quickly degraded by nucleases and cleared from the body [58]. In a study, liposome was modified with aptamers that specifically bind to

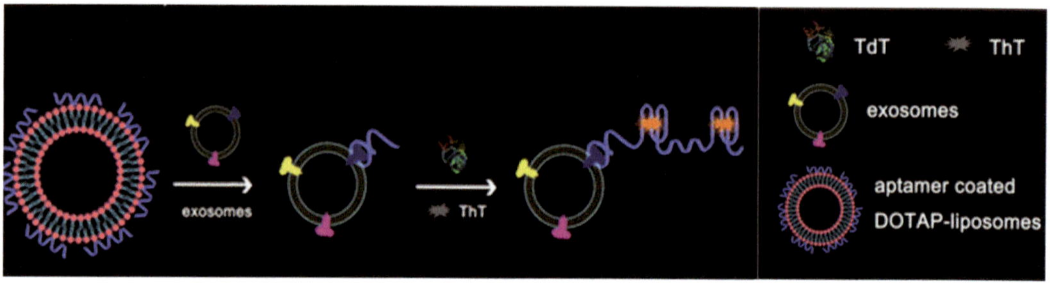

FIGURE 3.2 Fluorescence signal generation process of the reaction after aptamers bind with exosomes [60].

osteoblasts and loaded with a siRNA to silence osteogenic pleckstrin homology domain-containing family O member 1 (Plekho1) as a potential bone anabolic strategy. Using this nanoconjugate leads to siRNA delivery into osteoblasts and Plekho1-silenced targets. It causes bone formation, microarchitecture improvement, and eventually, bone mass increment [59]. As a promising biomarker, the exosome can carry different types of membrane proteins with high heterogeneity; thus, the sensitive and multiple analyses of exosomes are vital for diagnosing disease and their biological functions' detection. To this aim, an aptamer-coated liposome complex coupled with terminal deoxynucleotidyl transferase (TdT)-mediated polymerization was designed and fabricated. These immobilized aptamers select exosomal membrane proteins due to their high affinity. Also, this method is applied to reach a fingerprint map of different cancer cell-derived exosomes by using corresponding aptamers clusters. According to Fig. 3.2, the presence of thioflavin T (ThT) can give rise to strong fluorescence [60].

3.4.2 Aptamers and chitosan

Since listeria monocytogenes is among the top three causes of death among foodborne illnesses globally, its diagnosis is very important. Despite selective and accurate technologies, this diagnosis is laborious and needs extensive user training, the addition of reagents/labels, careful control of environmental conditions, and at least 8–24 hours for confirmation. Due to these technological problems, several biosensors and immunoassays have been developed to enhance detection rate and speed. Based on the results, maximum cell capture happens when aptamers conjugated to the nanobrush bind cells in the extended conformation. So, a sensing mechanism using the stimulation of chitosan-aptamer nanobrush borders was applied for fast detecting Listeria monocytogenes in food samples [61]. As another application of aptamers in drug delivery, liposomes anchored with anti-EGFR aptamer (Apt) conjugated chitosan (Apt-Cs) as stable carriers for erlotinib delivery to the targets in lung cancer therapy [62].

In order to have a selective extraction of ochratoxin A (OTA), chitosan was coated on a magnetic nanoparticle (NP) for stability and biocompatibility improvement. OTA special aptamers were coupled onto the magnetic chitosan NPs, and an extraction procedure was enhanced in an optimization procedure. Based on the results, this method was impressive for aptamer functionalization and reached a quick and effective OTA extraction and detection method in food samples [63]. Due to poor specificity of the target site and a lot of side effects of chemotherapy in cancer treatment, chitosan-coated silica (SiO_2@CS) NPs attached to epigallocatechin gallate were synthesized [64]. In another study, an anti-Mucin1 aptamer (Apt)-conjugated chitosan NP for targeted codelivery of insulin-like growth factor receptor 1 (IGF-1R) silencer siRNA and docetaxel to SKBR3 cells was designed [65].

Protein adsorption is a crucial step in cell-biomaterial interaction at their interface, whose accurate control may be helpful to trigger suitable cell responses. To this aim, aptamers can be used to control selective protein adsorption to biomaterials. According to the studies, selected aptamers to identify fibronectin surprisingly raise chitosan's ability to boost cell proliferation and adhesion [66].

3.4.3 Aptamers and graphene

Ricin is one of the deadliest poisons worldwide due to its extremely low lethal dose. Since there is no efficient treatment for ricin poisoning, there are immediate needs to extend fast and trustworthy methods for its detection in different fields, including medical diagnostics, food or water safety testing, and biodefense. So, fast and reliable ricin detection methods development is pivotal to comfort timely warning and decrease the mortality rate. In a study, aptamer-modified graphene micromotors showed good potential to detect ricin for biological threats detection in diverse biodefense applications [67].

Aptamers' affinity is adjustable depending on the application; so that they can be designed against a variety of targets, like metal ions, metabolites, proteins, and even whole cells. As a capturing reagent, an aptamer has distinguished advantages, such as small size, nontoxicity, modifiability, and unchallenging surface immobilization. These unique properties increase the possibility of a better function of aptamers than other affinity reagents. Extracting and detecting platform analytes from complex biological media is another application of aptamer-conjugated graphene oxide. This composite had apparent advantages in target enrichment and producing highly effective ionization of target molecules for mass spectrometry. These results indicate the potential of this approach for the analysis of small molecules in real biological samples [68].

Escherichia coli is the most common foodborne bacteria, detection of which is critical. This bacterium causes severe illnesses such as diarrhea, fever, and death if left undiagnosed and untreated. Aptamers have been widely used as biosensor receptors to recognize bacterial contamination. SsDNA aptamer is a stable, sensitive, and selective biomolecule used extensively for this kind of detection. Since binding aptamers to bacteria interact directly with the cell surface of the target rather than nucleic acids, they have a good potential for whole-bacteria detection. In some cases, gold NPs (AuNPs) were used to provide naked eye visible detection, and AuNPs were covered with graphene oxide to increase the aptamer conjugation (Fig. 3.3) [69].

Mercury, one of the most toxic heavy metals, threatens the environment and human health even in small concentrations due to its nonbiodegradability. It can enter the food chain and threaten human health. Because of the mercury's toxic effects, monitoring the level of mercury in the aquatic environment is essential. In a study to detect Hg^{2+},

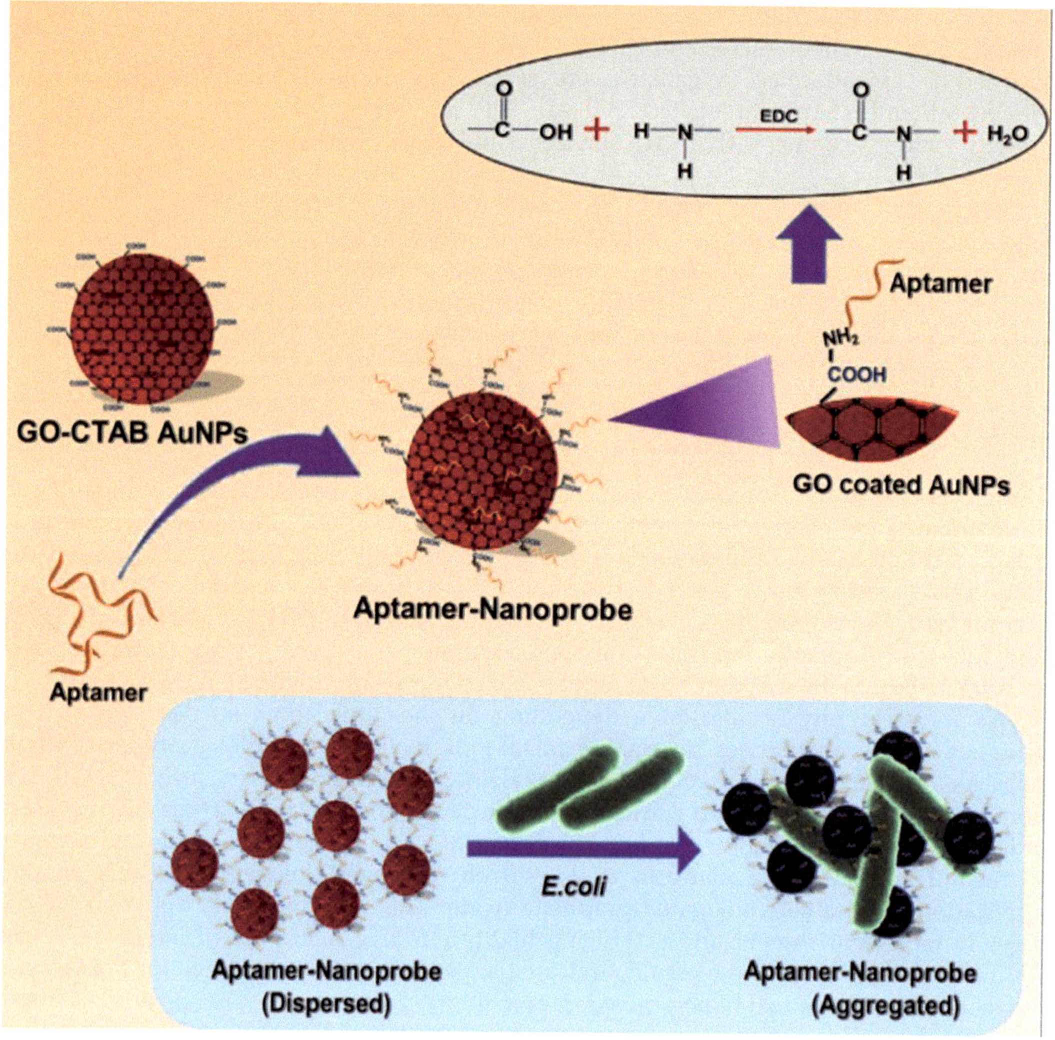

FIGURE 3.3 Screened aptamers conjugates with graphene oxide-coated CTAB-AuNPs via $COOH-NH_2$ linkage using EDC. Aptamer nanoprobe binds with its target *Escherichia coli* and aggregates, thus changing the color of AuNPs from *red* to *blue* [69].

a simple GO-based fluorescent sensor with high sensitivity and selectivity was used, so there was no complicated, high-cost, and time-consuming labeling. An SsDNA aptamer served as the molecular recognition probe with the ability to bind to Hg^{2+} ions selectively, and GO acted as a fluorophore [70].

A critical and challenging task in many fields of health analysis, environmental, and food control is label-free, highly sensitive, direct, and real-time-enabled optical biosensors developed for small molecules (less than 1 kDa in size). Aptamers can be applied for dealing with this task. For example, graphene was functionalized by the aptamer as the bioreceptor, in conjunction with spectral-phase interferometry to detect OTA. The composite was highly efficient in detecting the small molecules in competitive assays [71].

3.4.4 Aptamers and magnetic manoparticles

Risk assessment of emergency department heart failure (HF) patients is possible with brain natriuretic peptide (BNP) detection, a biologically active natural hormone. Due to the high importance of accurate HF diagnosis, various methods are suggested and evaluated to detect BNP. In a study, a triple detection strategy based on target-induced magnetic gold nanocomposite was proposed. Apt-MB, which is modified on AuNPs, specifically binds to the C-terminal of BNP in the Mag NP-Ab@BNP complex, and a large nanocomposite is formed by cascade conjugation in this process. Separation and fixing of the nanocomposite in solution after magnetic separation is possible on the gold electrode surface by hybridizing Apt and complementary DNA (cDNA). For quantitative determination of the BNP contents, electrochemical signals of MB molecules on Au NP Apt-MB were measured. This method showed high sensitivity and a wide dynamic detection range, explaining practical possibilities in clinical testing applications. This process can be seen in Fig. 3.4 [72].

Enrofloxacin (ENR), an important fluoroquinolone, is a high-potency antibacterial agent affecting mycoplasma, gram-positive, and gram-negative pathogens by inhibiting DNA synthesis. It has been widely used to prevent and treat disease in poultry and livestock breeding and aqua culture practices. However, residual ENR left over after its use may cause many side effects like drug-resistant bacteria development or, worse, resistant bacterial strains transference from animals to humans in the food chain and environmental contamination. Many countries and organizations established maximum residue limits for ENR usage to ensure consumer health. Because of the low cost and high effectiveness of ENR, developing countries still are using it illegally or limitedly; so, ENR residue detection in foods needs high sensitivity and accuracy. Liu et al. constructed a novel hybrid probe with several benefits, such as unique trace ENR selectivity, strong antiinterference ability with upconversion luminescence, and an excellent magnetic property by using aptamers as specific recognition elements, upconversion NPs as signal sources, and Fe_3O_4 NPs as magnetic substrates for aptamer immobilization. As a novel sensing material, the probe was used for ENR quantification in real samples, and its sensing behavior was investigated [73].

Zearalenone (ZEN) is a nonsteroidal estrogenic mycotoxin produced by fungi on stored grains. The former ZEN detection methods depend on expensive equipment, time-consuming sample preparation, and temperature-sensitive antibodies. A new strategy based on ZEN aptamer labeled with amine-functionalized magnetic NPs (MNPs) was used as a capture probe. Also, time-resolved fluorescence NPs labeled with cDNA were applied as signal probes. The bioassay was more efficient in sensitive, high throughput detection and less time-consuming than prior analytical approaches for laboratory and ZEN determination in cereal and feed samples [74].

In order to overcome the conventional cancer treatment and diagnosis limitation, using theranostic nanoplatforms (diagnostic and therapy combination) has globally emerged as a

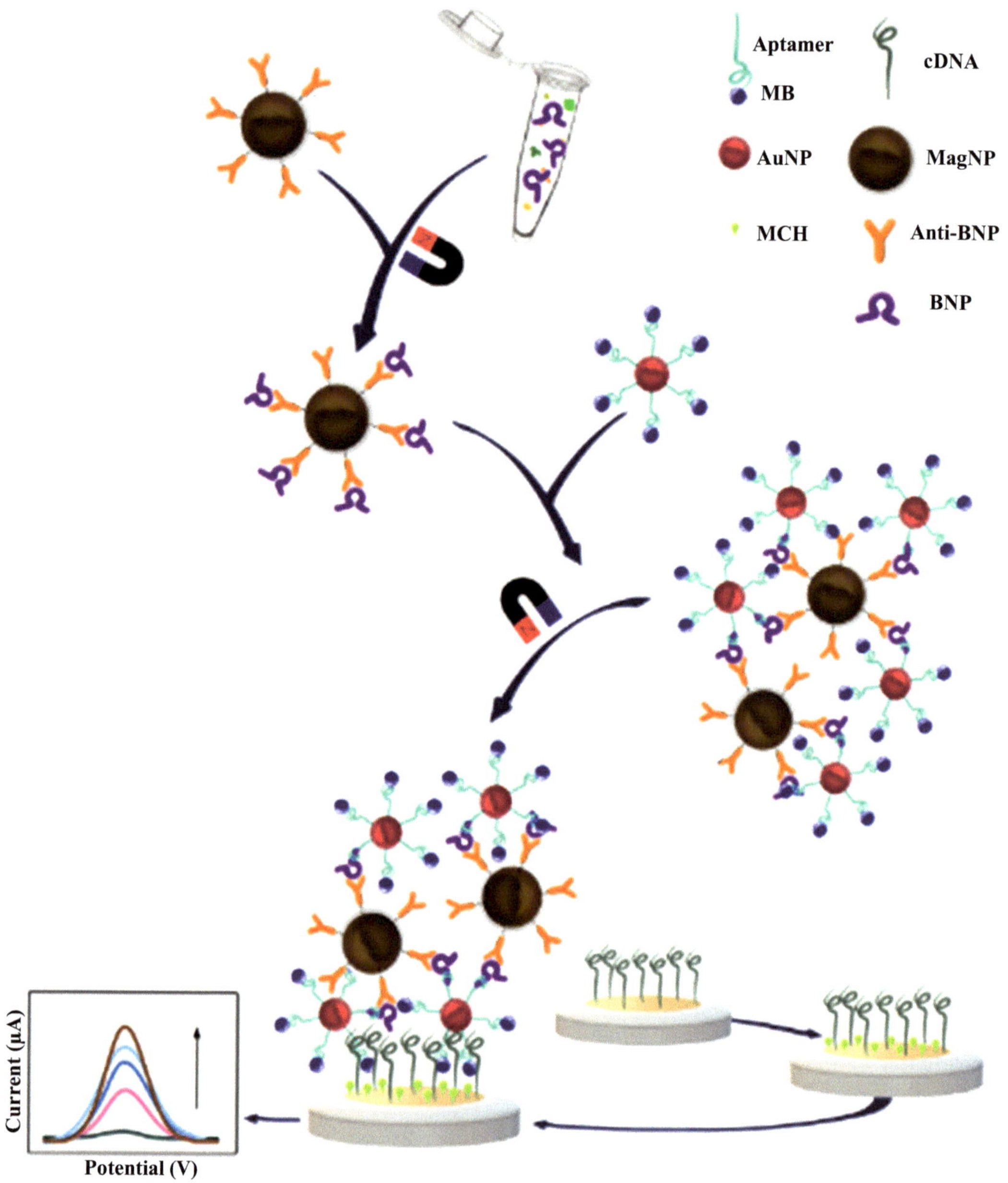

FIGURE 3.4 Schematic of triple recognition electrochemical immunoassay based on functional nanoparticles for brain natriuretic peptide [72].

promising approach for cancer treatment. In a study, a new theranostic nanoprobe was designed to treat hepatocellular carcinoma (HCC), specially HBV-associated HCC. A nanoprobe combined a nontoxic cellulose-derivative polymer potential delivery, epithelial cell adhesion molecule EpCAM aptamer cancer-specific capability, and NPs imaging capability [75].

The highly specific recognition of aptamers with magnetic separation to develop an upconversion luminescent nanoprobe-based bioassay for the detection of trace OTA was combined in another study. For avidin immobilization, surface NH_2 group-functionalized Fe_3O_4 MNPs were synthesized and linked to a biotinylated aptamer. The aptamer-functionalized MNPs acted as recognition elements to identify and capture the target substance. Also, the composition favors the fast separation and purification of the bound target and the fabrication of a simple assay in a homogeneous solution using an external magnet. The biotinylated OTA aptamer was conjugated onto the MNPs, and its hybridized complementary strand was linked to upconversion NPs and used as signal probes. This system could dissociate from the OTA aptamer [76].

References

[1] Kim YS, Raston NHA, Gu MB. Aptamer-based nanobiosensors. Biosens Bioelectron 2016;76:2–19.

[2] Bazak R, Houri M, El Achy S, Kamel S, Refaat T. Cancer active targeting by nanoparticles: a comprehensive review of literature. J Cancer Res Clin Oncol 2015;141:769–84.

[3] Srisawat C, Engelke DR. Selection of RNA aptamers that bind HIV-1 LTR DNA duplexes: strand invaders. Nucleic Acids Res 2010;38:8306–15.

[4] Marangoni K, Neves AF, Rocha RM, Faria PR, Alves PT, Souza AG, et al. Prostate-specific RNA aptamer: promising nucleic acid antibody-like cancer detection. Sci Rep 2015;5:1–13.

[5] Li S, Xu H, Ding H, Huang Y, Cao X, Yang G, et al. Identification of an aptamer targeting hnRNP A1 by tissue slide-based SELEX. J Pathol A J Pathol Soc Gt Br Irel 2009;218:327–36.

[6] Kimoto M, Yamashige R, Matsunaga K, Yokoyama S, Hirao I. Generation of high-affinity DNA aptamers using an expanded genetic alphabet. Nat Biotechnol 2013;31:453–7.

[7] Kraemer S, Vaught JD, Bock C, Gold L, Katilius E, Keeney TR, et al. From SOMAmer-based biomarker discovery to diagnostic and clinical applications: a SOMAmer-based, streamlined multiplex proteomic assay. PLoS One 2011;6:e26332.

[8] Parekh P, Kamble S, Zhao N, Zeng Z, Portier BP, Zu Y. Immunotherapy of CD30-expressing lymphoma using a highly stable ssDNA aptamer. Biomaterials 2013;34:8909–17.

[9] Keefe AD, Pai S, Ellington A. Aptamers as therapeutics. Nat Rev Drug Discov 2010;9:537–50.

[10] Toh SY, Citartan M, Gopinath SCB, Tang T-H. Aptamers as a replacement for antibodies in enzyme-linked immunosorbent assay. Biosens Bioelectron 2015;64:392–403.

[11] Sun H, Zu Y. A Highlight of recent advances in aptamer technology and its application. Molecules 2015;20:11959–80.

[12] Group Thees. Preclinical and phase 1a clinical evaluation of an anti-vegf pegylated aptamer (Eye001) for the treatment of exudative age-related macular degeneration. Retina 2002;22.

[13] Ireson CR, Kelland LR. Discovery and development of anticancer aptamers. Mol Cancer Ther 2006; 5:2957 LP – 2962.

[14] Zhou J, Rossi J. Aptamers as targeted therapeutics: current potential and challenges. Nat Rev Drug Discov 2017;.

[15] Dowdy SF. Overcoming cellular barriers for RNA therapeutics. Nat Biotechnol 2017;35:222–9.

[16] Odeh F, Nsairat H, Alshaer W, Ismail MA, Esawi E, Qaqish B, et al. Aptamers chemistry: chemical modifications and conjugation strategies. Mol 2020;25.

[17] Campbell MA, Wengel J. Locked vs. unlocked nucleic acids (LNA vs. UNA): contrasting structures work towards common therapeutic goals. Chem Soc Rev 2011;40:5680–9.

[18] Ni X, Castanares M, Mukherjee A, Lupold SE. Nucleic acid aptamers: clinical applications and promising new horizons. Curr Med Chem 2011;18:4206–14.

[19] Lee CH, Lee S-H, Kim JH, Noh Y-H, Noh G-J, Lee S-W. Pharmacokinetics of a cholesterol-conjugated aptamer against the hepatitis C virus (HCV) NS5B protein. Mol Ther Acids 2015;4:e254.
[20] Potyrailo RA, Murray AJ, Nagraj N, Pris AD, Ashe JM, Todorovic M. Towards maintenance-free biosensors for hundreds of bind/release cycles. Angew Chem Int Ed 2015;54:2174–8.
[21] Haruta K, Otaki N, Nagamine M, Kayo T, Sasaki A, Hiramoto S, et al. A novel PEGylation method for improving the pharmacokinetic properties of anti-interleukin-17A RNA aptamers. Nucleic Acid Ther 2017;27:36–44.
[22] Xiong X, Lv Y, Chen T, Zhang X, Wang K, Tan W. Nucleic acid aptamers for living cell analysis. Annu Rev Anal Chem 2014;7:405–26.
[23] Cho EJ, Lee J-W, Ellington AD. Applications of aptamers as sensors. Annu Rev Anal Chem 2009;2:241–64.
[24] Ng EWM, Adamis AP. Anti-VEGF aptamer (pegaptanib) therapy for ocular vascular diseases. Ann N Y Acad Sci 2006;1082:151–71.
[25] Jenison RD, Gill SC, Pardi A, Polisky B. Insight into the functional versatility of RNA through model-making with applications to data fitting. Science (80-) 1994;263:1425–9.
[26] Thomas H, Dinshaw JP. Adaptive recognition by nucleic acid aptamers. Science (80-) 2000;287:820–5.
[27] Zhang P, Zhao N, Zeng Z, Chang C-C, Zu Y. Combination of an aptamer probe to CD4 and antibodies for multicolored cell phenotyping. Am J Clin Pathol 2010;134:586–93.
[28] Sun H, Zu Y. Aptamers and their applications in nanomedicine. Small 2015;11:2352–64.
[29] Sun H, Zhu X, Lu PY, Rosato RR, Tan W, Zu Y. Oligonucleotide aptamers: new tools for targeted cancer therapy. Mol Ther Acids 2014;3:e182.
[30] Xu W, Siddiqui IA, Nihal M, Pilla S, Rosenthal K, Mukhtar H, et al. Aptamer-conjugated and doxorubicin-loaded unimolecular micelles for targeted therapy of prostate cancer. Biomaterials 2013;34:5244–53.
[31] Hoinka J, Zotenko E, Friedman A, Sauna ZE, Przytycka TM. Identification of sequence–structure RNA binding motifs for SELEX-derived aptamers. Bioinformatics 2012;28:i215–23.
[32] Buglak AA, Samokhvalov AV, Zherdev AV, Dzantiev BB. Methods and applications of in silico aptamer design and modeling. Int J Mol Sci 2020;21.
[33] Lee G, Jang GH, Kang HY, Song G. Predicting aptamer sequences that interact with target proteins using an aptamer-protein interaction classifier and a Monte Carlo tree search approach. PLoS One 2021;16:e0253760.
[34] Chen Z, Hu L, Zhang B-T, Lu A, Wang Y, Yu Y, et al. Artificial intelligence in aptamer–target binding prediction. Int J Mol Sci 2021;22:3605.
[35] Lee W, Han K. Constructive prediction of potential RNA aptamers for a protein target. IEEE/ACM Trans Comput Biol Bioinforma 2019;17:1476–82.
[36] Zhang L, Zhang C, Gao R, Yang R, Song Q. Prediction of aptamer-protein interacting pairs using an ensemble classifier in combination with various protein sequence attributes. BMC Bioinforma 2016;17:1–13.
[37] Bashir A, Yang Q, Wang J, Hoyer S, Chou W, McLean C, et al. Machine learning guided aptamer refinement and discovery. Nat Commun 2021;12:1–11.
[38] Hasegawa H, Savory N, Abe K, Ikebukuro K. Methods for improving aptamer binding affinity. Molecules 2016;21:421.
[39] Navien TN, Thevendran R, Hamdani HY, Tang T-H, Citartan M. In silico molecular docking in DNA aptamer development. Biochimie 2021;180:54–67.
[40] Li Z, Zhu J, Xu X, Yao Y. RDense: a protein-RNA binding prediction model based on bidirectional recurrent neural network and densely connected convolutional networks. IEEE Access 2019;8:14588–605.
[41] Song J, Zheng Y, Huang M, Wu L, Wang W, Zhu Z, et al. A sequential multidimensional analysis algorithm for aptamer identification based on structure analysis and machine learning. Anal Chem 2019;92:3307–14.
[42] Heredia FL, Roche-Lima A, Parés-Matos EI. A novel artificial intelligence-based approach for identification of deoxynucleotide aptamers. PLoS Comput Biol 2021;17:e1009247.
[43] Emami N, Pakchin PS, Ferdousi R. Computational predictive approaches for interaction and structure of aptamers. J Theor Biol 2020;497:110268.
[44] Alipanahi B, Delong A, Weirauch MT, Frey BJ. Predicting the sequence specificities of DNA-and RNA-binding proteins by deep learning. Nat Biotechnol 2015;33:831–8.
[45] Gandhi S, Lee LJ, Delong A, Duvenaud D, Frey BJ. cDeepbind: a context sensitive deep learning model of RNA-protein binding. BioRxiv 2018;345140.

[46] Hassanzadeh H.R., Wang M.D. DeeperBind: enhancing prediction of sequence specificities of DNA binding proteins. In: Proceedings of the IEEE international conference on bioinformatics and biomedicine, 2016, p. 178–83.

[47] Qin J, Huo J, Zhang P, Zeng J, Wang T, Zeng H. Improving the photocatalytic hydrogen production of Ag/gC_3N_4 nanocomposites by dye-sensitization under visible light irradiation. Nanoscale 2016;8:2249–59.

[48] Torkamanian-Afshar M, Nematzadeh S, Tabarzad M, Najafi A, Lanjanian H, Masoudi-Nejad A. In silico design of novel aptamers utilizing a hybrid method of machine learning and genetic algorithm. Mol Divers 2021;1–13.

[49] Yang Q, Jia C, Li T. Prediction of aptamer–protein interacting pairs based on sparse autoencoder feature extraction and an ensemble classifier. Math Biosci 2019;311:103–8.

[50] Hauser-Kawaguchi AMN, Luyt LG. Nanomedicine—nanoparticles in cancer imaging and therapy. Cancer Metastasis - Biol Treat 2015;20:205–44 Springer.

[51] Guo J, Gao X, Su L, Xia H, Gu G, Pang Z, et al. Aptamer-functionalized PEG-PLGA nanoparticles for enhanced anti-glioma drug delivery. Biomaterials 2011;32:8010–20.

[52] Sefah K, Shangguan D, Xiong X, O'Donoghue MB, Tan W. Development of DNA aptamers using cell-selex. Nat Protoc 2010;5:1169–85.

[53] Moosavian SA, Abnous K, Akhtari J, Arabi L, Gholamzade Dewin A, Jafari M. 5TR1 aptamer-PEGylated liposomal doxorubicin enhances cellular uptake and suppresses tumour growth by targeting MUC1 on the surface of cancer cells. Artif Cells. Nanomed Biotechnol 2018;46:2054–65.

[54] Martínez O, Bellard E, Golzio M, Mechiche-Alami S, Rols M-P, Teissié J, et al. Direct validation of aptamers as powerful tools to image solid tumor. Nucleic Acid Ther 2014;24:217–25.

[55] Melancon MP, Zhou M, Zhang R, Xiong C, Allen P, Wen X, et al. Selective uptake and imaging of aptamer- and antibody-conjugated hollow nanospheres targeted to epidermal growth factor receptors overexpressed in head and neck cancer. ACS Nano 2014;8:4530–8.

[56] Osborne SE, Matsumura I, Ellington AD. Aptamers as therapeutic and diagnostic reagents: problems and prospects. Curr Opin Chem Biol 1997;1:5–9.

[57] Zeng Z, Parekh P, Li Z, Shi Z-Z, Tung C-H, Zu Y. Specific and sensitive tumor imaging using biostable oligonucleotide aptamer probes. Theranostics 2014;4:945–52.

[58] Zhu G, Chen X. Aptamer-based targeted therapy. Adv Drug Deliv Rev 2018;134:65–78.

[59] Liang C, Guo B, Wu H, Shao N, Li D, Liu J, et al. Aptamer-functionalized lipid nanoparticles targeting osteoblasts as a novel RNA interference–based bone anabolic strategy. Nat Med 2015;21:288–94.

[60] Wang L, Pan Y, Liu Y, Sun Z, Huang Y, Li J, et al. Fabrication of an aptamer-coated liposome complex for the detection and profiling of exosomes based on terminal deoxynucleotidyl transferase-mediated signal amplification. ACS Appl Mater Interfaces 2020;12:322–9.

[61] Hills KD, Oliveira DA, Cavallaro ND, Gomes CL, McLamore ES. Actuation of chitosan-aptamer nanobrush borders for pathogen sensing. Analyst 2018;143:1650–61.

[62] Li F, Mei H, Xie X, Zhang H, Liu J, Lv T, et al. Aptamer-conjugated chitosan-anchored liposomal complexes for targeted delivery of erlotinib to EGFR-mutated lung cancer cells. AAPS J 2017;19:814–26.

[63] Wang S, Niu R, Yang Y, Zhou X, Luo S, Zhang C, et al. Aptamer-functionalized chitosan magnetic nanoparticles as a novel adsorbent for selective extraction of ochratoxin A. Int J Biol Macromol 2020;153:583–90.

[64] Alizadeh L, Alizadeh E, Zarebkohan A, Ahmadi E, Rahmati-Yamchi M, Salehi R. AS1411 aptamer-functionalized chitosan-silica nanoparticles for targeted delivery of epigallocatechin gallate to the SKOV-3 ovarian cancer cell lines. J Nanopart Res 2020;22:5.

[65] Jafari R, Majidi Zolbanin N, Majidi J, Atyabi F, Yousefi M, Jadidi-Niaragh F, et al. Anti-mucin1 aptamer-conjugated chitosan nanoparticles for targeted co-delivery of docetaxel and IGF-1R siRNA to SKBR3 metastatic breast cancer cells. Iran Biomed J 2019;23:21–33.

[66] Parisi L, Toffoli A, Bianchi MG, Bergonzi C, Bianchera A, Bettini R, et al. Functional fibronectin adsorption on aptamer-doped chitosan modulates cell morphology by integrin-mediated pathway. Materials 2019;12.

[67] Esteban-Fernández de Ávila B, Lopez-Ramirez MA, Báez DF, Jodra A, Singh VV, Kaufmann K, et al. Aptamer-modified graphene-based catalytic micromotors: off–on fluorescent detection of ricin. ACS Sens 2016;1:217–21.

[68] Gulbakan B, Yasun E, Shukoor MI, Zhu Z, You M, Tan X, et al. A dual platform for selective analyte enrichment and ionization in mass spectrometry using aptamer-conjugated graphene oxide. J Am Chem Soc 2010;132:17408–10.

[69] Gupta R, Kumar A, Kumar S, Pinnaka AK, Singhal NK. Naked eye colorimetric detection of Escherichia coli using aptamer conjugated graphene oxide enclosed Gold nanoparticles. Sens Actuators B Chem 2021;329:129100.
[70] Li M, Zhou X, Ding W, Guo S, Wu N. Fluorescent aptamer-functionalized graphene oxide biosensor for label-free detection of mercury(II). Biosens Bioelectron 2013;41:889–93.
[71] Nekrasov N, Yakunina N, Pushkarev AV, Orlov AV, Gadjanski I, Pesquera A, et al. Spectral-phase interferometry detection of ochratoxin a via aptamer-functionalized graphene coated glass. Nanomaterials 2021;11:226.
[72] Zhao J, Zhu Z-Z, Huang X, Hu X, Chen H. Magnetic gold nanocomposite and aptamer assisted triple recognition electrochemical immunoassay for determination of brain natriuretic peptide. Microchim Acta 2020;187:231.
[73] Liu X, Su L, Zhu L, Gao X, Wang Y, Bai F, et al. Hybrid material for enrofloxacin sensing based on aptamer-functionalized magnetic nanoparticle conjugated with upconversion nanoprobes. Sens Actuators B Chem 2016;233:394–401.
[74] Niazi S, Wang X, Pasha I, Khan IM, Zhao S, Shoaib M, et al. A novel bioassay based on aptamer-functionalized magnetic nanoparticle for the detection of zearalenone using time resolved-fluorescence NaYF4: Ce/Tb nanoparticles as signal probe. Talanta 2018;186:97–103.
[75] Pilapong C, Sitthichai S, Thongtem S, Thongtem T. Smart magnetic nanoparticle-aptamer probe for targeted imaging and treatment of hepatocellular carcinoma. Int J Pharm 2014;473:469–74.
[76] Wu S, Duan N, Wang Z, Wang H. Aptamer-functionalized magnetic nanoparticle-based bioassay for the detection of ochratoxin a using upconversion nanoparticles as labels. Analyst 2011;136:2306–14.

CHAPTER

4

Monoclonal antibodies: recent development in drug delivery

Sumel Ashique[1], Prathap Madeswara Guptha[2], Jovita Kanoujia[2], Ashish Garg[3], Afzal Hussain[4], S. Mohana Lakshmi[2] and Neeraj Mishra[2]

[1]Department of Pharmaceutics, Pandaveswar School of Pharmacy, Pandaveswar, West Bengal, India [2]Amity Institute of Pharmacy, Amity University Madhya Pradesh (AUMP), Gwalior, Madhya Pradesh, India [3]Department of Pharmaceutics, Guru Ramdas Khalsa Institute of Science and Technology (Pharmacy), Jabalpur, Madhya Pradesh, India [4]Department of Pharmaceutics, College of Pharmacy, King Saud University, Riyadh, Saudi Arabia

4.1 Introduction

Monoclonal antibody (mAbs) are manufactured by cloning a distinctive white blood cell and having a unique affinity toward the specific epitope. Therapeutic mAbs are basically gamma-immunoglobulin (or IgG) isotype in nature. mAbs are prepared by a unique clone of B cells and myeloma cells and mainly attack the specific antigens. mAbs are composed of four polypeptide chains (two similar heavy chains and two alike light chains) having a molecular weight of ~150 kD. mAbs are classified into five types (e.g., IgA, IgG, IgD, IgM, and IgE), and the most active therapeutics is IgG, which has the greater site-specific quality and affinities from nano to picomolar. The chains are bound together by disulfide linkages and fold to form a "Y"-shaped tetramer (Fig. 4.1A). Scientists Köhler and Milstein successfully developed hybridoma in 1975 [1] to produce pure mAbs in bulk quantity, considerably increasing the research and significant clinical utilization, and depending on their inception, mAbs are classified into four types [e.g., murine, chimeric, humanized, and human (Fig. 4.1B)]. Because of advancements in scientific and technological advances, mAbs have successfully been introduced into different health care centers. At present, in the world, around 570 therapeutic mAbs have been developed in clinical trials by various trading companies [2], and around 79 therapeutic mAbs have been

Molecular Pharmaceutics and Nano Drug Delivery
DOI: https://doi.org/10.1016/B978-0-323-91924-1.00014-9

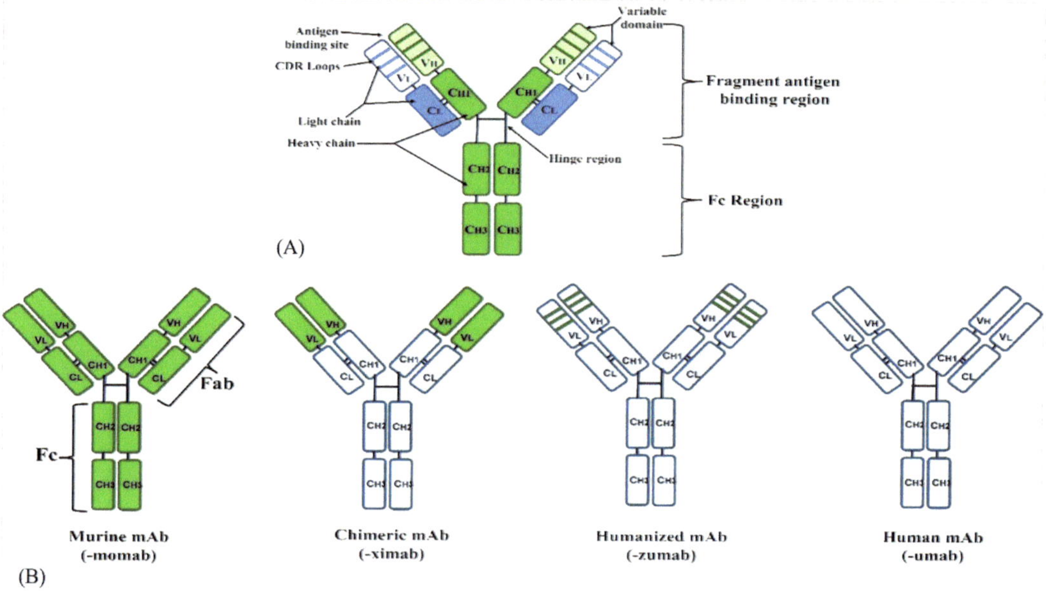

FIGURE 4.1 (A) Basic structure of mAbs and (B) classification of mAb murine, chimeric, humanized, and human.

approved by the United States Food and Drug Administration (US FDA) and now are available on the market (Table 4.1) [3]. The first monoclonal antibody named Orthoclone OKT-3 (muromonab-CD3) (murine originated) was approved in the year 1985, by the FDA for applying clinically in humans as an antirejection agent.

The significant upgrowing of therapeutic mAbs has been developed for several disease conditions in the last three decades. Currently, the chief technical developments have made the advancement of mAb therapies faster and more effective. Antigen-specific targeting offers efficient therapeutic treatment, and the incidence of molecular targeting therapy is indicating the progression of a novel initiation of bioactives. However, there is one limitation: a majority of the approved therapeutic mAbs have selectivity toward the primary assembly of definite antigens, though all proteins have original inherent structures for their own well-defined response [4]. mAbs mediate their functions by different types of direct or indirect effects by binding with cell surface receptors, membrane-associated proteins, growth factors, and so forth. By binding to the targeted antigen, antibodies can alter the cells also [5,6]. Antibody-based therapeutics have shown minimum adverse effects because of their greater selectivity; thus, therapeutic mAbs are considered as the potent category of new bioactives used currently. To overcome the issues of inhibited immunogenic viewpoint and efficiency, during the preparation of mAbs for a long time, researchers planned to use several methods to change rodent antibodies into structures similar to human antibodies, without changing targeting features [7]. For active targeting, physically or covalently conjugated ligands, such as mAb and their components, are constantly utilized and evaluated for targeted delivery designs in various chronic diseases also (Table 4.2) [7] (Table 4.3 and Table 4.4).

TABLE 4.1 List of recently Food and Drug Administration approved antibody drug conjugate [3].

Drug	Maker	Condition	Indication	Route	Does	Target	Approval year
Tisotumab vedotin	Seagen & Genamb	Recurrent or metastatic cervical cancer	Tivdak	i.v.	40 mg/vial	Tissue factor	2021
Loncastuximab tesirin	ADC Therapeutics	Large B-cell lymphoma	Zynlonta	i.v.	10 mg/vial	CD19	2021
Belantamab mafodotin	GlaxoSmithKline (GSK)	Adult patients with relapsed or refractory multiple myeloma	Blenrep	i.v.	100 mg/vial	BCMA	2020
Trastuzumab deruxtecan	AstraZeneca/Daiichi Sankyo	Treatment of adult patients with unresectable or metastatic HER2-positive breast cancer who have received two or more prior anti-HER2-based regimens in the metastatic setting	Enhertu	i.v.	100 mg/vial	HER2	2019
Enfortumab vedotin	Astellas/Seattle Genetics	Adult patients with locally advanced or metastatic urothelial cancer who have received a PD-1 or PD-L1 inhibitor, and a Pt-containing therapy	Padcev	i.v. infusion	20/30 mg/vial	Nectin-4	2019
Polatuzumab vedotin	Genentech, Roche	Relapsed or refractory (R/R) diffuse large B-cell lymphoma (DLBCL)	Polivy	i.v. infusion	140 mg/vial	CD79	2019
Moxetumomab pasudotox	Astrazeneca	For the treatment of adult patients with relapsed or refractory hairy cell leukemia	Lumoxiti	i.v. infusion	1 mg/vial	CD22-directed cytotoxin	2018
Inotuzumab ozogamicin	Pfizer/Wyeth	Relapsed or refractory CD22-positive B-cell precursor acute lymphoblastic leukemia	Besponsa	i.v. infusion	0.9 mg /vial	CD22-directed antibody-drug	2017
Trastuzumab emtansine	Genentech, Roche	HER2-positive metastatic breast cancer (mBC) following treatment with trastuzumab and a maytansinoid	Kadcyla	i.v. infusion	100 mg/vial	HER2-positive, metastatic breast cancer	2013

4.2 The molecular mechanisms of therapeutic antibody

The efficiency of mAb therapy can be determined via various mechanisms, such as direct effects of the antibody on cell action, for example, by hindering or the initiation of signaling mechanisms transported by the target molecule, in some cases initiating apoptosis directly. The additional significant mechanism is the targeting of the immune effector process to the tumor. The mAb can also be used for targeting payloads to the cell of interest. One of the novel findings in mAb therapy includes using the specificity of a mAb for a tumor-linked target in the development of chimeric antigen receptor (CAR) T-cell therapies [10]. Various treatment strategies applying unmodified mAbs have shown to be efficient in the management of several cancers, which acts by binding to the antigen on cancer cells or an antigen on other cells or proteins or by initiating the immune response process [11,12].

4.3 Advantages and disadvantages of mAbs

mAbs are now the highly effective biotherapeutics for the treatment of a variety of cancers and autoimmune diseases. They have various benefits over other antineoplastic bioactives, including enhanced efficacy, safety, and lower toxicity, as well as less side effects and a higher patient survival rate. Antibodies have a biorecognition mechanism designed to be able to improve the immune response by preventing intracellular and extracellular threats [13]. As a result of its specificity and accuracy, it is reminiscent of the "Ehrlich's magic bullet" concept, which involves addressing a particular infection for clinical intervention while limiting collateral harm to the patient. Surprisingly, it may provoke an antibody reaction and has been extensively utilized in microbiological investigation, diagnosis, and, more importantly, for therapy purposes. A mAb is a type of antibody that has a greater affinity for specific antigens and is increasingly used as a targeted treatment for a variety of diseases [14]. By establishing an "Ab-drug combination", the mAbs may specifically deliver the bioactive to the designated target [15]. This method has a promising future because of the high specificity with which they adhere to specific antigens [16]. Although there have been promising studies, this strategy faces various obstacles that prevent its widespread implementation as a therapy. There are a few limitations to clinical mAbs, including limited pharmacokinetic statistics and tissue reachability, as well as decreased immune system interactions, and these deficiencies highlight the need for additional research.

Costs of production: mAbs are huge (150 kDa) "multimeric proteins" that were generated passively using complex eukaryotic apparatus. Thus, the production of therapeutic monoclonal antibodies needed a large number of mammalian cells accompanied by numerous refinement steps, resulting in prohibitively expensive production expenditures and limiting the clinical mAb's use [17,18].

4.4 Pharmacokinetics versus tumor targeting

In mouse xenograft models, mAbs controlled against malignant cells antigens are highly retained in the systemic circulation, with less than 20% of the injected generally reacting

TABLE 4.2 List of Therapeutic mAb approved by Food and Drug Administration for treatment of chronic diseases [7].

MAb	Brand Name	Company	Target	Format	Technology	Condition	Approval year
Alemtuzumab	Campath, Lemtrada	Berlex Inc./Genzyme Corp./Millennium Pharmaceuticals Inc.	CD52-protein present on the surface of mature lymphocytes	Recombinant humanized immunoglobulin G1-IgG1	Hybridoma	B-cell chronic lymphocytic leukemia	2001
Adalimumab	Humira	AbbVie Inc.	inactivating tumor necrosis factor-alpha (TNFα)	Human IgG1	Phage display	Rheumatoid arthritis	2002
Ibritumomab Tiuxetan	Zevalin	Biogen Inc./Schering AG/Spectrum Pharmaceuticals Inc	CD20	Murine IgG1	Hybridoma	Non-Hodgkin Lymphoma	2002
Omalizumab	Xolair	Roche, F. Hoffmann-La Roche, Ltd.	IgE	Human IgG1	Hybridoma	Asthma	2003
Cetuximab	Erbitux	Bristol-Myers Squibb	Binds epidermal-growth-factor-receptor	Chimeric IgG1	Hybridoma	Advanced bowel cancer	2004
Bevacizumab	Avastin	Roche, F. Hoffmann-La Roche, Ltd./Genentech Inc	VEGF-A (vascular endothelial growth factor-VEGF)	(IgG1)	Hybridoma	Brain tumor	2004
Natalizumab	Tysabri	Biogen Inc./Elan Pharmaceuticals International, Ltd.	ITGA4	Humanized IgG4	Hybridoma	Multiple sclerosis	2004
Panitumumab	Vectibix	Amgen	EGFR	Human IgG2	Transgenic mice	Colorectal cancer	2006
Ranibizumab	Lucentis	Ovartis Pharmaceuticals Corp	VEGF-A	Humanized IgG1 Fab	Hybridoma	Macular degeneration	2006
Eculizumab	Soliris	Alexion Pharmaceuticals Inc	C5-gene complement component	Humanized IgG2/4	Hybridoma	prevents the breakdown of RBC in adults with paroxysmal nocturnal hemoglobinuria (PNH)	2007

(*Continued*)

TABLE 4.2 (Continued)

MAb	Brand Name	Company	Target	Format	Technology	Condition	Approval year
Ofatumumab	Arzerra	Genmab A/S /GlaxoSmithKline/ Novartis.	CD20- A protein found on B cells (a type of white blood cell)	Human IgG1	Transgenic mice	Chronic lymphocytic leukemia	2009
Ipilimumab	Yervoy	Bristol-Myers Squibb/ Medarex	CTLA-4(cytotoxic T-lymphocyte-associated protein 4)	Human IgG1	Transgenic	Metastatic melanoma	2011
Pertuzumab	Perjeta	Roche, F. Hoffmann-La Roche	HER2	Humanized IgG1	Hybridoma	Breast cancer	2012
Ramucirumab	Cyramza	Eli Lilly/ImClone Systems Inc	VEGFR2	Human IgG1	Phage display	Gastric cancer	2014
Nivolumab	Opdivo	Bristol-Myers Squibb/ Ono Pharmaceutical Co., Ltd	Programmed cell death protein 1	Human IgG4	Transgenic mice	Melanoma, non-small cell lung cancer	2014
Daratumumab	Darzalex	Genmab A/S/Janssen Biotech Inc	CD38-protein Coding gene	Human IgG1	Transgenic mice	Multiple myeloma	2015
Atezolizumab	Tecentriq	Roche, F. Hoffmann-La Roche, Ltd./Genentech Inc	PD-L1	Humanized IgG1	Hybridoma	Bladder cancer	2016
Inotuzumab ozogamicin	Besponsa	Wyeth Pharmaceuticals/Pfizer	CD22	Humanized IgG4	Hybridoma	Acute lymphoblastic leukemia	2017
Durvalumab	Imfinzi	MedImmune/ AstraZeneca	PD-L1-programmed death-ligand 1	Human IgG1	Transgenic mice	Bladder cancer	2017
Moxetumomab pasudodox	Lumoxiti	MedImmune/ AstraZeneca	CD22	Murine IgG1 dsFv	Phage display	Hairy cell leukemia	2018
Tisotumab vedotin	TIVDAK	Tissue factor	Disrupting agent monomethyl auristatin E	Tissue Factor (TF) specific human IgG1	Human IgG1 ADC	Cervical cancer	2021
Dostarlimab	Jemperli	PD-1	binds to the PD-1 receptor and blocks its interaction with PD-L1 and PD-L2	Humanized IgG4	Humanized monoclonal antibody	Endometrial cancer	2021

TABLE 4.3 Top 10 best-selling monoclonal antibody drugs in 2021 [8].

Rank	Generic name	Brand Name	Manufacturer	Condition/pharmacology class	Dosage form/strength	2021 worldwide sales (US $million)
1	Adalimumab	Humira	AbbVie	Rheumatoid and psoriatic arthritis, ankylosing spondylitis, Crohn's disease, ulcerative colitis	40 mg/0.8 mL in a single-use prefilled glass syringe	19,963
2	Pembrolizumab	Keytruda	Merck	Anti PD1-mAb	100 mg/4 mL (25 mg/mL) solution in a single-dose vial	16,825
3	Lenalidomide	Revilmid	Beigene	Multiple myeloma, Immunomodulator	Capsules: 2.5, 5, 10, 15 and 25 mg	12,710
4	Apixaban	Eliquis	Pfizer	Factor Xa inhibitor anticoagulant	2.5 and 5 mg orally twice daily	10,546
5	Aflibercept	Eylea	Regeneron Pharmaceuticals/Bayer	Age-Related Macular Degeneration	40 mg/mL solution for intra vitreal injection	8,872
6	Nivolumab	Opdivo	Ono Pharmaceutical	Anti-PD1 mAb	40, 100, and 240 mg/24 mL solution in a single-dose vial	8,759
7	Ustekinumab	Stelara	Johnson & Johnson	Human interleukin-12 and -23 antagonist- plaque psoriasis, active psoriatic arthritis	45 mg/0.5 mL or 90 mg/mL in a single-dose prefilled syringe	8.445
8	Bictegravir, emtricitabine, and tenofovir alafenamide	Biktarvy	Gilead Sciences	HIV INSTI/NTRI-nucleotide reverse transcriptase inhibitors	One tablet: 50 mg of bictegravir 200 mg of emtricitabine 25 mg of tenofovir alafenamide	
9	Ibrutinib	Imbruvica	AbbVie/Johnson & Johnson	BTK inhibitor	Capsules: 70 and 140 mg Tablets: 140 mg, 280, 420, and 560 mg	7,607
10	Rivaroxaban	Xarelto	Bayer/Johnson & Johnson	Factor Xa inhibitor anticoagulant	Tablets: 10, 15, and 20 mg	7,605

TABLE 4.4 List of US Food and Drug Administration approved human mAbs [9].

S. No	Antibody	Brand Name	Manufacturer	Target	Technology	Dosage form/strength	Approval year	US FDA Ref ID
1.	Adalimumab	Humira	Abbott Laboratories	TNFα	Phage display	40 mg/0.8 mL in a single-use prefilled glass syringe	2002	Reference ID: 4359269
2	Panitumumab	Vectibix	Amgen	EGFR	Xeno Mouse	Single-use vials (20 mg/mL): 100 mg/5 mL, 200 mg/10 mL, 400 mg/20 mL	2006	Reference ID: 3618836
3	Ustekinumab	Stelara	Johnson & Johnson	IL-12	HuMabMouse	Injection: 45 mg/0.5 mL or 90 mg/mL in a single-dose	2009	Reference ID: 3990240
4	Canakinumab	Ilaris	Novartis	IL-1β	HuMabMouse	single-use 6-mL, glass vial containing 180 mg of ILARIS as a lyophilized powder for reconstitution	2009	Reference ID: 3109737
5	Ofatumumab	Arzerra	GlaxoSmithKline (Genmab)	CD20	HuMabMouse	100 mg/5 mL single-use vial	2009	Reference ID: 3490691
6	Denosumab	Prolia, Xgeva	Amgen	RANKL	XenoMouse	60 mg in a 1 mL solution	2010	Reference ID: 3324257
7	Belimumab	Benlysta	GlaxoSmithKline	BCAF	Phage display	120 mg per vial, 400 mg per via	2011	Reference ID: 3109129
8	Ramucirumab	Cyramza	Eli Lilly	VEGFR2	Phage display	100 mg/10 mL (10 mg/mL) or 500 mg/50 mL (10 mg/mL) solution in a single-dose vial	2014	Reference ID: 4615930
9	Nivolumab	Opdivo	Bristol-Myers Squibb	PD-1	HuMabMouse	40 mg/4 mL, 100 mg/10 mL, and 240 mg/24 mL solution in a single-dose via	2015	Reference ID: 4844290
10	Alirocumab	Praluent	Sanofi and Regeneron	PCSK9	Veloclmmune Mouse	75 mg/mL or 150 mg/mL solution in a single dose	2015	Reference ID: 3797282
11	Daratumumab	Darzalex	Johnson & Johnson (Genmab)	CD38	HuMabMouse	100 mg/5 mL solution in a single-dose vial • 400 mg/20 mL solution in a single-dose via	2015	Reference ID: 4016996

12	Necitumumab	Portrazza	Eli Lilly (ImClone)	EGFR	Phage display	Injection: 800 mg/50 mL (16 mg/mL) solution in a single-dose via	2015	Reference ID: 3851135
13	Secukinumab	Cosentyx	Novartis	IL-17α	XenoMouse	Injection: 50 mg/mL solution in a single-use	2015	Reference ID: 3874646
14	Atezolizumab	Tecentriq	Roche, F. Hoffmann-La Roche, Ltd./ Genentech Inc.	PD-L1	Phage display	Injection: 40 mg/14 mL (60 mg/mL) and 1200 mg/20 mL (60 mg/mL) solution in a single-dose vial	2016	Reference ID: 4872883
15	Avelumab	Bavencio	Pfizer	PD-L1	Phage display	200 mg/10 mL (20 mg/mL) solution in single-dose vial.	2017	Reference ID: 41711121
16	Dupilumab	Dupixent	Sanofi and Regeneron	IL-4R	VelocImmune Mouse	Injection: 300 mg/2 mL solution in a single-dose	2017	Reference ID: 4075926
17	Guselkumab	Tremfya	Jassen Biotech	IL-23	Phage display	Injection: 100 mg/mL in a single-dose prefilled syringe.	2017	Reference ID 4123919
18	Erenumab	Aimovig	Novartis and Amgen	CGRPR	XenoMouse	Injection: 70 mg/mL solution in a single-dose	2018	Reference ID: 4264882
19	Emapalumab	Gamifant	NovImmune	IFNγ	Phage display	Injection: 10 mg/2 mL (5 mg/mL) solution in a single-dose vial 50 mg/10 mL (5 mg/mL) solution in a single-dose vial	2018	Reference ID: 4352133
20	Moxetumomab pasudodox	Lumoxiti	MedImmune/ AstraZeneca	CD22	Phage display	Injection:1 mg lyophilized cake or powder in a single-dose vial	2018	Reference ID: 4320135
21	Ravulizumab	Ultomiris	Alexion Pharmaceuticals	C5; humanized IgG2/4	Recombinant DNA technology	Injection: 300 mg/30 mL (10 mg/mL) in a single-dose vial	2019	Reference ID: 4367173
22	Isatuximab	Sarclisa	Sanofi-aventis U.S. LLC	CD38	Chimeric IgG1	Injection: 100 mg/5 mL (20 mg/mL) solution in single-dose vial 500 mg/25 mL (20 mg/mL) solution in single-dose vial	2020	Reference ID: 4568826
23	Dostarlimab	Jemperli	GlaxoSmithKline	PD-1, Endometrial cancer	Humanized IgG4	Injection: 500 mg/10 mL (50 mg/mL) solution in a single-dose via	2021	Reference ID: 4783636

with the tumor, which is the most difficult portion encountered by mAbs [19]. Large specific antibodies, which firmly bind their antigen during the first attack at the tumor's margin, cannot penetrate deeper within the cancer until enough antigen molecules in the periphery have been saturated. Therapeutic antibodies are also restricted by the affinity of these molecules for inhibitory Fc receptors, including FcRIIb, B-cells, macrophages, dendritic cells, and neutrophils that express it [20]. Over 99% of the cells will not survive because the process of fusing prevents the production of antibodies directed against specific antigens. A higher pH level can alter the surface charges of antibodies, causing them to buildup and cause an increase in viscosity due to electrostatic attraction, especially at higher concentrations [21]. mAbs confront the same hurdles as all proteinaceous treatments due to their protein structure [22], namely, the drug stability issue. It has been reported that a number of structural, colloidal, and chemical factors can hinder the development of good mAb formulations (such as oxidation, isomerization, deamidation, clumping, degradation, and fragmentation) [23,24]. As mAbs come into interaction with a wide range of temperatures, moisture, ionic strength, and stress levels, their structure changes, primarily in the hypervariable region, resulting in a series of unwanted products, many of them inhibiting the activity and enhancing the immunogenicity of the protein, potentially putting patients at risk [25]. Therefore, it is very challenging to find optimal adjuvants to prevent destabilization of mAbs. Furthermore, mAbs suffer other significant restrictions due to ambiguity and a significant reduction in their capacity to bypass biological blockage. Poor collaboration and high clinical adaptation costs are the two major impediments to mAb use universally. The viscosity and injection pressure for subcutaneous administration are influenced by the concentration of mAb, which results in a shorter half-life in low molecular weight compounds and changes in immunological reactions.

4.5 Approaches for developing targeted monoclonal antibodies

Human, humanized, hybrid, and mouse antibodies represent 51%, 34.7%, 12.5%, and 2.8% of all mAbs in clinical utilization, respectively; in therapeutic applications, human and humanized mAbs have become the dominant modality. In this segment, we address antibody humanization and methodological frameworks for generating completely human Abs (phage display, transgenic mice, and single B cell antibody isolation) [8].

4.5.1 XenoMouse hybridoma technology

Gene-targeted removal of the mouse immunoglobulin genes (heavy and light chain) has initially been used to immobilize these loci within embryonic stem (ES) cells in order to create homogeneous animals for the requisite alterations (Fig. 4.2). Mice resulting from hybridizing were in animals homozygous for these deletions being incapable of producing mouse immunoglobulin. Then, either human heavy- or light-chain DNA-carrying yeast artificial chromosomes were inserted into ES cells. Genetic recombination of mouse resulting from these ES cells caused in transgenic animals that produced both human and murine antibodies (Abs). Genetic recombination mouse unable of producing mouse

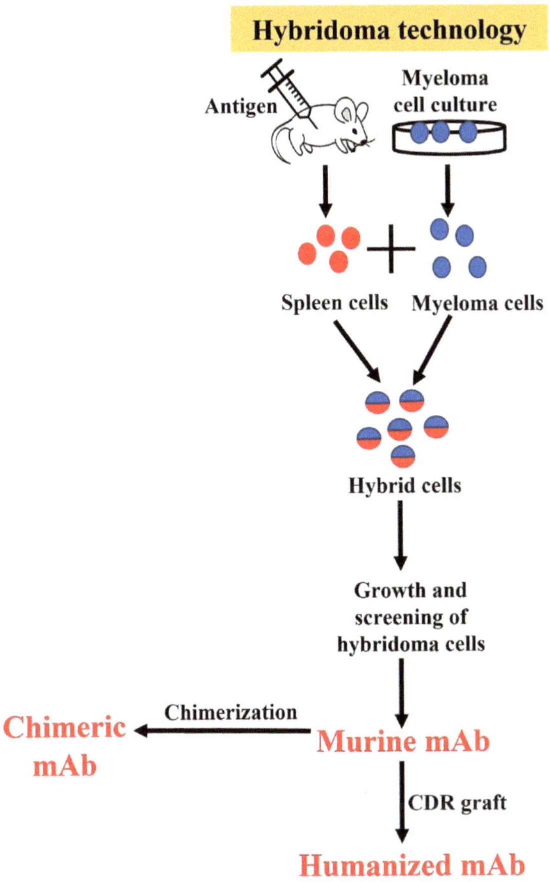

FIGURE 4.2 Hybridoma technology for mAb production.

immunoglobulin with genetically-engineered mice (carrying both human and mouse Abs) resulted in the Xeno Mouse strain, which carries only human Abs and is incapable of producing mouse antibodies. Antibody-producing B cells taken from an immunized XenoMouse's spleen are utilized to create hybridomas, in which the B cells merge with an immortal cell line. Finally, the hybridoma technique is used to generate completely human mAbs. The results of this technology are handy in terms of production since each hybridoma may produce larger amounts of identical totally human Abs that can be cultivated indefinitely and screened to detect antibodies of the desired specificity and sensitivity, besides targeting activities [26].

4.5.2 Phage display for the production of human mAbs

The first and most commonly utilized approach for in vitro antibody selection was phage display (Fig. 4.3). The surface of peptides should be able to display these peptides of bacteriophages. George P. Smith fused external peptides with pIII, a coat protein of bacteriophage

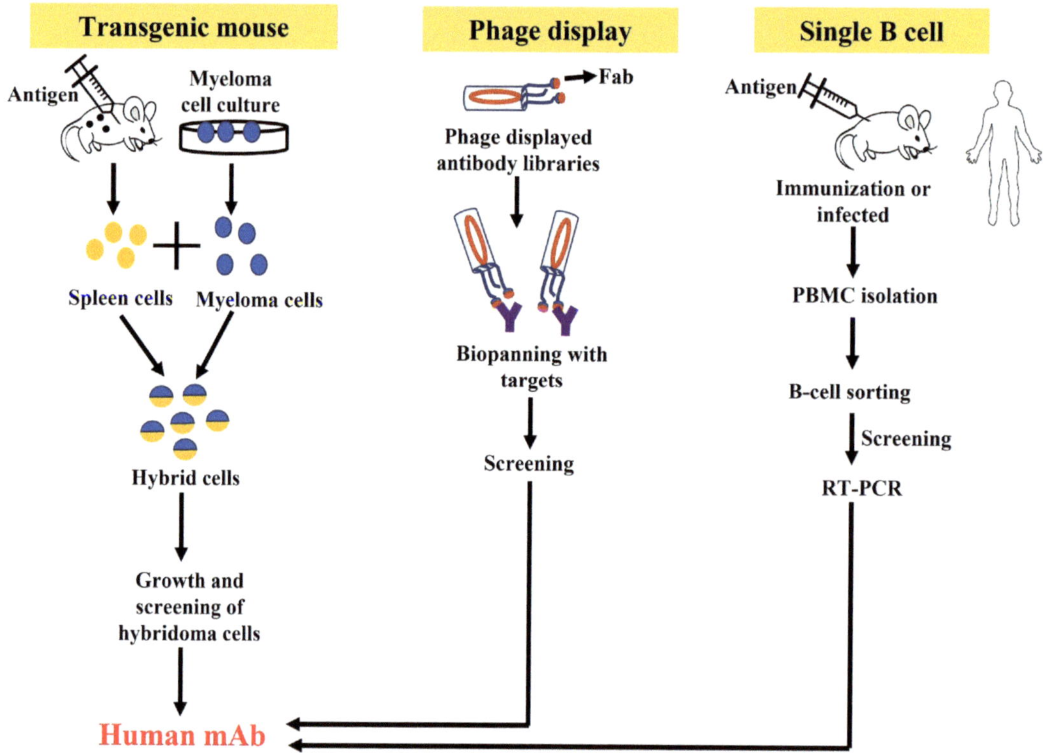

FIGURE 4.3 Transgenic animals, phase display, and single B cell approaches utilized in the production of mAb.

M13 using recombinant DNA techniques in 1985 [27]. In order to identify mAbs from phage display libraries, an antibody library must be created. Variable heavy and variable light polymerase chain reaction (PCR) products, representing the repertoire of Ig genes, are integrated into a phage display vector (phagemid). Reverse transcription of high-quality mRNA is carried out from human peripheral blood mononuclear cells (PBMCs) into cDNA. Following that, the chain-region genes of VH and VL are replicated using specialized primers to replicate all transcribed variable areas within the Ig repertoire [28]. Fab fragments can be found in phage-displayed libraries, while scFvs are composed of two domains linked by a flexible linker. A phage coat protein containing antibody Fab fragments showed increase; their structure is stable, and they can be converted into whole IgG antibodies without affecting their function [29]. Apparently, rearranged V genes of IgM repertoires are used to create naive antibody libraries. The human antibody germline is closely related to the sequences of the naive libraries since each sequence is generated from human B cells. This means that immunogenicity risks are very low. Today, practically all publicly available marketable collections are constructed on very varied nonimmunized gene repertoires, allowing the Abs selected for detection a potentially infinite number of targets [30]. Phage display provides the benefit of allowing researchers to customize essential properties of effective antibody medicines (e.g., affinity, specificity, cross-reactivity, and stability). A total of nine human antibodies derived from phage display are now in use, because US FDA has approved the use of this medication to treat humanoid diseases, confirming the technique's dependability as a foundation for antibody development.

4.5.3 Transgenic mice that produce human monoclonal antibodies

Transgenic mice (Fig. 4.3) offer a dependable platform for antibody drug development. Transgenic animals have various benefits over conventional human antibody manufacturing systems, including less requirement for humanization, more variety, a clonal selection approach to optimize antibody affinity through in vivo maturation. Human antibodies were first produced in transgenic mice by Alt et al. [31] in 1985, when they recommended inserting a human antibody gene into the mouse genome. This concept was novel and provided a fresh path for the advancement of human antibody production. A human heavy chain construct was cloned for the first time by Brüggemann et al. [32] in 1989, which had two different VH genes for diversity segments (D) coupled to the human heavy chain connecting clusters (CH) and the constant region. This transgenic strain might possibly be used to create hybridomas of human IgM antibodies. Several murine Ig knockout mouse strains were developed. Chen et al. used gene-targeted deletion to knockout murine JH and JK genes, inactivating mouse Ig [33]. Human IgH and IgL transgenic mice were then mated with murine IgH and IgL knockout mice to establish lines capable of producing more varied human antibodies. Longberg et al. created the first human Ig transgenic mouse strain, HuMab-Mouse [34], in 1994. Green et al. [35] used yeast spheroplast-ES cell fusion to successfully introduce human IgK (170 kb) and IgH (220 kb) genome YACs into mouse ES cells. Mendez et al. [36] subsequently established XenoMouse [37] by crossing human YACs with murine IgH and IgL knockout mice and introducing them into the mouse ES cells, resulting in larger human IgK (*700 KB) or IgH (* 1 Mb) YACs. Unlike mouse antibodies, XenoMouse only expresses human antibodies [38].

4.5.4 Antibody technique based on single B cells

It is well-known that body's immune system responds robustly to antibodies, which are highly precise, counteracting, and self-tolerating. Antibodies that can be used as therapeutics via the standard hybridoma process or utilizing transgenic mice might cause severe immunogenic responses, in addition to long-term vaccination protocols and screening [such as human antimouse antibodies (HAMAs)] [39]. Human B cells were immortalized with Epstein–Barr virus to overcome these challenges [40]. Micromanipulation, laser capture microdissection, and fluorescence-activated cell sorting (Fig. 4.3) can be used to isolate single B cells from either PBMCs or lymphoid tissues. Further, each Ig heavy chain and its corresponding light chain must be cloned directly [41] besides single B cell sorting [42]. By using nested or semi-nested reverse transcription-PCR, the variable heavy and light chains of each identified B cell are amplified [43]. Forward primers are usually targeted at the variable leader sequences of IgH and IgL, whereas reverse primers complement the Ig constant region [44]. The VH and VL recoveries might be increased by adjusting different primer-set compositions [45]. In order to generate recombinant mAbs, a mammalian cell is then used to express the cloned genes. A profile of each generated mAb is determined after it has been detected that it is reactive. The use of microarray chips and microengraving techniques is notable for screening secreted mAbs with high throughput [46,47] and evaluating their ideal reactivity.

Using the immunospot array test on a chip and a cell-based microarray chip technology and by covering a chip with an anti-Ig antibody, a chip can trap secreted antibodies and is therefore used to detect and recuperate particular antibody-secreting cells. Human mAbs have previously been produced for bacterial, parasitic, virus-infected, or autoimmune illnesses using the single B cell approach. A yeast infection can be treated with monoclonal anti-Candida mAb antibodies developed by single human B cells, which can boost protection against disseminated candidiasis through phagocytosis [48]. Antiviral mAbs have also been successfully produced using the single B cell method. Several studies have reported identifying dengue-neutralizing antibodies in memory B cells cultured from human antigens [49] and identifying antigen-specific B cells in the peripheral blood of DENV-immune individuals [50]. It was observed that rotavirus antibody gene repertoires in naive and memory B cell subsets were analyzed with the single B cell method [51] and that human rotavirus-specific mAbs could be generated by isolating single B cells from the intestinal tract mucosal [52]. A single human B cell method plus mAbs for bacterial and viral infections has also resulted in antibodies against the complement factor H that are therapeutic for cancer.

4.5.5 Humanization of mAbs

The humanization of mouse mAbs is considered on bulk quantities due to the ease of obtaining, low cost, and rapid development of mouse mAbs. Typical nonhumanized murine mAbs have a number of limitations as therapy, such as prompt HAMAs when patients are medicated with them. When humanized mAbs are used to reduce the immunogenicity of murine antibodies, they can effectively show effector responses.

4.5.6 Generation of humanized mAbs

In humanized mAbs, only the complementary-determining region (CDRs) of the light and heavy chains are murine, which were authorized in clinical trials in early 1988 [53]. CDR grafting is a well-known approach for producing humanized mAbs that was first proposed by Gregory P. Winter in 1986 [54]. Nonhuman CDR sequences are added to human framework sequences using this method, allowing the antibody to maintain its target-specific antigen response. It was the development of daclizumab in 1997, which attaches to the IL-2 receptor and inhibits transplant rejection [55], which was the first CDR-grafted humanized monoclonal antibody to be approved by the FDA. Various approaches have been developed to measure the quality of human mAbs in changing environments. An assessment of antibody sequence humanness known as the H-score has been developed by Abhinandan and Martin [56], which compares subset human variable region sequence databases with mean value specifications. mAb-based drugs are clinically more effective when humanized antibodies are used. It has created a new era in which mAbs can be engineered to have a greater range of potential uses in the biomedical field due to this complex control over antibody sequences. Recent developments have seen most mAbs used to treat various diseases being chimeric or humanized.

4.5.7 Human and humanized mAbs

There is already a plethora of antibodies that are therapeutic on the market for the treatment of a variety of medical problems, including immune-mediated chronic inflammation. Numerous clinical systems have been implemented, and the insufficiency of head-to-head comparative trials in distinguishing the relative clinical efficiency and safety profiles of one monoclonal antibody vs another can be a difficult problem. The ability to determine whether a monoclonal antibody is entirely human or humanized is one distinguishing feature of dermatologists when explaining clinical trial data. This finding illustrates the differences and similarities between totally human and humanized monoclonal antibodies in terms of nomenclature, engineering, and therapeutic prospects. While there are several variances among different types of monoclonal antibodies, recent research indicates that this categorization has little bearing on the overall clinical efficacy and safety profiles of a specific treatment. It is obvious from the molecular insights provided in this perspective that any monoclonal antibody, whether humanized or not, will have the same effect on cells, and must be examined separately for its medical influence in terms of safety and efficiency. Monoclonal antibodies will continue to be a potential treatment option for a wide range of disorders with dermatological consequences in the future [9].

4.5.8 Stereospecific monoclonal antibodies

Moreover, therapeutic mAbs can also be developed by one of the valuable approaches, in which mAbs are selected due to their greater affinity and selectivity toward definite antigens (Ag). It was discovered that mAbs can recognize two kinds of epitopes with great accuracy (linear epitope present on protein's primary structures and conformational epitopes present on protein's secondary and tertiary structures). As a result, identifying protein conformational configurations leads to increased specificity and affinity for therapeutic treatments. Usually, linear epitope-specific mAbs accept 2D configuration. However, stereospecific mAbs can recognize 3D molecule configurations. Because of their specificity and selectivity for target antigens, mAbs can be utilized as bioactives, and conformational epitope-specific mAbs have been demonstrated to be superior to linear epitope-specific mAbs. Because proteins are full conformational assemblies in nature, stereospecific antigen identification brings up new treatment options [4].

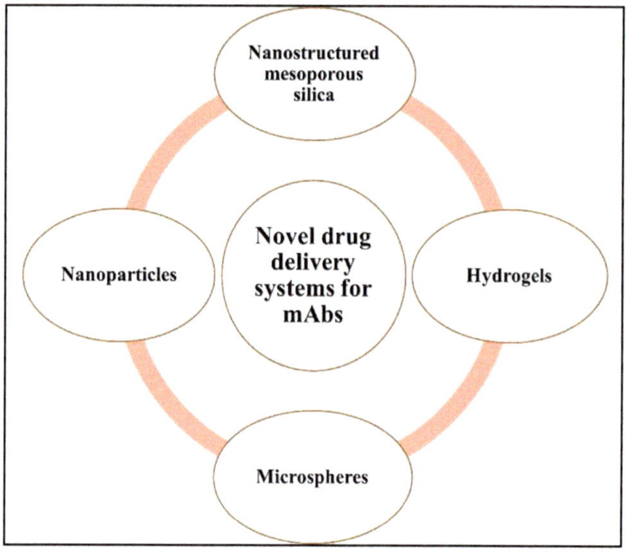

FIGURE 4.4 Novel drug delivery systems for mAbs.

4.6 Novel drug delivery systems for mAbs

Though mAbs have had a lot of success for therapeutic purposes over the last 40 years, some constraints such as deficient pharmacokinetics, poor pharmacodynamics, and systemic toxicity have limited their prospective usage. Advanced research is being directed toward numerous new techniques, including changed Fc function antibodies, bispecific antibodies, intrabodies, and antibody fragments, to achieve superior pharmacokinetics, improved selectivity, and increased efficiency [57]. In clinical application, both patients as well as health professionals need additional competent and more secured mAbs to initiation improved concurrence. The following section discusses a variety of novel drug delivery approaches that have been used to solve obstacles encountered during the development of mAb-based medicines (Fig. 4.4).

4.6.1 Nanoparticles

Nanoparticles (NPs) are a type of particulate delivery system that come in sizes ranging from 10 to 1000 nm and are widely used in pharmaceutical drug delivery systems [58]. There are numerous polymers accessible for creating NPs, one of which being poly lactic-co-glycolic acid (PLGA), which is a popular biodegradable polymer. This polymer hydrolysates into glycolic acid and lactic acid, which are easily metabolized in-vivo. Because the EMA and FDA have approved this polymer for a variety of uses in the development of drug delivery systems, PLGA-conjugated NPs are frequently employed in clinical trials [59]. When compared to free anti-OX40 mAbs, PLGA-based NPs loaded with mAbs are able to target tumor necrosis factor (TNF) receptor OX40, which is predominantly expressed on activated T cells, and are found to be more efficient.

Furthermore, it can persuade the development of cytotoxic T lymphocytes (CTLs), cytokine development, and tumor antigen-specific cytotoxicity [60]. It was also reported that mAb fragments (3D8 scFv) were loaded into PLGA-NPs, resulting in increased cellular uptake via cellular endocytosis. Self-analogous bevacizumab NPs were shown to be three times more readily taken up in A549 cells than in MRC-5 cells. Cancer cells prefer to take up uncoated mAb-NPs over normal cells [61].

4.6.2 Microspheres

Microspheres are being evaluated as a viable drug delivery carrier for IgGs or monoclonal antibodies, as they enable consistent therapeutic release and extended stability in the systemic circulation. IgG-MPEG-PCL-MPEG microspheres (6 m) were developed utilizing the double emulsion solvent evaporation technique, using copolymer of poly(ethylene glycol)-poly(-caprolactone) (PEG-PCL). At the time of irradiation, it was found that IgG-MPEG-PCL-MPEG microspheres had lower IgG destabilization rates and higher entrapment efficacy than IgG-PCL microspheres [62]. The s/o/w (solid-in-oil-in-water) method was established and optimized to prepare microspheres without compromising the stability issues of IgG or mAb. The combination of the s/o/w emulsion method and spray-drying leads to successful entrapment of IgG microparticles into the PLGA microsphere core. This new combination process resulted in improved entrapment efficiency (60% w/w) and drug loading (6% w/w) [63]. The full length anti-human TNF-α mAb-entrapped microspheres of PLGA were positively prepared by the s/o/s process with capability to load bioactives as well as single mAbs in microspheres.

The combination of mesenchymal stem cells and anti-BMP2 mAbs, as well as their entrapment in alginate microspheres, significantly boosted the osteogenesis associated with human bone marrow mesenchymal stem cells [64]. Ethylene-vinyl acetate copolymer (EVAc) was used to load IgG in the form of dry powder and characterized for efficient polymer-fabricated antigen delivery strategy [65]. EVAc microspheres can also be used for topical administration, sustained release injectables, and extended-release IgG. Another example of polymer-based vaginal delivery system was a vaginal ring, which delivers an Ab in the mouse model [66]. Direct, local delivery of Abs by applying aqueous gels made up of carboxymethyl cellulose may be effective antiinfective technique after surgical procedures. Abs have been delivered to the CNS for a long time using a hyaluronic acid-bound Ab hydrogel with a covalent link [67].

4.6.3 Hydrogels

Using a novel drug-loaded hydrogel system, the stability of epidermal growth factor was successfully enhanced [68]. The porous architecture and higher water content are ideal for encapsulating mAbs. Furthermore, three dimensional structures of hydrogel were capable of entrapping the mAbs in complex networking of hydrogel networks [69]. For the construction of therapeutically safe hydrogels capable of prolonged release of mAbs, a lot of research has been done on both natural materials (chitosan) and synthetic polymers (PLGA-PEG-PLGA). mAb delivery can be improved by applying the thermosensitive hydrogels with the character of transforming from solution to gel at body temperature. A modified biocompatible triblock copolymer of poly(2-ethyl-2-oxazoline)-bpoly(ε-caprolactone)-b-poly(2-ethyl-2-oxazoline) (PEOz-PCL-PEOz) was designed to prepare a biodegradable thermosensitive hydrogel, and it was able to delay the release of bevacizumab for several days (20 days) [70]. When delivered through subcutaneous injection, a trastuzumab-loaded hydrogel containing vitamin E-functionalized polycarbonate and poly(ethylene glycol) triblock copolymers was found to be effective in the treatment of breast cancer.

4.6.4 Other delivery systems

The degradation of mAbs during prolonged release has been measured using several innovative mAb-based delivery techniques. Using electrostatic forces (pH 7.4 solution), bevacizumab-loaded nanosized mesoporous silica (SiO_2) was created and found to have a delayed release of up to 30 days with protected functionality of released molecules [71].

4.7 Formulation challenges of mAbs

The structural changes in mAbs can happen at any stage of the development steps due to the presence of the tertiary structure of biologics. These biologics are highly susceptible to physical stress, which can cause alterations in mAbs throughout the process of protein synthesis, processing, and storage. Structural modifications can be linked to the presence of nonphysiological conditions during processing, which may cause structural alternatives to adapt in the final formulation. This is a significant constraint and hurdle in biopharmaceutical development, which is distinct from the creation of small molecule medicines, where such issues do not arise; nonetheless, pressures such as buffer selection, evolving processes, and container selection might raise this issue. Furthermore, any finished mAb-dependent biopharmaceutical formulations containing nonnative proteins should be overlooked. While taking protein solutions from vials, accumulation may result in nonuniform dosage [72,73]. Because of their proteinaceous composition, mAbs suffer stability concerns when exposed to pH, higher temperatures, stress and humidity [22]. The formulations rich in concentration are facing the problem of concentration-based decomposition of accumulated mAbs [74]. The development of highly viscous concentrated mAb is mostly dependent on molecular interactions and protein self-association. Typical difficulties encountered during the development of mAb-based therapeutics as well as mAbs are constrained to intravenous and subcutaneous administration of lyophilized and liquid formulations. The main issue is mAb stability, which has a detrimental impact on yield due to product loss due to buildup in downstream processing steps. Unwanted byproducts created during manufacturing procedures can accumulate in HEK 293 exposed mAbs. Immunogenic mAbs are made using hybriddoma technology, and CHO-expressed mAbs have an immunogenic glycosylation profile. Biologics with instability issues may produce less therapeutic response or sometimes adverse events too. The buildup of IFN, for example, can affect the production of neutralizing anti-drug Abs (NAb) capable of blocking IFN receptor binding, lowering clinical efficacy [75].

4.8 Future trends of mAbs

The approach of therapeutic antibodies is currently becoming an eye-catching option in the therapeutic purpose. Though there is still important growth likely for the therapeutic antibody field. Traditionally, antibodies are utilized to manage the cancer, autoimmune disorders, and infectious disorders. The mAbs may offer a potent therapeutic approach if the molecular mechanisms of a disease can be clearly described and the distinct proteins can be linked in pathogenesis. For example, anti-CGRP receptor antibodies such as erenumab, galcanezumab, or fremanezumab have been progressed for the management of migraine. Anti-proprotein convertase subtilisin/kexin type 9 (PCSK9) antibodies (evolocumab or alirocumab) are used for the treatment of hypercholesterolemia. Anti-fibroblast growth factor 23 (FGF23) antibody (burosumab) is utilized to treat X-linked hypophosphatemia. Anti-IL6R antibody (sarilumab and tocilizumab) can be used to treat rheumatoid arthritis. Anti-factor IXa/Xa antibody (emicizumab) is a promising treatment for hemophilia A. Anti-von Willebrand factor antibody (caplacizumab) is considered for the treatment of thrombotic thrombocytopenic purpura, and other antibodies will be accepted for new considerations in the future. Therapeutic mAbs can readily be classified into two broad categories. In the first one, the naked antibody is directly applied for disease therapy. Cancer treatments from this category may work by various mechanisms, such as mediated pathways like ADCC/CDC, direct targeting of cancer cells to induce apoptosis, targeting the tumor microenvironment, or targeting immune checkpoints. In altered pathways, the antibody kills cancer cells by recruiting natural killer cells or other immune cells. Currently, various novel methods have been employed to improve the therapeutic efficacy of ADCC or CDC, like antibody Fc point mutations or alteration of glycosylation to enhance the cancer cell killing rate [76,77]. The direct induction apoptosis in cancer cells has traditionally been the considered mechanism for therapeutic antibodies. For targeting the tumor microenvironment, antibodies can reduce tumorigenesis by targeting factors linked in cancer cell progression. Findings have measured the synergistic actions of antibodies and chemotherapeutic bioactives, radiotherapy, and other biologic components, which will greatly benefit the further progression of antibody drugs. Thereafter, the identification of novel biomarkers may augment the efficiency and specificity of antibody-based therapy for human disorders. In the second type of antibody therapeutics, additional alterations are made to the antibody in order to advance its therapeutic efficacy. To create an immunocytokine, a selected cytokine is fused to an antibody to improve the delivery specificity. Antibody drug conjugates (ADCs) are made up of an antibody that targets a cancer-specific marker combined to the small molecule drug; the antibody developments the delivery to the target site, attractive the efficiency of the small molecule while decreasing side effects by inhibiting nonspecific toxicity to nontarget tissues [78,79]. The antibody may also be fused to a radionuclide for direct radiotherapy specifically to the tumor site [80,81]. Antibody-engaged effector cell functions may increase the therapeutic potential of bispecific antibodies. With regard to immunoliposomes, the coupling site of the antibody (Fab) is cleaved from the constant area and eventually conjugated to different nanodrug delivery systems like liposomal drugs to provide more specific targeting [82] (Fig. 4.5).

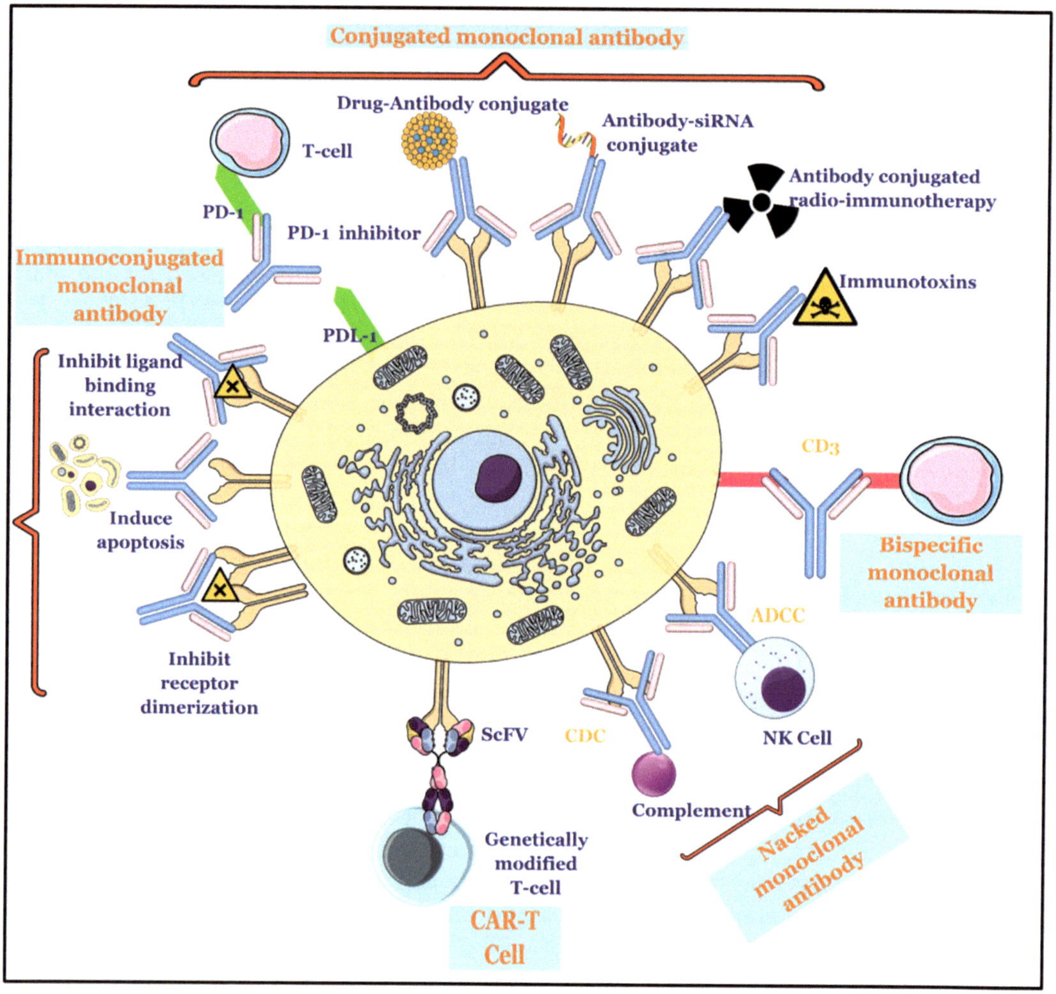

FIGURE 4.5 Molecular mechanism of therapeutic monoclonal antibody (mechanism of action of mAb therapy). (A) Naked mAb can function through various mechanisms, including antibody-dependent cellular cytotoxicity, using immune effector cells such as natural killer cells. Complement-mediated cytotoxicity (CMC) functions through the membrane attack complex and by inhibition of the receptor dimerization, inducing an apoptotic signal or through effecting target cells by blocking the binding of ligands. Immune checkpoint inhibitors, including PD-1, function by blocking the T-cell-inhibitory receptors and CTLA-4, which function through activation of the T-cell function. (B) Conjugated mAb includes payload antibody for delivery of specific drugs or chemotherapy agents directly to the tumor cells, radioimmunoconjugates to deliver radioisotopes to the cancer cells, immunotoxins to deliver highly toxic drugs to the target cells, and siRNA particles to downregulate a target gene. (C) CAR T-cell therapy uses a genetically engineered T cell to target a specific antigen on tumor cells. (D) Bispecific mAbs consists of two arms, with one arm recognizing cancer cells and the other activating antigens on immune effector cells including CD3.

4.9 Conclusion

There is a diverse variety of mAbs currently on the marketplace that have been extensively employed in clinics for diagnosis, treatment, and prognosis. Biotechnology-derived bioactives, such as antibody-dependent therapeutics, are on the forefront of innovation when it comes to treating a wide range of clinical conditions. In addition to conduct clinical studies, substances must be developed into stable formulations that may be utilized for targeted delivery. Since the mAbs have shown excellent clinical and commercial results, several scientists and pharmaceutical industry are now focusing on additional mAbs for delivery strategies. An enhancement in the efficiency of antibody therapeutics may be achieved by the use of transgenic organisms and "second-generation human chimeric mice." In the global pharmaceutical sector, the continual processing and refining of transgenic animals gives new avenues for the creation of antibody drugs. Because of the tremendous breakthroughs in the field of antibody medications, the use of mAbs has evolved as a crucial category of pharmacological compounds for a wide range of human conditions such as metabolic disorders, immunological conditions, infection, malignancies, and brain disease.

References

[1] Kohler G, Milstein C. Continuous cultures of fused cells secreting antibodies of predefined specificity. Nature 1975;256:495–7.

[2] Kaplon H, Reichert JM. Antibodies to watch in 2019. MAbs 2019;11:219–38.

[3] Tong JT, Harris PW, Brimble MA, Kavianinia I. An insight into FDA approved antibody-drug conjugates for cancer therapy. Molecules 2021;26(19):5847.

[4] Tsumoto K, Isozaki Y, Yagami H, Tomita M. Future perspectives of therapeutic monoclonal antibodies. Immunotherapy 2019;11(2):119–27.

[5] Carden CP, Arkenau HT, de Bono JS. Optimising the development of antibodies as treatment for cancer. In: Hidalgo M, Eckhardt SG, Garrett-Mayer E, Clendeninn NJ, editors. Principles of anticancer drug development. 1st ed New York, NY: Springer; 2011. p. 534–68.

[6] Charmsaz S, Scott AM, Boyd AW. Targeted therapies in hematological malignancies using therapeutic monoclonal antibodies against Eph family receptors. Exp Hematol 2017;54:31–9.

[7] Lu RM, Hwang YC, Liu IJ, Lee CC, Tsai HZ, Li HJ, et al. Development of therapeutic antibodies for the treatment of diseases. J Biomed Sci 2020;27(1):1–30.

[8] Wang H, Zheng X, Jin J, Zheng L, Guan T, Huo Y, et al. LncRNA MALAT1 silencing protects against cerebral ischemia-reperfusion injury through miR-145 to regulate AQP4. J Biomed Sci 2020;27(1):1–2.

[9] USFDA website i.e. https://www.accessdata.fda.gov.

[10] Batlevi CL, Matsuki E, Brentjens RJ, Younes A. Novel immunotherapies in lymphoid malignancies. Nat Rev Clin Oncol 2016;13(1):25–40.

[11] Scott AM, Wolchok JD, Old LJ. Antibody therapy of cancer. Nat Rev cancer 2012;12(4):278–87.

[12] Scott AM, Allison JP, Wolchok JD. Monoclonal antibodies in cancer therapy. Cancer Immun Archive 2012;12(1).

[13] Mallery DL, McEwan WA, Bidgood SR, Towers GJ, Johnson CM, James LC. Antibodies mediate intracellular immunity through tripartite motif-containing 21 (TRIM21). Proc Natl Acad Sci 2010;107(46):19985–90.

[14] Rodgers KR, Chou RC. Therapeutic monoclonal antibodies and derivatives: historical perspectives and future directions. Biotechnol Adv 2016;34(6):1149–58.

[15] Subramani K, Pathak Y. Antibody-mediated drug delivery systems: general review and applications. Antibody-Mediated Drug Deliv Syst: Concepts Technol Appl 2013;11:1.
[16] Dillman RO. Monoclonal antibody therapy. Principles of cancer biotherapy. Dordrecht: Springer; 2003. p. 329–90.
[17] Giritch A, Marillonnet S, Engler C, van Eldik G, Botterman J, Klimyuk V, et al. Rapid high-yield expression of full-size IgG antibodies in plants coinfected with noncompeting viral vectors. Proc Natl Acad Sci 2006;103 (40):14701–6.
[18] Graumann K, Premstaller A. Manufacturing of recombinant therapeutic proteins in microbial systems. Biotechnol J: Healthc Nutr Technol 2006;1(2):164–86.
[19] Beckman RA, Weiner LM, Davis HM. Antibody constructs in cancer therapy: protein engineering strategies to improve exposure in solid tumors. Cancer 2007;09(2):170–9.
[20] Nimmerjahn F, Ravetch JV. Antibodies, Fc receptors and cancer. Curr Opimmunol 2007;19(2):239–45.
[21] Tomar DS, Kumar S, Singh SK, Goswami S, Li L. Molecular basis of high viscosity in concentrated antibody solutions: strategies for high concentration drug product development in. MAbs 2016;8(2):216–28 *Taylor & Francis.*
[22] Frokjaer S, Otzen DE. Protein drug stability: a formulation challenge. Nat Rev Drug Discov 2005;4(4):298–306.
[23] Razinkov VI, Treuheit MJ, Becker GW. Accelerated formulation development of monoclonal antibodies (mAbs) and mAb-based modalities: a review of methods and tools. J Biomol Screen 2015;20(4):468–83.
[24] Uchiyama S. Liquid formulation for antibody drugs. Biochim Biophys Acta 2014;1844:2041–52.
[25] Pineda C, Castañeda Hernández G, Jacobs IA, Alvarez DF, Carini C. Assessing the immunogenicity of biopharmaceuticals. Bio Drugs 2016;30(3):195–206.
[26] Michnick SW, Sidhu SS. Submitting antibodies to binding arbitration. Nat Chem Biol 2008;4(6):326–9.
[27] Smith GP. Filamentous fusion phage: novel expression vectors that display cloned antigens on the virion surface. Science 1985;228:1315–17.
[28] Sheets MD, Amersdorfer P, Finnern R, Sargent P, Lindqvist E, Schier R, et al. Efficient construction of a large nonimmune phage antibody library: the production of high-affinity human single-chain antibodies to protein antigens. Proc Natl Acad Sci 1998;95(11):6157–62.
[29] Bradbury AR, Sidhu S, Dübel S, McCafferty J. Beyond natural antibodies: the power of in vitro display technologies. Nat Biotechnol 2011;29(3):245–54.
[30] Chan CE, Lim AP, MacAry PA, Hanson BJ. The role of phage display in therapeutic antibody discovery. Int Immunol 2014;26(12):649–57.
[31] Alt FW, Keith Blackwell T, Yancopoulos GD. Immunoglobulin genes in transgenic mice. Trends Genet 1885;1:231–6.
[32] Brüggemann M, Caskey HM, Teale C, Waldmann H, Williams GT, Surani MA, et al. A repertoire of monoclonal antibodies with human heavy chains from transgenic mice. Proc Natl Acad Sci 1989;86(17):6709–13.
[33] Chen J, Trounstine M, Alt FW, Young F, Kurahara C, Loring JF, et al. Immunoglobulin gene rearrangement in B cell deficient mice generated by targeted deletion of the JH locus. Int Immunol 1993;5(6):647–56.
[34] Lonberg N, Taylor LD, Harding FA, Trounstine M, Higgins KM, Schramm SR, et al. Antigen-specific human antibodies from mice comprising four distinct genetic modifications. Nature 1994;368:856–9.
[35] Green LL, Hardy MC, Maynard-Currie CE, Tsuda H, Louie DM, Mendez MJ, et al. Antigen-specific human monoclonal antibodies from mice engineered with human Ig heavy and light chain YACs. Nat Genet 1994;7 (1):13–21.
[36] Mendez MJ, Green LL, Corvalan JR, Jia XC, Maynard-Currie CE, Yang XD, et al. Functional transplant of megabase human immunoglobulin loci recapitulates human antibody response in mice. Nat Genet 1997;15 (2):146–56.
[37] Kashyap AK, Steel J, Oner AF, Dillon MA, Swale RE, Wall KM, et al. Combinatorial antibody libraries from survivors of the Turkish H5N1 avian influenza outbreak reveal virus neutralization strategies. Proc Natl Acad Sci 2008;105(16):5986–91.
[38] Jakobovits A, Amado RG, Yang X, Roskos L, Schwab G. From XenoMouse technology to panitumumab, the first fully human antibody product from transgenic mice. Nat Biotechnol 2007;25(10):1134–43.
[39] Legouffe E, Liautard J, Gaillard JP, Rossi JF, Wijdenes J, Bataille R, et al. Human anti-mouse antibody response to the injection of murine monoclonal antibodies against IL-6. Clin Exp Immunol 1994;98(2):323–9.
[40] Aman P, Ehlin-Henriksson B, Klein GE. Epstein-Barr virus susceptibility of normal human B lymphocyte populations. J Exp Med 1984;159(1):208–20.

[41] Küppers R, Zhao M, Hansmann ML, Rajewsky K. Tracing B cell development in human germinal centres by molecular analysis of single cells picked from histological sections. EMBO J 1993;12(13):4955–67.
[42] Pascual V, Liu YJ, Magalski A, De Bouteiller O, Banchereau J, Capra JD. Analysis of somatic mutation in five B cell subsets of human tonsil. J Exp Med 1994;180(1):329–39.
[43] Tiller T, Meffre E, Yurasov S, Tsuiji M, Nussenzweig MC, Wardemann H. Efficient generation of monoclonal antibodies from single human B cells by single-cell RT-PCR and expression vector cloning. J Immunol Methods 2008;329(1–2):112–24.
[44] Coronella JA, Telleman P, Truong TD, Ylera F, Junghans RP. Amplification of IgG VH and VL (Fab) from single human plasma cells and B cells. Nucleic acids Res 2000;28(20):e85.
[45] Wrammert J, Smith K, Miller J, Langley WA, Kokko K, Larsen C, et al. Rapid cloning of high-affinity human monoclonal antibodies against influenza virus. Nature 2008;453:667–71.
[46] Jin A, Ozawa T, Tajiri K, Obata T, Kondo S, Kinoshita K, et al. A rapid and efficient single-cell manipulation method for screening antigen-specific antibody-secreting cells from human peripheral blood. Nat Med 2009;15(9):1088–92.
[47] Love JC, Ronan JL, Grotenbreg GM, van der Veen AG, Ploegh HL. A microengraving method for rapid selection of single cells producing antigen-specific antibodies. Nat Biotechnol 2006;24(6):703–7.
[48] Rudkin FM, Raziunaite I, Workman H, Essono S, Belmonte R, MacCallum DM, et al. Single human B cell-derived monoclonal anti-Candida antibodies enhance phagocytosis and protect against disseminated candidiasis. Nat Commun 2018;9(1):1–6.
[49] Cox KS, Tang A, Chen Z, Horton MS, Yan H, Wang XM, et al. Rapid isolation of dengue-neutralizing antibodies from single cell-sorted human antigen-specific memory B-cell cultures. MAbs 2016;8:129–40.
[50] Woda M, Friberg H, Currier JR, Srikiatkhachorn A, Macareo LR, Green S, et al. Dynamics of dengue virus (DENV)–specific B cells in the response to DENV serotype 1 infections, using flow cytometry with labeled virions. J Infect Dis 2016;214(7):1001–9.
[51] Tian C, Luskin GK, Dischert KM, Higginbotham JN, Shepherd BE, Crowe JE. Immunodominance of the VH1–46 antibody gene segment in the primary repertoire of human rotavirus-specific B cells is reduced in the memory compartment through somatic mutation of nondominant clones. J Immunol 2008;180 (5):3279–88.
[52] Di Niro R, Mesin L, Raki M, Zheng NY, Lund-Johansen F, Lundin KE, et al. Rapid generation of rotavirus-specific human monoclonal antibodies from small-intestinal mucosa. J Immunol 2010;185(9):5377–83.
[53] Gorman SD, Clark MR. Humanisation of monoclonal antibodies for therapy. Semin Immunol 1990;2:457–66.
[54] Maloney DG, Grillo-López AJ, Bodkin DJ, White CA, Liles TM, Royston I, et al. IDEC-C2B8: results of a phase I multiple-dose trial in patients with relapsed non-Hodgkin's lymphoma. J Clin Oncol 1997;15(10):3266–74.
[55] Tsurushita N, Hinton PR, Kumar S. Design of humanized antibodies: from anti-Tac to Zenapax. Methods 2005;36:69–83.
[56] Abhinandan KR, Martin AC. Analyzing the "degree of humanness" of antibody sequences. J Mol Biol 2007;369(3):852–62.
[57] Morales JO, McConville JT. Novel strategies for the buccal delivery of macromolecules. Drug Dev Ind Pharm 2014;40(5):579–90.
[58] Leleux J, Williams RO. Recent advancements in mechanical reduction methods: particulate systems. Drug Dev Ind Pharm 2014;40(3):289–300.
[59] Danhier F, Ansorena E, Silva JM, Coco R, Le Breton A, Préat V. PLGA-based nanoparticles: an overview of biomedical applications. J Contr Rel 2012;161(2):505–22.
[60] Chen M, Ouyang H, Zhou S, Li J, Ye Y. PLGA-nanoparticle mediated delivery of anti-OX40 monoclonal antibody enhances anti-tumor cytotoxic T cell responses. Cell Immunol 2014;287(2):91–9.
[61] Srinivasan AR, Lakshmikuttyamma A, Shoyele SA. Investigation of the stability and cellular uptake of self-associated monoclonal antibody (MAb) nanoparticles by non-small lung cancer cells. Mol Pharm 2013;10 (9):3275–84.
[62] Erdemli Ö, Usanmaz A, Keskin D, Tezcaner A. Characteristics and release profiles of MPEG-PCL-MPEG microspheres containing immunoglobulin G. Colloids Surf B: Biointerfaces 2014;117:487–96.
[63] Marquette S, Peerboom C, Yates A, Denis L, Goole J, Amighi K. Encapsulation of immunoglobulin G by solid-in-oil-in-water: effect of process parameters on microsphere properties. Eur J Pharm Biopharm 2014;86 (3):393–403.

[64] Moshaverinia A, Ansari S, Chen C, Xu X, Akiyama K, Snead ML, et al. Co-encapsulation of anti-BMP2 monoclonal antibody and mesenchymal stem cells in alginate microspheres for bone tissue engineering. Biomaterials 2013;34(28):6572–9.
[65] Wang CH, Sengothi K, Lee T. Controlled release of human immunoglobulin G. 1. Release kinetics studies. J Pharm Sci 1999;88(2):215–20.
[66] Saltzman WM, Sherwood JK, Adams DR, Haller P. Long-term vaginal antibody delivery: delivery systems and biodistribution. Biotechnol Bioeng 2000;67(3):253–64.
[67] Tian WM, Zhang CL, Hou SP, Yu X, Cui FZ, Xu QY, et al. Hyaluronic acid hydrogel as Nogo-66 receptor antibody delivery system for the repairing of injured rat brain: in vitro. J Contr Rel 2005;102(1):13–22.
[68] Li X, Ye X, Qi J, Fan R, Gao X, Wu Y, et al. EGF and curcumin co-encapsulated nanoparticle/hydrogel system as potent skin regeneration agent. Int J Nanomed 2016;11:3993.
[69] Vermonden T, Censi R, Hennink WE. Hydrogels for protein delivery. Chem Rev 2012;112(5):2853–88.
[70] Wang CH, Hwang YS, Chiang PR, Shen CR, Hong WH, Hsiue GH. Extended release of bevacizumab by thermosensitive biodegradable and biocompatible hydrogel. Biomacromolecules 2012;13(1):40–8.
[71] Andrew JS, Anglin EJ, Wu EC, Chen MY, Cheng L, Freeman WR, et al. Sustained release of a monoclonal antibody from electrochemically prepared mesoporous silicon oxide. Adv Funct Mater 2010;20(23):4168–74.
[72] Manning MC, Chou DK, Murphy BM, Payne RW, Katayama DS. Stability of protein pharmaceuticals: an update. Pharm Res 2010;27(4):544–75.
[73] Angkawinitwong U, Sharma G, Khaw PT, Brocchini S, Williams GR. Solid-state protein formulations. Ther Deliv 2015;6(1):59–82.
[74] Connolly BD, Petry C, Yadav S, Demeule B, Ciaccio N, Moore JM, et al. Weak interactions govern the viscosity of concentrated antibody solutions: high-throughput analysis using the diffusion interaction parameter. Biophys J 2012;103(1):69–78.
[75] Farrell RA, Marta M, Gaeguta AJ, Souslova V, Giovannoni G, Creeke PI. Development of resistance to biologic therapies with reference to IFN-β. Rheumatology 2012;51(4):590–9.
[76] Saunders KO. Conceptual approaches to modulating antibody effector functions and circulation half-life. Front Immunol 2019;10:1296.
[77] Monnet C, Jorieux S, Souyris N, Zaki O, Jacquet A, Fournier N, et al. Combined glyco-and protein-Fc engineering simultaneously enhance cytotoxicity and half-life of a therapeutic antibody. MABs. 2014;6(2):422–36 *Taylor & Francis.*
[78] Neri D. Antibody–cytokine fusions: versatile products for the modulation of anticancer immunity. Cancer Immunol Res 2019;7(3):348–54.
[79] Beck A, Goetsch L, Dumontet C, Corvaïa N. Strategies and challenges for the next generation of antibody–drug conjugates. Nat Rev Drug Discov 2017;16(5):315–37.
[80] Larson SM, Carrasquillo JA, Cheung NK, Press OW. Radioimmunotherapy of human tumours. Nat Rev Cancer 2015;15(6):347–60.
[81] Labrijn AF, Janmaat ML, Reichert JM, Parren PW. Bispecific antibodies: a mechanistic review of the pipeline. Nat Rev Drug Discov 2019;18(8):585–608.
[82] Lu RM, Chang YL, Chen MS, Wu HC. Single chain anti-c-Met antibody conjugated nanoparticles for in vivo tumor-targeted imaging and drug delivery. Biomaterials 2011;32(12):3265–74.

CHAPTER

5

Hormonal delivery systems

Shivani Rai Paliwal[1], *Kunjbihari Sulakhiya*[2], *Pramod Kumar*[3], *Sabyasachi Maiti*[4] *and Rishi Paliwal*[5]

[1]Department of Pharmacy, Guru Ghasidas Vishwavidhyalaya (A Central University), Bilaspur, Chhattisgarh, India [2]Neuro Pharmacology Research Laboratory, Department of Pharmacy, Indira Gandhi National Tribal University, Amarkantak, Madhya Pradesh, India [3]Pulmonary Aerosol Delivery Group, Institute of Lung Health and Immunity (LHI), Helmholtz Zentrum, München, Bayern, Germany [4]Department of Pharmacy, Indira Gandhi National Tribal University, Amarkantak, Madhya Pradesh, India [5]Nanomedicine and Bioengineering Research Laboratory, Department of Pharmacy, Indira Gandhi National Tribal University, Amarkantak, Madhya Pradesh, India

5.1 Introduction

Hormones are the chemical messengers secreted in the circulation by endocrine glands. These hormones transported through blood, and at the target site, it interacts with specific receptors to regulate various cellular activities. On the basis of composition, hormones are divided into three categories: amine hormones, the peptides, and the steroids. The amino acid analogs include epinephrine and thyroid hormones. The peptide hormones may be single or double chain peptide and subclassified on the basis of size or glycosylation state. The steroid hormones may be adrenal steroids, synthesized in the adrenal cortex, or sex steroids, synthesized in ovaries or testes.

The longer circulation time and longer duration of effect distinguish hormones from neurotransmitters. Generally, hormones are associated with transport proteins while in circulation, but to elucidate the response or binding with the receptor, it must dissociate from protein. The receptors can be present on the cell surface like for peptide hormones or intracellular, as in the case of steroid or thyroid hormones. On receptor binding, secondary signaling pathways activated, which ultimately shows the physiological effect of the hormone.

Hormones are the widely explored therapeutics, as they are physiologically associated with various diseases, and they are used in therapy of several diseases. The most common

Molecular Pharmaceutics and Nano Drug Delivery
DOI: https://doi.org/10.1016/B978-0-323-91924-1.00001-0

hormone therapy includes oncologic hormone therapy, hormone replacement therapy (HRT), androgen replacement therapy, usage of oral contraceptive pills, and insulin and thyroxin treatment for diabetes and hypothyroidism. The delivery of hormones through a conventional delivery system like tablet, capsule, and so forth suffers from poor bioavailability and variation in the plasma level. Therapeutic hormones have been entrapped in nanocarriers for effective administration through several pathways, overcoming physiochemical and biological limitations. Novel drug delivery systems can be used to solve the problems associated with conventional delivery systems along with providing sustained, controlled, and targeted delivery of hormones for maximum efficacy and safety. Several novel drug delivery systems such as microparticles, liposomes, polymeric nanoparticles, lipid nanoparticles, inorganic nanoparticles, microemulsion, dendrimers, and so forth have been developed for the delivery of hormones.

5.2 Hormones as pharmacotherapeutics

Hormones are important chemical messengers secreted by the endocrine glands, and they play a crucial role in regulating many physiological processes and functions, including growth and development, metabolism, reproduction, and stress response in the body. Hormones can also be used as pharmacotherapeutics to treat various diseases and medical conditions. These are used either for restoration of missing hormones (decreased) or for bringing the increased hormonal levels to their normal levels through HRT and hormonal antagonists. Hormones can be administered in various forms, including oral pills, injections, patches, gels, and creams. HRT is a common form of hormone pharmacotherapy used to replace hormones that are no longer produced by the body or are produced in insufficient amounts. However, hormone therapy can have potential side effects and risks and should be prescribed and monitored by a qualified healthcare professional. Hormones used as pharmacotherapeutics include insulin, glucagon, thyroid hormones, corticosteroids, growth hormones (GHs), estrogens, progesterone, testosterone, follicle-stimulating hormone (FSH), luteinizing hormone-releasing hormone (LHRH), human chorionic gonadotropin (hCG), and so forth (Table 5.1). These are just a few examples; however, there are many other hormones used in medicine, and the use of hormones as pharmacotherapeutics continues to evolve with ongoing research and clinical trials [42].

5.2.1 Insulin

Insulin is a hormone produced by the pancreas that regulates blood glucose levels. In pharmacotherapy, insulin is used to treat diabetes, a condition characterized by high blood glucose levels due to either insufficient insulin production or ineffective insulin action [43]. Pharmacotherapy options for insulin include rapid-acting, short-acting, intermediate-acting, long-acting, and ultra-long-acting varieties. Because the onset and duration of action of these various insulin types differ, a variety of treatment options are possible based on the specific needs of the patient. The duration of action for rapid-acting insulin analogs, such as insulin lispro (Humalog), insulin aspart (NovoLog), and insulin glulisine

TABLE 5.1 Clinical applications of various hormones as hormonal therapy.

Disease/medical condition	Pharmacotherapeutic application	Advantages	Disadvantages	References
Insulin hormone				
Type 1 diabetes	Basal-bolus insulin therapy	Provides both basal and postprandial glucose control, can be customized for individual patient needs.	Requires multiple injections per day, increases the risk of hypoglycemia.	[1]
Type 2 diabetes	Basal insulin therapy	Provides basal glucose control, can be used in combination with oral antidiabetic drugs.	May require additional rapid-acting insulin for postprandial glucose control, may increase the risk of hypoglycemia.	[2]
Gestational diabetes	Insulin therapy as needed	Provides glucose control for mother and fetus, can be adjusted as needed during pregnancy.	May increase the risk of hypoglycemia, may require multiple injections per day.	[3]
Diabetic ketoacidosis	Insulin infusion therapy	Rapidly lowers blood glucose and ketone levels, reduces the risk of serious complications such as cerebral edema.	May increase the risk of hypoglycemia, requires close monitoring in an intensive care setting.	[4]
Hyperkalemia	Insulin infusion therapy	Rapidly lowers serum potassium levels.	May increase the risk of hypoglycemia, requires close monitoring in an intensive care setting.	[5]
Hyperglycemia in critical care	Insulin infusion therapy	Provides glucose control in critically ill patients, reduces the risk of serious complications such as infection and renal failure.	May increase the risk of hypoglycemia, requires close monitoring in an intensive care setting.	[6]

(Continued)

TABLE 5.1 (Continued)

Disease/medical condition	Pharmacotherapeutic application	Advantages	Disadvantages	References
Hypertriglyceridemia	Insulin therapy	Lowers serum triglyceride levels.	May increase the risk of hypoglycemia, requires close monitoring of glucose levels.	[7]
Lipodystrophy	Insulin therapy	Corrects metabolic abnormalities associated with lipodystrophy, improves quality of life.	May increase the risk of hypoglycemia, requires close monitoring.	[8]
Glucagon hormone				
Type 1 diabetes	Adjunctive therapy for severe hypoglycemia when intravenous glucose is not available	Rapidly increases blood glucose levels	Nausea and vomiting, rebound hypoglycemia	[9–11]
Beta-blocker overdose	Reversal of beta-blocker overdose-induced hypotension and bradycardia	Increases heart rate and blood pressure	Nausea and vomiting, may cause tachycardia and hypertension	[12–14]
Calcium channel blocker overdose	Reversal of calcium channel blocker overdose-induced hypotension and bradycardia	Increases heart rate and blood pressure	Nausea and vomiting, may cause tachycardia and hypertension	[15–17]
Gastrointestinal imaging	Relaxation of the smooth muscle of the stomach and duodenum to enhance imaging	Enhanced imaging of the GIT	Nausea and vomiting, may cause abdominal discomfort	[18–20]
Anaphylaxis	Adjunctive therapy for anaphylaxis to improve blood pressure and cardiac output	Increases blood pressure and cardiac output	Nausea and vomiting, may cause tachycardia and hypertension	[21–23]
Thyroid hormones				
Hypothyroidism	Replacement therapy with levothyroxine (T4)	Effective in restoring normal thyroid function	Requires long-term adherence to treatment	[24,25]

(*Continued*)

TABLE 5.1 (Continued)

Disease/medical condition	Pharmacotherapeutic application	Advantages	Disadvantages	References
Thyroid cancer	Suppression therapy with levothyroxine (T4)	Inhibits growth of residual or metastatic cancer cells	Can cause thyrotoxicosis if dosage is too high	[26,27]
Graves' disease	Adjunct therapy with antithyroid drugs	Reduces thyroid hormone levels and symptoms	May take several months to achieve remission	[28,29]
Myxedema coma	High-dose intravenous levothyroxine (T4)	Rapidly restores thyroid hormone levels	Risk of cardiac arrhythmias and other complications	[30,31]
Infertility	Adjunct therapy with levothyroxine (T4)	Improves ovulation and fertility in women with subclinical hypothyroidism	May require long-term treatment	[32]
Depression	Adjunct therapy with triiodothyronine (T3)	May enhance response to antidepressant therapy	Can cause cardiac side effects	[33]
Obesity	Adjunct therapy with levothyroxine (T4) or triiodothyronine (T3)	Increases metabolic rate and energy expenditure	May not be effective in long-term weight loss	[34]
Cardiovascular disease	Adjunct therapy with levothyroxine (T4)	Improves lipid profile and cardiac function	May increase risk of atrial fibrillation in older patients	[35]
Cognitive impairment	Adjunct therapy with levothyroxine (T4) or triiodothyronine (T3)	Improves cognitive function and memory	May not be effective in all patients	[36]
Thyroid storm	Intravenous thyroxine and supportive care	Effective in improving symptoms and reducing mortality	Can cause adverse effects such as arrhythmias and hypotension	[37]
Congenital hypothyroidism	Levothyroxine	Essential for normal growth and development	Can cause adverse effects if not monitored closely, such as overtreatment and growth retardation	[38]

(Continued)

TABLE 5.1 (Continued)

Disease/medical condition	Pharmacotherapeutic application	Advantages	Disadvantages	References
Corticosteroid hormones				
Asthma	Prednisone, fluticasone, budesonide	Reduces inflammation, improves lung function	Increased risk of infections, osteoporosis, diabetes, cataracts, weight gain	Retrieved from https://www.lung.org/lung-health-diseases/lung-disease-lookup/asthma/treatment-management/pharmacological-treatment/corticosteroids
Rheumatoid arthritis	Prednisone, methylprednisolone	Reduces inflammation, relieves pain and stiffness	Increased risk of infections, osteoporosis, diabetes, cataracts, weight gain	https://www.arthritis.org/drug-guide/prednisone
Multiple sclerosis	Methylprednisolone	Reduces inflammation, improves symptoms during relapses	Increased risk of infections, osteoporosis, diabetes, cataracts, weight gain	Retrieved from https://www.nationalmssociety.org/Treating-Ms/Medications
Inflammatory bowel disease	Prednisone, budesonide	Reduces inflammation, improves symptoms	Increased risk of infections, osteoporosis, diabetes, cataracts, weight gain	Retrieved from https://www.niddk.nih.gov/health-information/digestive-diseases/inflammatory-bowel-disease
Dermatological conditions	Hydrocortisone, betamethasone	Reduces inflammation, relieves itching	Skin thinning, increased risk of infections, striae, acne	Retrieved from https://www.aad.org/public/everyday-care/itchy-skin/ Retrieved from https://nationaleczema.org/eczema/treatment/topical-corticosteroids/
Allergies	Prednisone, methylprednisolone	Reduces inflammation, relieves symptoms	Increased risk of infections, osteoporosis, diabetes, cataracts, weight gain	Retrieved from https://acaai.org/allergies/types/hay-fever-rhinitis
Adrenal insufficiency	Hydrocortisone, Fludrocortisone	Replaces deficient hormones, improves symptoms	Increased risk of infections, osteoporosis, diabetes, cataracts, weight gain	Retrieved from https://www.niddk.nih.gov/health-information/endocrine-diseases/adrenal-insufficiency-addisons-disease

(Continued)

TABLE 5.1 (Continued)

Disease/medical condition	Pharmacotherapeutic application	Advantages	Disadvantages	References
Cushing's syndrome	Metyrapone, ketoconazole, mifepristone	Reduces cortisol production, relieves symptoms	Adrenal insufficiency, liver toxicity, fetal abnormalities	Retrieved from https://www.niddk.nih.gov/health-information/endocrine-diseases/cushings-syndrome
Organ transplantation	Prednisone, methylprednisolone	Prevents rejection, improves outcomes	Increased risk of infections, osteoporosis, diabetes, cataracts, weight gain	Retrieved from https://www.kidney.org/atoz/content/immunosuppressive-medication
Autoimmune disorders	Prednisone, methylprednisolone	Reduces inflammation, relieves symptoms	Increased risk of infections, osteoporosis, diabetes, cataracts, weight gain	Retrieved from https://www.rheumatology.org/I-Am-A/Patient-Caregiver/ Diseases-Conditions/Glucocorticoid-Induced-Osteoporosis
Cancer	Dexamethasone, prednisone	Reduces inflammation, relieves symptoms, enhances chemotherapy	Increased risk of infections, osteoporosis, diabetes, cataracts, weight gain	[39]; https://www.cancer.gov/about-cancer/treatment/drugs/prednisone/accessed on March 4, 2023
Shock	Hydrocortisone	Improves blood pressure, reduces inflammation	Increased risk of infections, osteoporosis, diabetes, cataracts, weight gain	[40,41]

(Apidra), is between 2 and 4 hours. These insulins are typically used to cover meals and correct high blood glucose levels. Regular insulin (Humulin R, Novolin R), for example, has a short-acting start of action and a 5–8 hours duration of action. This type of insulin is used to cover meals and correct high blood glucose levels. NPH insulin (Humulin N, Novolin N) is an example of intermediate-acting insulin with a 12–16 hours duration of action and a start of action of 1–3 hours. This type of insulin is typically used as a basal insulin to provide background insulin coverage throughout the day. Long-acting insulin analogs have an onset of action of 1–2 hours and an action duration of 18–24 hours. Examples include insulin glargine (Lantus), insulin detemir (Levemir), and insulin degludec (Tresiba). These insulins are typically used as a basal insulin to provide background insulin coverage throughout the day. Insulin degludec (Tresiba) and insulin glargine U300 (Toujeo), two ultra-long-acting insulin analogs, have a start of action of 1–4 hours and an action duration of up to 42 hours. These insulins are used as once-daily basal insulin to provide background insulin coverage throughout the day. A rapid- or short-acting insulin and an intermediate-acting insulin are combined to provide both basal and bolus coverage in the combo formulations insulin lispro protamine/insulin lispro (Humalog Mix 75/25) and insulin aspart protamine/insulin aspart (NovoLog Mix 70/30) [44,45].

Insulin is a hormone that is primarily used to manage diabetes, but it may also be used as a treatment for other medical conditions. Here are some examples of insulin as hormone therapy for diseases and medical conditions.

5.2.1.1 *Diabetes mellitus*

For those with type 1 diabetes, insulin is the main form of treatment; those with type 2 diabetes who are unable to control their blood glucose levels through other methods may also use insulin. Lowering blood glucose levels and delaying or preventing diabetes complications are the goals of insulin treatment.

5.2.1.2 *Diabetic ketoacidosis*

A severe diabetes complication known as diabetic ketoacidosis (DKA) happens when the body produces excessive amounts of ketone bodies as a result of low insulin levels. Insulin therapy is a key component of DKA treatment, as it helps to lower blood glucose levels and suppress ketone production [46].

5.2.1.3 *Hyperglycemic hyperosmolar state*

A potentially fatal diabetes complication known as hyperglycemic hyperosmolar state (HHS) is marked by excessively elevated blood glucose levels and severe dehydration. Insulin therapy is a crucial part of HHS treatment, as it helps to lower blood glucose levels and correct dehydration [47].

5.2.1.4 *Cystic fibrosis-related diabetes*

Diabetes caused by cystic fibrosis is a common complication of the disease and develops when the pancreas is unable to make enough insulin. Insulin therapy is the primary treatment for CFRD and aims to control blood glucose levels and prevent complications [48].

5.2.1.5 *Insulinoma*

Insulinoma is a rare tumor of the pancreas that produces too much insulin, leading to hypoglycemia. Insulin therapy may be used to manage hypoglycemia in people with insulinoma until the tumor can be surgically removed [49].

5.2.1.6 *Growth hormone deficiency*

A hormone called insulin-like growth factor 1 (IGF-1) is created as a result of GH activation. As insulin and IGF-1 share structural similarities, insulin therapy can be used to increase IGF-1 production in individuals with GH deficiency [50].

5.2.1.7 *Hyperkalemia*

Insulin therapy may be used to treat hyperkalemia by stimulating the uptake of potassium into cells, thus reducing blood potassium levels. This effect is due to insulin's ability to activate the Na^+/K^+ ATPase pump, which moves potassium from the bloodstream into cells [51].

5.2.1.8 *Diabetic gastroparesis*

Gastroparesis is a condition where there is delayed emptying of the stomach, often as a result of nerve damage. Insulin therapy may be used to improve gastric emptying in people with diabetic gastroparesis by reducing the levels of blood sugar that can contribute to delayed emptying [52].

5.2.1.9 *Hypertriglyceridemia*

Insulin therapy may be used to lower triglyceride levels in people with hypertriglyceridemia. Insulin helps to reduce the production of triglycerides in the liver by inhibiting the enzyme responsible for their synthesis [53].

5.2.1.10 *Lipodystrophy*

Lipodystrophy is a rare condition characterized by the loss of adipose tissue. Insulin therapy may be used to improve insulin resistance and glucose metabolism in people with lipodystrophy, as well as to prevent the development of diabetes [54].

5.2.1.11 *Other conditions*

Insulin may be used to treat other conditions, such as acromegaly (excess GH) and polycystic ovary syndrome (PCOS) [55].

It is important to note that insulin therapy should only be used under the guidance of a healthcare provider, as proper monitoring and dosage adjustments are crucial to avoid potential side effects and ensure effective treatment.

5.2.2 Glucagon

The pancreas secretes the hormone glucagon, which is essential for controlling blood sugar levels. By encouraging the breakdown of liver glycogen and triggering the release of glucose into the circulation, it functions counter to insulin and raises blood glucose levels. In addition to its use in the treatment of hypoglycemia, glucagon has been investigated for its potential therapeutic uses in various diseases and medical conditions. Glucagon is primarily used as a pharmacotherapeutic to address hypoglycemia, a condition marked by low blood glucose levels. By encouraging the liver to release glucose that has been held in the body, glucagon increases blood glucose levels. Glucagon can be administered via injection or nasal spray to rapidly raise blood glucose levels in people with diabetes who experience severe hypoglycemia, which can lead to unconsciousness or seizures if left untreated [56].

In addition to its use in treating hypoglycemia, glucagon has also been studied as a potential treatment for other conditions, such as obesity and type 1 diabetes. In obesity, glucagon has been shown to reduce appetite and increase energy expenditure, making it a potential target for weight loss interventions. In type 1 diabetes, glucagon has been investigated as an adjunct therapy to insulin, with some studies suggesting that the combination of insulin and glucagon may improve glucose control and reduce the risk of hypoglycemia [57].

However, the use of glucagon as a weight loss therapy is still in the early stages of research and its safety and efficacy have not been fully established.

However, more research is needed to determine the safety and efficacy of glucagon as a pharmacotherapeutic for these conditions and to develop new formulations and delivery methods that improve its usability and patient compliance.

Glucagon has been studied as a potential treatment for various gastrointestinal disorders, such as gastroparesis (delayed stomach emptying) and constipation [58,59].

However, further research is needed to determine its effectiveness in these conditions.

Recent studies have suggested that glucagon may play a role in the development of cardiovascular disease and that targeting glucagon signaling may be a potential therapeutic strategy [60].

5.2.3 Thyroid hormones

A group of pharmacotherapeutics known as thyroid hormones are used to address various thyroid disorders. Thyroxine (T4) and triiodothyronine (T3), the thyroid gland's two primary hormones, are essential for controlling the body's metabolism and energy production. Hypothyroidism, a condition in which the thyroid gland does not generate enough thyroid hormone, is treated with thyroid HRT. The purpose of therapy is to reduce symptoms like fatigue, weight gain, and depression while restoring the body's normal thyroid hormone levels. When the thyroid gland produces too much thyroid hormone, the disease is known as hyperthyroidism. While thyroid hormone therapy is not typically used as a first-line treatment for hyperthyroidism, it may be used in certain cases to help normalize thyroid hormone levels after treatment with antithyroid drugs or radioactive iodine. In some cases of thyroid cancer, thyroid hormone therapy may be used to suppress the production of thyroid-stimulating hormone, which can promote the growth of cancer cells. In cases where thyroid nodules produce excess thyroid hormone, thyroid hormone therapy may suppress hormone production and shrink the nodules. Some common thyroid hormone pharmacotherapeutic agents include levothyroxine (T4), liothyronine (T3), and desiccated thyroid extract. It is important to note that the use of thyroid hormones as therapeutic agents requires careful monitoring of thyroid hormone levels and proper dosage adjustments to avoid potential side effects and complications. Overall, thyroid hormones have a wide range of therapeutic applications and play a crucial role in maintaining overall health and well-being [25].

5.2.4 Corticosteroids

Corticosteroids are a class of hormones that are naturally produced in the adrenal cortex of the human body. They are involved in a wide range of physiological processes, including the regulation of metabolism, inflammation, and the immune response.

Synthetic corticosteroids, such as prednisone, prednisolone, and dexamethasone, are commonly used as pharmacotherapeutics in the treatment of various medical conditions due to their potent antiinflammatory and immunosuppressive properties [61]. Some of the clinical applications of corticosteroids are given below.

5.2.4.1 *Inflammatory conditions*

Corticosteroids are often used to treat inflammatory conditions such as arthritis, asthma, and inflammatory bowel disease. They work by suppressing the immune system and reducing inflammation, which can help to alleviate symptoms such as pain, swelling, and difficulty breathing (https://www.mayoclinic.org/steroids/art-20045692/accessed on March 4, 2023).

5.2.4.2 *Autoimmune disorders*

Corticosteroids can also be used to treat autoimmune disorders such as lupus, multiple sclerosis, and rheumatoid arthritis. These conditions occur when the immune system attacks healthy tissues in the body, and corticosteroids can help to suppress this response and reduce inflammation [62].

5.2.4.3 *Allergic reactions*

Corticosteroids can be used to treat allergic reactions, such as severe allergic reactions to food or insect bites and allergic rhinitis (hay fever). They can help to reduce inflammation and swelling and relieve symptoms such as itching and redness.

5.2.4.4 *Cancer*

Corticosteroids can be used as part of cancer treatment to reduce inflammation and swelling around tumors and to help manage symptoms such as nausea and vomiting [63].

5.2.4.5 *Adrenal insufficiency*

In cases where the adrenal gland is not producing enough corticosteroids, synthetic corticosteroids can be used to replace the missing hormone [64].

While corticosteroids can be highly effective in treating various medical conditions, they are not without side effects. Weight gain, mood swings, increased appetite, high blood pressure, and an increased chance of infections are just a few of the typical side effects of corticosteroids. Corticosteroid use over an extended period of time may also result in more severe adverse effects like osteoporosis, cataracts, and diabetes [65]. In conclusion, corticosteroids are powerful pharmacotherapeutics that have a wide range of clinical applications in the treatment of various medical conditions. While they can be highly effective in managing symptoms and reducing inflammation, they can also have significant side effects that need to be carefully monitored and managed by healthcare professionals.

5.2.5 Growth hormone

Somatotropin, also referred to as GH, is a peptide hormone that is crucial for human growth and development. It is created by the pituitary gland and works on specific body tissues to promote cell growth and reproduction [66].

GH deficiency can lead to a variety of clinical conditions, including short stature, delayed puberty, and reduced bone density. As a result, GH has been developed as a pharmacotherapeutic agent for the treatment of these conditions [67].

Recombinant human GH (rhGH), which is made using recombinant DNA technology, is one of many GH drugs on the market. The US Food and Drug Administration has approved RhGH for the treatment of a number of conditions, including Prader-Willi syndrome, Turner syndrome, chronic renal insufficiency, and GH deficiency [68].

RhGH has been shown to be effective in increasing growth velocity in children with GH deficiency and in improving height in children with Turner syndrome. It has also been shown to improve bone density in adults with GH deficiency [69]. In addition to its role in growth and development, GH has other physiological effects, including anabolic and metabolic effects. As a result, GH has been investigated as a potential treatment for various conditions, including muscle wasting, osteoporosis, and obesity. However, the use of GH as a pharmacotherapeutic agent is not without its risks. GH therapy can cause side effects such as fluid retention, insulin resistance, and increased risk of diabetes. Long-term use of GH may also increase the risk of developing certain cancers [70]. Therefore the use of GH as a pharmacotherapeutic agent should be carefully considered on a case-by-case basis, and patients should be closely monitored for potential side effects.

5.2.6 Estrogen hormone

Estrogen is a group of hormones that play crucial roles in various physiological processes, including sexual development and reproductive functions, as well as bone metabolism and cardiovascular health. Estrogen-based pharmacotherapeutics are widely used for the management of various medical conditions, including menopausal symptoms, osteoporosis, and hormone-sensitive cancers. Here are some examples of estrogen-based pharmacotherapeutics and their references.

5.2.6.1 Hormone replacement therapy

In order to treat menopausal symptoms like hot flashes, vaginal dryness, and mood changes, HRT uses estrogen and/or progestin hormones. HRT has also been demonstrated to strengthen bones and lower the chance of osteoporosis [71].

5.2.6.2 Selective estrogen receptor modulators

A class of medications known as selective estrogen receptor modulators (SERMs) affects some tissues in a way that mimics estrogen, while having an antiestrogenic impact on others. They are employed in the control of hormone-sensitive breast cancer as well as the prevention and treatment of osteoporosis. Tamoxifen, raloxifene, and bazedoxifene are examples of SERMs [72].

5.2.6.3 *Aromatase inhibitors*

Aromatase inhibitors are a class of drugs that block the production of estrogen in postmenopausal women. They are used for the treatment of hormone-sensitive breast cancer and have also been investigated for the prevention of breast cancer. Examples of aromatase inhibitors include anastrozole, letrozole, and exemestane [73]. *Estrogen Therapy for Gender-Affirming Treatment* states that Estrogen therapy is a crucial component of gender-affirming treatment for transgender women. It helps to feminize the body by inducing breast development, reducing body hair growth, and redistributing fat to a more feminine pattern [74].

Overall, estrogen-based pharmacotherapeutics have a significant impact on women's health and play a critical role in the management of various medical conditions.

5.2.7 Progesterone hormone

Progesterone is a hormone primarily produced by the ovaries in females, but it is also produced by the testes and adrenal glands in males. It plays a vital role in the menstrual cycle, pregnancy, and the development of the embryo and fetus. Progesterone deficiency can lead to several health issues, including menstrual irregularities, infertility, and miscarriage [75]. Therefore, progesterone replacement therapy is often used as a pharmacotherapeutic approach to manage these conditions. Here are some of the pharmacotherapeutic uses of progesterone hormone along with their references.

5.2.7.1 *Menstrual irregularities*

Progesterone replacement therapy is commonly used to regulate menstrual cycles and treat conditions such as irregular periods, heavy bleeding, and premenstrual syndrome. Progesterone helps to balance estrogen levels and promote normal menstrual cycles [76].

5.2.7.2 *Infertility*

Progesterone is essential for successful pregnancy, and its deficiency can lead to infertility. Progesterone supplementation during the luteal phase of the menstrual cycle can improve fertility and increase the chance of successful pregnancy [77].

5.2.7.3 *Miscarriage*

Progesterone supplementation is also used to reduce the risk of miscarriage in women with a history of recurrent miscarriage. Progesterone helps to support the pregnancy and maintain the lining of the uterus [78].

5.2.7.4 *Endometrial cancer*

Progesterone therapy is used to treat endometrial hyperplasia and endometrial cancer. Progesterone helps to reduce the growth and proliferation of endometrial cells and prevent the development of cancer [79].

5.2.8 Testosterone hormone

Male reproductive organs and secondary sexual traits are mainly developed and maintained by the hormone testosterone. It controls red blood cell production, muscular mass, bone density, and fat distribution. Testosterone therapy is a commonly used pharmacotherapeutic approach for conditions associated with low testosterone levels, such as hypogonadism, infertility, and delayed puberty. Various studies have demonstrated the therapeutic applications of testosterone as pharmacotherapeutics in hypogonadism or andropause. In a research that looked at the long-term effects of testosterone therapy on the metabolic syndrome in hypogonadal men, it was found that the condition's various symptoms, such as insulin resistance, dyslipidemia, and obesity, were improved [80].

A study looked into the connection between ageing and risk factors that can be changed, like smoking and obesity, as well as the disruption of the hypothalamic–pituitary–testicular axis in older males. The research discovered that testosterone therapy may be useful in improving testosterone levels and associated symptoms in older men and that low testosterone levels were linked to modifiable risk factors [81].

The effects of transdermal testosterone gel on sexual function, mood, muscle strength, and body composition parameters in hypogonadal men was investigated. The study found that testosterone therapy improved all of these parameters in hypogonadal men [82].

Endocrine Society recommends using testosterone therapy in men with androgen deficiency syndromes, including hypogonadism and andropause. The guideline provides guidance on diagnosing, monitoring, and treating these conditions using testosterone therapy [83].

5.2.9 Follicle stimulating hormone

The hormone FSH is crucial for the growth of follicles in the testicles and ovaries. FSH is a drug that can be used to treat some fertility problems in both males and women. In women, FSH is used to stimulate the growth of ovarian follicles, which contain the eggs. This is often used in fertility treatments such as in vitro fertilization (IVF) to help increase the number of eggs that can be retrieved [84].

FSH is also used to treat certain types of ovulation disorders, such as PCOS. In men, FSH can be used to stimulate the production of sperm in the testes. This is often used in combination with other hormones, such as hCG, to treat infertility [85].

FSH can be administered as an injection, and the dosage and timing of the injections will vary depending on the individual's condition and treatment plan. However, FSH therapy is not without risks and potential side effects, such as ovarian hyperstimulation syndrome in women and testicular enlargement in men. Overall, FSH can be an effective pharmacotherapeutic option for certain fertility issues, but it should only be used under the guidance of a qualified healthcare professional [86].

5.2.10 Luteinizing hormone-releasing hormone

A naturally produced hormone called LHRH is essential for controlling the reproductive system. LHRH stimulates the release of LH and FSH from the pituitary gland, which in turn stimulate the creation of estrogen and testosterone. LHRH agonists and antagonists are drugs that are used as pharmacotherapeutics in a number of conditions related to the reproductive system, including the following:

Prostate cancer: LHRH agonists (leuprolide acetate) and antagonists (Firmagon) are used to treat advanced prostate cancer. By reducing the levels of testosterone in the body, these drugs can slow the growth of cancer cells [87].

Endometriosis: LHRH agonists can be used to treat endometriosis, a condition where tissue that normally lines the uterus grows outside of it. By suppressing estrogen production, LHRH agonists can alleviate the symptoms of endometriosis [88].

In vitro fertilization: LHRH agonists are sometimes used as part of IVF treatment to prevent premature ovulation and improve the chances of success [89].

Delayed puberty: LHRH agonists can be used to treat delayed puberty by stimulating the production of FSH and LH [90].

LHRH agonists and antagonists are typically administered via injection or implantation. Common examples of LHRH agonists include leuprolide, goserelin, and triptorelin, while degarelix is an example of an LHRH antagonist. As with any medication, LHRH agonists and antagonists can have side effects, including hot flashes, fatigue, and sexual dysfunction [91]. However, they are generally considered safe and effective for their intended uses when used under the guidance of a healthcare professional.

5.2.11 Human chorionic gonadotropin hormone

In the course of pregnancy, the placenta spontaneously produces the hormone known as hCG [92].

However, it can also be used as a pharmacotherapeutic agent for various medical purposes. It is important to note that hCG should only be used under a healthcare professional's supervision and not for off-label purposes or without a prescription. Additionally, hCG can have side effects, including headaches, fatigue, irritability, and swelling or pain at the injection site.

Here are some of the ways in which hCG can be used as a pharmacotherapeutic:

Fertility treatment: hCG is commonly used in combination with other hormones (such as a FSH) to help women with fertility issues ovulate and conceive. It can also be used in men to stimulate the production of testosterone and improve fertility [93].

Weight loss: hCG is sometimes used as part of a weight loss program, although its effectiveness for this purpose is controversial. Some studies suggest that hCG injections can help suppress appetite and promote fat loss, but others have found no significant benefits [94].

Cryptorchidism: hCG can be used to treat boys with cryptorchidism (undescended testes) by stimulating the testes to descend into the scrotum [95].

Hypogonadism: In men with hypogonadism (low testosterone), hCG can be used to stimulate the testes to produce more testosterone [96].

Pituitary gland disorders: hCG can be used to treat some pituitary gland disorders, such as hypogonadotropic hypogonadism, and delayed puberty [97].

Ovarian cysts: hCG can be used to treat ovarian cysts by stimulating the corpus luteum to produce progesterone, which can help shrink the cysts [98].

5.3 Novel drug delivery systems for hormones

Novel drug delivery systems are used as controlled drug delivery systems for several classes of therapeutics including small molecules, proteins/peptide, gene, and hormones too. They offer numerous advantages including reduction in dosing frequency, less toxicity, and avoidance of exposure to unwanted organs/tissues (Fig. 5.1). In this section, we will discuss some of these novel drug delivery systems used for hormone delivery.

5.3.1 Microparticles

Microparticles are spherical particles in the size range of 1–250 μm in diameter. They may be microspheres in which the drug is dispersed in the matrix or microcapsule, where drug is in the core surrounded by a polymeric membrane. Various methods are used for the preparation of microparticles, including organic phase separation, solvent evaporation, emulsion polymerization, and spray drying. However, physicochemical properties of hormones restrict the use of several methods because inactivation, intermolecular interaction, and sensitivity to process parameters make their formulation difficult. Parameters like stability, solubility, interaction

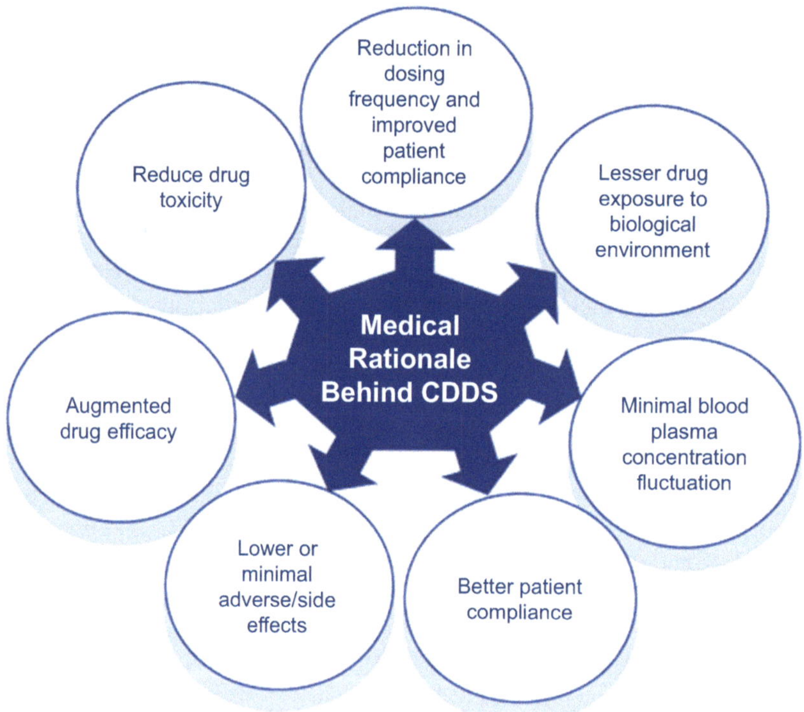

FIGURE 5.1 Medical rationale behind controlled release drug delivery systems. *Source: Adopted from Adepu S, Ramakrishna S. Controlled drug delivery systems: current status and future directions. Molecules. 2021 Sep 29;26(19):5905 under the terms and conditions of the Creative Commons Attribution (CC BY) license.*

with excipients, heat sensitivity, and pH of these agents should be studied for the preparation of stable microparticulate formulation. Microparticles provide protection to loaded pharmacotherapeutics against enzymatic degradation and sustained or controlled delivery up to several weeks. Although implants can also offer longer delivery profile, microparticles are easy to administer when compared to implants (Siepmann and Siepmann, 2006), and they provide flexibility of selection of different polymers, particle size, and drug loading to alter the release profile. A number of biodegradable polymers such as poly (lactic-co-glycolic acid), poly (ε-caprolactone), polyanhydrides, and polyalkyl cyanoacrylates have been used for microparticle preparation (Strobel et al., 2020).

Mukharjee et al. (2007) reported poly(ε-caprolactone) microspheres for noninvasive controlled delivery of insulin for management of diabetes with better patient compliance. The double emulsion solvent evaporation method was used for the preparation and demonstrated that the developed microsphere showed controlled release of insulin for the prolonged period (Mukharjee et al., 2007). Leong et al. (2011) developed lectin-functionalized pH-sensitive carboxy methylated kappa-carrageenan microparticles for oral insulin delivery. Lectin modification improved intestinal mucoadhesion, and the release profile showed that the hypoglycemic effect lasted up to 24 hours in diabetic rats. Bowey et al. (2013) prepared insulin-loaded alginate microparticles by spray-drying technology to improve stability and pharmacokinetics. The in vitro bioactivity assay demonstrated that the developed microparticles contain bioactive insulin that can be potentially used for oral drug delivery. 88% of the released insulin from the microparticles was bioactive, showing spray drying can be effectively used for producing microparticles (Bowey et al., 2013). El-Kamel et al. (2007) reported testosterone-loaded solid lipid microparticles (SLMs) for transdermal delivery. The SLMs containing different lipid glyceryl monostearate, glyceryl distearate, stearic acid, and glyceryl behenate were prepared using emulsion melt homogenization. They demonstrated that the morphology and particle size are affected by type of lipid and drug release can also be controlled. The results showed that SLMs are the promising carrier for transdermal drug delivery (El-Kamel et al., 2007).

Knowles et al. developed PLGA microparticles for sustained delivery of gonadotropin-releasing hormone analogs (GnRHa) for induction of ovulation in Coregonus peled [99]. The prolonged administration of GnRHa by multiple injection is required for ovulation and spawning. Sustained drug release preparations provide controlled release and are convenient to use with low toxicity and greater effectiveness [100]. Authors reported that the single GnRHa injection of microparticulate preparation showed successful induction and synchronization of ovulation [99]. These studies demonstrated that entrapment of bioactives in microparticle-preserved bioactivity protects the bioactives from a harsh environment, improves biodistribution, provides sustained or controlled release, and ultimately enhances therapeutic potential of pharmacotherapeutics.

5.3.2 Liposomes

Liposomes are the well-investigated phospholipid vesicles consisting of lipid bilayers with aqueous core. They can encapsulate both hydrophilic and hydrophobic therapeutic moieties. Liposomes are widely explored nanocarriers for delivery of various hormones, as they stabilize the therapeutic compound, improve biodistribution, and overcome various obstacles to cellular and tissue uptake and so forth. The therapeutic benefits of liposomes over other drug delivery systems are their biocompatibility and biodegradability, different sizes and morphologies based on composition, easy modification of surface properties, low toxicity, nonimmunogenicity, and low cost [101]. Moreover, several modifications have been tried to control their biological properties and pharmacokinetic properties and make them suitable for targeted delivery of hormones [102]. However, they have some drawbacks like limited stability, low encapsulation of hydrophilic drugs, and rapid clearance by reticuloendothelial cells.

As discussed above, liposomes represent a useful drug delivery system, but oral delivery of the therapeutic molecule is difficult due to poor stability of these vesicles in harsh gastrointestinal tract (GIT) conditions and they have to be stabilized by the use of phospholipids with high phase transition temperature or polymer coating. There are several reports that utilized liposomes for delivery of hormones to enhance the bioavailability and for targeted delivery. Parmentier et al. reported hGH-loaded liposomes for oral delivery [103]. They incorporated bioenhancer and tetraether lipids to enhance stability and permeation. The liposomal formulation showed enhanced bioavailability of hGH [103].

Several reports described the successful encapsulation of the triiodothyronine (T3) hormone in liposomal vesicles to improve stability and cellular uptake; for example, Fountain et al. developed multivesicular liposomal vesicles consisting of dimyristoylphophatidylcholine, cholesterol, and dicetylphosphate with 60% loading efficiency [104]. Similarly, Pireddu et al. reported three different liposomal formulations such as plain liposomes, pegylated liposomes, and lactoferrin-modified stealth liposomes with 90% loading efficiency [105]. The results of these studies showed that liposomal formulations improve the T3 delivery and its accumulation to the receptor site [105]. Lamparelli et al. also reported that these are extremely good carriers for T3 delivery, as they showed higher cellular uptake and also maintained biological activity [106].

Liposomes have been used for insulin delivery to enhance oral absorption and prolong its action. Several reports are available for oral delivery of insulin using the liposomal drug delivery system [107–109]. Choudhari et al. reported that the hypoglycemic effect of liposomal insulin depends on the lipid composition and surface charge [107]. However, variability in the glycemic response and a high dose of liposomes entrapped insulin requirement are some of the key limits of the peroral liposomal insulin therapy.

5.3.3 Polymeric nanoparticles

Nanoparticles can be defined as a particulate structure in the size range of 1–100 nm and are widely explored for drug delivery and other biomedical applications. Synthetic polymers like polyvinyl alcohol, poly-L-lactic acid, polyethylene glycol, and poly(lactic-co-glycolic acid) as well as natural polymers like alginate and chitosan can be used to create nanoparticulate delivery systems [110,111]. Polymeric nanoparticles are classified in two categories: nanospheres and nanocapsules. The performance of polymeric nanoparticles is influenced by size, surface charge, molecular weight, and so forth. Size affects the ability to cross the physiological barrier, surface charge affects the circulation time, and high molecular weight polymer is required for sustained drug release. Nanoparticles could help to overcome the limitation of a conventional delivery system for hormone delivery such as biodistribution and intracellular trafficking through targeted delivery with a controlled release [112]. Nanoparticles improve the stability and solubility of encapsulated hormones, facilitate transport across the cell membrane, and prolong circulation to potentiate the safety and efficacy. Many polymeric nanoparticle delivery systems have been developed for delivery of therapeutic hormones due to their versatility, for targeted delivery, to improve bioavailability, for sustained drug release, to increase solubility, and to increase the stability of hormones against degradation. Summarizes some strategies used in insulin delivery using polymeric approaches/systems.

For effective hormone delivery, polymeric nanoparticles have also been extensively researched. Lin and colleagues reported chitosan nanoparticles for oral delivery of insulin and studied their transport on caco-2 cells. Chitosan nanoparticles demonstrated enhanced paracellular permeability and improved stability of insulin. The results showed the sustained release of insulin with a decreased glucose level for 10 hours [100]. In another study, biodegradable polymer PLGA and Eudragit RS were used to prepare insulin-loaded nanoparticles to improve the penetration of insulin through the intestinal mucosa. The developed nanoparticles were enclosed in enteric-coated hydroxypropyl methylcellulose phthalate capsules for oral administration and showed a decreased glucose level for a prolonged period of time [113]. Similarly, when folate-conjugated pegylated PLGA nanoparticles were used for oral delivery, the bioavailability of insulin was increased by two-fold compared to subcutaneous injection of insulin [114]. Ghasemi et al. reported mPEG-PLA and PLA-PEG-PLA copolymeric nanoparticles for the delivery of rhGH, and the results showed that rhGH was stable during encapsulation and these nanoparticles provide safe and efficient sustained release for more than a month [115].

Estrogens are organic substances that play a part in the growth and upkeep of the female reproductive system and sexual traits. Estradiol, a primary and powerful estrogen, is used to treat menopausal symptoms, provide HRT, manage menopausal symptoms, prevent postmenopausal osteoporosis, and reduce the chance of breast cancer [116,117]. Estradiol's limited bioavailability and extensive hepatic metabolism need frequent administration, which causes a variety of adverse effects. To enhance oral bioavailability, and for sustained release of estradiol, PLGA nanoparticles were developed [118]. The nanoparticles demonstrated sustained release of estradiol for more than 30 days with effective intestinal uptake [118]. Similarly, estradiol-loaded PLGA nanoparticles were developed for the treatment of menopause-associated symptoms [119]. The result showed that the encapsulation improved the bioavailability and sustained release of estradiol was observed [119].

Chitosan nanoparticles have been created for nasal administration of insulin, and prolonged insulin release with a constant plasma concentration and improved therapeutic effectiveness was demonstrated [120]. Mansourpour et al. developed chitosan, and alginate complex, for oral delivery of insulin. The complex successfully encapsulated insulin and showed enhanced permeability for oral absorption [121]. Similarly, Liu et al. also reported hyaluronic acid-coated calcium carbonate nanoparticles for oral administration of insulin [122]. These formulations demonstrated an effective blood glucose lowering effect in diabetic rats.

By blocking calcium efflux from the bone, the peptide hormone calcitonin regulates calcium homeostasis and lowers blood calcium levels. Although calcitonin is therapeutically used to treat osteoporosis, its oral bioavailability is low because of proteolytic degradation in the GIT. To overcome this problem, chitosan-modified PLGA nanoparticles were prepared, which showed sustained release and improved oral absorption of this hormone [123].

5.3.4 Lipid nanoparticles

Lipid nanoparticles are a small spherical nanocarrier made up of physiologically compatible and nontoxic lipids. Therapeutic compounds are encapsulated within lipid coating comprised of phospholipids, cholesterol, polyethylene glycol-conjugated lipids, and cationic lipids. Lipid nanoparticles have attracted significant interest as carriers for the delivery of therapeutic molecules with low bioavailability due to their remarkable benefits including low toxicity, affordable scale-up manufacturing, good biocompatibility, and high drug loading efficiency. These nanocarriers have the potential to enhance the gastrointestinal stability, solubility, and permeability of the medications they carry [110]. Solid lipid nanoparticles (SLNs) and nanostructured lipid carriers (NLCs) are the two main categories of lipid nanoparticles. SLNs are composed of a lipid core made up of lipids such as triglycerides, fatty acids, phospholipids or waxes with a monolayer surfactant like polaxamers, lecithin, bile salts etc which stabilize lipid core in aqueous dispersions [124]. SLNs consist of solid hydrophobic cores of glycerides, esters, or waxes, while NLCs' core contains a mixture of solid and liquid lipids, making it an amorphous structure [125]. NLCs are also known as second-generation SLNs, and their amorphous core reduces mobility of loaded drugs, thereby enhancing drug loading and controlled release properties.

SLNs can be used for the delivery of both hydrophilic and hydrophobic molecules including anticancer drugs, cardiovascular drugs, and hormones. They have demonstrated the potential to protect encapsulated hormones from GIT degradation and to enhance transmucosal transport through mucoadhesion, internalization, and absorption enhancement mechanisms [126]. As an example, lectin-modified SLNs were developed to protect insulin from enzymatic degradation and enhanced oral absorption. The developed system showed 7.11% higher bioavailability than that after subcutaneous injection, indicating the role of SLNs in facilitation of oral absorption of insulin [127]. Similarly, they also reported octaarginine-modified SLNs for oral insulin delivery, and the result showed that uptake was increased by 18-fold as compared to insulin solution [128]. SLNs were also developed for pulmonary delivery of insulin, and it was shown that improved stability and prolonged hypoglycemic effect resulted in enhanced bioavailability [129]. These studies suggested that SLNs have remarkable potential for oral delivery of hormones, as they are able to bypass barriers such as proteolytic enzymes and harsh GIT pH and due to their biocompatibility and cost-effectiveness.

NLCs have advantages such as small size, high loading capacity, and reduction in drug leakage during storage. They are biocompatible, safe due to the absence of organic solvents, economically cost-effective, and scalable to larger batches. These properties make NLCs an ideal delivery system for hydrophobic drugs and hormones. Melatonin-loaded olive oil-based NLCs were developed for application in IVF media [130]. It was reported that incorporation of melatonin in NLCs reduced the dosage and can be a superior option for application in IVF media [130].

5.3.5 Nanoemulsion

Nanoemulsions are drug delivery carriers having an average droplet size ranging from 50 to 500 nm, consisting of emulsified oil or water droplets finely dispersed in the opposite phase. They are made from emulsifiers that are generally regarded as safe. Nanoemulsions can be either oil in water (o/w) or water in oil (w/o). The properties that make nanoemulsion different from other emulsions are its stability, easy penetration, and different patterns of physical and rheological characteristics on the basis of droplet size. The very fine particle size and less surface tension make them stable by reducing the possibility of creaming or sedimentation. On the basis of these properties, nanoemulsion can be a promising carrier for delivery of various hormones with the advantages of spontaneous formation, thermodynamic stability, and facilitated administration. Several studies have reported the use of nanoemulsion for delivery of hormones to improve permeation and bioavailability.

Generally, protein and peptide hormones are administered parenterally not orally due to enzymatic degradation in GIT and poor permeation across the intestinal epithelium. Nanoemulsions have been explored to enhance oral bioavailability due to their protective ability and transient opening of cellular junction by lipid constituent and surfactants. However, w/o emulsion transformed to o/w emulsion in the presence of gastric juice and exposed the entrapped therapeutics to degradative enzymes. Therefore if these systems protected and safely transported through the stomach by coating them with polyelectrolyte polymers such as alginates or chitosan, they can improve oral bioavailability of various hormones like insulin [131]. Alginate/chitosan crosslinked w/o/w nanoemulsion was developed for oral delivery of insulin to improve permeability, bioadhesion, and hence bioavailability [132].

The transdermal route is a better choice for hormone delivery, as oral administration leads to rapid degradation and low bioavailability. The Biolipid/B2 is a nanoemulsion that can be directly applied to the skin by a metered pump for systemic hormone delivery through the transdermal route. Biolipid/B2-based nanoemulsion formulation with estriol and estradiol was reported for transdermal HRT [133]. Biolipid/B2 is a colloidal system that is used as a transdermal penetration enhancer vehicle. The developed formulation restored the estradiol serum level and may be used for HRT in postmenopausal symptoms [133]. A similar formulation for testosterone transdermal delivery was also developed [134], and it was shown that they can be used as a potential therapeutic agent in andropause therapy [134].

5.3.6 Self-emulsifying drug delivery systems

Self-emulsifying drug delivery systems (SEDDS) have the capacity to solubilize hydrophobic drugs in aqueous media. SEDDS are an isotropic system consisting of drug, lipid/oil, cosolvent, and surfactants. Generally, triglycerides oils and ethoxylated nonionic surfactants at the concentration greater than 25% are used for formulation of these systems. Upon dilution by aqueous phase, they form oil/water emulsion like when they reach to GIT. The size of droplets is approximately around 100 nm [135]. The small droplet size provides a large interfacial area for the drug absorption and the drug is available in a dissolved form. SEDDS have several advantages, including consistent drug absorption, protection of drugs from GIT, high drug loading efficiency, and more uniform and reproducible bioavailability [136]. The oil droplets provide mucus penetration characteristics to hydrophobic drugs and make them ideal delivery vehicles for them. SEDDS produce emulsion of the droplet size in the range of 200 nm to 5 μm, with turbid appearance, while self-microemulsifying drug delivery systems (SMEDDS) have a droplet size less than 100 nm with translucent appearance and self-nano drug delivery systems form nanoemulsion with a droplet size less than 100 nm having clear or transparent appearance [137].

SEDDS can be used for oral delivery of insulin, as they preserve the bioactivity and provide protection against enzymatic hydrolysis, like SMEDDS [138]. Several SEDDS have been reported to improve oral bioavailability of insulin [139,140]; however, the hydrophilic nature of insulin makes its incorporation in a lipophilic system difficult. An insulin–lipid complex such as Labrasol, Kolliphor RH40, and so forth was used for better loading and improved oral absorption [141].

The steroidal hormone testosterone belongs to class IV of the biopharmaceutical classification system, that is, it has low solubility and limited permeability. It also undergoes hepatic first pass metabolism, leading to very low bioavailability after oral administration [142]. SEDDS can be used to improve oral bioavailability of testosterone, as they increase the solubility of lipophilic molecules. Additionally, due to the presence of a surfactant and lipid it, absorbed through the lymphatic route, avoiding first pass metabolism. However, the formulation excipients play a crucial role on therapeutic efficacy and safety of SEDDS formulation. It was reported that SEDDS improve the dissolution profile and oral bioavailability of testosterone undecanoate [143]. Further, the role of various excipients for the development of SEDDS for oral delivery of testosterone was studied [144].

5.3.7 Nanogels

Aqueous dispersions of hydrogel particles known as nanogels are made up of nanoscale (less than 200 nm) cross-linked polymer networks [145]. They are swollen chemically cross-linked networks of natural or synthetic polymers, and they have a high degree of flexibility of their size, shape, surface modification, and degradation mechanisms. Due to unique properties provided by their small size, nanogels are a significant class of drug delivery systems that have attracted considerable research interest [146,147]. Nanogels have the tunable size and surface characteristics to prevent fast clearance, high drug loading capacity, controlled and sustained drug release at the target site, and the capacity to pass through tiny capillary vessels, which make them superior drug delivery systems. Nanogels have the ability to encapsulate both hydrophilic and hydrophobic molecules including proteins, DNA, RNA, oligonucleotides, and so forth within their polymer matrix. Nanogels are widely explored as drug delivery carriers as they protect the entrapped drug during storage and circulation, controlled drug delivery can be achieved by making them stimuli-responsive, and they can be easily functionalized with targeting ligands for site-specific delivery. Because of their biodegradability, abundance, and biocompatibility, nanogels derived from natural polysaccharides are of considerable interest for drug delivery and controlled release. For use in biomedical applications, nanogels with hydrophilic functional groups like hydroxyl (–OH), carboxyl (–COOH), amino

($-NH_2$), amide, and sulfonic ($-SO_3H$) groups are also being used. Antisense oligonucleotides can also be delivered using copolymers like the branched PEG-cl-PEI derived from poly (ethylene glycol) (PEG) and poly (ethylenimine) (PEI) [146]. However, their use in vivo has frequently been constrained by stability and quick systemic circulation periods. The nanogels are widely explored for oral insulin delivery due to their characteristic features such as presence of hydrophilic groups, biocompatibility, and opportunities for development of stimuli, that is, temperature, pH, glucose, and electric and magnetic field responsive delivery system. Several authors reported the use of stimuli-responsive nanogels for oral delivery of insulin [148,149]. A nanogel consisting of a temperature- and pH-sensitive polymer was developed [149]. The swelling and deswelling of nanogel depends on the pH at the site, for example, at pH below the pKa, polymers remain protonated and form a collapsed network to entrap insulin inside the network. However, above the pKa, the polymer becomes deprotonated, resulting in the swelling of the network and expulsion of loaded content [149]. According to the study, negative CS-based nanogels may also be utilized to deliver insulin orally due to their mucoadhesive and permeation enhancing properties [150].

Peptide hormones like hGH, calcitonin, and melatonin get inactivated due to aggregation or precipitation when exposed to different pH and ionic strengths. To alleviate this problem, pH-responsive, pH-dependent, or thermosensitive nanocarriers can be formulated to stabilize the hormones. The frequent intravenous administration of the hGH is required due to short plasma half-life, which leads to poor outcomes, increased toxicity, and reduced patient compliance. Dual ionic thermosensitive nanogels were formulated for sustained delivery of hGH, and a 13-fold increase in the area under the curve and enhanced bioavailability compared with free hormone solution was demonstrated [151]. Similarly, chitosan-based nanogel formulation was developed for pulmonary delivery of calcitonin. Reportedly, the developed nanogel showed a higher hypocalcemic effect for a longer period of time [152].

5.3.8 Dendrimers

Dendrimers are branched, well-defined, symmetrical structures of polymers, and they are characterized by globular shape. Functional groups are found at the end of the arms, which can be easily modified to alter their physical and chemical properties. A full generation with a hydroxyl or amine surface group and a half generation with a carboxyl surface group are the two different types of dendrimer generation. Dendrimers also have internal cavities, which can be used to entrap various therapeutic molecules. They provide a significant degree of flexibility in drug loading, as therapeutics can be either noncovalently trapped inside dendrimer or covalently attached to the dendrimer surface. Dendrimers have several advantages such as small size (1–100 nm), and drugs can be entrapped within the core or attached to the surface functional group and easily modified for stimuli-responsive drug release and targeted drug delivery.

Extensive research has been carried out for dendrimer-based drug delivery; however, it is challenging to construct a dendrimer for hormone delivery as only few polar functional groups are available for conjugation. Several types of dendrimers like poly (amidoamine)

(PAMAM), poly (propylene imine), tecto, chiral, hybrid, and so forth are explored for drug/gene delivery. The PAMAM dendrimers are hydrophilic, biocompatible, and nonimmunogenic systems that are mostly employed for hormone therapy. It was reported that positively charged PAMAM dendrimers were often used for mucosal delivery of insulin due to absorption-enhancing effects [153]. Researchers also demonstrated that dendrimers could also improve insulin bioavailability via nasal administration [154]. Thus, dendrimers can be used by various routes for successful hormone delivery.

Because it is a key regulator of the reproductive system, LHRH is frequently used to treat a broad range of illnesses, including breast cancer, prostate cancer, and other reproductive disorders. The continuous use of LHRH may lead to decrease in androgens and estrogens due to downregulation of LHRH receptors. It was reported that LHRH dendrimers enhance stability and bioavailability, while maintaining the biological activity of hormones for oral delivery [155]. Apart from various advantages, dendrimers have a few limitations: cationic dendrimers may cause cytotoxicity, and higher generation dendrimers show toxicity and hemolytic activities.

5.3.9 Inorganic nanoparticles

Several organic nanoparticulate systems have been developed, such as polymeric nanoparticles, liposomes, micelles, and so forth, for the delivery of hormones. However, these systems suffer from some drawbacks like chemical stability, presence of undesirable organic solvents, and microbial contamination. Inorganic nanoparticles are more stable, nontoxic, hydrophilic, and biocompatible compared to organic nanoparticles. Due to their great capacity for cellular absorption, lack of immunogenic reaction, and low toxicity, inorganic nanoparticles have drawn a lot of attention as medication or gene delivery vehicles. Inorganic nanoparticles include calcium phosphate nanoparticles, iron oxide nanoparticles, fullerenes, gold nanoparticles, silver nanoparticles, carbon nanotubes, quantum dots, and so forth. The inorganic nanoparticles have been widely used for hormone delivery.

Calcium phosphates are biocompatible, resorbable, and porous, and several attempts have been made to use them as drug, chemical, hormone, and biological delivery systems. Calcium phosphate nanoparticles have been reported for oral delivery of insulin (Paul and Sharma, 2001). Insulin-loaded calcium phosphate nanoparticles have been processed through the lymphatic route and significantly reduced the first pass metabolism of insulin. BioSanta Pharmaceutical has also developed these nanoparticles, and in preclinical trials, two formulations, BioOral and BioAir, showed sustained delivery of insulin. For the oral or inhaled delivery of other proteins, such as hGH, similar formulations may be utilized.

Gold nanoparticles are the most stable metal nanoparticles, which can be of various shapes or structures like nanospheres, nanorod, nanocubes, nanoshells, nanowires, and so forth. They have characteristic advantages such as size-related electrical, magnetic, and optical properties. The size- and shape-dependent optical properties of gold nanoparticles have been widely explored for the delivery of therapeutic molecules, including drug, peptide, protein, DNA, and hormones. Gold nanoparticles are biocompatible and nontoxic, and they provide a large surface for adsorption of several biomolecules and for functionalization. These colloidal nanoparticles have shown promising results in the delivery of many hormones. Joshi et al. in 2006, prepared gold nanoparticles for transmucosal delivery of insulin for the treatment of diabetes mellitus and studied the effectiveness of the developed systems by oral and nasal routes. The findings showed that nasal insulin absorption was superior to oral insulin absorption, and gold nanoparticles could be used as superior insulin delivery vehicles to reduce blood glucose levels (Joshi et al., 2006).

5.3.10 Transferosomes

Transferosomes are the deformable flexible vesicles, and they resemble the natural cell vesicle. These elastic vesicles are widely used for targeted and controlled drug delivery due to their penetrating power through pores. Transferosome membrane flexibility can be changed by combining the right surface-active agents in the right proportions. The resulting flexible and permeability-optimized transferosome vesicle can quickly and easily change its shape in response to surrounding stress by adjusting the local concentration of each bilayer component to the local stress experienced by the bilayer. When used under nonocclusive conditions, this flexibility also reduces the chance of a full vesicle rupture in the skin and enables transferosomes to follow the natural water gradient through the epidermis. When applied to the skin, they easily penetrate stratum corneum through pores via deforming vesicles without losing integrity and can be successfully used for transdermal delivery of various biomolecules including hormones. The large molecules such as protein and peptide hormones that are unable to diffuse into skin can be delivered by using these flexible vesicles. For example, transferosomes were reported for the noninvasive delivery of insulin through the transdermal route. The large size of insulin makes it inappropriate for transdermal distribution using the conventional method and show only 50% bioavailability when compared to subcutaneous injection. The encapsulation of insulin in transferosomes called transfersulin increases the bioavailability and overcomes the inconvenience associated with invasive subcutaneous injection [156]. Shamshiri and colleagues also developed hGH-loaded transferosomes for noninvasive transdermal delivery. The transferosomes demonstrated more pronounced release of the GH as compared to the hormone delivered alone. The authors concluded that the vesicular system was better for encapsulating and delivering hormones via the transdermal route [157]. Similarly, many reports are available for transferosomes-mediated estradiol delivery [158,159].

5.4 Conclusion and future perspectives

Therapeutic hormones have been a delicate class of molecules that require specialized drug delivery systems. Hormone delivery systems like microparticles, nanoparticles, lipid-based systems (liposome and lipid nanoparticles), nanoemulsion, dendrimer, nanogels, and so forth have been successfully explored. Various routes of delivery such as topical, oral, and parenteral are tested using such novel drug delivery systems. Primary literature review of preclinical evaluation indicates suitability of these carriers in hormone delivery. However, limited marketed success of these products has led to the progress and clinical translational perspective of the approach.

References

[1] DeWitt DE, Hirsch IB. Outpatient insulin therapy in type 1 and type 2 diabetes mellitus: scientific review. JAMA. 2003;289(17):2254–64.

[2] Lankisch MR, Ferlinz KC, Leahy JL, Scherbaum WA. Intensive insulin therapy in critically ill patients. N Engl J Med 2013;368(3) 253-252.

[3] Kitzmiller JL, Block JM, Brown FM, et al. Managing preexisting diabetes for pregnancy: summary of evidence and consensus recommendations for care. Diabetes Care 2008;31(5):1060–79.

[4] Kitabchi AE, Umpierrez GE, Murphy MB, et al. Management of hyperglycemic crises in patients with diabetes. Diabetes Care 2001;24(1):131–53.

[5] Kovesdy CP, Regidor DL, Mehrotra R, et al. Serum and dialysate potassium concentrations and survival in hemodialysis patients. Clin J Am Soc Nephrol 2007;2(5):999–1007.

[6] Wiener RS, Wiener DC, Larson RJ. Benefits and risks of tight glucose control in critically ill adults: a meta-analysis. JAMA. 2008;300(8):933–44.

[7] Haffner SM. Management of dyslipidemia in adults with diabetes. Diabetes Care 2004;27(Suppl 1):S68–71.

[8] Brown RJ, Araujo-Vilar D, Cheung PT, et al. The diagnosis and management of lipodystrophy syndromes: a multi-society practice guideline. J Clin Endocrinol Metab 2016;101(12):4500–11.

[9] Cryer PE. The barrier of hypoglycemia in diabetes. Diabetes 2008;57(12):3169–76. Available from: https://doi.org/10.2337/db08-1084.

[10] Fitchett DH. Glucagon-like peptide 1: physiology and potential therapeutic applications. Am J Med 2010;123 (1 Suppl):S4–16. Available from: https://doi.org/10.1016/j.amjmed.2009.09.031.

[11] Seaquist ER, Anderson J, Childs B, et al. Hypoglycemia and diabetes: a report of a workgroup of the American Diabetes Association and the Endocrine Society. Diabetes Care 2013;36(5):1384–95. Available from: https://doi.org/10.2337/dc12-2480.

[12] St-Onge M, Anseeuw K, Cantrell FL, et al. Experts consensus recommendations for the management of calcium channel blocker poisoning in adults. Crit Care Med 2017;45(3):e306–15. Available from: https://doi.org/10.1097/CCM.0000000000002169.

[13] Vahedian-Azimi A, Hajibeygi B, Azizi-Fini I, et al. Efficacy of glucagon in the treatment of beta-blocker overdose. Exp Clin Cardiol 2013;18(4):e246–9.

[14] Watson WA, Litovitz TL, Rodgers Jr GC, et al. 2004 Annual report of the American Association of Poison Control Centers toxic exposure surveillance system. Am J Emerg Med 2005;23(5):589–666.

[15] Bismuth-Evenzal Y, Becker Y, Billan S, et al. Glucagon treatment for calcium channel blocker overdose. Clin Toxicol (Phila) 2015;53(5):410–15. Available from: https://doi.org/10.3109/15563650.2015.1033614.

[16] Hoeffner EG, Pickhardt PJ, Kim DH, et al. Gastrointestinal imaging with CT: applications of 3D reconstruction algorithms. Radiographics. 2006;26(4):1059–76. Available from: https://doi.org/10.1148/rg.264055168.

[17] Lee CM, Stewart RL. Gastrointestinal imaging for inflammatory bowel disease. World J Gastroenterol 2015;21(5).

[18] Hoeffel C, Nguyen K, Mambrini A, et al. Bowel preparation before MR imaging of the abdomen: comparison of three methods. Radiology 2005;236(1):89–94. Available from: https://doi.org/10.1148/radiol.2361040243.

[19] Kondo H, Kanematsu M, Goshima S, et al. Gadolinium ethoxybenzyl diethylenetriamine pentaacetic acid-enhanced magnetic resonance imaging for colorectal cancer: a preliminary study. J Comput Assist Tomogr 2016;40(2):294–7. Available from: https://doi.org/10.1097/RCT.0000000000000346.

[20] McAlindon ME, Plevris JN, McNeill JG, Garden OJ. Pharmacological agents in radiology: gastrointestinal tract. Gut. 1994;35(3):438–42. Available from: https://doi.org/10.1136/gut.35.3.438.

[21] Schwartz J, Raveh D, Toker S, et al. Treatment of anaphylactic shock with glucagon. Am J Emerg Med 1984;2 (4):301–3. Available from: https://doi.org/10.1016/0735-6757(84)90082-8.

[22] Simmons JW, Hartman CR, Seki SM, et al. Efficacy of high-dose glucagon in a porcine model of bupivacaine-induced cardiac arrest. Ann Emerg Med 1999;33(4):396–404. Available from: https://doi.org/10.1016/s0196-0644(99)70328-8.

[23] White JR, Campbell RK. Glucagon for the treatment of hypotension and shock. Ann Pharmacother 2011;45 (3):388–96. Available from: https://doi.org/10.1345/aph.1P500.

[24] Biondi B, Wartofsky L. Treatment of hypothyroidism: an evidence-based approach. Nat Rev Endocrinol 2014;10(2):111–21.

[25] Jonklaas J, Bianco AC, Bauer AJ, Burman KD, Cappola AR, Celi FS, et al. Guidelines for the treatment of hypothyroidism: prepared by the american thyroid association task force on thyroid hormone replacement. Thyroid 2014;24(12):1670–751. Available from: https://doi.org/10.1089/thy.2014.0028.
[26] Haugen BR, Alexander EK, Bible KC, et al. 2015 American Thyroid Association Management guidelines for adult patients with thyroid nodules and differentiated thyroid cancer: the American Thyroid Association guidelines task force on thyroid nodules and differentiated thyroid cancer. Thyroid 2016;26(1):1–133.
[27] Durante C, Haddy N, Baudin E, et al. Long-term outcome of 444 patients with distant metastases from papillary and follicular thyroid carcinoma: benefits and limits of radioiodine therapy. J Clin Endocrinol Metab 2006;91(8):2892–9.
[28] Cooper DS. Antithyroid drugs. N Engl J Med 2005;352(9):905–17.
[29] Ross DS, Burch HB, Cooper DS, et al. 2016 American Thyroid Association guidelines for diagnosis and management of hyperthyroidism and other causes of thyrotoxicosis. Thyroid 2016;26(10):1343–421.
[30] Popoveniuc G, Chandra T, Sud A, Sharma M, Blackman MR, Burman KD, et al. A diagnostic scoring system for myxedema coma. EndocrPract 2014;20(8):808–17. Available from: https://doi.org/10.4158/EP13460.OR PMID: 24518183.
[31] Wartofsky L. Myxedema coma. Endocrinol Metab Clin North Am 2006;35(4):687–98.
[32] Kim CH, Ahn JW, Kang SP, Kim SH, Chae HD, Kang BM. Effect of levothyroxine treatment on in vitro fertilization and pregnancy outcome in infertile women with subclinical hypothyroidism undergoing in vitro fertilization/intracytoplasmic sperm injection. Fertil Steril 2011;95(5):1650–4.
[33] Bauer M, et al. World J Biol Psychiatry 2019;20(9):669–83.
[34] Cao Y, et al. Front Endocrinol (Lausanne) 2020;11:166.
[35] Biondi B, et al. Nat Rev Endocrinol 2019;15(6):323–38.
[36] Samaraweera L, et al. Front Endocrinol (Lausanne) 2020;11:611.
[37] Chiha M, Samarasinghe S, Kabaker AS. Thyroid storm: an updated review. J Intensive Care Med 2017;32(4):187–94.
[38] Rose SR, Brown RS, Foley T, Kaplowitz PB, Kaye CI, Sundararajan S, et al. Update of newborn screening and therapy for congenital hypothyroidism. Pediatrics 2014;133(2):161–72.
[39] Cook AM, McDonnell AM, Lake RA, Nowak AK. Dexamethasone co-medication in cancer patients undergoing chemotherapy causes substantial immunomodulatory effects with implications for chemo-immunotherapy strategies. Oncoimmunology. 2015;5(3):e1066062. Available from: https://doi.org/10.1080/2162402X.2015.1066062 PMID: 27141331; PMCID: PMC4839331.
[40] Labib HA, Hassan AI, Kamaly AM, Wahba SS, Ammar MA. Evaluation of the role of hydrocortisone either alone or combined with fludrocortisone in the outcome of septic shock in adults. Ain-Shams J Anesthesiol 2022;14(1):60.
[41] Sprung CL, Annane D, Keh D, Moreno R, Singer M, Freivogel K, et al. Hydrocortisone therapy for patients with septic shock. N Engl J Med 2008;358(2):111–24.
[42] Hyman Paul, Kelner Paul. Pharmacotherapeutic uses of hormones. Nurs Clin North Am 2007;42(1):1–18. Available from: https://doi.org/10.1016/j.cnur.2006.11.002.
[43] Insulin Basics | ADA. https://diabetes.org/healthy-living/medication-treatments/insulin-other-injectables/insulin-basics; n.d. [accessed 10.03.23].
[44] Buse JB, Wexler DJ, Tsapas A, Rossing P, Mingrone G, Mathieu C, et al. 2021 Update to the American Diabetes Association standards of medical care in diabetes. Diabetes Care 2021;44(1):S1–232.
[45] Heinemann L, Home PD. Insulin delivery devices: technology update. Med Dev (Auckland, NZ) 2018;11:43–52. Available from: https://doi.org/10.2147/MDER.S146869).
[46] Kitabchi AE, Umpierrez GE, Miles JM, Fisher JN. Hyperglycemic crises in adult patients with diabetes. Diabetes Care 2009;32(7):1335–43.
[47] Pasquel FJ, Umpierrez GE. Hyperosmolar hyperglycemic state: a historic review of the clinical presentation, diagnosis, and treatment. Diabetes Care 2014;37(11):3124–31.
[48] Moran A, Brunzell C, Cohen RC, et al. Clinical care guidelines for cystic fibrosis-related diabetes: a position statement of the American Diabetes Association and a clinical practice guideline of the Cystic Fibrosis Foundation, endorsed by the Pediatric Endocrine Society. Diabetes Care 2010;33(12):2697–708.
[49] Service FJ. Hypoglycemic disorders. N Engl J Med 1995;332(17):1144–52.
[50] Guler HP, Zapf J, Froesch ER. Short-term metabolic effects of recombinant human insulin-like growth factor I in healthy adults. N Engl J Med 1987;317(3):137–40.

[51] Palmer BF. Potassium homeostasis and clinical implications. Am J Med 2010;123(4):292–9.
[52] Kashyap P, Farrugia G. Diabetic gastroparesis: what we have learned and had to unlearn in the past decade. Gut. 2010;59(12):1716–26.
[53] Ginsberg HN, Zhang YL, Hernandez-Ono A. Metabolic syndrome: focus on dyslipidemia. Obes (Silver Spring) 2006;14(Suppl 1):41S–9S.
[54] Misra A, Peethambaram A, Garg A. Clinical features and metabolic derangements in acquired generalized lipodystrophy: case reports and review of the literature. Med (Baltim) 2004;83(1):18–34.
[55] Melmed S, Polonsky KS, Larsen PR, Kronenberg HM. Williams Textbook of Endocrinology. 13th ed. Philadelphia, PA: Elsevier Saunders; 2016.
[56] Dungan K, et al. Glucagon-like peptide-1 receptor agonists compared with basal insulins for the treatment of type 2 diabetes mellitus: a systematic review and meta-analysis. Diabetes ObesMetab 2016;18(1):89–101.
[57] Finan B, et al. Unimolecular dual incretins maximize metabolic benefits in rodents, monkeys, and humans. Sci Transl Med 2013;5(209) 209ra151.
[58] Camilleri M, et al. Effect of glucagon-like peptide-1 receptor agonist on gastric emptying and meal-related symptoms in idiopathic gastroparesis. Aliment PharmacolTher 2008;27(10):990–9.
[59] Chey WD, et al. Linaclotide for irritable bowel syndrome with constipation: a 26-week, randomized, double-blind, placebo-controlled trial to evaluate efficacy and safety. Am J Gastroenterol 2012;107(4):1702–12.
[60] Lee YH, et al. The role of glucagon in cardiovascular disease: good, bad, or indifferent? Rev EndocrMetabDisord 2021;22(2):343–53.
[61] Ramamoorthy S, Cidlowski JA. Corticosteroids: mechanisms of action in health and disease. Rheum Dis Clin North Am 2016;42(1):15–31. Available from: https://doi.org/10.1016/j.rdc.2015.08.002 PMID: 26611548; PMCID: PMC4662771.
[62] Hall BM, Head H, Neurology HO. Corticosteroids in autoimmune diseases. Aust Prescr 1999;22:9–11. Available from: https://doi.org/10.18773/austprescr.1999.008).
[63] Lossignol D. A little help from steroids in oncology. J Transl Int Med 2016;4(1):52–4. Available from: https://doi.org/10.1515/jtim-2016-0011 Epub 2016 Apr 14. PMID: 28191519; PMCID: PMC5290916).
[64] Younes AK, Younes NK. Recovery of steroid induced adrenal insufficiency. TranslPediatr 2017;6(4):269–73. Available from: https://doi.org/10.21037/tp.2017.10.01 PMID: 29184808; PMCID: PMC5682381).
[65] Yasir, M., A. Goyal, S. Sonthalia. Corticosteroid adverse effects (2018).
[66] Juul A, et al. Growth hormone treatment in adults. N Engl J Med 2019;381(26):2486–98.
[67] Högler W, et al. Diagnosis and management of growth hormone deficiency in childhood and adolescence. Horm Res Paediatr 2016;86(6):361–97.
[68] Rosenfeld RG, et al. Recombinant human growth hormone (somatropin) in children with growth hormone deficiency. Pituitary. 2017;20(2):180–8.
[69] Davenport ML, et al. Growth hormone treatment of early growth failure in toddlers with Turner syndrome: a randomized, controlled, multicenter trial. J Clin Endocrinol Metab 2007;92(8):3406–16.
[70] Copeland KC. The National Cooperative Growth Study experience with long-term growth hormone therapy. Horm Res. 2002;58(Suppl 3):63–9.
[71] Rossouw JE, et al. Risks and benefits of estrogen plus progestin in healthy postmenopausal women: principal results From the Women's Health Initiative randomized controlled trial. JAMA. 2002;288(3):321–33.
[72] Cummings SR, et al. Effect of raloxifene on risk of breast cancer in postmenopausal women: results from the MORE randomized trial. JAMA. 1999;281(23):2189–97.
[73] Coates AS, et al. A randomized trial of exemestane after two to three years of tamoxifen therapy in postmenopausal women with primary breast cancer. N Engl J Med 2004;350(11):1081–92.
[74] Wierckx K, et al. Hormone therapy in transgender people. Endocr Rev 2019;40(1):97–117.
[75] Tal R, Taylor HS. Endocrinology of pregnancy. [Updated 2021 Mar 18]. In: Feingold KR, Anawalt B, Blackman MR, et al., editors. Endotext [Internet]. South Dartmouth (MA): MDText.com, Inc. 2000. https://www.ncbi.nlm.nih.gov/books/NBK278962/.
[76] Prior JC. Progesterone for treatment of symptomatic menopausal women. Climacteric. 2018;21(4):345–51.
[77] Pandian Z, McTavish AR, Aucott L, et al. Interventions for luteal phase support in assisted reproduction cycles. Cochrane Database Syst Rev 2015;7:CD009154.
[78] Coomarasamy A, Devall AJ, Brosens JJ, et al. Micronized vaginal progesterone to prevent miscarriage: a critical evaluation of randomized evidence. Am J Obstet Gynecol 2016;214(3):318–29.

[79] Leone Roberti Maggiore U, Ferrero S, Candiani M, et al. Progestins and progesterone in hormone replacement therapy and the risk of endometrial hyperplasia. Best Pract Res Clin ObstetGynaecol 2018;53:63–73.

[80] Traish AM, Haider A, Doros G, Saad F. Long-term testosterone therapy in hypogonadal men ameliorates elements of the metabolic syndrome: an observational, long-term registry study. Int J Clin Pract 2014;68 (3):314–29. Available from: https://doi.org/10.1111/ijcp.12321.

[81] Wu FC, Tajar A, Pye SR, et al. Hypothalamic-pituitary-testicular axis disruptions in older men are differentially linked to age and modifiable risk factors: the European Male Aging Study. J Clin Endocrinol Metab 2008;93(7):2737–45. Available from: https://doi.org/10.1210/jc.2007-1972).

[82] Wang C, Swerdloff RS, Iranmanesh A, et al. Transdermal testosterone gel improves sexual function, mood, muscle strength, and body composition parameters in hypogonadal men. J Clin Endocrinol Metab 2000;85 (8):2839–53. Available from: https://doi.org/10.1210/jcem.85.8.6736).

[83] Bhasin S, Cunningham GR, Hayes FJ, et al. Testosterone therapy in men with androgen deficiency syndromes: an Endocrine Society clinical practice guideline. J Clin Endocrinol Metab 2010;95(6):2536–59. Available from: https://doi.org/10.1210/jc.2009-2354.

[84] Bosch E, Simon C. Follicle-stimulating hormone (FSH) therapy in assisted reproduction: a review. Fertil Steril 2016;105(3):719–26. Available from: https://doi.org/10.1016/j.fertnstert.2015.12.131.

[85] Lisi F, Rinaldi L, Fishel S, Lisi R. Use of follicle stimulating hormone in infertility treatment: an overview of protocol options, efficacy and safety. Expert Opin drug Saf 2018;17(6):575–84. Available from: https://doi.org/10.1080/14740338.2018.1474793).

[86] Wang JG, Douglas NC, Nakhuda GS. Gonadotropin-releasing hormone analogs for the prevention of ovarian hyperstimulation syndrome in IVF: a systematic review and meta-analysis. Fertil Steril 2020;113(5):956–67. Available from: https://doi.org/10.1016/j.fertnstert.2020.02.103).

[87] Gittelman M, Pommerville P, Persson BE, et al. A 12-Month, open-label, multicenter study of the safety and tolerability of leuprolide acetate 22.5 mg 6-month depot formulation for suppression of testosterone in patients with prostate cancer. Adv Ther 2020;37(2):691–703. Available from: https://doi.org/10.1007/s12325-019-01191-w.

[88] Cakmak H, Taylor HS, Yazici G. Medical treatment of endometriosis: emerging strategies. Best practice & research. Clinical Obstetr Gynaecol 2020;66(16–30). Available from: https://pubmed.ncbi.nlm.nih.gov/32798157/).

[89] Guerriero S, Condorelli M. Luteinizing hormone-releasing hormone agonists in ovarian stimulation for in vitro fertilization In Vitro Fertilization. 2019. p. 89–103. Springer, Cham. Available from: https://link.springer.com/chapter/10.1007/978-3-030-21150-0_7.

[90] Bozzola M, Bozzola E, Montalbano C, Stamati FA, Ferrara P, Villani A. Delayed puberty versus hypogonadism: a challenge for the pediatrician. Ann Pediatr Endocrinol Metab 2018;23(2):57–61. Available from: https://doi.org/10.6065/apem.2018.23.2.57 Epub 2018 Jun 20. PMID: 29969875; PMCID: PMC6057016).

[91] Meani D, Solarić M, Visapää H, Rosén RM, Janknegt R, Soče M. Practical differences between luteinizing hormone-releasing hormone agonists in prostate cancer: perspectives across the spectrum of care. Ther Adv Urol 2017;10(2):51–63. Available from: https://doi.org/10.1177/1756287217738985 PMID: 29434673; PMCID: PMC5805008.

[92] Betz D., Fane K. Human Chorionic Gonadotropin. [Updated 2022 Aug 8]. In: StatPearls [Internet]. Treasure Island (FL): StatPearls Publishing. Available from: https://www.ncbi.nlm.nih.gov/books/NBK532950/); 2022 January.

[93] Vlahos N., et al. (2016). Human chorionic gonadotropin in ovulation induction and ovarian. https://www.ncbi.nlm.nih.gov/pmc/articles/PMC5024212/).

[94] Greenway et al. (2015). Human chorionic gonadotropin (HCG) for the treatment of obesity: a review of the literature. https://www.ncbi.nlm.nih.gov/pmc/articles/PMC4670012/).

[95] Gendrel et al. (2012). Cryptorchidism: medical treatment with human chorionic gonadotropin. https://www.ncbi.nlm.nih.gov/pmc/articles/PMC3321432/).

[96] Bouloux P.M., et al. (2003). Induction of spermatogenesis by recombinant follicle-stimulating hormone (rFSH) and human chorionic gonadotropin (hCG) in gonadotropin-deficient men with hypothalamic-pituitary damage. https://www.ncbi.nlm.nih.gov/pubmed/12727959).

[97] Kirschner M.A., et al. (1973). Human chorionic gonadotropin treatment of delayed puberty and related disorders of pituitary function. https://www.ncbi.nlm.nih.gov/pubmed/4351105).

[98] Tulandi T., et al. (1990). Human chorionic gonadotropin decreases the size of simple ovarian cysts: a randomized, placebo-controlled trial. https://www.ncbi.nlm.nih.gov/pubmed/2297898).

[99] Knowles J, Vysloužil J, Muselík J, Stejskal V, Kouřil J, Podhorec P. Efficacy of poly (lactic-co-glycolic acid) microparticles as a gonadotropin-releasing hormone analogue delivery system to stimulate ovulation of peled Coregonus peled. Czech J Anim Sci 2021;66(8):331–8.

[100] Lin Y-H, Chen C-T, Liang H-F, Kulkarni AR, Lee P-W, Chen C-H, et al. Novel nanoparticles for oral insulin delivery via the paracellular pathway. Nanotechnology 2007;18:105102.

[101] Paliwal SR, Paliwal R, Agrawal GP, Vyas SP. Liposomal nanomedicine for breast cancer therapy. Nanomedicine. 2011;6(6):1085–100.

[102] Paliwal SR, Paliwal R, Vyas SP. pH-sensitive liposomes in drug delivery. Smart Mater Drug Delivery 2013;1:80 Apr 25.

[103] Parmentier J, Hofhaus G, Thomas S, Cuesta LC, Gropp F, Schröder R, et al. Improved oral bioavailability of human growth hormone by a combination of liposomes containing bio-enhancers and tetraether lipids and omeprazole. J Pharm Sci 2014;103(12):3985–93.

[104] Fountain MW, Ganjam VK, Schultz RD. Liposome carrier vehicle for triiodothryonine. Clin Exp Pharmacol Physiol 1982;9(1):101–5.

[105] Pireddu R, Pibiri M, Valenti D, Sinico C, Fadda AM, Simbula G, et al. A novel lactoferrin-modified stealth liposome for hepatoma-delivery of triiodothyronine. Int J pharmaceutics 2018;537(1–2):257–67.

[106] Lamparelli EP, Ciardulli MC, Scala P, Scognamiglio M, Charlier B, Di Pietro P, et al. Lipid nano-vesicles for thyroid hormone encapsulation: a comparison between different fabrication technologies, drug loading, and an in vitro delivery to human tendon stem/progenitor cells in 2D and 3D culture. Int J Pharm 2022;624:122007.

[107] Choudhari KB, Labhasetwar V, Dorle AK. Liposomes as a carrier for oral administration of insulin: effect of formulation factors. J Microencapsul 1994;11(3):319–25.

[108] Muramatsu K, Maitani Y, Nagai T. Dipalmitoylphosphatidylcholine liposomes with soybean-derived sterols and cholesterol as a carrier for the oral administration of insulin in rats. Biol Pharm Bull 1996;19(8):1055–8.

[109] Spangler RS. Insulin administration via liposomes. Diabetes care 1990;13(9):911–22.

[110] Kurmi BD, Paliwal R, Paliwal SR. Dual cancer targeting using estrogen functionalized chitosan nanoparticles loaded with doxorubicin-estrone conjugate: a quality by design approach. Int J Biol macromolecules 2020;164:2881–94 Dec 1.

[111] Vyas S.P., Paliwal R., Paliwal S.R. Chapter 25: Chitosan/chitosan derivatives as carriers and immunoadjuvants in vaccine delivery. Chitin, chitosan, oligosaccharides and their derivatives: biological activities and applications. CRC Press/Taylor & Francis Group LLC, Boca Raton. 2011:339-356.

[112] Tekchandani P, Kurmi BD, Paliwal SR. Nanomedicine to deal with cancer cell biology in multi-drug resistance. Mini Rev Med Chem 2017;17(18):1793–810.

[113] Wu ZM, Zhou L, Guo XD, Jiang W, Ling L, Qian Y, et al. HP55-coated capsule containing PLGA/RS nanoparticles for oral delivery of insulin. Int J Pharm 2012;425(1–2):1–8.

[114] Jain S, Rathi VV, Jain AK, Das M, Godugu C. Folate-decorated PLGA nanoparticles as a rationally designed vehicle for the oral delivery of insulin. Nanomedicine 2012;7:1311–37.

[115] Ghasemi R, Abdollahi M, Emamgholi Zadeh E, Khodabakhshi K, Badeli A, Bagheri H, et al. mPEG-PLA and PLA-PEG-PLA nanoparticles as new carriers for delivery of recombinant human Growth Hormone (rhGH). Sci Rep 2018;8(1):1–3.

[116] Paliwal SR, Paliwal R, Agrawal GP, Vyas SP. Targeted breast cancer nanotherapeutics: options and opportunities with estrogen receptors. Crit Rev Ther Drug Carr Syst 2012;29(5).

[117] Rai S, Paliwal R, Vaidya B, Gupta PN, Mahor S, Khatri K, et al. Estrogen (s) and analogs as a non-immunogenic endogenous ligand in targeted drug/DNA delivery. Curr Med Chem 2007;14(19):2095–109.

[118] Hariharan S, Bhardwaj V, Bala I, Sitterberg J, Bakowsky U, Ravi Kumar MN. Design of estradiol loaded PLGA nanoparticulate formulations: a potential oral delivery system for hormone therapy. Pharm Res 2006;23:184–95 Jan.

[119] Prakapenka AV, Quihuis AM, Carson CG, Patel S, Bimonte-Nelson HA, Sirianni RW. Poly (lactic-co-glycolic acid) nanoparticle encapsulated 17β-estradiol improves spatial memory and increases uterine stimulation in middle-aged ovariectomized rats. Front. Behav Neurosci 2020;14:597690 Dec 16.

[120] Mishra SS, Sharma A. Preparation and characterization of chitosan nanoparticles of insulin for nasal delivery. J Drug Deliv Therapeutics 2018;8(5-s):400–6.

[121] Mansourpour M, Mahjub R, Amini M, Ostad SN, Shamsa ES, Rafiee-Tehrani M, et al. Development of acid-resistant alginate/trimethyl chitosan nanoparticles containing cationic β-cyclodextrin polymers for insulin oral delivery. AAPS Pharmscitech 2015;16:952–62 Aug.

[122] Liu C, Kou Y, Zhang X, Dong W, Cheng H, Mao S. Enhanced oral insulin delivery via surface hydrophilic modification of chitosan copolymer based self-assembly polyelectrolyte nanocomplex. Int J Pharmaceutics 2019;554:36–47 Jan 10.

[123] Lee MJ, Seo DY, Lee HE, Choi GJ. Therapeutic effect of chitosan modification on salmon-calcitonin-loaded PLGA nanoparticles. Korean J Chem Eng 2011;28:1406–11 Jun.

[124] Paliwal R, Paliwal SR, Kenwat R, Kurmi BD, Sahu MK. Solid lipid nanoparticles: a review on recent perspectives and patents. Expert Opin Ther Pat 2020;30(3):179–94.

[125] Vyas SP, Rai S, Paliwal R, Gupta PN, Khatri K, Goyal AK, et al. Solid lipid nanoparticles (SLNs) as a rising tool in drug delivery science: one step up in nanotechnology. Curr Nanosci 2008;4(1):30–44.

[126] Sarmento B, Martins S, Ferreira D, Souto EB. Oral insulin delivery by means of solid lipid nanoparticles. Int J Nanomed 2007;2(4):743–9.

[127] Zhang N, Ping Q, Huang G, Xu W, Cheng Y, Han X. Lectin-modified solid lipid nanoparticles as carriers for oral administration of insulin. Int J Pharm 2006;327(1–2):153–9.

[128] Zhang Z, Lv H, Zhou J. Novel solid lipid nanoparticles as carriers for oral administration of insulin. Die Pharm-An Int J Pharm Sci 2009;64(9):574–8.

[129] Yang X, Liu Y, Liu C, Zhang N. Biodegradable solid lipid nanoparticle flocculates for pulmonary delivery of insulin. J Biomed Nanotechnol 2012;8(5):834–42.

[130] Siahdasht FN, Farhadian N, Karimi M, Hafizi L. Enhanced delivery of melatonin loaded nanostructured lipid carriers during in vitro fertilization: NLC formulation, optimization and IVF efficacy. RSC Adv 2020;10(16):9462–75.

[131] Sarmento B, Ribeiro A, Veiga F, Sampaio P, Neufeld R, Ferreira D. Alginate/chitosan nanoparticles are effective for oral insulin delivery. Pharm Res 2007;24:2198–206.

[132] Li X, Qi J, Xie Y, Zhang X, Hu S, Xu Y, et al. Nanoemulsions coated with alginate/chitosan as oral insulin delivery systems: preparation, characterization, and hypoglycemic effect in rats. Int J Nanomed 2012;23–32 Dec 28.

[133] Gonzaga LW, Botelho MA, Queiroz DB, Fechine P, Freire R, Azevedo E, et al. Nanotechnology in hormone replacement therapy: safe and efficacy of transdermal estriol and estradiol nanoparticles after 5 years follow-up study. Lat Am J Pharm 2012;31(3):442–50.

[134] Botelho MA, Queiroz DB, Freitas A, Guerreiro S, Umbelino S, Barros G. Effects of a new testosterone transdermal delivery system, Biolipid B2-testosterone in healthy middle aged men: a Confocal Raman Spectroscopy Study. J Pharm Sci Innov 2013;2(2):1–7.

[135] Kumar S, Gupta SK, Sharma PK. Self-emulsifying drug delivery systems (SEDDS) for oral delivery of lipid based formulations-a review. African J Basic Appl Sci 2012;4:7–11.

[136] Sachan R, Khatri K, Kasture SB. Self-emulsifying drug delivery system a novel approach for enhancement of bioavailability. Int J Pharm Tech Res 2010;2(3):1738–45.

[137] Balakumar K, Raghavan CV, Abdu S. Self nanoemulsifying drug delivery system (SNEDDS) of rosuvastatin calcium: design, formulation, bioavailability and pharmacokinetic evaluation. Colloids Surf B: Biointerfaces 2013;112:337–43.

[138] Ma EL, Ma H, Liu Z, Zheng CX, Duan MX. In vitro and in vivo evaluation of a novel oral insulin formulation. Acta Pharm Sin 2006;27(10):1382–8.

[139] Hintzen F, Perera G, Hauptstein S, Müller C, Laffleur F, Bernkop-Schnürch A. In vivo evaluation of an oral self-microemulsifying drug delivery system (SMEDDS) for leuprorelin. Int J Pharm 2014;472(1–2):20–6.

[140] Leonaviciute G, Zupančič O, Prüfert F, Rohrer J, Bernkop-Schnürch A. Impact of lipases on the protective effect of SEDDS for incorporated peptide drugs towards intestinal peptidases. Int J Pharm 2016;508 (1–2):102–8.

[141] Eaimtrakarn S, Rama Prasad YV, Ohno T, Konishi T, Yoshikawa Y, Shibata N, et al. Absorption enhancing effect of labrasol on the intestinal absorption of insulin in rats. J Drug Target 2002;10(3):255–60.

[142] Frey H, Aakvaag A, Saanum D, Falch J. Bioavailability of oral testosterone in males. Eur J Clin Pharmacol 1979;16:345–9 Sep.

[143] Liang X, Hua Y, Liu Q, Li Z, Yu F, Gao J, et al. Solid self-emulsifying drug delivery system (solid SEDDS) for testosterone undecanoate: in vitro and in vivo evaluation. Curr. Drug Deliv 2021;18(5):620–33.

[144] Ribeiro BC, Cintra ER, Lima EM, Silva LA, Diniz DG. Evaluation of testosterone compatibility with different excipients for the development of a self-emulsifying drug delivery system. J Therm Anal Calorim 2023;148 (1):159–68.

[145] Kesharwani D, Mishra S, Paul SD, Paliwal R, Satapathy T. The functional nanogel: an exalted carrier system. J Drug Deliv Ther 2019;9(2-s):570–82.

[146] Kabanov AV, Vinogradov SV. Nanogels as pharmaceutical carriers: finite networks of infinite capabilities. Angew Chem Int Ed 2009;48(30):5418–29.

[147] Kesharwani D, Paul SD, Paliwal R, Satapathy T. Exploring potential of diacerin nanogel for topical application in arthritis: formulation development, QbD based optimization and pre-clinical evaluation. Colloids Surf B: Biointerfaces 2023;223:113160. Available from: https://doi.org/10.1016/j.colsurfb.2023.113160.

[148] Bai Y, Zhang Z, Zhang A, Chen L, He C, Zhuang X, et al. Novel thermo-and pH-responsive hydroxypropyl cellulose-and poly (l-glutamic acid)-based microgels for oral insulin controlled release. Carbohydr Polym 2012;89(4):1207–14.

[149] Ramkissoon-Ganorkar C, Liu F, Baudyš M, Kim SW. Modulating insulin-release profile from pH/thermo-sensitive polymeric beads through polymer molecular weight. J Contr Rel 1999;59(3):287–98.

[150] Wang J, Xu M, Cheng X, Kong M, Liu Y, Feng C, et al. Positive/negative surface charge of chitosan based nanogels and its potential influence on oral insulin delivery. Carbohydr Polym 2016;136:867–74 Jan 20.

[151] Park MR, Seo BB, Song SC. Dual ionic interaction system based on polyelectrolyte complex and ionic, injectable, and thermosensitive hydrogel for sustained release of human growth hormone. Biomaterials. 2013;34(4):1327–36.

[152] Makhlof A, Werle M, Tozuka Y, Takeuchi H. Nanoparticles of glycol chitosan and its thiolated derivative significantly improved the pulmonary delivery of calcitonin. Int J Pharm 2010;397(1–2):92–5.

[153] Kesharwani P, Gorain B, Low SY, Tan SA, Ling EC, Lim YK, et al. Nanotechnology based approaches for anti-diabetic drugs delivery. Diabetes Res Clin Pract 2018;136:52–77 Feb 1.

[154] Dong Z, Katsumi H, Sakane T, Yamamoto A. Effects of polyamidoamine (PAMAM) dendrimers on the nasal absorption of poorly absorbable drugs in rats. Int J Pharm 2010;393(1–2):245–53.

[155] Rafiee A, Mansfeld FM, Moyle PM, Toth I. Synthesis and characterization of luteinizing hormone-releasing hormone (lhrh)-functionalized mini-dendrimers. Int J Org Chem 2013;3:51–7.

[156] Cevc G. Transdermal drug delivery of insulin with ultradeformable carriers. Clin Pharm 2003;42:461–74 Apr.

[157] Kateh Shamshiri M, Momtazi-Borojeni AA, Khodabandeh Shahraky M, Rahimi F. Lecithin soybean phospholipid nano-transfersomes as potential carriers for transdermal delivery of the human growth hormone. J Cell Biochem 2019;120(6):9023–33.

[158] El Maghraby GM, Williams AC, Barry BW. Oestradiol skin delivery from ultradeformable liposomes: refinement of surfactant concentration. Int J Pharm 2000;196(1):63–74.

[159] Maghraby GM, Williams AC, Barry BW. Skin delivery of oestradiol from deformable and traditiona liposomes: mechanistic studies. J Pharm Pharmacol 1999;51(10):1123–34.

CHAPTER

6

Vesicular drug delivery systems: a novel approach in current nanomedicine

Elisabetta Mazzotta, Martina Romeo and Rita Muzzalupo

Department of Pharmacy, Health and Nutritional Sciences, University of Calabria, Rende, Italy

6.1 Introduction

The last century has witnessed unprecedented growth of nanotechnology applications in medicine with the aims to advance medical treatments, both for diagnostics and therapy, and improve health care quality. The design at the nanoscale range allows for the development of scaffolding systems able to overcome the limitations of conventional drug delivery. The reasons why nanoscale particles are attractive for medical purposes are their important and unique features, such as the small size and large functional surface that can be engineered to bind, adsorb, and carry compounds with targeting, imaging, and/or therapeutic properties. Various types of nanostructure materials have been developed by researchers for pharmaceutical applications. Among them, vesicular systems have caught increasing attention. Vesicular systems are core–shell structures consisting of one or more concentric bilayers formed as a result of self-assembling of amphiphilic molecules in aqueous environments. In aqueous media, indeed, amphiphilic molecule polar groups line up to form a water-attracting surface, while their lipophilic chains form a water-free zone (Fig. 6.1).

Their architecture makes them a versatile platform for the delivery of both hydrophilic and hydrophobic therapeutic agents. Hydrophilic drugs can be included in the core, whereas the lipid bilayer offers space for integration of hydrophobic drugs. They have been largely used, indeed, as a carrier of anticancer, antimicrobial drug, protein, gene, and imaging agents [1]. Many studies have demonstrated that vesicular systems improve drug pharmacokinetics and protect it against dilution and degradation or inactivation in the bloodstream. Interestingly, targeted delivery of drugs at the desired pathological tissue can also be achieved, thereby lowering its concentration at the other sites in the body and reducing toxic side effects [2].

Molecular Pharmaceutics and Nano Drug Delivery
DOI: https://doi.org/10.1016/B978-0-323-91924-1.00002-2

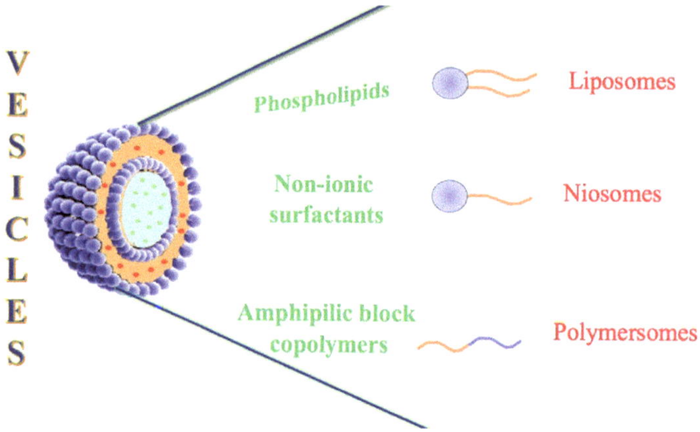

FIGURE 6.1 Sketch of different types of vesicular nanocarriers.

Key advantages of vesicular delivery systems are versatility and plasticity. Vesicle composition is, indeed, an important parameter affecting physicochemical characteristics including particle size, surface charge, bilayer fluidity and permeability, stability and drug loading, and release rate [3]. Therefore, composition may vary and be chosen depending on the desired application. Source materials may be natural compounds such as phospholipids and polymers or have a "chemical" origin such as nonionic surfactants. Some of the most used amphiphilic molecules employed in the design of a vesicle structure are reported in Fig. 6.2. In addition, some drugs may be formulated as nanoscale vesicles and then function as their own "carrier." In addition, some drugs can be formulated as nanoscale vesicles and act as vectors of themselves. These types of drugs, known as surfadrug, have in their structure one or more flexible and hydrophobic aromatic nuclei, to which an ester group or a charge-bearing N atom is directly linked, or which include a pyridine-like N atom [4]. The direct use of drugs for vesicle preparation offers the possibility to bypass the use of additional excipients, improve formulation safety, and increase the amount of loaded drugs.

The pioneer formulations of vesicles made up of a drug, known as diclosomes, were developed by Tavano and coworkers [5]. The authors proposed the use of antiflammatory drug, diclofenac sodium, as the main component of the vesicular bilayer and it was observed that diclosomes exhibit the best performance with respect to traditional niosomes loaded with the diclofenac sodium aqueous core.

6.2 Type of vesicles

Vesicles for drug delivery purposes are categorized based on the amphiphilic component of the bilayer in liposome, niosomes, and polymersomes (Fig. 6.1). The nature of the amphiphilic molecule affects vesicle properties, and some of the main differences are summarized in Table 6.1. In the next paragraph, we will describe in detail the most interesting advantages and application of every vesicular aggregate.

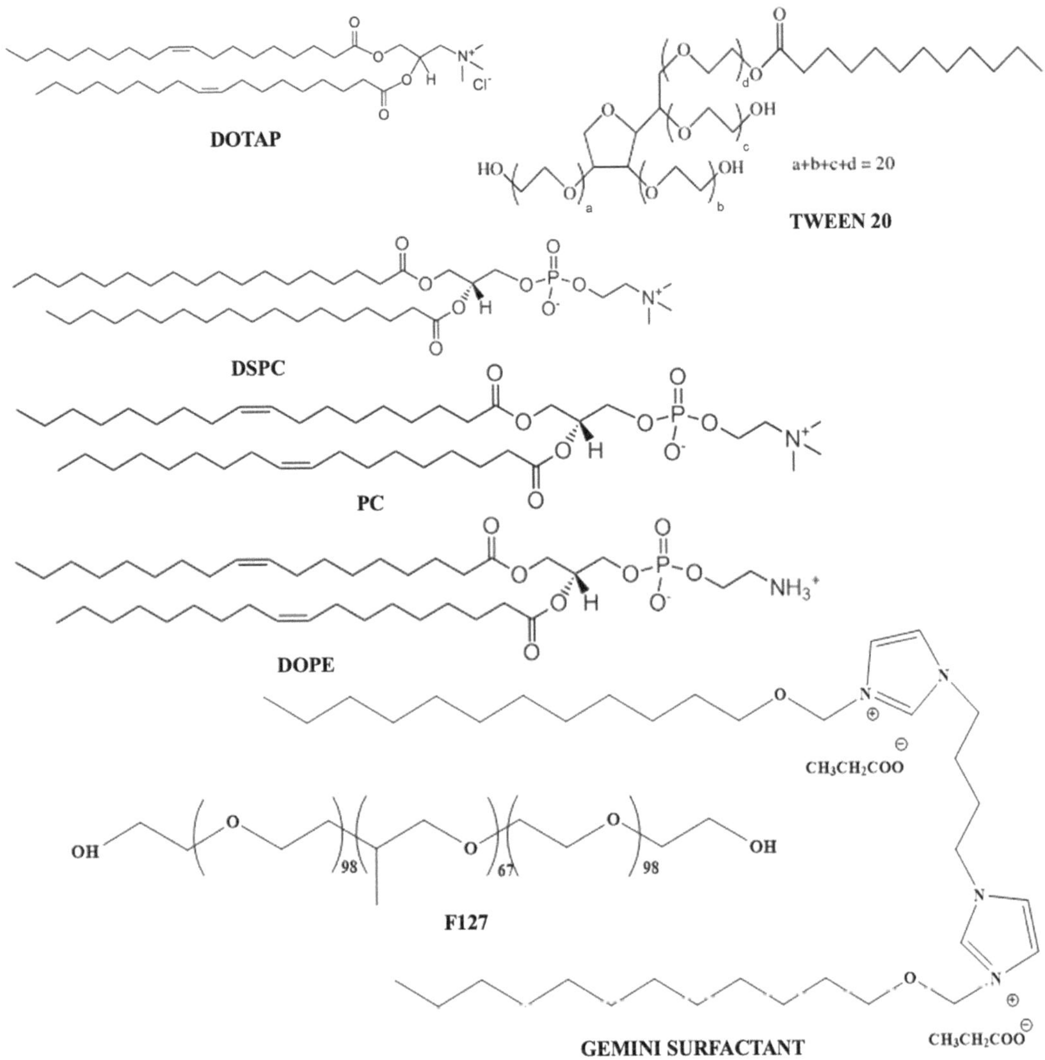

FIGURE 6.2 Common amphiphilic molecules employed in the design of vesicular drug delivery systems.

6.2.1 Liposomes

Liposomes are the oldest vesicles used as drug carriers and depict the first example of a clinically approved nanomedicine [6,7]. Actually, there are, indeed, more than 40 liposomal products either on the market or in various phases of clinical trials (Doxil, AmBisome, and Myocet) [8]. The main reasons of their wide translation in clinical therapy are their low immunogenicity, toxicity, and better therapeutic efficacy [9]. Liposomes are concentric bilayer vesicles composed of natural or synthetic lipids. A large variety of lipids with different head groups, chain saturation, chain lengths, and charge are available for

TABLE 6.1 Comparative features of liposomes, niosomes, and polymersomes.

Liposomes	Niosomes	Polymersomes
Phospholipids	Nonionic surfactants	Amphiphilic block copolymer
Chemically unstable	Chemically stable	Chemically stable
High permeability	Tunable permeability	Low permeability
Special storage condition	No special storage conditions	No special storage conditions
Expensive	Inexpensive	Inexpensive
Limited versatility	Wide chemical versatility	Wide chemical versatility

their synthesis. Common phospholipids used are phosphatidylcholines, phosphatidylethanolamines, phosphatidylserines, and phosphatidylglycerols [10].

From their first description in 1960, several improvements of liposome technology have been pursued evolving various formulations with distinctive characteristics such as conventional liposomes, sterically stabilized liposomes, ligand-targeted liposomes, and multifunctional liposomes [11].

Conventional liposomes are composed of anionic, cationic, or neutral phospholipids. Despite their ability to improve drug pharmacokinetics, conventional liposomes exhibit many problems such as fast macrophage uptake, chemical instability, and high membrane permeability, resulting in poor retention efficiency and drug leakage during blood circulation. Many approaches have been addressed to enhance in vivo performance, and one of them was the surface modification with hydrophilic polymers such as polyethylene glycol (PEG) developing stealth liposomes.

The hydrophilic polymer is able to establish a steric barrier reducing rapid recognition and uptake by reticuloendothelial system (RES) and in vivo opsonization remaining, therefore, in circulation longer than conventional liposomes [12]. Anyway, the stealth strategy shows several drawbacks such as poor targeting efficiency. To overcome this limitation, liposomes conjugated on their surface with molecules selectively overexpressed at the disease target site such as antibodies, peptides, and carbohydrates, glycoproteins or specific receptors ligands have been developed. Ligand-targeted liposomes increase drug selectivity, achieving a narrow distribution and accumulation at the site of interest with minimal deposition in healthy tissues. Finally, a new generation of liposomes, which incorporate multiple complementary targeting strategies, have been developed to further improve liposomal targeting and maximize therapeutic outcomes.

6.2.2 Niosomes

Niosomes are structurally similar to liposomes and have attracted increasing interest as a better alternative to liposomes, thanks to their higher stability and lower production cost. Niosomes and liposomes display almost similar behavior in sustained and targeted drug delivery. The only difference is their composition and chemical properties related to the material used in their preparation. Nonionic surfactants are the main constituent of niosomes and show better chemical stability with respect to phospholipids. Moreover, niosomes do not require a special storage condition, handling, and purification, which are necessary for liposome preparation. A variety of nonionic surfactants, such as polysorbates, alkyl esters, and alkyl ethers, are typically used for niosome preparation. In the last few years, attention has been focused on the development of newer classes of surface-active agents such as gemini surfactants to prepare innovative devices.

Gemini surfactants are composed of two hydrophobic chains and two polar head groups covalently connected by a covalently spacer group at the level of the head groups. Compared to corresponding single-chain surfactants, gemini surfactants exhibit superior aggregation capacity and, thus, lower CMC value [13]. Gemini surfactants based on amino acid have attracted increasing interest for the ability to combine the advantages of gemini surfactants in terms of efficiency with the higher biodegradability and lower toxicity of amino acids [14]. Specifically, gemini surfactants derived from lysine and arginine are very interesting since in addition to their better physicochemical properties, they showed an important antibacterial activity against a broad spectrum of gram-positive and gram-negative microorganisms [15].

6.2.3 Polymersomes

Polymersomes are artificial vesicles based on the self-assembly of amphiphilic copolymers. Block copolymers are macromolecules similar to lipids composed of a combination of hydrophilic and hydrophobic portions, which tend to self-assemble into various supramolecular structures. Amphiphilic block copolymers can be composed of two and three types of monomers with different structures like ABA, BAB, or ABC formats, where A and C are hydrophilic blocks with diverse chemical composition and B is the hydrophobic block and also complex multiblock copolymers with linear or grafted blocks [16].

Typical hydrophilic blocks are nonionic polyethylene oxide or PEG, anionic polymethylacrylic acid or polyacrylic acid (PAA), cationic poly(2-vinyl pyridine) or poly(4-vinyl pyridine), and so forth. Instead, common hydrophobic blocks are polystyrene, polypropylene oxide, polybutadiene, and polylactic acid. Molecular composition and length of the hydrophobic and hydrophilic blocks, indeed, influence different physicochemical properties such as membrane rigidity, size, and stability.

Owing to the material used to prepare them, polymersomes present countless advantages such a high stability [17], extended blood circulation, drug loading capacity, and membrane versatility due to the great variability of the starting materials. Compared to liposomes, polymersomes exhibit a greater life span and are generally more stable due to low membrane permeability; therefore, they can retain drugs with greater efficiency.

An interesting feature of these type of vesicles is the large versatility of polymer chemistry. Unlike phospholipids that exhibit a large limitation of functionalization, polymers can be functionalized in countless ways, and so, they are easily tunable for the desired therapeutic application [18]. This capability allows to design a variety of polymersomes with adjustable fluidity, permeability, stability, responsiveness, and targeting and imaging properties.

6.3 Engineered vesicles for therapeutic purposes

The main goal of nanoscale vesicles as delivery agents is to deliver drugs with high selectivity to target tissues. Various approaches have been explored by researchers to develop smarter, safer, and more effective therapeutic nanovesicles systems. Advances in nanomedicine to achieve personalized therapy include targeted drug delivery, responsiveness to specific stimuli, and multifunctional approaches. The main goal of nanomedicine is to enable nanosystems to deliver the cargo (drugs, genes, radioisotopes, etc.) in a specific manner to avoid systemic toxicity and accurately measure the therapeutic efficacy delivered.

6.3.1 Transformable drug delivery vesicles

One strategy to improve the therapeutic index of nanoparticles is to engineer them to be transformable in response to the given stimuli. Nanovesicles, indeed, can be engineered to be sensitive and release their cargo under the action of specific stimuli. Taking advantage of the abnormal environment of pathological site, nanosized vesicles can be tailor-made by making their structure moieties sensitive to a specific environmental stimuli. These smart vesicles may selectively localize drug release in a specific disease tissue and represent good tools to achieve controlled or on-demand release [19]. Two main strategies are widely exploited in the design of nanodevices with personalized release kinetics. In one approach, internal stimuli related to the intrinsic difference between healthy and pathological tissue may be used to trigger drug release. Changes in pH, enzymatic expression, and concentration of the redox agent are common internal triggers used to provide an intrinsic, autonomous, and targeted drug release pattern [20]. Conversely, the second approach used to improve drug selectivity relies on the use of physical stimuli externally applied. These include temperature, light, ultrasound, and electric or magnetic fields (Fig. 6.3). The use of external stimuli allows to achieve a pulsatile drug release profile and provide also a high control over temporal and spatial drug release into the targeted site [21–23].

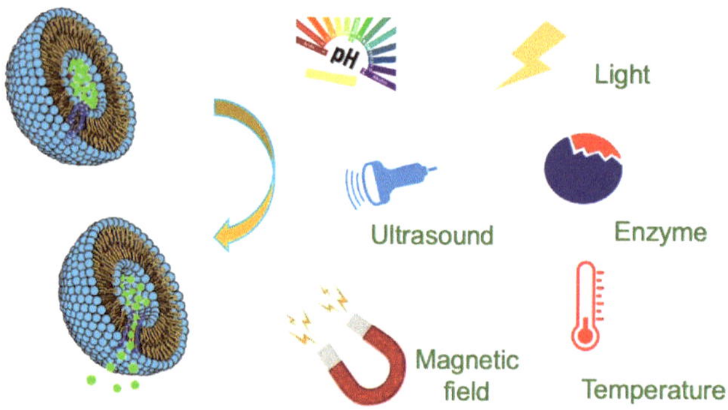

FIGURE 6.3 Schematic representation of main exogenous and endogenous stimuli involved in the design of transformable vesicles.

6.3.2 Actively targeted vesicles

A further approach applied to improve drug selectivity is the active strategy that relies on the covalent attachment on the nanocarrier surface of ligands highly specific for target cells. These devices, so engineered, recognize and bind to receptors overexpressed on the pathological targeting site, inducing their internalization via receptor-mediated endocytosis. This specific molecular recognition offers the opportunity to address and deliver drugs to a specific site and to decrease cytotoxicity and side effects of drugs on healthy cells and organs, which are common drawbacks of traditional therapy. Various receptors have been recognized as a potential target for treatment of several diseases, and a large number of ligands such as antibodies aptamers, peptide, polysaccharide, and small molecules have been studied to promote binding to themselves [24] (Table 6.2). Folic acid [41], epidermal growth factor [42], and transferrin [27] are common target moieties widely employed in the design of a target drug delivery system for cancer therapy. In the last few years, particularly appealing results have led to the employment of antibodies, aptamers, and peptides in the design of tumor-targeting nanoparticles for their low immunogenicity and high specificity and affinity to their biomarker [43]. Moreover, the simultaneous conjugation of more than one targeting moiety on the nanocarrier surface has been proposed to prevent receptor saturation and allows for a sufficient concentration of nanocarriers in the intracellular environment of pathological cells [44]. The high surface-area-to-volume ratio of nanosized vesicles allows, indeed, to achieve high ligand density on the surface and to bypass the activity of multidrug resistance transporter cells. To achieve better clinical outcomes, one of the last challenges of nanomedicine is the targeting of subcellular organelles such as nucleus or mitochondria [45]. Common drugs act, in fact, at the nucleus or mitochondria level, and so, the direct release at the subcellular site/organelle is necessary to enhance therapeutic efficacy. The simultaneous conjugation on the nanocarrier surface of cellular and subcellular targeting allows for nanovesicle internalization via endocytosis in disease cells and then nanoparticle delivery to a specific intracellular compartment by organelle-targeting moieties on their surface. Typical moieties widely used to mediate nuclear and mitochondrial targeting are, respectively, transactivator of transcription (TAT) peptide [46] and triphenylphosphonium (TPP) moiety [47].

6.3.3 Multifunctional vesicles

A further advance of nanotechnology relies on the development of vesicles that integrate multiple complementary targeting approaches in the same systems to optimally perform delivery functions and so improve drug efficacy.

The ability to engineer nanoscale vesicles to possess multiple functions represents the greatest remaining challenges in the field of drug delivery, opening a new avenue in clinical therapy. The design of the drug delivery platforms by combining passive, active, and stimuli-responsive targeting enhances their safety and efficacy resulting tools able to interact with a high degree of specificity with a specific cell or tissue [48].

Various combinations of targeting strategies have been investigated in the design of smart functional vesicles and have shown exciting results in preclinical studies, demonstrating their potential as therapeutics carriers [49]. Vesicles engineered to exhibit

TABLE 6.2 Diverse targeting ligands used for active and specific cell recognition of nanovesicles for cancer therapy.

	Ligand	Target	Formulation	Drug	Cells	References
Small molecules	Folic acid	FR	Span 80 niosomes	Curcumin	MCF-7, MDA-MB 231	[25]
	Folic acid	FR	FA-PEG-DSPE liposomes	5-Fluorouracil	CT26	[26]
	Transferrin	Tf-R	L64ox/Chol niosomes	Doxorubicin	MCF-7, MDA-MB-231	[27]
Peptides	ApoE	LDLR	ApoE-PS-DOX	Doxorubicin	U-87 MG	[28]
	Stearyl-H16 peptide	Lysosome	H16-Liposomes DOPC, CHOL	α-GAL (lysosomal enzyme)	HT1080	[29]
	Peptide R8	Brain	EPC, CHOL, DSPE-PEG2000 liposomes	Doxorubicin	U87-MG	[30]
	MPP Peptide	Cytochrome C reductase	CHOL, DOPE Liposomes	Antimycin A	A549	[31]
Antibodies	Anti-ER-antibody	ER	SPC, CHOL, DSPE-PEG2000 liposomes	Doxorubicin	MCF-7	[32]
	Cetuximab	EGFR	DPPC, CHOL, DSPE-PEG2000 liposomes	Doxorubicin	A431-A549	[33]
	Anti-CD123 antibodies	IL3R	Span-80, cholesterol niosomes	Daunorubicin hydrochloride	NB4, THP-1	[34]
Aptamers	TLS1c	Biotin	BioTL-Cab/ liposomes	Cabazitaxel	Caco-2, HepG2, MEAR cell lines	[35]
	AS1411	Nucleolin	Aptamer-Doxorubicin Liposomes	Doxorubicin	MCF-7	[36]
	AS1411	MMP2	PEG-Peptide-PLA polymersomes	SN38	CHO, C26	[37]
	AS1411	Nucleolin	Tween-80 niosomes	Nucleolipidic Ru (III)-complex HoThyRu	HeLa, HTB-38, HCC2998, HEK-293T	[38]
Carbohydrates	Hyaluronic acid	CD44	HA-PEG-BMLs liposomes	Doxorubicin	MEF, LLC1, U87	[39]
	Hyaluronic acid	CD44	Egg yolk lecithin, DOPE, Chol liposome	Paclitaxel	A549, MCF-7	[40]

multifunctionality and smart release provide better control of cargo release and reduced toxicity on normal tissue [50]. Moreover, nanovesicles that integrate various functionalities may perform imaging, drug monitoring, targeted delivery, and controlled release simultaneously, enhancing accurate disease diagnosis and prognosis.

6.4 Pharmaceutical application of vesicles

6.4.1 Cancer therapy

Exploiting the unique characteristics of the tumor microenvironment, vesicular systems can be smartly designed to be high selective to cancer cells. To this purpose, several strategies are used, such as active and passive targeting and stimuli-responsiveness. Passive targeting relies on the spontaneous nanodevice accumulation to the tumor site by the enhanced permeability and retention effect. Vesicles with a diameter range of 60–500 nm commonly extravasate the leaky vessels of tumor vasculature [51,52]. Anyway, this tendency is significantly limited by RES uptake in liver and spleen. To bypass this problem and extent vesicle half-life, long-circulating vesicles by surface coating with PEG have been developed [53].

Active targeting consists of covalent attachment to the vesicle surface of targeted ligands, the receptors of which are overexpressed in tumor tissue [54]. This approach promotes specific binding and cellular uptake, achieving high targeting specificity and drug delivery efficiency, avoiding the nonspecific toxic effect on healthy tissue. A large variety of molecules have been employed in the design of cancer-targeted vesicles (Table 6.2). Specific targets include growth factor receptors, G protein-coupled receptors, and integrin receptors ($\alpha v\beta 3$ and $\alpha v\beta 5$) [55]. Sometimes, vesicle constituents may possess intrinsic targeting properties as with sugar-based surfactants that exhibit glycan moieties able to address insulin-independent glucose transporter, being widely overexpressed in human tumors enhancing targeted delivery of anticancer drugs [56]. More interesting biological moieties for target drug delivery are antibodies and peptides, which exhibit improved selectivity and specificity toward overexpressed cell membrane receptors [57]. Many novel peptides have been discovered to act as ligands with high affinity of various receptors such as transferrin, epidermal growth factor (EGFR/HER1 and HER2), gastrin-releasing peptide, aminopeptidase N, vascular endothelial growth factor 2, and integrin receptors overexpressed in many tumor phenotypes [58]. In 2021, Ouyang et al. [28] demonstrated that the functionalization of polymersomes with apolipoprotein E derived peptide results in eightfold higher enrichment of doxorubicin intratumoral concentration, effectively inhibiting glioblastoma and representing a safe chemotherapy. A further advance in drug targeting was carried out by researchers developing the concept of dual targeting based on the simultaneous conjugation of various targeting ligands exploiting the synergist effect and reducing receptor saturation [59]. Folic acid was widely used for the design of dual ligand-endowed vesicles: promising results consisting of an improved cellular uptake and enhanced tumor killing effect have been observed when combined with transferrin [60], glutamic hexapeptide [61], and TAT peptide [62].

After internalization in cancer cells, it may be ideal that the nanocarrier undergoes transformation, releasing entrapped drugs in response to a given local stimulus. In light of this, smart stimulus-sensitive vesicles have been designed to achieve a specific controlled release, avoiding drug leakage in healthy tissue and subsequent toxic effects [63]. Typically, tumors have a lower pH than healthy tissues, so labile bonds based on diorthoesters, vinyl esters, cisterine-cleavable lipopolymers, double esters, and hydrazones have been proposed for the design of pH-sensitive vesicles [64]. In addition, some molecules with pH-titratable groups such as phospholipids, cholesterol derivative, and polymers [64–66] are also employed for constructing pH-sensitive tools. A further stimulus largely investigated to achieve target cancer therapy is redox potential, which takes advantage of the higher GSH intracellular concentration in tumor cells, which are able to cleave redox-cleavable groups and trigger drug release. In light of this, introduction of disulfide bonds (–S–S–), diselenide bonds (–Se–Se–), thioether bonds (–C–S–S–C–), and thioketal linkers have been actively pursued [67,68].

The use of multifunctional vectors that simultaneously possess more than one useful targeting property in the same system has been proposed as a further evolution in the field of nanomedicine [69]. Multifunctional nanoparticle systems can integrate imaging, targeting, and treatment modalities for simultaneous delivery of multiple treatment agents, applying effective combinatorial therapeutic regimens against cancer. It has been reported that stealth vesicles equipped with the targeting part possess several pharmacokinetic advantages over traditional ligand-targeted vesicles [70,71]. In 2021, Peng et al. [72] designed multitarget redox-sensitive liposomes comodified with glucose and TPP to ensure effective delivery of doxorubicin and lonidine for antiglioma therapy. Antiglioma evaluation showed that the two drugs have a synergistic effect and their delivery into liposomes could enhance their cooperation. In vitro antiglioma efficacy showed that multifunctional liposomes can inhibit tumor cell proliferation and induce apoptosis. In addition, the devices have significant interference on mitochondria, such as reducing intracellular ATP production, inducing ROS generation, and promoting depolarization of mitochondrial membrane potential. Moreover, the introduction of PEGylation through glutathione-sensitive disulfide bonds confers to the vesicle-favorable in vivo pharmacokinetic properties, brain targeting ability, low toxicity, and high antiglioma efficacy. A fascinating attempt was carried out by Baradan et al. [73], who coated liposomes encapsulating 5-fluoruracil using hyaluronic acid having not only pH sensitivity but also targeting properties to colorectal cancer cells expressing CD44 receptors. These modified liposomes showed optimal targeted delivery and drug release into colorectal cancer cells, rendering them susceptible to apoptosis, cell cycle arrest, and decreased colony formation.

A revolutionary method to fight cancer has recently emerged and is focused on the use of immune vesicles to boost immune response against tumor cells. This approach is the main strategy pursued in cancer treatment and is discussed in the paragraph below.

6.4.2 Diagnostic

Early diagnosis is a crucial factor influencing disease survival and clinical outcome [74]. Conventional diagnostics systems carry several disadvantages, such as untargeted biodistribution, low bioavailability, and delayed detection [75]. Nanoparticles hold great promise as diagnostic tools since they may be engineered to achieve high specificity toward a target, delivering a large payload amount in a single dose and simultaneously delivering both imaging agents and therapeutics, resulting in nanosystems that can simultaneously diagnose, treat, and monitor therapeutic response (nanotheranostic) [76]. Fluorescent molecules or contrast agents like gadolinium chelates and superparamagnetic iron oxide nanoparticles (SPIONs) are typically loaded in vesicles to improve their half-life and stability [77], developing nanosensors for detecting and grading diseases at the early stage. The spatial orientation of molecular cargos such as magnetic resonance imaging (MRI) contrast agents, fluorescent dyes, and drug molecules is influenced by the physicochemical properties of vesicles. Consequently, physicochemical properties could be engineered to increase the diagnostic and therapeutic efficacy of molecular cargos [78]. For example, gadolinium relaxivity depends on the ability to interact with water protons. Liposomes are not suitable devices for the gadolinium derivative due to the slower water diffusion across the lipid bilayers [79]. Polymersomes with a porous structure were prepared using a chemical initiator and phospholipids that were subsequently extracted with a surfactant, generating a highly porous outer membrane, which showed an R1 relaxivity that is threefold higher than that of nonporous polymersomes [80]. Another strategy relies on the immobilization of the chelated gadolinium on the polymersome surface that decreases the distance between the gadolinium ions and the surrounding water [81].

A niosomal formulation of methyl aminolevulinate was developed for the encapsulation of radionuclides to achieve an improved PDD/PDT (photodynamic diagnosis/therapy) system [82]. To do so, the surface of these liposomes was decorated with folate and the resulting devices demonstrated superior activities compared to the free compound. In another study, folate-targeted and radiolabeled liposomes were used for the codelivery of paclitaxel (PTX) and vinorelbine, aiming to design a theranostic system. Data obtained highlighted higher uptake in the tumor tissue, stronger antitumoral effect, and imaging potential, suggesting their promising role as a nanotheranostic agent [83].

Peptides are also employed to selectively address diagnostic nanovesicles [84]. Song et al. [85] proposed the simultaneous functionalization with two peptides targeted for angiogenesis of liposomes for the delivery of a gadolinium derivative. From the results obtained, it can be found that the simultaneous presence of two targeting moieties exerts a synergistic effect in delivering the contrast agent to the tumor site with specificity, enhancing the signal rate in in vivo MRI and resulting in a good system for molecular imaging of tumors. A pH-responsive peptide able to produce targeting activity at low pH such as that of tumor tissue was proposed for the design of theranostic devices based on liposomal formulation containing PTX and SPIONPs. The resulting nanovesicles showed effective antitumor activity with an MRI effect by producing dual functionality with a single therapeutic dosage form [86]. Demir and coworkers [87] encapsulated gold nanoparticles and a photosensitizer, protoporphyrine IX, in FA-modified targeted Tween 80/Chol niosomes to develop a theranostic tool for cancer therapy. The resulting nanovesicles, thanks to their targeting capability, exhibited therapeutic efficacy in HeLa and A549 cell lines for radiotherapy and photodynamic therapy as well as for combined therapy (PDT + RT) and cell imaging applications. An innovative tool to support COVID-19 diagnosis was developed by Hu and coworkers [88] combining two different technologies: antibody-mediated capture and liposome-mediated delivery. In the assay, extracellular vesicles directly captured from plasma through the interaction of an antibody with the surface protein CD81 were then fused with reagent-loaded liposomes to sensitively amplify and detect a SARS-CoV-2 gene target. This approach accurately identified patients with COVID-19, and its major utility is the ability to detect plasma extracellular vesicles-derived SARS-CoV-2 RNA as an early and durable sign of systemic infection and could be used as a secondary test for suspected COVID-19 cases that are negative with quantitative polymerase chain reaction with reverse transcription.

6.4.3 Gene delivery

The delivery of nucleic acids to mammalian cells (transfection) has emerged as a new frontier of molecular medicine for the genetic treatment of hereditary diseases, cancers, and some viral infections [89–92]. Although naked nucleic acid administration is considered the safest way to transfect cells, such a process is sadly ineffective. To overcome this limitation, researchers have focused on developing and using vectors as a vehicle for safe and effective gene delivery, such as nanovesicles. In 2018, the first gene nanomedicine based on liposomes (Patisiran, ONPATTRO) has been approved by the US Food and Drug Administration for the treatment of the polyneuropathy of hereditary TTR-mediated amyloidosis, enhancing the translation of gene therapy from concept to clinical application [93]. More recently, liposome technology to formulate mRNA vaccines to treat the devastating COVID-19 disease has received the approval by regulatory agencies. The main feature vesicles used to develop efficient gene delivery systems must have is the presence of a positive charge on the vesicle surface. In fact, the presence in the vesicle bilayer of cationic polymers (e.g., poly-l-lysine, polyethylenimine, poly(starchamine), and chitosan) [94] or lipids [95–97] enhances the formation of complexes with anionic nucleic acids through simple electrostatic interactions improving intracellular transfer [98]. Moreover, several studies have suggested that the type and amount of cationic lipid or surfactant significantly affects the transfection efficiency. Specifically, some helper and neutral lipids such as 1, 2-dioleoyl-sn-glycero-3-phosphoethanolamine (DOPE), dioleoylphosphatidylcholine (DOPC), monoolein (MO), and cholesterol are commonly employed in the design of gene delivery vesicles for their ability to significantly improve transfection efficiency [99]. Nonionic surfactants such as Span and Tween have been also recognized to act as a helper component, improving transfection efficiency and the stability and bilayer fluidity [100,101]. Recently, chloroquine and sphingolipids have been proposed as an interesting material for gene delivery due to their ability to act as a biophysical properties enhancer and to improve deoxyribonucleic acid (DNA) binding affinity and so transfection efficiency of niosomal formulations [102,103]. Acyl chain length and saturation influence also the efficacy of gene therapy. Abumanhal-Masarweh et al. [104] found that liposomes with longer acyl chains and monounsaturated phospholipid performed much better than shorter tails and saturated phospholipid on cellular uptake.

Transfection efficiency resulted in dependence on vesicle size and surface charge. Sakai-Kato et al. [105] investigated the effect of particle size (100–200 nm) on transfection efficiency that enhanced with the increase of particle size, which was due to the strong electrostatic interaction between cationic liposomes and plasma membrane. Conversely, fusion efficiency was reduced as the size of lipoplexes increased because larger lipoplexes were more stable than their smaller counterparts during the process of endosomal membrane fusion [106]. For efficient and targeted gene delivery to brain cells, Singhs et al. [107] developed surface-modified liposomes with a cell-penetrating peptide and transferrin loaded with chitosan-complexed plasmid DNA. Transfection efficiency in neuronal cells has been reported to be higher using bifunctional liposomes (PenTf-liposomes) compared to Plain-, Tf-, and Pen-liposomes. The efficient cellular internalization and endosomal escape properties resulted in transfection enhancement, suggesting the potentiality of the dual-targeting liposome gene delivery system to provide better brain targeting ability and therapeutic efficacy for treatment of neurodegenerative disease. More advanced approaches to augment effectiveness of gene therapy are based on the codelivery of biotherapeutic molecules along with traditional drugs in smart vesicles [108]. Saad et al. [109] formulated cationic liposomes loaded with doxorubicin complexed with siRNA for the treatment of multiresistant lung cancer cells that revealed a higher apoptosis index than each of the therapeutics when used individually. Similar results were manifested by Shim et al. [110], in whose study trilysinoyl oleylamide-based cationic liposomes were prepared for systemic codelivery of siRNA and an anticancer drug. The advantages of chemotherapeutic and biological drugs were also combined in a pH-sensitive liposome-based platform by Swami et al. [111], achieving a notably elevated tumor cell toxicity compared to individual counterparts. Maurer and coworkers [112] designed magnetic cation niosomes for siRNA delivery in combination with either erlotinib or trastuzumab against BT-474 cells. The noisome mediated downregulation of the antiapoptotic LFG gene in BT-474 cells, increasing the activity of the targeted antineoplastic agents more profoundly as compared to their combination with free siRNA.

6.4.4 Immunotherapy and vaccines

Nowadays, immunotherapy and vaccines, both aiming to boost the human immune system, represent the mainstream and efficacious strategies for the prevention and treatment of a variety of diseases, including infectious and cancer.

The first vaccines based on killed microorganisms or viruses, live attenuated organisms, and inactivated toxins drastically reduced the morbidity and mortality of numerous diseases over the past two centuries [113]. Despite the progress and wide use of these conventional vaccines, they still have the risk that attenuated antigens may revert to full virulence and there will be limited immune response [114]. Recent advances in vaccinology have led to the development of nanovaccines that have advantages of lymph node accumulation and antigen presentation compared with conventional vaccines. One of the main advantages of using nanovesicles for antigen delivery is the ability to protect it from nonspecific degradation, to control the delivery profile, and to codeliver other chemotherapeutics for a potential synergic therapy [115]

Strategies employed to design vesicles for immunotherapy application involve mainly the activation of antigen-presenting cells (APCs) or the amelioration of the cell microenvironment from immunosuppressive to immunoactive [116].

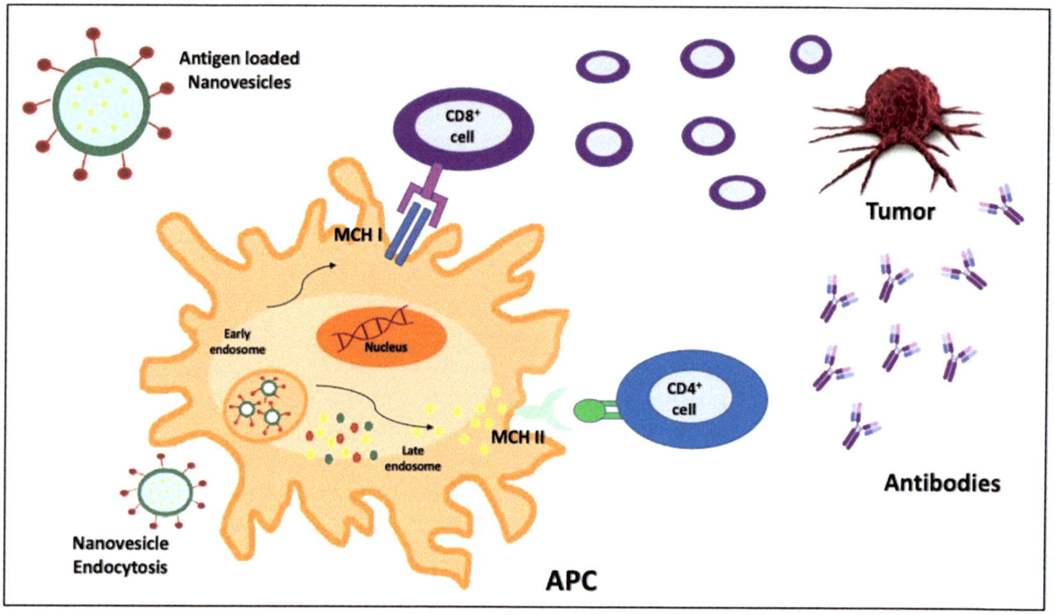

FIGURE 6.4 **Schematic representation of cancer immunotherapy mediated by nanovesicles.** Nanovesicles loaded with antigens or mRNA-encoding antigen proteins are recognized by APC-inducing antigen presentation by two major pathways. In the first, the exogenous antigen is degraded via the endosome pathway and is loaded onto major histocompatibility complex (MHC) class II, activating the helper ($CD4^+$) cell and thus inducing humoral immunity. This interaction promotes the activation of B cells that produce proinflammatory cytokines and antibodies that trigger tumor apoptosis. In the second pathway, the endogenous antigen is degraded in proteasomes and is loaded onto MHC class I molecules, thereby inducing the activation of $CD8^+$ lymphocytes that subsequently attack tumor cell inducing cytotoxicity.

To this goal, nanovesicles can be loaded with several immune modulators (cytokines, interleukins, chemokines, antibodies, and toll-like receptor (TLR) agonists) or antigens (proteins, peptides, DNA, etc.).

In the first strategy, vesicles loaded with antigens are recognized and uptaken by APCs that present the captured antigens on major histocompatibility complex (MHC) molecules to T cells by two different pathways. In the first, the exogenous antigen is degraded via the endosome pathway and is loaded onto MHC class II molecules, activating B cells and thus inducing humoral immunity. In the second pathway, the endogenous antigen is degraded in proteasomes and is loaded onto MHC class I molecules, thereby inducing cellular immunity via the proliferation and differentiation into specific cytotoxic T cells, thus more effectively exerting the cell killing effect (Fig. 6.4).

Liposomes represent ideal devices for the cytosolic pathway for their intrinsic membrane fusion ability [117]. Furthermore, different studies highlight the ability of the cation lipid to increase the deposition of antigen at the injection site and prolong the presence of antigen depot in the draining lymph nodes, resulting in sustained antigen uptake and APC activation [118].

It has been shown that surface charge is the crucial factor affecting immune response activation and that positively charged (cationic) liposomes are more effective as vaccine adjuvants than negatively charged (anionic) and zwitterionic (neutral) liposomes [119,120] This superiority is due to the ability of cationic liposomes to promote the effective uptake by APCs due to the electrostatic interaction between the cationic liposomal parts and the negatively charged molecules on the surface of APCs [121]. This facilitates fusion with APCs, with subsequent intracellular localization of the liposomes and release of their antigen payload.

For instance, in 2018, Sailor and coworkers [122] used positively charged fusogenic siRNA-loaded liposomes to enhance immune responses to Staphylococcus aureus infection, resulting in the knock down of proinflammatory marker IRF5 in macrophages and increased elimination capacity and accelerate healing.

The immunostimulatory effect of cationic liposomes depends on the composition of the phospholipid used, including the type of lipid head groups, hydrophobic acyl tails, and their degree of saturation. Cationic liposomes based on ethylphosphocholine derivatives (1,2-dioleoyl-sn-glycero-3-ethylphosphocholine) are more effective in stimulating the maturation of DCs than those prepared using 1,2-dioleoyl-3-trimethylammonium-propane (DOTAP) lipids. A variety of cationic liposomes have been shown to mediate immunostimulatory effects. The most commonly used cationic liposomes are those prepared with dimethyl dioctadecylammonium, 3β-[N-(N′, N′-dimethylaminoethane)-carbamoyl] cholesterol, and DOTAP [123].

To increase antigen cross-presentation, nanovesicles have been rationally designed in multiple ways. One strategy relies on surface modifications using pH-responsive or fusogenic materials that lead to cross-presentation of exogenous antigens via the cytosolic pathway. Conversely, the targeting of receptors on APCs has been pursued to selectively release exogenous antigen in early endosomes, activating the vacuolar pathway.

In the cytosolic pathway, surface conjugation with a pH-sensitive polymer or fusogenic peptide has been proposed to induce a vesicular destabilization in the acidic cytosol environment, resulting in the cytosolic delivery of encapsulated immunostimulating agents and enhanced therapeutic effect. Cell-penetrating peptides such as octaarginine (R8) and fusogenic peptides (e.g., GALA and KALA) are commonly use to achieve them [124]. Similarly, synthetic polymers based on poly(carboxyl acid) having pH-responsive membrane-disruptive ability such as poly(ethyl acrilic acid) and poly(propyl acrylic acid), and carboxyl group-introduced poly(glycidol)s that are able to induce membrane fusion after protonation of their carboxyl groups are also employed [125]. Innovative tools for cancer immunotherapy were developed by Pithchamaini et al. [126] that synthetize fusogenic NKsome made up of activated natural killer membranes fused with the cationic liposome capable of directly target tumor cells, thanks to the abnormal expression of NK-92 cell membrane receptors. The engineered NKsome loaded with doxorubicin can recognize tumor cells with the help of NK cell markers and fused with the tumor cells more efficiently than normal cells, thereby showing its antitumor potential by releasing the chemotherapeutic drug. NKsome shows a higher affinity toward cancer than normal cells and exhibits enhanced tumor homing efficiency in vivo with an extended circulation half-life. Moreover, liposomes showed excellent antitumor potential against human breast cancer cells and MCF-7 in vitro and in vivo.

As already cited, another strategy used in immunotherapy is the targeting of APCs by conjugation on the vesicle surface of the molecule that is able to specifically target receptors overexpressed on APCs. In light of this, glycan molecules that exhibit a high specificity toward C-type lectin receptors (CLRs) are widely used, which enhance loading and presentation of antigen through MHC class I and II, induce antigen-specific $CD4^+$ and $CD8^+$ T-cell proliferation, and skew T-helper cells [127]. In 2019, Liu et al. [128] designed drug-free mannosylated liposomes that are able to target macrophage phenotypes, enhancing tumor growth inhibition compared to bare liposomes. An interesting result was achieved using glycoliposomes obtained by coating liposomes with glycan Lewis(Le)X, which is highly specific for CLR. The obtained liposomes when loaded with the adjuvant monophosphoryl lipid A induced dendritic cell maturation and a potent antitumor response [129].

Inclusion of methoxypoly(ethyleneglycol), mPEG-phospholipid, into the liposomal bilayer successfully enhanced lymph node accumulation [130]. In a recent study, Truong et al. [131] investigated the effect of Tween 80 and Tween 20 incorporation in the lipid bilayer on size, charge, stability, DNA encapsulation, and in vivo transfection efficiency.

Tweens belong to a family of PEG surfactants with branched PEG chains attached to lipid tails with different lengths, and so, this difference could affect immune response. Indeed, in vivo transfection studies demonstrated that particles with the shorter Tween 20 were able to target the lymph nodes more efficiently and achieved highly specific transfection better than the longer Tween 80.

The second strategy used in the development of immunovesicles is turning the immunosuppressive environment immunoactive by upregulation of immunoactive signaling pathways (e.g., the stimulator of interferon genes [STING] pathway), inhibition of immune checkpoints (e.g., PD-1, PD-L1, and cytotoxic T-lymphocyte antigen 4 [CTLA-4]), and polarization of M2 TAMs to M1 macrophages.

A cytosolic pattern recognition receptor utilized for spontaneous induction of antitumor T-cell immunity is used to activate STING. Wilson J. T. et al. [132]. designed pH-sensitive polymersomes for efficient cytosolic delivery of 2′,5–3′5′ cyclic guanosine monophosphate–adenosine monophosphate, agonists of STING. The incorporation of pH-sensitive, cationic 2-(diethylamino) ethyl methacrylate groups in the polymersome structure mediates the intracellular release of GAMP via an endosomal escape mechanism enhancing its immunomodulatory potency and therapeutic efficacy, resulting in tumor growth inhibition and inducing a immunological memory that protects against tumor rechallenge. In 2020, Chang H. C. et al. [133]. constructed pH-induced transformable nanovesicles based on poly(e-caprolactone)-hydrazone-PEG for the codelivery of tumor endogenous antigens HCP and immunological adjuvants CpG ODNs. Nanovesicles were also modified with CD80 antibody for APC targeting, and after APC-targeted delivery inside immune organs (spleen and lymph nodes), they remarkably are degraded in the acidic environment of endosome/lysosome, resulting in a stronger cargo release. Subsequently, CpG ODNs activate TLR9 signaling, while HCPs were presented by MHC I and II molecules, and these two routes induce a synergistic T cell-mediated antitumor immune response.

Another strategy to enhance antitumor immunoresponse involves the use of antibodies or inhibitor that block programmed death ligand-1 (PD-L1)/PD-1 pathways. In light of this, the research group of Guo [134] developed pH-sensitive liposome coloaded with docetaxel and PD-L1 antibody to kill tumor cell directly, while switching off immunosuppression. This smart platform exhibited effective tumor inhibition and prolonged survival time due to activation of the tumor-specific $CD8^+$ T cell, highly selective tumor killing, and decreased systemic toxicity. Another checkpoint inhibitor widely used to enhance nanoparticle immune response is CD47. For instance, Zhou and coworkers [135] designed MMP-2/pH dual-activable prodrug vesicle for cancer immunotherapy combining CD induction and CD47 blockade via the loading with a photosensitizer and oxaliplatin. The obtained nanoplatform efficiently suppressed the growth of both primary tumors and distant metastasis. Moreover, a specific antitumor immune memory effect to prevent autologous tumor recurrence was also observed. Using monoclonal antibodies is also one of the main ongoing clinical approaches to enhance immune responses against cancer cells. For instance, Irvine et al. [136] engineered, with anti-CD137 and an IL-2Fc fusion protein, the surfaces of PEGylated liposomes to activate tumor-specific T lymphocytes and tumor-draining lymph nodes and, thus, antitumor immune response. PEGylated liposomes containing CTLA-4-blocking monoclonal antibodies were prepared and their therapeutic effect and biodistribution were evaluated in mice bearing colon carcinoma tumors. PEGylated liposomes had prolonged blood half-lives and higher accumulation at the tumor site than non-PEGylated liposomes and free CTLA-4 blockade antibody. According to these results, improved therapeutic response consisting of lowest tumor volume and highest survival time were also observed, suggesting their great potentiality to be translated to clinical trials [137].

In the last few years, using nucleic acid vaccines has become an innovative and interesting strategy for combatting infectious diseases and cancers. Compared with traditional vaccines, nucleic acid-based vaccines have the advantages of being safe, easy to produce, scalable, modifiable, and inexpensive and exhibiting a shorter production cycle [138]. Notably, the application of mRNA as vaccine has long been hampered by instability, innate immunogenicity, and low delivery efficiency in vivo. To overcome these hurdles, appropriate delivery systems have been studied and the emerging of SARS-COV-2 infection in 2019 accelerated the development of mRNA vaccines [139]. In December 2020, FDA approved the first mRNA drugs (Pfizer/BioNTech COVID-19 vaccines) for use in humans. Nucleic acid loaded in nanocarriers contain instructions to guide the host cells to produce antigenic proteins, which, subsequently, stimulate specific immune responses. Vaccines are cationic nanoparticles, consisting of a cholesterol, an ionizable cationic lipid, a PEGylated lipid, a phospholipid (distearoylphosphatidylcholine) helper lipid, and entrapped mRNA coding for the protein spike of the coronavirus. The mRNA will then be expressed as the spike protein, in turn promoting an immune response to it that will kill or inactivate the invading virus. The mechanism by which liposomes act as an immunological adjuvant to augment the immune response to the spike protein is not clear at present.

Richner et al. [140] developed mRNA nanovesicles vaccine encoding Zika structural genes to protect against Zika virus infection for intramuscular delivery to induce high levels of protein expression in vivo. The results showed that it conferred protection and sterilized immunity in several strains of immunocompetent mice and the protective response was durable; even 14 weeks after boosting, challenged mice showed no morbidity or mortality. In one of the first proof-of-concept study, researchers compared the efficacy to boost mice's immune response of mRNA vaccine based on liposomes consisting of ionizable amino lipid, phospholipid, cholesterol, and PEG containing lipid and commercial vaccines by inactivated virus against rabies and influenza [141]. A strong immune response in mice were achieved, which was similar to or even higher than that achieved after a single intramuscular injection of nonreplicating mRNA vaccines, which induced functional antibody titers comparable to vaccination with a full human dose of licensed vaccines based on inactivated virus. The efficacy remained stable during an observation period of up to 1 year after one single booster dose, opening new avenues for accelerated vaccine development in the field of infectious diseases. More recently [142], a first-in-human study focused on mRNA vaccine encapsulated in liposomes using as antigen rabies virus glycoprotein was carried out to assess the safety, reactogenicity, and immunogenicity potential of this new vaccine model in comparison with a licensed rabies vaccine formulation in adult human volunteers. The authors observed a high reactogenicity at the initial tested doses of 5 μg, while when tested at 1 and 2 μg doses, no vaccine-related serious adverse events or withdrawals occurred. Moreover, liposomal formulation had functional antibody responses after two doses that were comparable with three doses of licensed rabies vaccine up to 4 weeks after the second dose.

To date, in clinical trials of tumor immunotherapy applications, many studies have evaluated the antitumor effect of mRNA vaccines and indicated that it is feasible to use mRNA vaccines for the prevention and treatment of tumors.

In 2018, Guan et al. [143] developed immunostimulatory spherical nucleic acids consisting of liposomal cores functionalized with a dense shell of RNA inserted into the wall of the lipid core via hydrophobic cholesterol moieties. The resulting device was able to selectively target toll-like receptors TLRs and triggered an NF-κB pathway to activate dendritic cells greater than that of free or cationic lipid-transfected RNA of the same sequence selective for them.

In another work, Markov et al. [144] proposed the use of mannosilated liposomes for the delivery of plasmid DNA encoding EGFP and total tumor RNA to DC. The resulting device enhanced the antitumor response in a murine melanoma model reducing five- to sixfold the number of melanoma lung metastases.

Sayour and coworkers [145] designed RNA cancer vaccine based on nanoliposomes encapsulated with personalized tumor-derived mRNA (representing a tumor-specific transcriptome). The developed vaccine was shown to significantly increase percent expression of MHC class I/II, costimulatory molecules, and activation markers on tumor APCs and potentiate antitumor T cell immunity through endogenous host T-cell responses.

A promising vaccine platform for cancer treatment based on DPPP:Chol liposomes coencapsulating the pore-forming protein sticholysin II (StII) with ovalbumin (OVA) has been developed by Lanio et al. [146]. Resulting devices were able to induce OVA-specific cytotoxic T lymphocyte (CTL) activation and an antitumor response in vivo. Specifically, the study highlighted that liposomes were encapsulated by a phagocytic mechanism resulting in the cross-presentation of the encapsulated OVA by the vacuolar pathways, suggesting the vital role of macrophages in antigen cross presentation and inducing of immune response.

6.5 Conclusions and outlooks

Overall, vesicular systems are some of the best new delivery entities that have great potential for targeted drug delivery. Smart vesicles have already enhanced anticancer therapy and the delivery of vaccines, proteins, and DNA, and further benefits could be achieved soon, allowing for their translation in clinical practice. In addition to their biocompatibility and biodegradability, they provide an ideal opportunity for the development of versatile drug delivery platforms owing to possibility of using several kinds of material in the vesicular membrane, such as polymers, lipids, and nonionic surfactants. An accurate selection of different components could lead to the construction of tailor-made devices with desirable properties for the desired therapeutic purpose. Some liposome-based formulations are currently in clinical use, but despite extensive studies, there are still many hurdles to overcome before the full therapeutic potential of vesicular systems can be achieved. Reliable and reproducible fabrication processes and good scale-up properties must be developed. Moreover, the in vivo behavior of vesicle systems in terms of biodistribution, biological fate, and acute and subacute toxicity needs to be intensively investigated. We can hope to know more about it in the coming years.

References

[1] Kapoor B, Gupta R, Gulati M, Singh SK, Khursheed R, Gupta M. The why, where, who, how, and what of the vesicular delivery systems. Adv Colloid Interface Sci, 271. 2019. p. 101985.
[2] Kamboj S, Saini V, Magon N, Bala S, Jhawat V. Vesicular drug delivery systems: a novel approach for drug targeting. Int J Drug Deliv 2013;5(2):121–30.
[3] Liang CH, Chou TH. Effect of chain length on physicochemical properties and cytotoxicity of cationic vesicles composed of phosphatidylcholines and dialkyldimethylammonium bromides. Chem Phys Lipids 2009;158(2):81–90.
[4] Attwood D. The mode of association of amphiphilic drugs in aqueous solution. Adv Colloid Interface Sci 1995;55:271–303.
[5] Tavano L, Mazzotta E, Muzzalupo R. Innovative topical formulations from diclofenac sodium used as surfa-drug: the birth of diclosomes. Colloids Surf B: Biointerfaces 2018;164:177–84.
[6] Bangham AD, Horne RW. Nature 1962;196:952–3.
[7] Alibolandi M, Abnous K, Mohammadi M, Hadizadeh F, Sadeghi F, Taghavi S, et al. J Contr Rel 2017;264:228.
[8] Mathiyazhakan M, Wiraja C, Xu C. A concise review of gold nanoparticles-based photo-responsive liposomes for controlled drug delivery. Nano-micro Lett 2018;10(1):1–10.
[9] Mohammadi M, Shaegh SAM, Alibolandi M, Ebrahimzadeh MH, Tamayol A, Jaafari MR, et al. J Contr Rel 2018;274:35.
[10] Barenholz Y. Liposome application: problems and prospects. Curr Opcol interface Sci 2001;6(1):66–77.
[11] Sercombe L, Veerati T, Moheimani F, Wu SY, Sood AK, Hua S. Advances and challenges of liposome assisted drug delivery. Front Pharmacol 2015;6:286.
[12] Moghimi SM, Szebeni J. Stealth liposomes and long circulating nanoparticles: critical issues in pharmacokinetics, opsonization andprotein-binding properties. Prog Lipid Res 2003;42:463–78. Available from: https://doi.org/10.1016/S0163-7827(03)00033-X.
[13] Mahale NB, Thakkar PD, Mali RG, Walunj DR, Chaudhari SR. Niosomes: novel sustained release nonionic stable vesicular systems—an overview. Adv Colloid Interface Sci 2012;183:46–54.
[14] Pérez L, Pinazo A, Pons R, Infante M. Gemini surfactants from natural amino acids. Adv Colloid Interface Sci 2014;205:134–55.
[15] Pinazo A, Manresa MA, Marques AM, Bustelo M, Espuny MJ, Pérez L. Amino acid–based surfactants: new antimicrobial agents. Adv Colloid Interface Sci 2016;228:17–39.
[16] Kita-Tokarczyk K, Grumelard J, Haefele T, Meier W. Block copolymer vesicles—using concepts from polymer chemistry to mimic biomembranes. Polymer 2005;46(11):3540–63.
[17] Jang WS, Park SC, Kim M, Doh J, Lee D, Hammer DA. The effect of stabilizer on the mechanical response of double-emulsion-templated polymersomes. Macromol Rapid Commun 2015;36(4):378–84.

[18] Egli S, Schlaad H, Bruns N, Meier W. Functionalization of block copolymer vesicle surfaces. Polymers 2011;3 (1):252–80.
[19] Wang S, Hu X, Wei W, Ma G. Transformable vesicles for cancer immunotherapy. Adv Drug Deliv Rev 2021;179:113905.
[20] El-Sawy HS, Al-Abd AM, Ahmed TA, El-Say KM, Torchilin VP. Stimuli-responsive nano-architecture drug-delivery systems to solid tumor micromilieu: past, present, and future perspectives. ACS Nano 2018;12 (11):10636–64.
[21] Wang Y, Kohane DS. External triggering and triggered targeting strategies for drug delivery. Nat Rev Mater 2017;2(6):1–14.
[22] Kauscher U, Holme MN, Björnmalm M, Stevens MM. Physical stimuli-responsive vesicles in drug delivery: Beyond liposomes and polymersomes. Adv Drug Deliv Rev 2019;138:259–75.
[23] Thambi T, Lee DS. Stimuli-responsive polymersomes for cancer therapy. Stimuli responsive polymeric nanocarriers for drug delivery applications. Woodhead Publishing; 2019. p. 413–38.
[24] Kim JW, Cochran JR. Targeting ligand–receptor interactions for development of cancer therapeutics. Curr OpChem Biol 2017;38:62–9.
[25] Akbarzadeh I, Yaraki MT, Ahmadi S, Chiani M, Nourouzian D. Folic acid-functionalized niosomal nanoparticles for selective dual-drug delivery into breast cancer cells: an in-vitro investigation. Adv Powder Technol 2020;31(9):4064–71.
[26] Moghimipour E, Rezaei M, Ramezani Z, Kouchak M, Amini M, Angali KA, et al. Folic acid-modified liposomal drug delivery strategy for tumor targeting of 5-fluorouracil. Eur J Pharm Sci 2018;114:166–74.
[27] Tavano L, Muzzalupo R, Mauro L, Pellegrino M, Ando S, Picci N. Transferrin-conjugated pluronic niosomes as a new drug delivery system for anticancer therapy. Langmuir 2013;29(41):12638–46.
[28] Ouyang J, Jiang Y, Deng C, Zhong Z, Lan Q. Doxorubicin delivered via ApoE-directed reduction-sensitive polymersomes potently inhibit orthotopic human glioblastoma xenografts in nude mice. Int J Nanomed 2021;16:4105.
[29] Hayashi T, Shinagawa M, Kawano T, Iwasaki T. Drug delivery using polyhistidine peptide-modified liposomes that target endogenous lysosome. Biochem Biophys Res Commun 2018;501(3):648–53.
[30] Yuan BO, Zhao Y, Dong S, Sun Y, Hao F, Xie J, et al. Cell-penetrating peptide-coated liposomes for drug delivery across the blood–brain barrier. Anticancer Res 2019;39(1):237–43.
[31] Mallick S, Lee S, Park JI, Choi JS. Liposomes containing cholesterol and mitochondria-penetrating peptide (MPP) for targeted delivery of antimycin A to A549 cells. Colloids Surf B: Biointerfaces 2018;161:356–64.
[32] Wang Y, Wang Z, Qian Y, Fan L, Yue C, Jia F, et al. Synergetic estrogen receptor-targeting liposome nanocarriers with anti-phagocytic properties for enhanced tumor theranostics. J Mater Chem B 2019;7(7):1056–63.
[33] Liu KC, Arivajiagane A, Wu SJ, Tzou SC, Chen CY, Wang YM. Development of a novel thermal-sensitive multifunctional liposome with antibody conjugation to target EGFR-expressing tumors. Nanomed Nanotechnol Biol Med 2019;15(1):285–94.
[34] Liu FR, Jin H, Wang Y, Chen C, Li M, Mao SJ, et al. Anti-CD123 antibody-modified niosomes for targeted delivery of daunorubicin against acute myeloid leukemia. Drug Deliv 2017;24(1):882–90.
[35] Cheng Y, Ou Z, Li Q, Yang J, Hu M, Zhou Y, et al. Cabazitaxel liposomes with aptamer modification enhance tumor-targeting efficacy in nude mice. Mol Med Rep 2019;19(1):490–8.
[36] Xing H, Tang L, Yang X, Hwang K, Wang W, Yin Q, et al. Selective delivery of an anticancer drug with aptamer-functionalized liposomes to breast cancer cells in vitro and in vivo. J Mater Chem B 2013;1 (39):5288–97.
[37] Ramezani P, Abnous K, Taghdisi SM, Zahiri M, Ramezani M, Alibolandi M. Targeted MMP-2 responsive chimeric polymersomes for therapy against colorectal cancer. Colloids Surf B: Biointerfaces 2020;193:111135.
[38] Riccardi C, Fàbrega C, Grijalvo S, Vitiello G, D'Errico G, Eritja R, et al. AS1411-decorated niosomes as effective nanocarriers for Ru (III)-based drugs in anticancer strategies. J Mater Chem B 2018;6(33):5368–84.
[39] Jose G, Lu YJ, Chen HA, Hsu HL, Hung JT, Anilkumar TS, et al. Hyaluronic acid modified bubble-generating magnetic liposomes for targeted delivery of doxorubicin. J Magnetism Magnetic Mater 2019;474:355–64.
[40] Tian Y, Zhang H, Qin Y, Li D, Liu Y, Wang H, et al. Overcoming drug-resistant lung cancer by paclitaxel-loaded hyaluronic acid-coated liposomes targeted to mitochondria. Drug Dev Ind Pharm 2018;44(12):2071–82.

[41] Narmani A, Rezvani M, Farhood B, Darkhor P, Mohammadnejad J, Amini B, et al. Folic acid functionalized nanoparticles as pharmaceutical carriers in drug delivery systems. Drug Dev Res 2019;80(4):404–24.
[42] Grapa CM, Mocan T, Gonciar D, Zdrehus C, Mosteanu O, Pop T, et al. Epidermal growth factor receptor and its role in pancreatic cancer treatment mediated by nanoparticles. Int J Nanomed 2019;14:9693.
[43] Bazak R, Houri M, El Achy S, Kamel S, Refaat T. Cancer active targeting by nanoparticles: a comprehensive review of literature. J Cancer Res Clin Oncol 2015;141(5):769–84.
[44] Peiris PM, He F, Covarrubias G, Raghunathan S, Turan O, Lorkowski M, et al. Precise targeting of cancer metastasis using multi-ligand nanoparticles incorporating four different ligands. Nanoscale 2018;10 (15):6861–71.
[45] Chen WH, Luo GF, Zhang XZ. Recent advances in subcellular targeted cancer therapy based on functional materials. Adv Mater 2019;31(3):1802725.
[46] Pan L, He Q, Liu J, Chen Y, Ma M, Zhang L, et al. Nuclear-targeted drug delivery of TAT peptide-conjugated monodisperse mesoporous silica nanoparticles. J Am Chem Soc 2012;134(13):5722–5.
[47] Battogtokh G, Choi YS, Kang DS, Park SJ, Shim MS, Huh KM, et al. Mitochondria-targeting drug conjugates for cytotoxic, anti-oxidizing and sensing purposes: current strategies and future perspectives. Acta Pharm Sin B 2018;8(6):862–80.
[48] Choudhury H, Gorain B, Pandey M, Nirmal J, Kesharwani P. Surface engineering of nanoparticles for imparting multifunctionality. Nanoparticle therapeutics. Academic Press; 2022. p. 181–210.
[49] Tavano L, Muzzalupo R. Multi-functional vesicles for cancer therapy: the ultimate magic bullet. Colloids Surf B: Biointerfaces 2016;147:161–71.
[50] Meng S, Su B, Li W, Ding Y, Tang L, Zhou W, et al. Enhanced antitumor effect of novel dual-targeted paclitaxel liposomes. Nanotechnology 2010;21(41):415103.
[51] Maeda H, Nakamura H, Fang J. The EPR effect for macromolecular drug delivery to solid tumors: improvement of tumor uptake, lowering of systemic toxicity, and distinct tumor imaging in vivo. Adv Drug Deliv Rev 2013;65(1):71–9.
[52] Fang J, Nakamura H, Maeda H. The EPR effect: unique features of tumor blood vessels for drug delivery, factors involved, and limitations and augmentation of the effect. Adv Drug Deliv Rev 2011;63(3):136–51.
[53] Gabizon A, Catane R, Uziely B, Kaufman B, Safra T, Cohen R, et al. Prolonged circulation time and enhanced accumulation in malignant exudates of doxorubicin encapsulated in polyethylene-glycol coated liposomes. Cancer Res 1994;54(4):987–92.
[54] Frisch B, Hassane FS, Schuber F. Conjugation of ligands to the surface of preformed liposomes by click chemistry. Liposomes. Humana Press; 2010. p. 267–77.
[55] Vhora I, Patil S, Bhatt P, Gandhi R, Baradia D, Misra A. Receptor-targeted drug delivery: current perspective and challenges. Ther Deliv 2014;5(9):1007–24.
[56] Muzzalupo R, Tavano L, La Mesa C. Alkyl glucopyranoside-based niosomes containing methotrexate for pharmaceutical applications: evaluation of physico-chemical and biological properties. Int J Pharm 2013;458 (1):224–9.
[57] Mojarad-Jabali S, Farshbaf M, Walker PR, Hemmati S, Fatahi Y, Zakeri-Milani P, et al. An update on actively targeted liposomes in advanced drug delivery to glioma. Int J Pharm 2021;602:120645.
[58] Aronson MR, Medina SH, Mitchell MJ. Peptide functionalized liposomes for receptor targeted cancer therapy. APL Bioeng 2021;5(1):011501.
[59] Hare JI, Moase EH, Allen TM. Targeting combinations of liposomal drugs to both tumor vasculature cells and tumor cells for the treatment of HER2-positive breast cancer. J Drug Target 2013;21(1):87–96.
[60] Tavano L, Mauro L, Naimo GD, Bruno L, Picci N, Andò S, et al. Further evolution of multifunctional niosomes based on pluronic surfactant: dual active targeting and drug combination properties. Langmuir 2016;32(35):8926–33.
[61] Yang Y, Zhao Z, Xie C, Zhao Y. Dual-targeting liposome modified by glutamic hexapeptide and folic acid for bone metastatic breast cancer. Chem Phys Lipids 2020;228:104882.
[62] Zhao P, Wang H, Yu M, Cao S, Zhang F, Chang J, et al. Paclitaxel-loaded, folic-acid-targeted and TAT-peptide-conjugated polymeric liposomes: in vitro and in vivo evaluation. Pharm Res 2010;27(9):1914–26.
[63] Mura S, Nicolas J, Couvreur P. Stimuli-responsive nanocarriers for drug delivery. Nat Mater 2013;12 (11):991–1003.

[64] Ferreira DDS, Lopes SCDA, Franco MS, Oliveira MC. pH-sensitive liposomes for drug delivery in cancer treatment. Ther Deliv 2013;4(9):1099–123.
[65] Baranei M, Taheri RA, Tirgar M, Saeidi A, Oroojalian F, Uzun L, et al. Anticancer effect of green tea extract (GTE)-Loaded pH-responsive niosome Coated with PEG against different cell lines. Mater Today Commun 2021;26:101751.
[66] Kocak G, Tuncer C, Butun V. pH-responsive polymers. Polym Chem 2017;8:144–76.
[67] Scott EA, Stano A, Gillard M, Maio-Liu AC, Swartz MA, Hubbell JA. Dendritic cell activation and T cell priming with adjuvant- and antigenloaded oxidation-sensitive polymersomes. Biomaterials 2012;33:6211–19.
[68] Ong W, Yang Y, Cruciano AC, McCarley RL. Redox-triggered contents release from liposomes. J Am Chem Soc 2008;130(44):14739–44.
[69] Singh A, Talekar M, Tran TH, Samanta A, Sundaram R, Amiji M. Combinatorial approach in the design of multifunctional polymeric nano-delivery systems for cancer therapy. J Mater Chem B 2014;2(46):8069–84.
[70] Noble GT, Stefanick JF, Ashley JD, Kiziltepe T, Bilgicer B. Ligand-targeted liposome design: challenges and fundamental considerations. Trends Biotechnol 2014;32(1):32–45.
[71] Sapra P, Allen TM. Ligand-targeted liposomal anticancer drugs. Prog Lipid Res 2003;42(5):439–62.
[72] Peng Y, Lu J, Li R, Zhao Y, Hai L, Guo L, et al. Glucose and triphenylphosphonium co-modified redox-sensitive liposomes to synergistically treat glioma with doxorubicin and lonidamine. ACS Appl Mater Interfaces 2021;13(23):26682–93.
[73] Mansoori B, Mohammadi A, Abedi-Gaballu F, Abbaspour S, Ghasabi M, Yekta R, et al. Hyaluronic acid-decorated liposomal nanoparticles for targeted delivery of 5-fluorouracil into HT-29 colorectal cancer cells. J Cell Physiol 2020;235(10):6817–30.
[74] Stephen BJ, Suchanti S, Mishra R, Singh A. Cancer nanotechnology in medicine: a promising approach for cancer detection and diagnosis. Crit Rev Ther Drug Carr Syst 2020;37:375–405.
[75] Siegmund KD, Marjoram P, Woo YJ, Tavare S, Shibata D. Inferring clonal expansion and cancer stem cell dynamics from DNA methylation patterns in colorectal cancers. Proc Natl Acad Sci USA 2009;106:4828–33.
[76] Indoria S, Singh V, Hsieh MF. Recent advances in theranostic polymeric nanoparticles for cancer treatment: a review. Int J Pharm 2020;582:119314.
[77] Ahmad J, Ahmad MZ, Akhter H. Surface-engineered cancer nanomedicine: rational design and recent progress. Curr Pharm Des 2020;26:1181–90.
[78] Leong J, Teo JY, Aakalu VK, Yang YY, Kong H. Engineering polymersomes for diagnostics and therapy. Adv Healthc Mater 2018;7(8):1701276.
[79] Smith CE, Shkumatov A, Withers SG, Yang B, Glockner JF, Misra S, et al. ACS Nano 2013;7:9599.
[80] Cheng Z, Tsourkas A. Langmuir 2008;24:8169.
[81] Turner JL, Pan D, Plummer R, Chen Z, Whittaker AK, Wooley KL. Adv Funct Mater 2005;15:1248.
[82] Haran G, Cohen R, Bar LK, Barenholz Y. Transmembrane ammonium sulfate gradients in liposomes produce efficient and stable entrapment of amphipathic weak bases. Biochim Biophys Acta 1993;1151(2):201–15.
[83] Karpuz M, Silindir-Gunay M, Ozer AY, Ozturk SC, Yanik H, Tuncel M, et al. Diagnostic and therapeutic evaluation of folate-targeted paclitaxel and vinorelbine encapsulating theranostic liposomes for non-small cell lung cancer. Eur J Pharm Sci 2021;156:105576.
[84] Wang SH, Lee ACL, Chen IJ, Chang NC, Wu HC, Yu HM, et al. Structure-based optimization of GRP78-binding peptides that enhances efficacy in cancer imaging and therapy. Biomaterials 2016;94:31–44.
[85] Song Y, Li W, Meng S, Zhou W, Su B, Tang L, et al. Dual integrin αvβ 3 and NRP-1-targeting paramagnetic liposome for tumor early detection in magnetic resonance imaging. Nanoscale Res Lett 2018;13(1):1–9.
[86] Zheng XC, Ren W, Zhang S, Zhong T, Duan XC, Yin YF, et al. The theranostic efficiency of tumor-specific, pH-responsive, peptide-modified, liposome-containing paclitaxel and superparamagnetic iron oxide nanoparticles. Int J Nanomed 2018;13:1495.
[87] Demir B, Barlas F, Gumus ZP, Ünak P, Timur S. Theranostic niosomes as a promising tool for combined therapy and diagnosis: "All-in-One" approach. ACS Appl Nano Mater 2018;1(6):2827–35.
[88] Ning B, Huang Z, Youngquist BM, Scott JW, Niu A, Bojanowski CM, et al. Liposome-mediated detection of SARS-CoV-2 RNA-positive extracellular vesicles in plasma. Nat Nanotechnol 2021;16(9):1039–44.
[89] Lostalé-Seijo I, Montenegro J. Synthetic materials at the forefront of gene delivery. Nat Rev Chem 2018;2(10):258–77.
[90] Wirth T, Parker N, Ylä-Herttuala S. History of gene therapy. Gene 2013;525(2):162–9.

[91] Pan JJ, Zhang SW, Chen CB, Xiao SW, Sun Y, Liu CQ, et al. Effect of recombinant adenovirus-p53 combined with radiotherapy on long-term prognosis of advanced nasopharyngeal carcinoma. J Clin Oncol 2009;27 (5):799–804.

[92] Aied A, Greiser U, Pandit A, Wang W. Polymer gene delivery: overcoming the obstacles. Drug Discov Today 2013;18(21–22):1090–8.

[93] Hoy SM. Patisiran: first global approval. Drugs 2018;78:1625–31.

[94] Barua S, Ramos J, Potta T, Taylor D, Huang HC, Montanez G, et al. Discovery of cationic polymers for non-viral gene delivery using combinatorial approaches. Comb Chem High Throughput Screen 2011;14 (10):908–24.

[95] Hoekstra D, Rejman J, Wasungu L, Shi F, Zuhorn I. Gene delivery by cationic lipids: in and out of an endosome. Biochem Soc Trans 2007;35(1):68–71.

[96] Alvarez-Lorenzo C, Barreiro-Iglesias R, Concheiro A, Iourtchenko L, Alakhov V, Bromberg L, et al. Biophysical characterization of complexation of DNA with block copolymers of poly (2-dimethylaminoethyl) methacrylate, poly (ethylene oxide), and poly (propylene oxide). Langmuir 2005;21(11):5142–8.

[97] Simões S, Filipe A, Faneca H, Mano M, Penacho N, Düzgünes N, et al. Cationic liposomes for gene delivery. Expert Opin drug Deliv 2005;2(2):237–54.

[98] Ojeda E, Agirre M, Villate-Beitia I, Mashal M, Puras G, Zarate J, et al. Elaboration and physicochemical characterization of niosome-based nioplexes for gene delivery purposes. In *Non-viral gene delivery vectors*. New York, NY: Humana Press; 2016. p. 63–75.

[99] Tavano L, Mazzotta E, Muzzalupo R. Nanovesicular formulations for cancer gene therapy. Curr Pharm Des 2017;23(35):5327–35.

[100] Huang YZ, Gao JQ, Chen JL, et al. Cationic liposomes modified with non-ionic surfactants as effective non-viral carrier for gene transfer. Colloids Surf B: Biointerfaces 2006;49:158–64.

[101] Huang Y, Rao Y, Chen J, et al. Polysorbate cationic synthetic vesicle for gene delivery. J Biomed Mat Res 2011;96:513–19.

[102] Sainz-Ramos M, Villate-Beitia I, Gallego I, Al Qtaish N, Menéndez M, Lagartera L, et al. Correlation between biophysical properties of niosomes elaborated with chloroquine and different tensioactives and their transfection efficiency. Pharmaceutics 2021;13(11):1787.

[103] Qtaish NA, Gallego I, Villate-Beitia I, Sainz-Ramos M, Martínez-Navarrete G, Soto-Sánchez C, et al. Sphingolipid extracts enhance gene delivery of cationic lipid vesicles into retina and brain. Eur J Pharm Biopharm 2021;169:103–12.

[104] Abumanhal-Masarweh H, da Silva D, Poley M, Zinger A, Goldman E, Krinsky N, et al. Tailoring the lipid composition of nanoparticles modulates their cellular uptake and affects the viability of triple negative breast cancer cells. J Control Rel 2019;307:331–41.

[105] Sakai-Kato CK, Yoshida K, Izutsu KI. Effect of surface charge on the size-dependent cellular internalization of liposomes. Chem Phys Lipids 2019;224:104726–32.

[106] Bruininks BMH, Souza PCT, Ingolfsson H, Marrink S-JJ. A molecular view on the escape of lipoplexed DNA from the endosome. eLife 2020;9:52012–28.

[107] Dos Santos Rodrigues B, Banerjee A, Kanekiyo T, Singh J. Functionalized liposomal nanoparticles for efficient gene delivery system to neuronal cell transfection. Int J Pharm 2019;566:717–30.

[108] Abtahi NA, Naghib SM, Ghalekohneh SJ, Mohammadpour Z, Nazari H, Mosavi SM, et al. Multifunctional stimuli-responsive niosomal nanoparticles for co-delivery and co-administration of gene and bioactive compound: in vitro and in vivo studies. Chem Eng J 2022;429:132090.

[109] Saad M., Garbuzenko O.B., Minko T. Co-delivery of siRNA and an anticancer drug for treatment of multidrug-resistant cancer; 2008.

[110] Shim G, Han SE, Yu YH, Lee S, Lee HY, Kim K, et al. Trilysinoyl oleylamide-based cationic liposomes for systemic co-delivery of siRNA and an anticancer drug. J Contr Rel 2011;155(1):60–6.

[111] Swami R, Kumar Y, Chaudhari D, Katiyar SS, Kuche K, Katare PB, et al. pH sensitive liposomes assisted specific and improved breast cancer therapy using co-delivery of SIRT1 shRNA and Docetaxel. Mater Sci Eng C 2021;120:111664.

[112] Maurer V, Altin S, Ag Seleci D, Zarinwall A, Temel B, Vogt PM, et al. In-vitro application of magnetic hybrid niosomes: targeted siRNAdelivery for enhanced breast cancer therapy. Pharmaceutics 2021;13:394.

[113] De Gregorio E, Rappuoli R. From empiricism to rational design: a personal perspective of the evolution of vaccine development. Nat Rev Immunol 2014;14(7):505–14.
[114] Appay V, Douek DC, Price DA. CD8 + T cell efficacy in vaccination and disease. Nat Med 2008;14(6):623–8.
[115] Sahdev P, Ochyl LJ, Moon JJ. Biomaterials for nanoparticle vaccine delivery systems. Pharm Res 2014;31:2563–82.
[116] Shi Y. Clinical translation of nanomedicine and biomaterials for cancer immunotherapy: progress and perspectives. Adv Ther 2020;3(9):1900215.
[117] Yuba E. Design of pH-sensitive polymer-modified liposomes for antigen delivery and their application in cancer immunotherapy. Polym J 2016;48(7):761–71.
[118] Henriksen-Lacey M, Christensen D, Bramwell VW, Lin-denstrøm T, Agger EM, Andersen P, et al. Liposomal cationic charge and antigen adsorption are important properties for the efficient deposition of antigen at the injection site and ability of the vaccine to induce a CMI response. J Contr Rel 2010;145:102–8.
[119] Smith DM, Simon JK, Baker Jr JR. Applications of nanotechnology for immunology. Nat Rev Immunol 2013;13(8):592–605.
[120] Latin N, Bachhawat BK. The effect of liposome surface charges in immunopotentiation. Biosci Rep 1984;4:99–107.
[121] Nakanishi T, Kunisawa J, Hayashi A, Tsutsumi Y, Kubo K, Nakagawa S, et al. The positively charged liposome functions as an efficient immune adjuvant in inducing immune responses to soluble proteins. Biochem Biofis res Common 1997;240:793–7.
[122] Kim B, Pang HB, Kang J, Park JH, Ruoslahti E, Sailor MJ. Immunogene therapy with fusogenic nanoparticles modulates macrophage response to Staphylococcus aureus. Nat Commun 2018;9(1):1–13.
[123] Inglut CT, Sorrin AJ, Kuruppu T, Vig S, Cicada J, Ahmad H, et al. Immunological and toxicological considerations for the design of liposomes. Nanomaterials 2020;10:190.
[124] Yang Z, Ma Y, Zhao H, Yuan Y, Kim BY. Nanotechnology platforms for cancer immunotherapy. Wiley Interdiscip Rev Nanomed Nanobiotechnol 2020;12(2):e1590.
[125] Yuba E. Liposome-based immunity-inducing systems for cancer immunotherapy. Mol Immunol 2018;98:8–12.
[126] Pitchaimani A, Nguyen TDT, Aryal S. Natural killer cell membrane infused biomimetic liposomes for targeted tumor therapy. Biomaterials. 2018;160:124–37.
[127] Streng-Ouwehand I, Unger WW, Van Kooyk Y. C-type lectin receptors for tumor eradication: future directions. Cancers 2011;3(3):3169–88.
[128] Ye J, Yang Y, Dong W, Gao Y, Meng Y, Wang H, et al. Drug-free mannosylated liposomes inhibit tumor growth by promoting the polarization of tumor-associated macrophages. Int J Nanomed 2019;14:3203.
[129] Boks MA, Ambrosini M, Bruijns SC, Kalay H, van Bloois L, Storm G, et al. MPLA incorporation into DC-targeting glycoliposomes favours anti-tumour T cell responses. J Control Rel 2015;216:37–46.
[130] Moghimi SM. The effect of methoxy-PEG chain length and molecular architecture on lymph node targeting of immuno-PEG liposomes. Biomaterials 2006;27:136–44.
[131] Zukancic D, Suys EJA, Pilkington EH, Algarni A, Al-Wassiti H, Truong NP. The importance of poly(ethylene glycol) andlipid structure in targeted gene delivery to lymph nodes by lipid nanoparticles. Pharmaceutics 2020;12:68.
[132] Shae D, Becker KW, Christov P, Yun DS, Lytton-Jean AKR, Sevimli S, et al. Endosomolytic polymersomes increase the activity of cyclic dinucleotide STING agonists to enhance cancer immunotherapy. Nat Nanotechnol 2019;14:269–78.
[133] Chang HC, Zou ZZ, Wang QH, Li J, Jin H, Yin QX, et al. Targeting and specific activation of antigen-presenting cells by endogenous antigen-loaded nanoparticles elicits tumor-specific immunity. Adv Sci 2020;7:1900069.
[134] Gu Z, Wang Q, Shi Y, Huang Y, Zhang J, Zhang X, et al. Nanotechnology-mediated immunochemotherapy combined with docetaxel and PD-L1 antibody increase therapeutic effects and decrease systemic toxicity. J Contr Rel 2018;286:369–80.
[135] Zhou F, Feng B, Yu H, Wang D, Wang T, Ma Y, et al. Tumor microenvironment-activatable prodrug vesicles for nanoenabled cancer chemoimmunotherapy combining immunogenic cell death induction and CD47 blockade. Adv Mater 2019;31(14):1805888.

[136] Kwong B, Gai SA, Elkhader J, Wittrup KD, Irvine DJ. Localized immunotherapy via liposome-anchored Anti-CD137 + IL-2 prevents lethal toxicity and elicits local and systemic antitumor immunity. Cancer Res 2013;73(5):1547–58.
[137] Nikpoor AR, Tavakkol-Afshari J, Sadri K, Jalali SA, Jaafari MR. Improved tumor accumulation and therapeutic efficacy of CTLA-4-blocking antibody using liposome-encapsulated antibody: in vitro and in vivo studies. Nanomedicine 2017;13:2671–82.
[138] Azad N, Rojanasakul Y. Vaccine delivery-current trends and future. Curr drug Deliv 2006;3(2):137–46.
[139] Wang Y, Zhang R, Tang L, Yang L. Nonviral delivery systems of mRNA vaccines for cancer gene therapy. Pharmaceutics 2022;14(3):512.
[140] Richner JM, Himansu S, Dowd KA, Butler SL, Salazar V, Fox JM, et al. Modified mRNA vaccines protect against zika virus infection. Cell 2017;168:1114–25.
[141] Lutz J, Lazzaro S, Habbeddine M, Schmidt KE, Baumhof P, Mui BL, et al. Unmodified mRNA in LNPs constitutes a competitive technology for prophylactic vaccines. NPJ Vaccines 2017;2(1):1–9.
[142] Aldrich C, Leroux-Roels I, Huang KB, Bica MA, Loeliger E, Schoenborn-Kellenberger O, et al. Proof-of-concept of a low-dose unmodified mRNA-based rabies vaccine formulated with lipid nanoparticles in human volunteers: a phase 1 trial. Vaccine 2021;39:1310–18.
[143] Guan C, Chernyak N, Dominguez D, Cole L, Zhang B, Mirkin CA. RNA-based immunostimulatory liposomal spherical nucleic acids as potent TLR7/8 modulators. Small 2018;14(49):1803284.
[144] Markov OV, Mironova NL, Shmendel EV, Serikov RN, Morozova NG, Maslov MA, et al. Multicomponent mannose-containing liposomes efficiently deliver RNA in murine immature dendritic cells and provide productive anti-tumour response in murine melanoma model. J Contr Rel 2015;213:45–56.
[145] Sayour EJ, De Leon G, Pham C, Grippin A, Kemeny H, Chua J, et al. Systemic activation of antigen-presenting cells via RNA-loaded nanoparticles. Oncoimmunology 2017;6(1):e1256527.
[146] Cruz-Leal Y, Grubaugh D, Nogueira CV, Lopetegui-González I, Del Valle A, Escalona F, et al. The vacuolar pathway in macrophages plays a major role in antigen cross-presentation induced by the pore-forming protein sticholysin II encapsulated into liposomes. Front Immunol 2018;2473.

CHAPTER

7

Polymeric micelles in drug delivery and targeting

Anchal Pathak, Teeja Suthar, Gautami Nirbhavane and Keerti Jain

Drug Delivery and Nanomedicine Research Laboratory, Department of Pharmaceutics, National Institute of Pharmaceutical Education and Research (NIPER)—Raebareli, Lucknow, Uttar Pradesh, India

Abbreviations

AFM	Atomic force microscopy
CD44	Cluster of differentiation 44
CMC	Critical micelle concentration
DiR	1,10-dioctadecyl-3,3,30,30-tetramethylindotricarbocyanine iodide
DOX	Doxorubicin
EPR	Enhanced permeability and retention
FA	Folic acid
FR	Folate receptors
FRET	Förster resonance energy transfer
GSH	Glutathione
HA	Hyaluronic acid
LCST	Lower critical solution temperature
MMP	Matrix metalloproteinases
PCL	Poly(ε-caprolactone)
PDC	Polymer–drug conjugates
PDI	Polydispersity index
PDT	Photodynamic therapy
PE	Poly(ester)
PEG	Polyethylene glycol
PEO	Poly(ethylene oxide)
PMs	Polymeric micelles
PNIPAM	Poly(N-isopropyl acrylamide)
TPGS	D-α-Tocopheryl polyethylene glycol 1000 succinate

Molecular Pharmaceutics and Nano Drug Delivery
DOI: https://doi.org/10.1016/B978-0-323-91924-1.00004-6

7.1 Introduction

Nanomedicine is one of the extensively researched fields that aims to improve the pharmaceutical and health care strategies. Advancement in nanotechnology has encouraged the fabrication of various nanocarriers like liposomes, micelles, carbon nanotubes, dendrimers, and nanoemulsions, which have been employed for several biomedical applications, including drug delivery and diagnostic imaging [1–4]. Nanomedicine can be explored to enhance the solubility of poorly soluble drugs, deliver large therapeutic molecules across biological barriers, and protect the therapeutic agents during systemic circulation [5,6]. In the recent years, amphiphilic block copolymers have been explored to formulate nanosystems to achieve controlled and targeted delivery of drugs, peptides, and genes.

Polymeric micelles (PMs) are core-shell type nanostructures, having a size between 10 and 100 nm. Amphiphilic block copolymers get assembled into organized core-shell structures in aqueous solution at the copolymer concentration above the critical micelle concentration (CMC) to form PMs (Fig. 7.1) [7]. The exceptional properties of PMs, including flexible structure, stimuli-responsive cargo release, and charge-switching ability enable them to overcome the limitations of the existing delivery systems such as poor bioavailability, rapid drug release, and drug efflux. PMs exhibit several advantages over other nanocarriers like narrow size range, high solubilizing capacity, low toxicity, longer half-life, and excellent targeting efficiency. The inner hydrophobic core acts as a nanochamber for the incorporation of lipophilic therapeutic agents, which can enhance the solubility up to 500-fold, and the outer hydrophilic shell protects them from the external environment (temperature, concentration, pH, etc.) [8].

The core-shell structure of PMs prevents the drug removal by the mononuclear phagocyte system and enables extended systemic circulation of the drug. PMs can be utilized to achieve drug accumulation at the targeted locus in chemotherapy, as its tunable size range could increase the localization of the therapeutic agent around the tumor microenvironment by the enhanced permeability and retention (EPR) effect. PMs also bestow the ability to encapsulate more than one type of therapeutic agent and modify its release. PMs have been explored as theranostic nanosystems for the chemotherapy mapping and imaging of the tumor site [9].

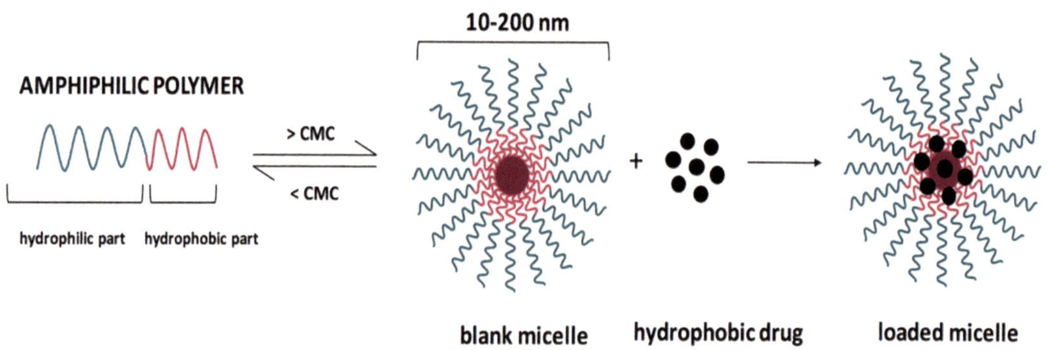

FIGURE 7.1 Schematic representation of polymeric micelle, where the hydrophobic drug is incorporated within the core of micelles. Reproduced with permission from [6].

This chapter summarizes the applicability of PMs as a drug delivery platform, integrated with smart functionalities to achieve enhanced solubility and improved targetability. Various techniques for characterization of PMs like CMC, morphology, drug loading, and drug release are discussed in the following sections. Considering the applicability of PMs in drug delivery and targeting, novel interactions in PMs can be elucidated and capitalized to improve therapeutic outcomes.

7.2 Polymeric micelles

Micellization is a spontaneous process, where the amphiphilic diblock or triblock copolymers assemble into nanosized aggregates above their CMC, through noncovalent interactions like hydrogen bonding or van der Waals interaction, and form self-organized molecular assembly called PMs. The formation of PMs is influenced by attractive and repulsive interactions, where attractive forces cause the molecules to associate, while the repulsive force prevents the micelles from expanding indefinitely [10]. At concentrations below their CMC, the polymer exists as a single entity, whereas on increasing the concentration toward the CMC, the polymer molecules assemble themselves in a micellar form so that the hydrophobic component is separated from the aqueous component [11].

Different types of PMs can be synthesized based upon the amphiphilic copolymer, polymer concentration, temperature, and the solvent parameters such as pH and solvent ratio. The drug can be incorporated within the PMs through polymer–drug conjugation, drug encapsulation, or development of polyion complex micelles [12]. Polyion complexes are formed *via* spontaneous assemblage of ionic copolymers with oppositely charged therapeutic agents or genetic materials.

7.2.1 Polymer–drug conjugates

Polymer–drug conjugates (PDCs) are formed between the drug and functional groups present over polymeric surface *via* hydrolysable chemical bonds [13]. The copolymers such as poly(ethylene oxide) (PEO)-b-poly(amino acid), PEO-b poly(ester) (PE), polyethylene glycol (PEG)-b-P(β-benzyl-L-aspartate), and (PEG)-b-P(γ-benzyl-L-glutamate) etc. have been explored till now for developing PDCs. These polymers contain numerous functional moieties, which allows for conjugation of therapeutic compounds to the polymeric chain. For example, reactive groups of drug molecules are conjugated covalently with PEO-b-PEs through the activated terminal hydroxyl group of the PE region. The poly(amino acid) block also contains several functional groups, which allow multiple drug molecules to be conjugated to a single polymeric chain [14]. There are two major approaches to develop PDCs; the first one is self-assembling of the amphiphilic copolymer incorporating both drugs as well as targeting moieties, and the second one is the coassembly of a block copolymer–drug conjugate and a block copolymer-targeting moiety conjugate forming mixed micelles [15].

With the continued advances in the development of PMs, "smart" PMs were introduced, which were responsive toward biological stimulus, such as, pH, temperature, or ionic strength. The polymers exploited in PMs, respond through conformational changes to enable the release of the therapeutic agent in response to biological stimulus. Rashidzadeh et al. synthesized glycidyl azide polymer-curcumin conjugate through pH-sensitive imine linkage. The fabricated conjugate self-assembled into a micellar system in aqueous media with a size of 180 nm. In vitro release studies indicated pH-triggered curcumin release in acidic conditions (64%), as compared to the normal physiological condition (13.5%) in 30 hours [16]. This study indicates the stability of the amphiphilic conjugate at normal physiological conditions, which can dissociate in the acidic microenvironment at the tumor site, suggesting that "smart PMs" could be an attractive approach to deliver the chemotherapeutic agents.

7.2.2 Drug-encapsulated polymeric micelles

Physical and chemical techniques are employed to achieve solubilization and stable encapsulation of drugs within PMs. The chemical method involves covalent cross-linking of the therapeutic agent with side chains of functionalized block copolymers. Monodisperse PMs are formed when the reactive moieties of the copolymer are aptly hydrophobic or low in number. The most common ways of cross-linked PMs fabrication are (1) radical polymerization (PMs with polymerizable moieties in the core), (2) bifunctional crosslinkers (PMs with reactive moieties in the core), and (3) disulfide bonds (PMs with thiol groups) [13].

PMs can be fabricated by physical methods, which involves (1) direct dissolution method, where copolymers and therapeutic agents are dispersed in the water followed by its self-assembly into PMs above the CMC [17]; (2) solvent evaporation (or solvent casting) method, which uses volatile organic solvents such as methanol or chloroform that can dissolve both the drug and the copolymer. Drug and copolymer are first solubilized in the solvent and then solvent is evaporated forming a thin polymeric film. Hydration of this film under constant stirring forms drug-loaded PMs [18]; (3) dialysis method, which is utilized to develop PMs for poorly water-soluble polymers or therapeutic agents. The mixture of therapeutic agent and copolymer is solubilized in water-miscible organic solvent, followed by dialysis against water, which replaces the organic solvent from the system and forms drug-loaded PMs [19]; (4) freeze-drying technique involves the development of PMs by preparing dispersion of drugs and copolymers in freeze-dryable organic solvents (i.e., tert-butyl alcohol or pentane), followed by freeze-drying and reconstitution with isotonic aqueous media [20]. (5) Cosolvent evaporation techniques involve the preparation of dispersion of polymers and drugs in a water-miscible organic solvent. The aqueous phase (nonsolvent for the core-forming copolymer) is added to the organic phase, which forms PMs after the evaporation of organic cosolvent in the final step [21].

7.2.3 Polyion complex micelles

A polyion complex system is fabricated by the electrostatic interaction between oppositely charged polymer and drug combinations. This method is suitable for DNA, peptides, and other charge-carrying therapeutic moieties. When the charge is neutralized, the block copolymer self-assembles into the polyion complex and stabilizes micelles [22]. The morphology of polyion complexes is determined by the topology of polyelectrolytes employed and the pattern of their assembly. The major limitation of these complexes is their probable instability during the self-assembly process, which is affected by polyelectrolyte concentration, mixing ratio, and polyion complexes cross-linking [23]. The polyion complex may incorporate various features manipulated by the addition of salt, change in temperature, and pH. For example, salt addition leads to the shielding of charges, which reduces the polyelectrolyte interactions and triggers for micelles disassembly. pH also manipulates the complexation and formation of polyion complex micelles. These features explain the utility of polyion micelles in biomedical applications such as delivery of nucleic acids and peptides [24].

7.3 Characterization and evaluation of polymeric micelles

The nanosize, ease of fabrication, and excellent solubilization properties make PMs a noteworthy carrier for various drug delivery applications. Improved bioavailability of drug and targeted/controlled drug release can be obtained *via* these nanocarriers. PMs can be characterized for morphology (particle size and shape), CMC, optical transmittance, thermodynamic and kinetic stability, critical solution temperature, and drug release kinetics (Fig. 7.2). These characteristics determine the fate of PMs and drug bioavailability. Various parameters for characterization of PMs are briefly discussed in the following subtopics.

7.3.1 Particle size, size distribution, and zeta potential

Dynamic light scattering can be utilized for determination of average particle size, polydispersity index (PDI), and surface charge of the PMs. The PDI monitors the physical stability of the PMs, where lower values indicate monodisperse particles and a PDI value of more than 0.7 represents polydispersity of the sample. The zeta potential can be utilized to predict the storage stability of the PMs, where the aggregation of PMs is less likely to happen if they possess sufficient surface charge density over the surface providing electric interparticulate repulsion. PMs with a zeta potential value of about ± 30 mV are electrostatically stable and represent a stable micellar nanosystem [25].

7.3.2 Morphology and shape

The morphology of the PMs can be determined by electron microscopy and atomic force microscopy (AFM). Electron microscopy generates images *via* electron beam interactions with the sample at various depths. Scanning electron microscopy utilizes a specific set of coils to scan the beam in the raster-like pattern and collect scattered electrons, while transmission electron microscopy uses the transmitted electrons from the sample and offers information regarding the inner structure, morphology, and stress state of the

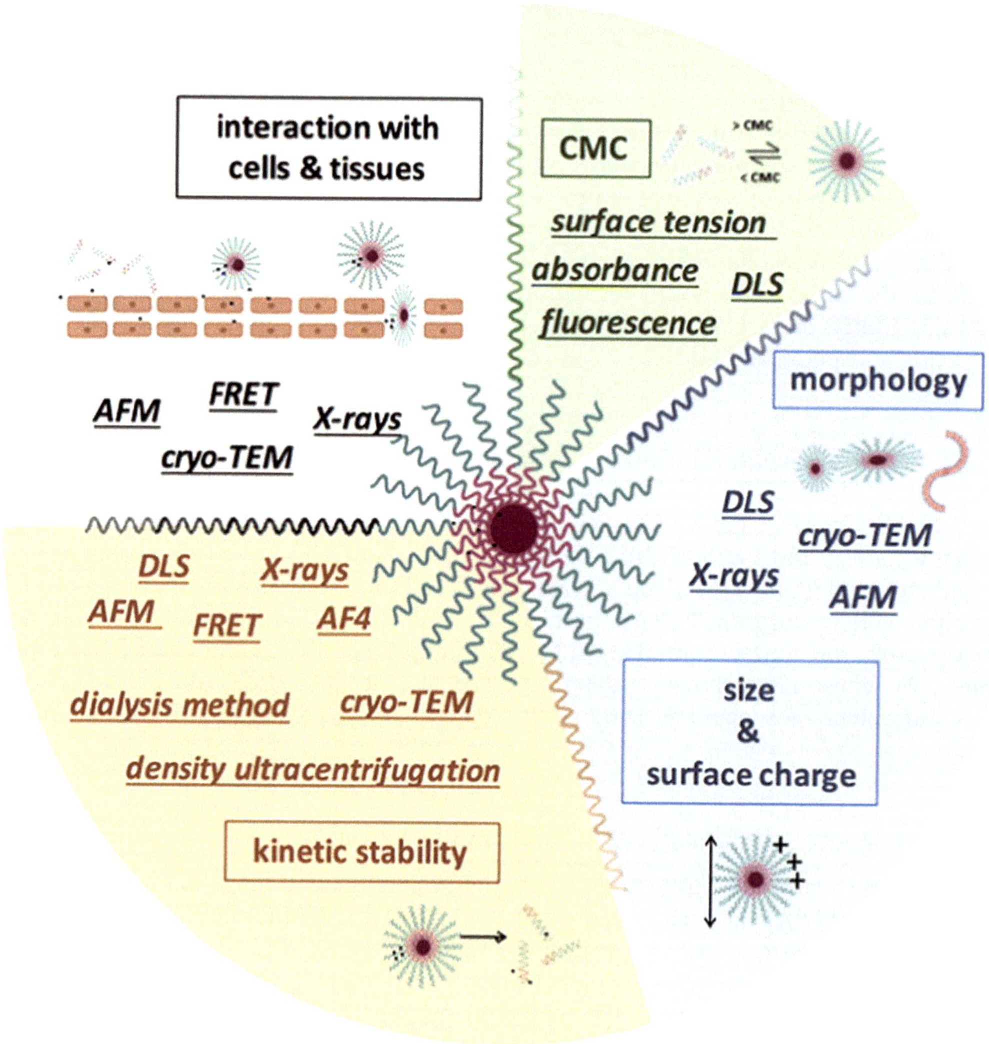

FIGURE 7.2 Characterization techniques of polymeric micelles. Reproduced with permission from [6]. *AFM*, Atomic force microscopy; *FRET*, Förster resonance energy transfer; *DLS*, dynamic light scattering; *AF4*, flow field-flow fractionation; *cryo-TEM*, cryo-transmission electron microscopy.

sample. AFM can be used for the determination of qualitative and quantitative aspects about physical properties of micellar systems [25]. Sipos et al. developed dexamethasone-loaded mixed PMs to enhance the solubility of drug. AFM was used to determine the morphology of the PMs, where planar AFM images showed aggregation of PMs, followed by formation of clusters around the cryoprotectant mannose, with the average size of PMs between 60 and 100 nm (Fig. 7.3) [26].

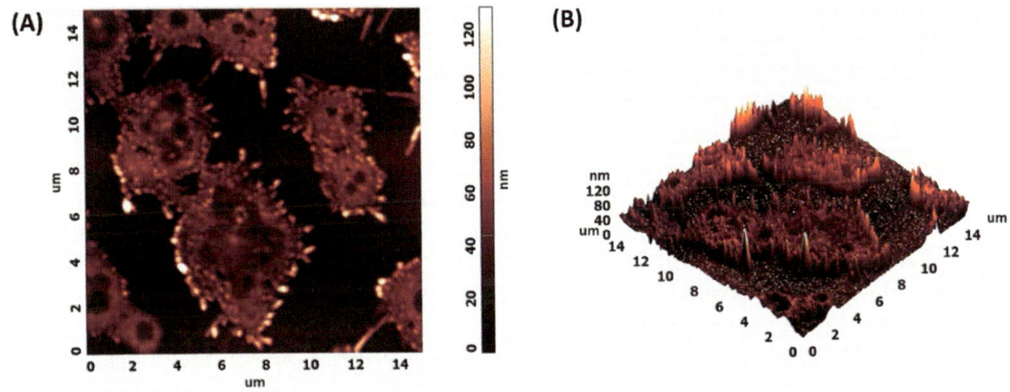

FIGURE 7.3 Atomic force microscopy images of dexamethasone loaded polymeric micelles: (A) planar image and (B) 3D topographical image. Reproduced with permission from [26].

7.3.3 Critical micelle concentration

The CMC determines the thermodynamic stability, where low values of CMC indicate better stability of PMs. CMC is affected by various factors like hydrophobicity, the glass transition temperature, and the hydrophilic/hydrophobic length blocks ratio. Low value of CMC of amphiphilic copolymers is desirable for long blood circulation, which is achieved by augmenting the hydrophobic segment of amphiphilic micelles. The measurement of conductivity, osmotic pressure, interfacial tension, and viscosity can be used to determine the CMC [6]. CMC can also be determined by the surface tension method, using the Wilhelmy plate or the Du Noüy ring [27,28].

7.3.4 Stability

The physical and kinetic stability of the PMs can be determined through Förster resonance energy transfer (FRET), resonance energy transfer, electronic energy transfer, and zeta potential. FRET is used to analyze the structure stability, micellar assembly, and the drug micelle association [29]. PMs should confer predetermined thermodynamic and kinetic stability that prevent the uncontrolled and premature drug release. The biodistribution, metabolism, and toxicity of PMs can be altered by the absorption of intracellular fluid proteins over the micellar surface and formation of corona [6].

7.3.5 In vitro drug release studies

The rate of drug release from the PMs can be determined through the in vitro release studies, where the dissolution media is selected on the basis of the drug solubility and stability in media, test sensitivity, and the test procedure. Several factors can affect drug release from PMs, including the amount of drug(s) loaded, the partition coefficient, core size, and the existence of cross-linking. The dialysis bag method can be used to carry out the drug release studies, where drug-loaded PMs are kept in the dialysis bag having an appropriate molecular weight cut-off and dialyzed against release media [30].

Several factors determine the release of drug from PMs, which is related to the rate of polymer degradation, construct of the copolymer and drug, fabrication methods used for PMs development, physicochemical characteristics of PMs, and the method of drug incorporation within the PMs. The drug release from the PMs is also affected by the rate of drug diffusion, rate of copolymer degradation, and partition coefficient [14]. Drugs can be released from the PMs *via* different mechanisms like (1) polymer protonation/deprotonation, followed by the dissociation of the amphipathic structure, (2) separation of the PM amphiphilic blocks, (3) disruption of the bond between the drug and polymer, and (4) reduced hydrophobicity of the hydrophobic segment of the PMs, which causes swelling of PMs and release of drug from the PMs [31]. The major difference in the mechanism of drug release from the PMs and polyion complexes is that drug release is preceded by diffusion in PMs, whereas exchange of ions in physiological media triggers the release of the drug from the polyion complex. Modification of the chemical assembly of the PM-forming block copolymer could alter the characteristics of the core-shell forming block and modify drug release patterns. For instance, the sustained drug release pattern can be attained by increasing the lipophilicity or rigidity of the micellar core, which confines the ion movements inside the micellar core in the PMs. Also, the reduced rate of micellar dissociation and sustained drug release can be achieved *via* introduction of strong hydrophobic interactions among core-forming blocks and drugs [13].

7.4 Application of polymeric micelles in drug delivery

Current therapeutic regimens of various ailments, including cancer, infectious disease, and neurodegenerative disorders necessitate the usage of targeted drug delivery to achieve the required drug concentration at the anticipated locus [32,33]. However, the existence of a blood–brain barrier, drug resistance, and presence of efflux pumps over the cell surface reduces the therapeutic efficiency of drugs. PMs are one of the most prominent nanocarriers that can improve the solubility of poorly soluble drugs, protect the cargo during in vivo transit, overcome the biological barriers, and provide controlled drug release with excellent target specificity. PMs have also been explored for the targeted delivery, where the fundamental concepts of EPR effect and utilization of targeting ligand enhance the preferential accumulation of drug at the target site [2,34]. The applications of PMs are described in the following subsections.

7.4.1 Solubility enhancement

PMs have been extensively investigated to enhance the solubility of poorly soluble drugs, improve the bioavailability, and eradicate erratic biodistribution patterns. The hydrophobic interior of PMs serves as a solubilization depot for the poorly soluble drugs that otherwise would precipitate in gastrointestinal fluid, while the hydrophilic shell assists in preventing opsonization of the PMs, leading to longer systemic circulation and good stability in vivo [35].

In an attempt to enhance the solubility of dasatinib for the treatment of proliferative vitreoretinopathy, Li at al. fabricated dasatinib-loaded PMs of PEG-b-poly(ε-caprolactone) (PCL) *via* the antisolvent method with an average size of 55 nm, 95.41% entrapment efficiency, and 1.94% drug loading. The results suggested that PMs improved the solubility of dasatinib up to 475 times the saturated solubility of the drug. Dasatinib-loaded PMs significantly inhibited cellular proliferation, adhesion, and migration in comparison to the pure drugs owing to the enhanced solubility of the drugs [36]. Mikhail and Allen coupled docetaxel to the hydrophobic segment of PEG-b-PCL and confirmed the formation of PDC by proton nuclear magnetic resonance spectroscopy and gel permeation chromatography studies. Encapsulation of docetaxel in PMs led to a 1840 times enhancement in the solubility of docetaxel [37].

Hussein et al. prepared self-assembled PMs from block copolymer poloxamer 407 and encapsulated tenoxicam within the core to enhance the solubility of the drug. The micellar system demonstrated the size of 33.07 nm, a low PDI of 0.155, and an entrapment efficiency 84.02%. Saturation solubility of the tenoxicam-loaded PMs lyophilized powder showed about 122-fold enhancement in aqueous solubility in comparison to the free drug, subsequently enhanced the oral bioavailability of tenoxicam [38]. These studies clearly indicate that PMs can be utilized to increase the solubility of hydrophobic drugs, which further improve the bioavailability and therapeutic efficacy of drugs.

7.4.2 Passive targeting

The term "passive targeting" has been widely utilized in the field of nanomedicine to enhance the accumulation of therapeutic agent at the targeted locus. The vasculature permeability is altered in the case of inflammation or tumors due to inflammatory stimuli such as cytokines and microbial toxins [39]. The defective leaky vasculature and diminished lymphatic drainage system in cancer could result in "passive targeting." PMs have been developed to achieve passive targeting by the EPR effect in cancer therapy, where the chemotherapeutic agent could attain entry and accumulation at the cancer site [40]. The physiochemical characteristics of PMs like particle size, molecular weight, and zeta potential can influence the tumor targeting property through a leaky vasculature. Positively charged nanocarriers undergo rapid clearance from blood as compared to the negatively charged ones; therefore, negatively charged nanocarriers are preferred in cancer targeting through the EPR effect [33].

The passive targeting by PMs is hindered either by premature release of the therapeutic agent from the nanocarrier, or inadequate delivery at the target site. Therefore, a major challenge in passive targeting by PMs is the selection of the appropriate polymeric micellar system that can constrain the premature drug release and promote cellular internalization to achieve adequate drug accumulation at the site of action [14]. Further, passive targeting approaches are nonselective, as they affect the healthy cells as well, thus necessitating the use of various ligands to achieve selective targeting at the site of action.

7.4.3 Active targeting

Active targeting or ligand-mediated targeting guides the nanosystem to the targeted locus and increases the cellular uptake. Targeting ligands have the affinity for receptors expressed over the target cells, which promotes specific ligand–receptor interactions. The ligand targeting is directed to enhance the interaction between nanocarrier and the cell, followed by increased concentration of drug at the target site [41].

PMs anchored with ligand mediates transmembrane-specific receptor–ligand interactions, which facilitate selective binding of carrier to the target receptors. Functionalization with targeting ligand facilitates transcytosis across the cells *via* several mechanisms including receptor-mediated, transporter-mediated, or cell-mediated transcytosis. The mechanism of active targeting involves the detection of representative moiety by its target substrate [42,43]. The ligands such as aptamer, antibodies, folic acid (FA), hyaluronic acid (HA), growth factors, and transferrin interact with intracellular or extracellular matrix components and promotes the internalization of PMs [44]. Some of the ligand-mediated active targeting approaches through PMs are discussed below.

7.4.3.1 *Aptamer-coupled polymeric micelles*

Aptamers are highly flexible, nonimmunoresponsive, nucleic acid-based targeting ligands with a molecular weight of 10–30 kDa having higher affinity and specificity toward the target [45]. Chemically, they are single-stranded oligonucleotides having a simple fabrication method and good stability in biological conditions. They are nucleotide analogs of antibodies, but they can be considered economical and flexible versions of monoclonal antibodies. The 3D structure of aptamer facilitates their binding at the specific target site *via* salt bridges, hydrogen bonding, electrostatic interaction, or aromatic ring stacking. The aptamers' features such as minimal toxicity, nanosize (1–2 nm), less chances of batch failure, and ease of substitution make them a suitable candidate for ligand-based active targeting [46]. Aptamer-functionalized PMs have emerged as an effective carrier system, specifically in cancer therapy where they have shown an enhanced drug uptake in cancer cells.

Researchers developed doxorubicin (DOX)-loaded aptamer-modified PMs using amphiphilic diblock copolymer PCL-b-PEO to improve the targeting efficiency of PMs. Cell viability studies suggested that DOX-loaded aptamer-modified PMs inhibited cancer cells proliferation more significantly as compared to nonmodified PMs. The flow cytometry studies showed that aptamers have significantly improved the targeting efficiency of micelles toward Panc-1 cells, instigating a higher apoptosis rate. The aptamer-decorated PMs exhibited improved tumor penetration into the three-dimensional spheroid of Panc-1 cells in comparison to the unmodified PMs [47]. The study suggested that the aptamer-anchored PMs could improve the therapeutic efficacy of the chemotherapeutic agent and reduce the toxic effects.

Jabbari et al. fabricated a nucleolin aptamer (AS1411)-functionalized camptothecin-loaded novel diblock β-cyclodextrin-{PCL-poly(2-aminoethylmethacrylate)}$_{21}$ PMs to increase the accumulation of camptothecin at the tumor locus. The flow cytometry and fluorescence imaging analyses revealed higher internalization of aptamer-conjugated PMs into the target cells in comparison to the nontarget cells. The in vivo studies in female

BALB/c mice (4–6 weeks old) bearing breast cancer suggested that the aptamer-anchored PMs showed high tumor inhibitory potential as compared to the free camptothecin [48]. These studies demonstrated the target specificity of aptamer-decorated PMs, which could be explored further to achieve site-specific delivery of antineoplastic drugs.

7.4.3.2 *Folic acid-coupled polymeric micelles*

FA-coupled PMs are employed in cancer therapy to target folate receptors (FRs), as these receptors are expressed 1000 times more over cancerous cells as compared to normal cells. FA is a small nonimmunogenic molecule, which binds to the FR selectively. FR-α helps in the uncontrolled and rapid proliferation of tumor cells [49]. Therefore, FA has been explored widely as a targeting ligand in the cancer therapy.

Wang et al. developed DOX-loaded FA-functionalized succinylated gelatin PMs to achieve folate targeted antitumor therapy. The FA-anchored PMs demonstrated higher cytotoxicity against FR-overexpressing MCF-7 cells as compared to nonfunctionalized PMs. FA-functionalized DOX-loaded PMs exhibited higher fluorescence intensity in MCF-7 cells in comparison to nonfunctionalized ones, indicating enhanced uptake of FA-modified conjugate. Also, PMs conjugated with FA exhibited superior antitumor activity in MCF-7 tumor-bearing mice than plain drug and DOX-encapsulated PMs without FA functionalization [50]. This report suggested that FA-succinylated gelatin PMs could be an efficient nanocarrier to achieve targeted therapy in cancer.

Moharil et al. developed gemcitabine-based PMs conjugated with FA for targeted delivery of DOX and gemcitabine to the cancer cells overexpressing FRα and FRβ (Fig. 7.4A). Biodistribution studies were performed in 4T1.2 tumor-bearing mice using 1,10-dioctadecyl-3,3,30,30-tetramethylindotricarbocyanine iodide (DiR) as a fluorescent probe. The results showed that PMs functionalized with FA increased the DiR signal intensities in the tumor section, while reduced signals were observed in the liver and spleen, indicating reduced nonspecific uptake (Fig. 7.4B). Cellular uptake studies on human oral epidermal carcinoma KB cells demonstrated significantly enhanced DOX uptake from the FA-conjugated system as compared to free DOX (Fig. 7.4C) [51]. The folate-conjugated nanotherapeutics have enormous potential for selective targeting of cancer, with improved internalization of therapeutic agents at the target site.

7.4.3.3 *Hyaluronic acid-coupled polymeric micelles*

HA, a natural polysaccharide made up of repeated disaccharide units, that is, N-acetyl glucosamine and D-glucuronic acid, has acquired much attention due to its excellent biocompatibility and tumor targeting ability. HA interacts with the cell-specific receptors that is, cluster of differentiation 44 (CD44), which is overexpressed over many tumor cells; therefore, HA-based PMs have been explored for CD44-mediated tumor targeting. HA shows excellent biocompatibility and ease of modification and readily undergoes enzymatic degradation, and thus, it is widely explored for CD44 targeting in cancer therapy [52].

The hydrophilic end of HA is conjugated with the hydrophobic agent to create an amphiphilic system, which further self-assembles in aqueous solutions, forming amphiphilic PMs with its hydrophilic end projecting outside and hydrophobic end inside. Such systems can be employed for CD44-mediated uptake (Fig. 7.5) as well as for EPR effect,

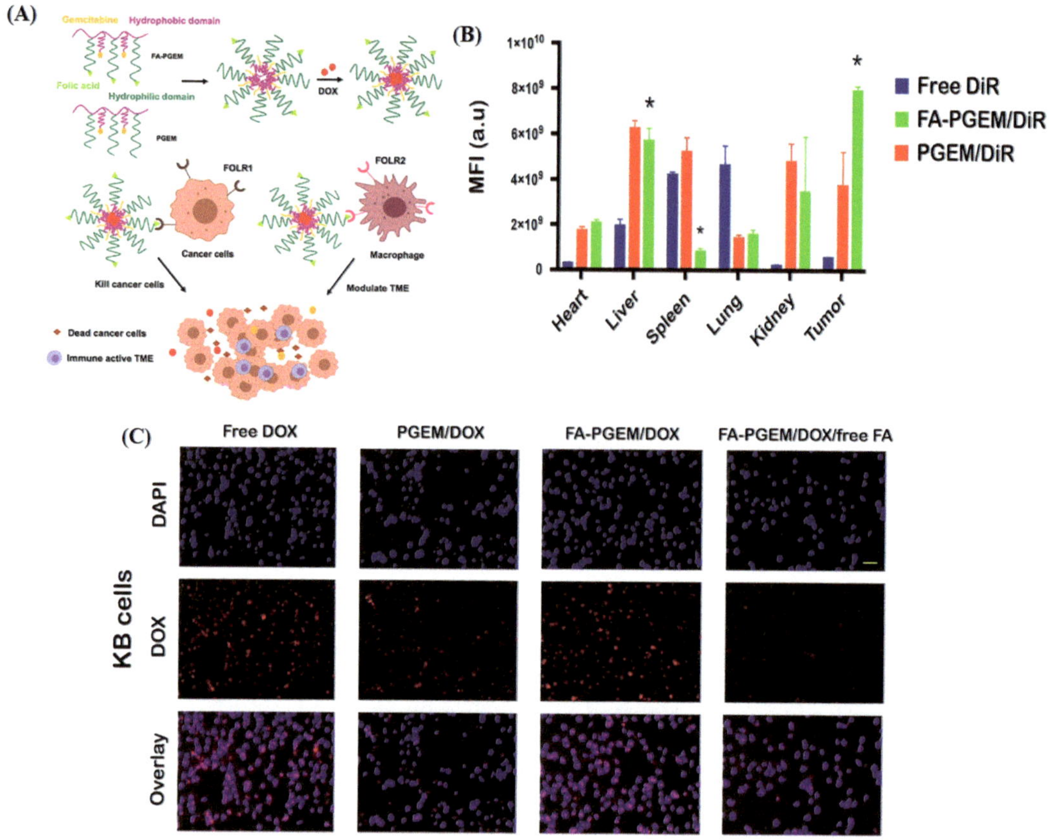

FIGURE 7.4 Folate-mediated active targeting; (A) fabrication of doxorubicin (DOX)-loaded folic acid-gemcitabine-based pro-drug polymeric micelles (PM), (B) tissue biodistribution of PMs in 4T1.2 tumor-bearing mice, and (C) fluorescence microscopic images representing cellular uptake of DOX loaded PMs in KB cells. Reproduced with permission from [51]. *MFI*, Mean fluorescence intensity.

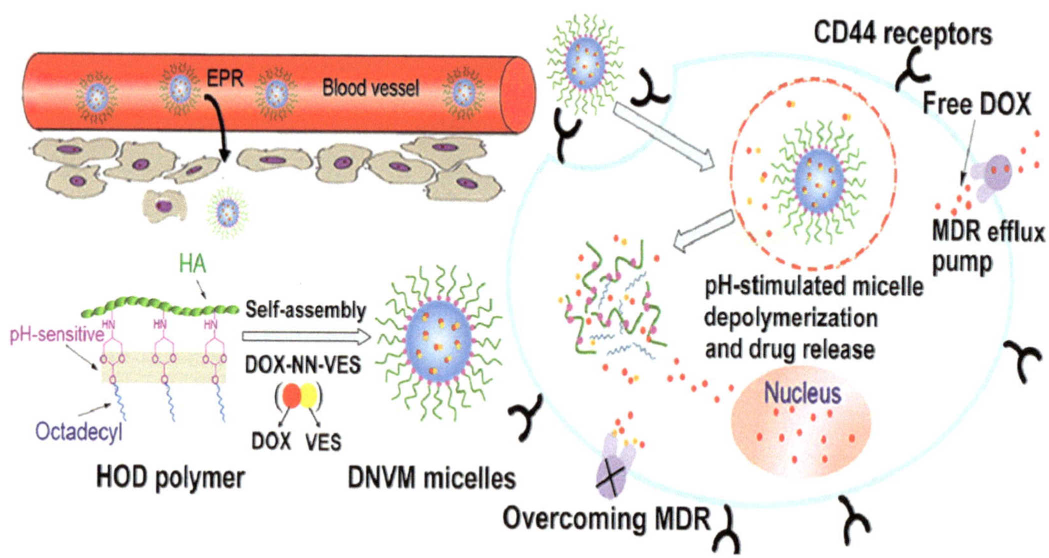

FIGURE 7.5 pH-responsive and CD44-targeted hyaluronic acid micelles to overcome doxorubicin resistance. Reproduced with permission from [55]. *VES*, Vitamin E succinate; *HOD*, hyaluronic acid-2-(octadecyloxy)-1,3-dioxan-5-amine; *DNVM*, hyaluronic acid-2-(octadecyloxy)-1,3-dioxan-5-amine PMs; *MDR*, multi-drug resistance.

which is an interesting approach for cancer therapy [53]. Researchers developed paclitaxel-loaded HA-deoxycholic acid-histidine micellar system to achieve CD44 receptor targeting and endosomal-pH triggered release of paclitaxel in cancer therapy. The paclitaxel incorporated within HA-deoxycholic acid-histidine micelles showed superior pharmacokinetic profiles with longer half-life than Taxol (marketed formulation of paclitaxel). In vivo studies in female nude mice suggested a more efficient tumor growth inhibition rate (64.9%) in HA-conjugated micelle-treated group as compared to Taxol (28.1%) owing to effective cellular internalization through CD44 receptor-mediated endocytosis and endosomal pH triggered release of paclitaxel [54].

Photodynamic therapy (PDT) for cancer treatment involves the exposure of photosensitizers and light of specific wavelength at the tumor site, which generates reactive oxygen species and induces intratumor cytotoxic reaction. Wang et al. used HA-b-poly(lactide-co-glycolide) copolymer to fabricate photosensitizer protoporphyrin IX-loaded PMs for active PDT in CD44 receptor-overexpressing cancer cells. Increased phototoxicity toward CD44-overexpressing A549 human lung adenocarcinoma cell lines was reported in 2D monolayer cell cultures and 3D tumor spheroids due to higher intracellular accumulation of the PMs through CD44-mediated endocytosis and deeper spheroid penetration [56]. This study paves a path toward exploration of HA as a targeting ligand for PDT in cancer treatment.

HA is emerging as a versatile building block ligand for cancer targeting due to the simplified fabrication process, biocompatibility, hydrophilicity, as well as CD44-targeting ability [57]. The studies demonstrated that HA serves as a main ligand for CD44 receptors, which is the hallmark of the tumor cell development. HA-based PMs can be further explored as a suitable gene/drug delivery platform in cancer therapy.

7.4.3.4 *Transferrin-coupled polymeric micelles*

The transferrin receptors are expressed in most of the human tissues, which serves as the entry port for iron in the cells. Despite the ubiquitous expression of transferrin receptors, they are overexpressed on the malignant cells and their expression can be correlated with tumor progression. The overexpression of this receptor on tumor cells, internalization ability, and the requirement of iron for cancer cell proliferation makes this receptor desirable for the delivery of chemotherapeutic agents. Transferrin and its conjugates (drug and antibodies) have been explored widely for cancer targeting. Utilization of transferrin can enhance the intracellular drug concentration, resulting in effective tumor targeting with reduced toxicity in the off-target cells [58].

Tf-conjugated curcumin-loaded methoxy-PEG-poly(lactide) PMs were fabricated to achieve localization of curcumin at the target site. In vitro cellular uptake studies in HeLa cells and HepG2 cells showed increased internalization of Tf-conjugated PMs within the cells as compared to the nontargeted PMs [59]. The PMs conjugated with Tf could be researched further for receptor-targeted, prolonged, and pH-triggered drug release in chemotherapy. In another study, Tf-mediated D-α-tocopheryl polyethylene glycol 1000 succinate (TPGS)-based ultrabright gold cluster and docetaxel-loaded theranostic PMs were synthesized for diagnosis and treatment of cancer. Docetaxel-loaded Tf-conjugated PMs showed 71.13-times decrease in the IC_{50} value in comparison to Taxotere (marketed formulation) in MDA-MB-231-luc breast cancer cells. In vivo studies of theranostic TPGS

PMs based on fluorescence and luciferase-induced bioluminescence imaging confirmed the Tf receptor targeted imaging and therapy [60]. Therefore, Tf-anchored PMs can be utilized in the cancer treatment owing to their ability to cross the blood–brain barrier as well as deliver chemotherapeutic agents intracellularly.

The studies demonstrated that the nanosized PMs with a large surface area showed enhanced binding to the target cells and thus, promoting the accumulation of drug. The functionalization of outer corona with aptamers, FA, HA, transferrin, antibodies, monosaccharides, biotin, and so forth could promote the binding affinity toward specific receptors. These functionalized PMs showed more effective internalization of therapeutic agents in comparison to nonfunctionalized PMs. Therefore, ligand-mediated PMs could be explored further to establish a proof of concept for targeted delivery of therapeutic agents.

7.4.4 Stimuli-responsive polymeric micelles

Stimuli-responsive PMs are fabricated from particular class of polymers that undergoes structural alteration in response to several exogenous and endogenous stimuli. Fig. 7.6 represents the drug release mechanism of PMs based on various stimuli. Stimuli-responsive

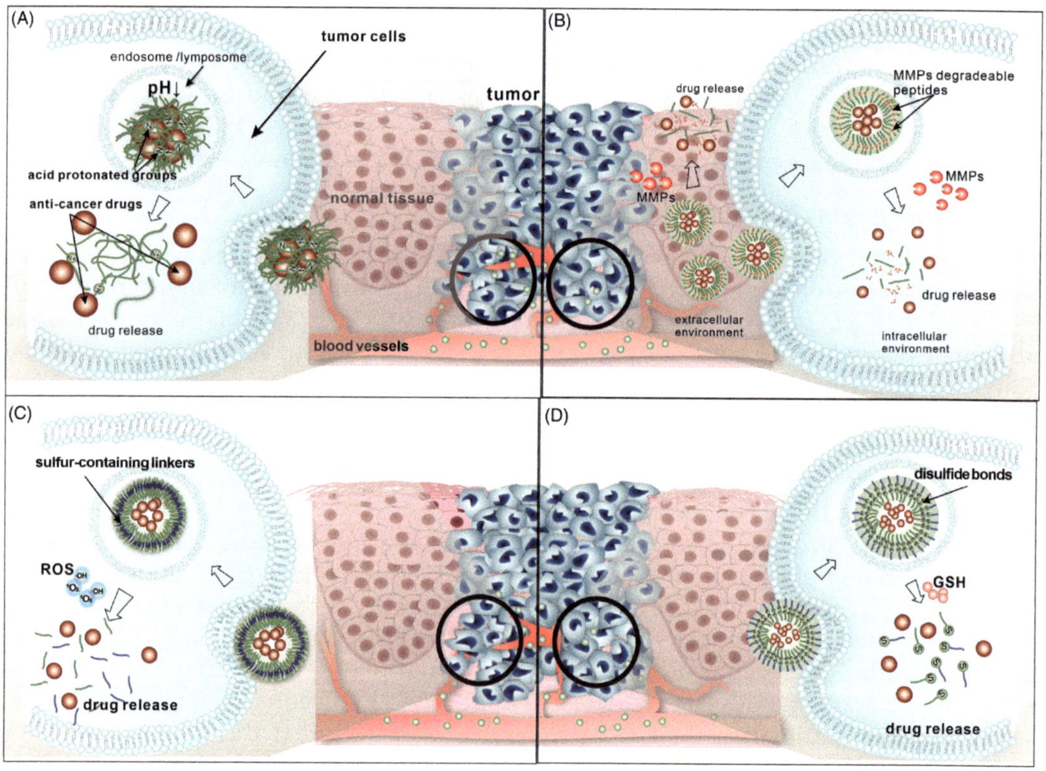

FIGURE 7.6 Transport of stimuli-responsive nanocarrier demonstrating controlled drug release based on endogenous factors; (A) pH, (B) MMP, (C) ROS, and (D) redox potential [63]. *ROS*, Reactive oxygen species.

nanocarriers induce the release of the therapeutic agent in response to endogenous factors such as pH, reactive oxygen species, specific enzyme like matrix metalloproteinases (MMP), and external activators like light, temperature, and ultrasound [61]. The external or internal stimuli cause destabilization, polymerization, isomerization, or disintegration of the micellar assembly. The conformation of PMs changes depending on the "stimulus sensitivity," which refers to the ability of micelles to destabilize in response to physiological or exogenous activators [62]. The following subsections discuss the application of stimuli-sensitive PMs in targeted therapy.

7.4.4.1 pH-responsive polymeric micelles

Among several intrinsic stimuli, pH-responsive PMs have been widely explored in chemotherapy owing to micellar destabilization and rapid drug release in the acidic environment. pH is an endogenous stimulus correlated with the malignant tissues, which results from hypoxia, cell death, and higher glycolysis rate, leading to accumulation of lactic acid [64]. Two major parameters that should be considered prior to the synthesis of pH-responsive micellar nanosystems are the stability of PMs in systemic circulation and rapid depolymerization of the micellar component at the tumor site. Depending on the PMs sensitivity toward pH, the therapeutic agent will be released from the carrier outside or inside the cancer cells [65].

Various chemical bonds like hydrazone, acetal, imine, and orthoester that remain intact at physiological pH but dissociate in acidic microenvironments are employed to fabricate drug-loaded pH-sensitive PMs. The pH-sensitive bonds are utilized to link the hydrophilic surface with the hydrophobic core of PMs, which disassembles and liberates the drug in the tumor microenvironment. Generally, pH-sensitive PMs are fabricated from polymers bearing ionizable moieties that can accept or donate the ionizable protons responding to the pH microenvironment. Anionic polymer bearing carboxylic acid moiety, that is, poly (acrylic acid) and poly(methacrylic acid) and cationic polymer containing tertiary amine group sidechains, that is, poly(N, N′-dimethyl aminoethyl methacrylate) are some of the pH-sensitive polymers used in fabrication of pH-responsive PMs [64].

Orthoester-based PEG-hydroxydodecanoic acid was used to develop PMs to achieve pH-sensitive release of DOX. The cellular uptake studies demonstrated that DOX-loaded PMs were internalized within the tumor cells *via* clathrin and macrophage-mediated endocytic pathways. The DOX was released from the PMs at pH 5.0, suggesting pH-sensitive drug release in the tumor microenvironment [66]. The study indicated that PMs with pH-sensitive chemical bonds remain stable in systemic circulation and rapidly release the drug in the acidic environment and such pH-sensitive PMs may be employed in the treatment of various cancers.

7.4.4.2 Redox-sensitive polymeric micelles

The difference in redox potential between cancerous and normal tissues is considered as a potential target for the development of redox-sensitive PMs. Glutathione (GSH) is abundantly found in cancer cells, where GSH concentration in tumor tissue is 100–1000 times more as compared to normal tissues. The redox-sensitive PMs are prepared using the amphiphilic polymer, where hydrophobic and hydrophilic components are attached through GSH-sensitive bonds, most commonly the disulfide bond [67]. The PMs undergo degradation due to the reduction of disulfide to the thiol group in response to increased intracellular GSH levels, followed by rapid release of drugs into the intracellular compartment of tumor cells [9].

Aminoglucose-conjugated redox-responsive PMs of PEG-ss-poly(D,L-lactide) were fabricated to achieve accumulation of paclitaxel at the tumor site. Intracellular drug release studies showed that paclitaxel release was accelerated significantly in response to GSH. In the absence of GSH, >30% paclitaxel release was observed, while >53% drug release was achieved in the presence of 5 mM GSH [68]. The functionalization of PMs promotes the uptake of the redox-responsive PMs inside the cancer cells to facilitate the drug release inside the tumor in response to GSH concentration.

7.4.4.3 *Enzyme-responsive polymeric micelles*

Enzymes play a very significant role in metabolic activities and can be utilized to trigger the release of drugs from enzyme-responsive PMs owing to their catalytic properties and specificity. The abnormal overexpression of numerous enzymes such as proteases, peptidases, and glycosidases is associated with many deadliest diseases including cancer. The level of various enzymes MMP, phospholipase A2, and cathepsin B rises in cancerous cells; hence, PMs can be functionalized with enzyme-labile linkages to provide on-demand enzyme-responsive release of therapeutic agents at the tumor site [65].

A copolymer of PEG2000-MMP2-sensitive peptide (pp)-transactivating transcription activator-PEG1000-phosphoethanolamine was developed for enzyme-sensitive paclitaxel delivery. In the absence of MMP2, the micelles were intact, while in the presence of MMP2 enzyme, the MMP2-sensitive peptide was catalyzed in the extracellular matrix, pp was cleaved, and the PEG shell was removed, thus releasing the drug inside the cancer cells. The in vivo tumor retention study demonstrated that MMP2-sensitive paclitaxel-loaded PMs showed significant MMP2-dependent cellular uptake and facilitated the tumor penetration and anticancer activity in cancer cells [69]. The enzyme-sensitive PMs incorporate specific functional groups in their structure that can be recognized and disintegrated by enzymes at the target site. Enzyme-responsive PMs are more specific and efficient in comparison to the pH or redox-responsive PMs, which makes them an attractive carrier to facilitate the drug accumulation at the target locus.

7.4.4.4 *Thermoresponsive polymeric micelles*

Thermoresponsive PMs are developed from thermoresponsive polymeric blocks that destabilize and release the drug in response to temperature variation. Poly(N-isopropyl acrylamide) (PNIPAM) is one of the most explored thermoresponsive polymers utilized in the fabrication of PMs. It has a lower critical solution temperature (LCST) at about 32°C, that is, the polymer retains the water *via* H-bond formation below 32°C, and the bond is disrupted above 32°C, making the polymer hydrophobic to precipitate out, followed by destabilization and release of drug from PMs [62].

Researchers fabricated FA-functionalized paclitaxel-loaded thermoresponsive PMs using PCL-b-2s(PNIPAM-co-acrylamide)-b′-mPEG/PEG-FA with LCST 39.6°C to obtain temperature-induced release at the target site. In vitro drug release studies suggested that about 50% drug was released at 37°C after 100 hours, while >80% of drug was released at 40°C in 40 hours. The intracellular uptake study of the formulation demonstrated that increasing the temperature enhanced the internalization of PMs [70]. The study showed that drug release from the PMs can be increased at the tumor site by utilizing thermoresponsive polymers, which can minimize the drug resistance and nonspecific distribution of the drug.

PNIPAM is one of the most investigated polymers to obtain thermoresponsive release of therapeutic agents; however, the disadvantages such as adherence to proteins and insignificant hysteresis constrains their utility. Temperature-sensitive PMs based on oligo(ethylene glycol) polymers are being explored due to their biocompatibility [71]. Pluronic and poly(hydroxypropyl methacrylamide-lactate) have also been explored for the synthesis of thermosensitive PMs [72].

The abovementioned studies showed that micellar systems have a huge potential for targeted delivery of cargo. PMs can be developed efficiently to disassemble in response to intrinsic or extrinsic stimuli to release the drugs. The specific polymers or ligands responding to pH, ROS, upregulated enzymes, temperature, and so forth could be employed to develop stimuli-responsive PMs. In the next section of this chapter, we have comprehensively discussed the challenges encountered in translation of PMs from bench to bedside.

7.5 Challenges associated with clinical translation

Despite the extensive ongoing research and vast array of advantages offered by PMs, there are certain challenges that hinder their clinical utility and commercialization such as poor uptake at the targeted site, inadequate drug release, and the scalability on industrial scale. PMs show adequate entrapment efficiency as well as drug loading at a lab scale, but it fails to achieve the same during large-scale production. Stability of PMs in systemic circulation is another issue, which occurs due to their infinite dilution in blood. Dilution of PMs lowers the CMC value that leads to reduced half-life of drug and dissociation of PMs, followed by leakage of encapsulated drugs from the polymeric assembly. The instability of these PMs may also arise due to the loss of hydrophobic and hydrophilic equilibrium when a large number of hydrophobic drugs are incorporated within the core region of PMs [73].

Therefore, remarkable efforts are required to develop an understanding regarding critical process parameters, that is, synthesis reaction, physicochemical characteristics of core-forming blocks, and degree of polymerization required for the fabrication of PMs. Besides, factors related to the preparation method of PMs such as type of organic solvent, cosolvent system composition, temperature, stirring speed, and time also influence the physiochemical properties of PMs. Despite the research that remains to be carried out, clinical and preclinical studies have demonstrated PMs as efficient nanocarriers for therapeutic, diagnostic, and theranostic agents [9].

7.6 Conclusion

PMs have emerged as promising nanocarriers for the targeted drug delivery due to their exceptional biocompatibility, reduced toxicity, drug solubilization in their hydrophobic core, and improved systemic circulation. The small size, ease of fabrication, and excellent solubilization properties make PMs remarkable carriers for various drug delivery applications. However, drug loading in the self-assembled micellar systems is not always optimum and off-target drug release remain an issue. Various efforts have been made by researchers to fabricate functionalized PMs to obtain targeted drug delivery and reduce off-target accumulation. The functionalization of PMs with targeting moieties like aptamer, antibodies, FA, HA, growth factors, transferrin, and so forth and fine-tuning of their structure *via* alteration of hydrophobic and hydrophilic segments improve the physicochemical properties and efficacy of drugs. The stimuli-responsive PMs based on endogenous stimuli (pH, enzymes, and redox potential) or exogenous stimuli (magnetic field and ultrasound) are also proving their potential by overcoming the limitations of conventional delivery systems. Several PMs are under clinical evaluation, although most of them are still under preclinical investigation. In conclusion, PMs, especially functionalized PMs, hold immense potential in targeted and controlled delivery of a vast number of drugs.

Acknowledgments

The authors are grateful to Department of Pharmaceuticals, Ministry of Chemicals and Fertilizers, Government of India, for providing facilities for writing this chapter. The authors, Dr. Keerti Jain and Ms. Anchal Pathak, acknowledge Indian council of Medical Research (ICMR), New Delhi, for the financial support in the form of ICMR Extramural Research Project (Project ID: 2020–4686; Ref. No. 5/13/34/2020/NCD-III). The NIPER–Raebareli communication number for this manuscript is NIPER-R/Communication/382.

Conflict of interest

The authors report no conflict of interest.

References

[1] Suthar T, Jain VK, Popli H, Jain K. Nanoemulsions as effective carriers for targeting brain tumors. Nanocarriers Drug-Target Brain Tumors 2022;347–63. Available from: https://doi.org/10.1016/B978-0-323-90773-6.00008-7.

[2] Gauro R, Nandave M, Jain VK, Jain K. Advances in dendrimer-mediated targeted drug delivery to the brain. J Nanopart Res 2021;23. Available from: https://doi.org/10.1007/s11051-021-05175-8.

[3] Sharma P, Jain K, Jain NK, Mehra NK, Jain K, Sharma P, et al. Ex vivo and in vivo performance of anti-cancer drug loaded carbon nanotubes. J Drug Deliv Sci Technol 2017;41:134–43. Available from: https://doi.org/10.1016/j.jddst.2017.07.011.

[4] Kaur S, Mehra NK, Jain K, Jain NK. Development and evaluation of targeting ligand-anchored CNTs as prospective targeted drug delivery system. Artif Cells, Nanomed Biotechnol 2017;45:242–50. Available from: https://doi.org/10.3109/21691401.2016.1146728.

[5] Juneja M, Suthar T, Pardhi VP, Ahmad J, Jain K. Emerging trends and promises of nanoemulsions in therapeutics of infectious diseases. Nanomedicine (London) 2022;17:793–812. Available from: https://doi.org/10.2217/NNM-2022-0006.

[6] Ghezzi M, Pescina S, Padula C, Santi P, Del Favero E, Cantù L, et al. Polymeric micelles in drug delivery: an insight of the techniques for their characterization and assessment in biorelevant conditions. J Control Rel 2021;332:312–36. Available from: https://doi.org/10.1016/j.jconrel.2021.02.031.

[7] Xu W, Ling P, Zhang T. Polymeric micelles, a promising drug delivery system to enhance bioavailability of poorly water-soluble drugs. J Drug Deliv 2013;2013:1–15. Available from: https://doi.org/10.1155/2013/340315.

[8] Deshmukh AS, Chauhan PN, Noolvi MN, Chaturvedi K, Ganguly K, Shukla SS, et al. Polymeric micelles: basic research to clinical practice. Int J Pharm 2017;532:249–68. Available from: https://doi.org/10.1016/j.ijpharm.2017.09.005.

[9] Kaur J, Gulati M, Jha NK, Disouza J, Patravale V, Dua K, et al. Recent advances in developing polymeric micelles for treating cancer: breakthroughs and bottlenecks in their clinical translation. Drug Discov Today 2022;. Available from: https://doi.org/10.1016/j.drudis.2022.02.005.

[10] Majumder N, Das NG, Das SK. Polymeric micelles for anticancer drug delivery. Ther Deliv 2020;11:613–35. Available from: https://doi.org/10.4155/tde-2020-0008.

[11] Grimm O, Wendler F, Schacher FH. Micellization of photo-responsive block copolymers. Polymers (Basel) 2017;9. Available from: https://doi.org/10.3390/polym9090396.

[12] Almeida M, Magalhães M, Veiga F, Figueiras A. Poloxamers, poloxamines and polymeric micelles: definition, structure and therapeutic applications in cancer. J Polym Res 2018;25. Available from: https://doi.org/10.1007/s10965-017-1426-x.

[13] Mandal A, Bisht R, Rupenthal ID, Mitra AK. Polymeric micelles for ocular drug delivery: from structural frameworks to recent preclinical studies. J Control Rel 2017;248:96–116. Available from: https://doi.org/10.1016/j.jconrel.2017.01.012.

[14] Croy S, Kwon G. Polymeric micelles for drug delivery. Curr Pharm Des 2006;12:4669–84. Available from: https://doi.org/10.2174/138161206779026245.

[15] Hu X, Jing X. Biodegradable amphiphilic polymer-drug conjugate micelles. Expert Opin Drug Deliv 2009;6:1079–90. Available from: https://doi.org/10.1517/17425240903158917.

[16] Rashidzadeh H, Rezaei SJT, Zamani S, Sarijloo E, Ramazani A. pH-sensitive curcumin conjugated micelles for tumor triggered drug delivery. J. Biomater. Sci. Polym. Ed. 2021;32:320–36. Available from: https://doi.org/10.1080/09205063.2020.1833815.

[17] Yokoyama M. Polymeric micelles as a new drug carrier system and their required considerations for clinical trials. Expert Opin Drug Deliv 2010;7:145–58. Available from: https://doi.org/10.1517/17425240903436479.

[18] Lavasanifar A, Samuel J, Kwon GS. The effect of fatty acid substitution on the in vitro release of amphotericin B from micelles composed of poly(ethylene oxide)-block-poly(N-hexyl stearate-L-aspartamide). J Control Rel 2002;79:165–72. Available from: https://doi.org/10.1016/S0168-3659(01)00537-5.

[19] Lavasanifar A, Kwon GS. Micelles of poly(ethylene oxide)-block-poly(N-alkyl stearate L-aspartamide): synthetic analogues of lipoproteins for drug delivery. J Biomed Mater Res 2000;52:831–5. Available from: https://doi.org/10.1002/1097-4636(20001215)52:4<831::aid-jbm29>3.0.co;2-k.

[20] Le Garrec D, Gori S, Luo L, Lessard D, Smith DC, Yessine MA, et al. Poly(N-vinylpyrrolidone)-block-poly(d,l-lactide) as a new polymeric solubilizer for hydrophobic anticancer drugs: in vitro and in vivo evaluation. J Control Rel 2004;99:83–101. Available from: https://doi.org/10.1016/j.jconrel.2004.06.018.

[21] Song R, Zhou Y, Li Y, Yang Z, Li F, Huang Q, et al. Preparation and characterization of mPEG-g-α-zein biohybrid micelles as a nano-carrier. J Appl Polym Sci 132 2015;. Available from: https://doi.org/10.1002/app.42555.

[22] Nishiyama N, Okazaki S, Cabral H, Miyamoto M, Kato Y, Sugiyama Y, et al. Novel cisplatin-incorporated polymeric micelles can eradicate solid tumors in mice. Cancer Res 2003;63:8977–83.

[23] Mignani S, Shi X, Zablocka M, Majoral JP. Dendritic macromolecular architectures: dendrimer-based polyion complex micelles. Biomacromolecules 2021;22:262–74. Available from: https://doi.org/10.1021/acs.biomac.0c01645.

[24] Shah S, Leon L. Structural dynamics, phase behavior, and applications of polyelectrolyte complex micelles. Curr Opin Colloid Interface Sci 2021;53. Available from: https://doi.org/10.1016/j.cocis.2021.101424.

[25] Joshi K, Chandra A, Jain K, Talegaonkar S. Nanocrystalization: an emerging technology to enhance the bioavailability of poorly soluble drugs. Pharm Nanotechnol 2019;7:259–78. Available from: https://doi.org/10.2174/2211738507666190405182524.

[26] Sipos B, Csóka I, Budai-Szűcs M, Kozma G, Berkesi D, Kónya Z, et al. Development of dexamethasone-loaded mixed polymeric micelles for nasal delivery. Eur J Pharm Sci 2021;166. Available from: https://doi.org/10.1016/j.ejps.2021.105960.

[27] Hamley I. Block copolymers in solution: fundamentals and applications; 2012. https://doi.org/10.1002/9780470016985.

[28] Scholz N, Behnke T, Resch-Genger U. Determination of the critical micelle concentration of neutral and ionic surfactants with fluorometry, conductometry, and surface tension—a method comparison. J Fluoresc 2018;28:465–76. Available from: https://doi.org/10.1007/s10895-018-2209-4.

[29] Chen T, He B, Tao J, He Y, Deng H, Wang X, et al. Application of Förster resonance energy transfer (FRET) technique to elucidate intracellular and in vivo biofate of nanomedicines. Adv Drug Deliv Rev 2019;143:177–205. Available from: https://doi.org/10.1016/j.addr.2019.04.009.
[30] Yu M, Yuan W, Li D, Schwendeman A, Schwendeman SP. Predicting drug release kinetics from nanocarriers inside dialysis bags. J Control Rel 2019;315:23–30. Available from: https://doi.org/10.1016/j.jconrel.2019.09.016.
[31] Wang Z, Deng X, Ding J, Zhou W, Zheng X, Tang G. Mechanisms of drug release in pH-sensitive micelles for tumour targeted drug delivery system: a review. Int J Pharm 2018;535:253–60. Available from: https://doi.org/10.1016/j.ijpharm.2017.11.003.
[32] Jain K, Mehra N, Jain N. Nanotechnology in drug delivery: safety and toxicity issues. Curr Pharm Des 2015;. Available from: https://doi.org/10.2174/1381612821666150901103208.
[33] Jain K, Verma AK, Mishra PR, Jain NK. Surface-engineered dendrimeric nanoconjugates for macrophage-targeted delivery of amphotericin B: formulation development and in vitro and in vivo evaluation. Antimicrob Agents Chemother 2015;. Available from: https://doi.org/10.1128/AAC.04213-14.
[34] Ghosh S, Mishra P, Dabke A, Pathak A, Bhowmick S, Misra A. Targeting approaches using polymeric nanocarriers. Appl Polym Drug Deliv 2021;393–421. Available from: https://doi.org/10.1016/b978-0-12-819659-5.00014-8.
[35] Lu Y, Park K. Polymeric micelles and alternative nanonized delivery vehicles for poorly soluble drugs. Int J Pharm 2013;453:198–214. Available from: https://doi.org/10.1016/j.ijpharm.2012.08.042.
[36] Li Q, Lai KL, Chan PS, Leung SC, Li HY, Fang Y, et al. Micellar delivery of dasatinib for the inhibition of pathologic cellular processes of the retinal pigment epithelium. Colloids Surf B Biointerfaces 2016;140:278–86. Available from: https://doi.org/10.1016/j.colsurfb.2015.12.053.
[37] Mikhail AS, Allen C. Poly(ethylene glycol)- b -poly(ε-caprolactone) micelles containing chemically conjugated and physically entrapped docetaxel: synthesis, characterization, and the influence of the drug on micelle morphology. Biomacromolecules 2010;11:1273–80. Available from: https://doi.org/10.1021/bm100073s.
[38] Abdul Hussein HA, Maraie NK. Tenoxicam-loaded polymeric micelles material: formulation, optimization, and evaluation. Mater Today Proc 2022;61:672–80. Available from: https://doi.org/10.1016/J.MATPR.2021.08.218.
[39] Mahmud A, Xiong XB, Aliabadi HM, Lavasanifar A. Polymeric micelles for drug targeting. J Drug Target 2007;15:553–84. Available from: https://doi.org/10.1080/10611860701538586.
[40] Raval N, Maheshwari R, Shukla H, Kalia K, Torchilin VP, Tekade RK. Multifunctional polymeric micellar nanomedicine in the diagnosis and treatment of cancer. Mater Sci Eng C 2021;126. Available from: https://doi.org/10.1016/j.msec.2021.112186.
[41] Bertrand N, Wu J, Xu X, Kamaly N, Farokhzad OC. Cancer nanotechnology: the impact of passive and active targeting in the era of modern cancer biology. Adv Drug Deliv Rev 2014;. Available from: https://doi.org/10.1016/j.addr.2013.11.009.
[42] Ahmad J, Rizwanullah M, Suthar T, Albarqi HA, Ahmad MZ, Vuddanda PR, et al. Receptor-targeted surface-engineered nanomaterials for breast cancer imaging and theranostic applications. Crit Rev Ther Drug Carr Syst 2022;39. Available from: https://doi.org/10.1615/CRITREVTHERDRUGCARRIERSYST.2022040686.
[43] Thanuja MY, Anupama C, Ranganath SH. Bioengineered cellular and cell membrane-derived vehicles for actively targeted drug delivery: so near and yet so far. Adv Drug Deliv Rev 2018;132:57–80. Available from: https://doi.org/10.1016/j.addr.2018.06.012.
[44] Zhong Y, Meng F, Deng C, Zhong Z. Ligand-directed active tumor-targeting polymeric nanoparticles for cancer chemotherapy. Biomacromolecules 2014;15:1955–69. Available from: https://doi.org/10.1021/bm5003009.
[45] Alshaer W, Hillaireau H, Fattal E. Aptamer-guided nanomedicines for anticancer drug delivery. Adv Drug Deliv Rev 2018;134:122–37. Available from: https://doi.org/10.1016/j.addr.2018.09.011.
[46] Keefe AD, Pai S, Ellington A. Aptamers as therapeutics. Nat Rev Drug Discov 2010;9(7):537–50. Available from: https://doi.org/10.1038/nrd3141.
[47] Tian L, Pei R, Zhong L, Ji Y, Zhou D, Zhou S. Enhanced targeting of 3D pancreatic cancer spheroids by aptamer-conjugated polymeric micelles with deep tumor penetration. Eur J Pharmacol 2021;894. Available from: https://doi.org/10.1016/j.ejphar.2020.173814.

[48] Jabbari A, Yaghoobi E, Azizollahi H, Shojaee S, Ramezani M, Alibolandi M, et al. Design and synthesis of a star-like polymeric micelle modified with AS1411 aptamer for targeted delivery of camptothecin for cancer therapy. Int J Pharm 2022;611. Available from: https://doi.org/10.1016/j.ijpharm.2021.121346.
[49] Jain K, Gupta U, Jain NK. Dendronized nanoconjugates of lysine and folate for treatment of cancer. Eur J Pharm Biopharm 2014;87(3):500–9. Available from: https://doi.org/10.1016/j.ejpb.2014.03.015.
[50] Wang Y, Ren J, Liu Y, Liu R, Wang L, Yuan Q, et al. Preparation and evaluation of folic acid modified succinylated gelatin micelles for targeted delivery of doxorubicin. J Drug Deliv Sci Technol 2018;46:400–7. Available from: https://doi.org/10.1016/j.jddst.2018.06.002.
[51] Moharil P, Wan Z, Pardeshi A, Li J, Huang H, Luo Z, et al. Engineering a folic acid-decorated ultrasmall gemcitabine nanocarrier for breast cancer therapy: dual targeting of tumor cells and tumor-associated macrophages. Acta Pharm Sin B 2022;12:1148–62. Available from: https://doi.org/10.1016/j.apsb.2021.09.024.
[52] Luo Z, Dai Y, Gao H. Development and application of hyaluronic acid in tumor targeting drug delivery. Acta Pharm Sin B 2019;9:1099–112. Available from: https://doi.org/10.1016/j.apsb.2019.06.004.
[53] Harrer D, Sanchez Armengol E, Friedl JD, Jalil A, Jelkmann M, Leichner C, et al. Is hyaluronic acid the perfect excipient for the pharmaceutical need? Int J Pharm 2021;601. Available from: https://doi.org/10.1016/j.ijpharm.2021.120589.
[54] Liu Y, Zhou C, Wei S, Yang T, Lan Y, Cao A, et al. Paclitaxel delivered by CD44 receptor-targeting and endosomal pH sensitive dual functionalized hyaluronic acid micelles for multidrug resistance reversion. Colloids Surf B Biointerfaces 2018;170:330–40. Available from: https://doi.org/10.1016/j.colsurfb.2018.06.024.
[55] Qiu L, Xu J, Ahmed KS, Zhu M, Zhang Y, Long M, et al. Stimuli-responsive, dual-function prodrug encapsulated in hyaluronic acid micelles to overcome doxorubicin resistance. Acta Biomater 2022;140:686–99. Available from: https://doi.org/10.1016/j.actbio.2021.11.050.
[56] Wang X, Wang J, Li J, Huang H, Sun X, Lv Y. Development and evaluation of hyaluronic acid-based polymeric micelles for targeted delivery of photosensitizer for photodynamic therapy in vitro. J Drug Deliv Sci Technol 2018;48:414–21. Available from: https://doi.org/10.1016/j.jddst.2018.10.018.
[57] Wickens JM, Alsaab HO, Kesharwani P, Bhise K, Amin MCIM, Tekade RK, et al. Recent advances in hyaluronic acid-decorated nanocarriers for targeted cancer therapy. Drug Discov Today 2017;22:665–80. Available from: https://doi.org/10.1016/j.drudis.2016.12.009.
[58] Agrawal P, Sonali RP, Singh G, et al. Bioadhesive micelles of D-α-tocopherol polyethylene glycol succinate 1000: synergism of chitosan and transferrin in targeted drug delivery. Colloids Surf B Biointerfaces 2017;152:277–88. Available from: https://doi.org/10.1016/j.colsurfb.2017.01.021.
[59] Kumari P, Rompicharla SVK, Muddineti OS, Ghosh B, Biswas S. Transferrin-anchored poly(lactide) based micelles to improve anticancer activity of curcumin in hepatic and cervical cancer cell monolayers and 3D spheroids. Int J Biol Macromol 2018;116:1196–213. Available from: https://doi.org/10.1016/j.ijbiomac.2018.05.040.
[60] Muthu MS, Kutty RV, Luo Z, Xie J, Feng SS. Theranostic vitamin E TPGS micelles of transferrin conjugation for targeted co-delivery of docetaxel and ultra bright gold nanoclusters. Biomaterials 2015;39:234–48. Available from: https://doi.org/10.1016/j.biomaterials.2014.11.008.
[61] Dai Y, Chen X, Zhang X. Recent advances in stimuli-responsive polymeric micelles: via click chemistry. Polym Chem 2019;10:34–44. Available from: https://doi.org/10.1039/c8py01174e.
[62] Biswas S, Kumari P, Lakhani PM, Ghosh B. Recent advances in polymeric micelles for anti-cancer drug delivery. Eur J Pharm Sci 2016;. Available from: https://doi.org/10.1016/j.ejps.2015.12.031.
[63] Liang J, Yang B, Zhou X, Han Q, Zou J, Cheng L. Stimuli-responsive drug delivery systems for head and neck cancer therapy. Drug Deliv 2021;28:272–84. Available from: https://doi.org/10.1080/10717544.2021.1876182.
[64] Gao GH, Li Y, Lee DS. Environmental pH-sensitive polymeric micelles for cancer diagnosis and targeted therapy. J Control Rel 2013;. Available from: https://doi.org/10.1016/j.jconrel.2012.11.012.
[65] Yang H, Khan AR, Liu M, Fu M, Ji J, Chi L, et al. Stimuli-responsive polymeric micelles for the delivery of paclitaxel. J Drug Deliv Sci Technol 2020;56. Available from: https://doi.org/10.1016/j.jddst.2020.101523.
[66] Long M, Liu S, Shan X, Mao J, Yang F, Wu X, et al. Self-assembly of pH-sensitive micelles for enhanced delivery of doxorubicin to melanoma cells. J Drug Deliv Sci Technol 2020;59. Available from: https://doi.org/10.1016/j.jddst.2020.101859.

[67] Mirhadi E, Mashreghi M, Faal Maleki M, Alavizadeh SH, Arabi L, Badiee A, et al. Redox-sensitive nanoscale drug delivery systems for cancer treatment. Int J Pharm 2020;589. Available from: https://doi.org/10.1016/j.ijpharm.2020.119882.

[68] Zhou Y, Wen H, Gu L, Fu J, Guo J, Du L, et al. Aminoglucose-functionalized, redox-responsive polymer nanomicelles for overcoming chemoresistance in lung cancer cells. J Nanobiotechnol 2017;15. Available from: https://doi.org/10.1186/s12951-017-0316-z.

[69] Yao Q, Dai Z, Hoon Choi J, Kim D, Zhu L. Building stable MMP2-responsive multifunctional polymeric micelles by an all-in-one polymer-lipid conjugate for tumor-targeted intracellular drug delivery. ACS Appl Mater Interfaces 2017;9:32520–33. Available from: https://doi.org/10.1021/acsami.7b09511.

[70] Rezaei SJT, Nabid MR, Niknejad H, Entezami AA. Folate-decorated thermoresponsive micelles based on star-shaped amphiphilic block copolymers for efficient intracellular release of anticancer drugs. Int J Pharm 2012;. Available from: https://doi.org/10.1016/j.ijpharm.2012.07.069.

[71] Cao H, Guo F, Chen Z, Kong XZ. Preparation of thermoresponsive polymer nanogels of oligo(ethylene glycol) diacrylate-methacrylic acid and their property characterization. Nanoscale Res Lett 2018;. Available from: https://doi.org/10.1186/s11671-018-2610-6.

[72] Talelli M, Hennink WE. Thermosensitive polymeric micelles for targeted drug delivery. Nanomedicine 2011;. Available from: https://doi.org/10.2217/nnm.11.91.

[73] Rani S, Sharma AK, Khan I, Gothwal A, Chaudhary S, Gupta U. Polymeric nanoparticles in targeting and delivery of drugs. Nanotechnology-based approaches for targeting and delivery of drugs and genes. Elsevier; 2017. p. 223–55. Available from: https://doi.org/10.1016/B978-0-12-809717-5.00008-7.

CHAPTER

8

Physicochemical characterization of drug delivery systems based on nanomaterials

Viviane Lucia Beraldo-de-Araújo, Victória Soares Soeiro, Marcelo Van Vliet Lima, Juliana Souza Ribeiro Costa and Laura de Oliveira-Nascimento

Faculty of Pharmaceutical Sciences, University of Campinas (UNICAMP), Campinas, SP, Brazil

8.1 Introduction

Active pharmaceutical ingredients (APIs) can be formulated in a variety of dosage forms and administered by many routes. This flexibility happens if excipients in the formulation fulfill physical, chemical, and biological requirements to allow the pharmacological effect to take place. Among powders, pastes, gels, liquids and patches, the formulation must sustain API stability and promote its local or systemic delivery. In turn, organoleptic and manufacturing aspects also depend on the set of ingredients. The simple content list is not enough to vehicle an active molecule: excipients must go through extensive characterization concerning chemical and physical aspects of the molecule, bulk material, and API compatibility [1].

Nanostructuration may enhance API properties or enable a new one. A broad range of nanosized dosage forms have been developed and some of them already became drug products. The commercial types include nanocrystals, nanoemulsions, dendrimers, polymeric nanoparticles, lipid-based nanoparticles, and iron-based ones (Fig. 8.1). Besides material diversity, there are also a variety of processes, from bottom up to top down nanostructuration, which employ high or low energy mixing methods, precipitation, centrifugation, comminution and sculpturing steps, among others [2].

Even nanomaterials (NMs) with the same chemical composition but with a different shape or internal structure bring the possibility of a different physicochemical stability,

Molecular Pharmaceutics and Nano Drug Delivery
DOI: https://doi.org/10.1016/B978-0-323-91924-1.00005-8

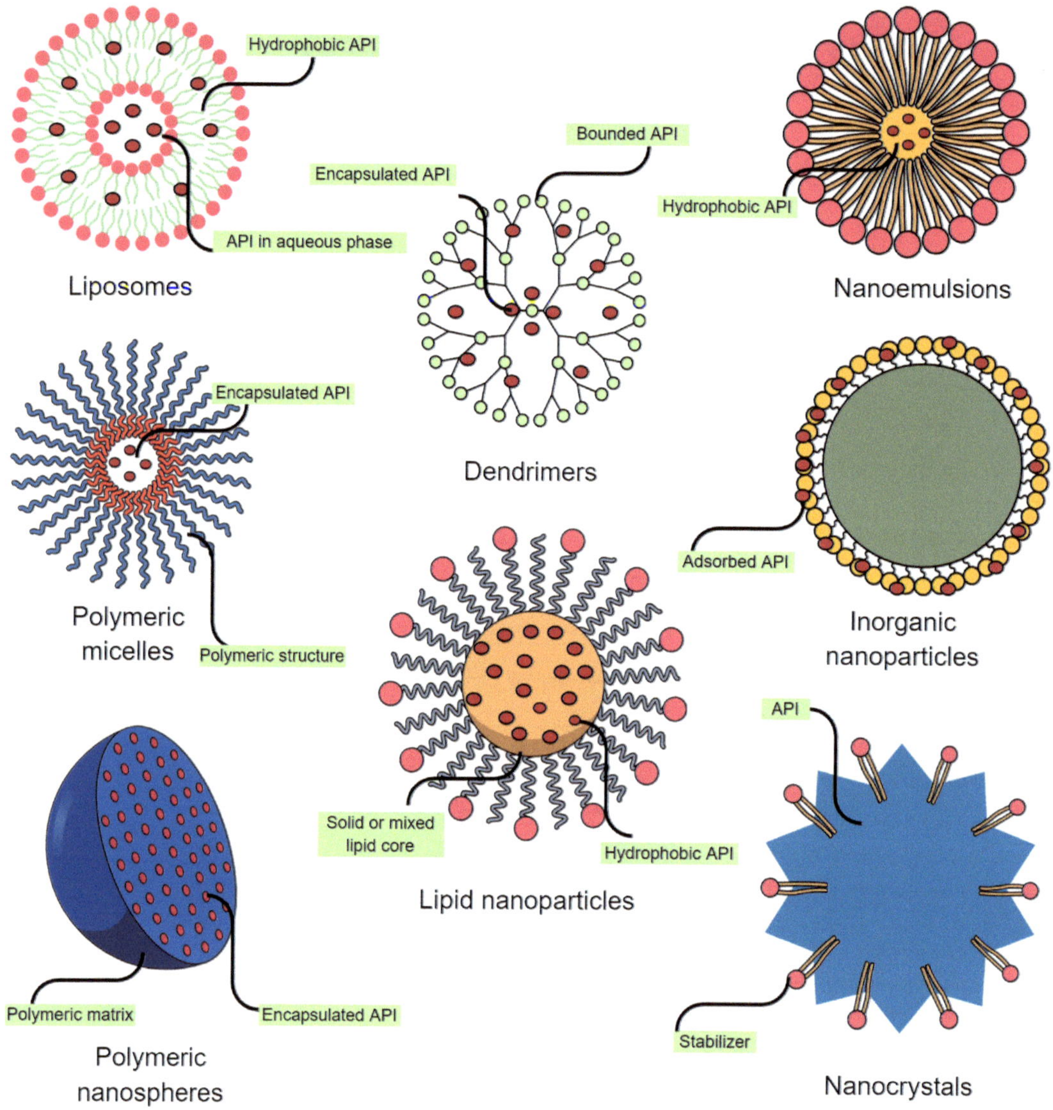

FIGURE 8.1 Examples of particulate nanostructures for active pharmaceutical ingredient (API) delivery. **Liposomes:** Vesicles formed by a hydrophobic lipid bilayer and a hydrophilic aqueous core with a nanometric size. **Polymeric micelles:** An aqueous core surrounded by an amphiphilic copolymer shell. **Polymeric nanospheres:** A solid hydrophobic and polymeric nucleus or a hydrated nucleus of crosslinked hydrophilic polymers, possibly with an excipient to stabilize the colloid (stabilizer). **Dendrimers:** Branched polymeric molecules that can carry API by loading or crosslinking. **Lipid nanoparticles:** A solid or mixed lipid core surrounded by stabilizers (nanostructured lipid carrier, NLC; solid lipid nanoparticles, SLN), but also structures with a lipid monolayer shell, surfactants, and internal lipid vesicles. **Nanoemulsions:** Metastable dispersions of immiscible phases joined by surfactant molecules. **Inorganic nanoparticles:** Solid inorganic cores surrounded by stabilizers. **Nanocrystals:** API crystal cores separated by stabilizers.

pharmacological performance, or toxicity/environmental impact. Thus, physicochemical characterization remains an essential milestone that drives risk assessment and precede efficacy studies of nanomedicines. To harmonize concepts and techniques, several institutions around the world publish standard documents and guidelines for nanostructures. The International Organization for Standardization (ISO), the Organization for Economic Cooperation and Development, the American Society for Testing and Materials (ASTM), and others have specific projects concerning NMs, regardless of their use. The European Medicines Agency (EMA), the Food and Drug administration Agency from United States (FDA), and other health governmental agencies have committees focused on NMs related with health products, including API delivery (which includes drug delivery).

As with any other pharmaceutical product, characterization of nanomedicines evaluates the critical quality attributes defined for the intended route of administration, dosage form, and specific properties of each composition. In 2022, the United States Pharmacopeia (USP) released a general chapter of "drug products containing nanomaterials" [3] that defines structures and list quality attributes. Fig. 8.2 relates general quality attributes of NMs, as described by the USP and FDA [4]. Obviously, size is an essential parameter since it defines if the material has nanosized dimensions. However, some measurement techniques rely on mathematical models that assume a certain shape, which requires the previous assessment of NM morphology. Size has been related with NM cell uptake, interaction, biodistribution, plasma half-life, and clearance outcomes [5], apart from drug solubility and colloidal stability.

The NM organization and chemical features can dictate its physiological role, as pointed before, but also determine the type of physicochemical analysis and stability concerns. NM composition should be described by its individual ingredients, such as polymer

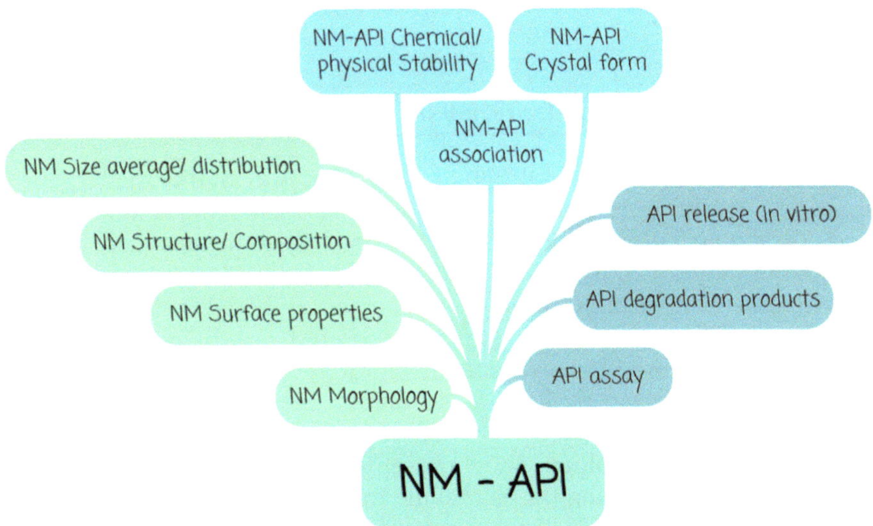

FIGURE 8.2 General attributes of nanomaterials associated with active pharmaceutical ingredients in medicines.

identity/molecular weight, but also by its structure, such as multilamellar vesicles, coated material, or crystalline content. In turn, the material surface contains valuable information for delivery systems. Surface topography, charge, and coating type, when present, influence carrier properties: the charge and coating modify NM interaction with cell membranes and physiological media, which may change targeting, toxicity, and clearance properties. Coating can provide cargo protection and retention in the way to the desired release site. Regarding formulation stability, charges do influence colloidal stability of dispersions and flow properties of solid bulk material.

Once in the body, another key point is how the active molecules will be related to the carrier though time and different body compartments. Dissolution/release in vitro assays can screen batch to batch inconsistencies that may bring changes in pharmacokinetics; furthermore, they can even predict the resultant API in vivo release and establish an in vitro/in vivo correlation.

Although there are more properties that can be evaluated, this chapter will focus on the USP-listed general attributes, so the reader can have a broader understanding. Each property can be assessed by more than one method; however, only a few are described in the guidelines. Standardization is paramount to reproducibility and interlaboratory/company robustness, in addition to offering proper product comparisons. Another important aspect of using standard methods comes from the need of accurate data to support manufacturing, toxicological, clinical, and environmental studies. So, this chapter will concentrate on techniques that are standardized by at least one of the previously cited institutions. Due to the stated relevance of physicochemical analysis, techniques will be briefly discussed in the next topics. They were organized by attribute and specific literature is related on the reference section. For an overall glance, Table 8.1 relates the techniques to evaluate nanostructured API attributes that have a standard protocol published by ISO or ASTM. Both are rich and tested sources of protocols and specific information for test application, comparison, and good practices.

8.2 Nanomaterial shape/morphology

NMs assume various shapes, with different assemblies like multivesicular units or solid cores with a fluid corona. It is essential to characterize their morphology to predict and comprehend API dynamics and biological interactions, which include cellular uptake, API release, surface-binding capability, "asbestos-like" behavior, and so forth. From the analytical point of view, several techniques rely on mathematical models based on spherical particles, so shape will influence the choice of method for NM size distribution [6,7].

The assessment of NM morphology depends on the sample state (dry or wet), conductibility, and particle sensitiveness to the technique. Shape characterization is mainly obtained from high-resolution microscopy techniques, providing meticulous and direct information on the NM morphology. They are settled in the interaction between the NM atomic structure with the scanning probe (atomic force microscopy, AFM), or the impinging electron beam. The electrons provide a relatively superficial scanning (scanning electron microscopy, SEM) or a more in-depth analysis in the transmission mode through ultrathin samples (transmission electron microscopy, TEM), providing information toward

TABLE 8.1 Techniques standardized by American Society for testing and materials and ISO that address directly nanomaterial attributes applicable to active pharmaceutical ingredient nanostructuration.

Technique	Attribute	ASTM guidelines	ISO guidelines
Atomic force microscopy (AFM)	Structure morphology	E2859-11(2017) - Standard Guide for Size Measurement of Nanoparticles Using Atomic Force Microscopy	ISO 13095:2014 Surface Chemical Analysis—Atomic force microscopy—Procedure for in situ characterization of AFM probe shank profile used for nanostructure measurement
Asymmetrical-flow (AF4) and centrifugal (CF3) field-Flow Field Fractionation	Size/NM concentration/ chemical composition (various detectors)	X	ISO/TS 21362:2018 - Nanotechnologies—Analysis of nano-objects using asymmetrical flow and centrifugal field-flow fractionation
Brunauer–Emmett–Teller method	Surface—area, porosity	X	ISO/TS 17200:2020 - Nanotechnology—Nanoparticles in powder form—Characteristics and measurements
Cryo-transmission electron microscopy	Structure morphology	E3143-18b - Standard Practice for Performing Cryo-Transmission Electron Microscopy of Liposomes	X
Circular dichroism	Structure (protein-based)	X	ISO/TS 23459:2021 - Nanotechnologies—Assessment of protein secondary structure during an interaction with nanomaterials using ultraviolet circular dichroism
Dynamic light scattering	Size	E2490-09(2021) - Standard Guide for Measurement of Particle Size Distribution of Nanomaterials in Suspension by Photon Correlation Spectroscopy; E3247-20 - Standard Test Method for Measuring the Size of Nanoparticles in Aqueous Media Using Dynamic Light Scattering	ISO 22412:2017 - Particle size analysis—Dynamic light scattering (DLS); ISO/TR 22814:2020 - Good practice for dynamic light scattering (DLS) measurements
Electroacoustic spectroscopy	Surface—charge	X	ISO 13099-3:2014 - Colloidal systems—Methods for zeta potential determination—Part 3: Acoustic methods

(*Continued*)

TABLE 8.1 (Continued)

Technique	Attribute	ASTM guidelines	ISO guidelines
Inductively coupled plasma mass spectrometry	Size, NM concentration, chemical composition (inorganic NM)	X	ISO/TS 19590:2017 - Nanotechnologies—Size distribution and concentration of inorganic nanoparticles in aqueous media via single particle inductively coupled plasma mass spectrometry
Nanoparticle tracking analysis	Size/NM concentration	E2834-12(2018) - Standard Guide for Measurement of Particle Size Distribution of Nanomaterials in Suspension by Nanoparticle Tracking Analysis (NTA)	X
Scanning electron microscopy	Size/shape/morphology/chemical composition	X	ISO 19749:2021 - Nanotechnologies—Measurements of particle size and shape distributions by scanning electron microscopy
Static multiple light scattering	Size/NM concentration	X	ISO/TS 21357:2022 - Nanotechnologies—Evaluation of the mean size of nano-objects in liquid dispersions by static multiple light scattering (SMLS)
Transmission electron microscopy	Size/shape/morphology	X	ISO 21363:2020 - Nanotechnologies—Measurements of particle size and shape distributions by transmission electron microscopy
X-ray diffraction	Crystal properties	X	ISO/TS 17200:2020 - Nanotechnology—Nanoparticles in powder form—Characteristics and measurements
Zeta potential (electrophoretic light scattering)	Surface charge	E2865-12(2018) - Standard Guide for Measurement of Electrophoretic Mobility and Zeta Potential of Nanosized Biological Materials	ISO 13099-2:2012 - Colloidal systems—Methods for zeta potential determination—Part 2: Optical methods

ASTM and ISO websites. OBS: "ISO/TR 18196:2016 Nanotechnologies—Measurement technique matrix for the characterization of nano-objects" describes several other methods, such as thermal and spectroscopy characterization, relating applicable standards that were not made for NM but are applicable to them. This table did not include specific carbon nanotube protocols because of their scarce use as a drug delivery tool. In vitro assessments with cells were not included. Standards have a life cycle, so always check if there is a newer version on the institution sites.

the physical dimension of a NM particle size, shape, and structure. AFM provides the same type of information, in addition to surface texture [3].

The classical electronic microscopy (TEM/SEM) is widely used, with the requirement of fixed, dehydrated, and conductive samples. Drying liquid samples can lead to NM agglomeration or aggregation, which alters shape information. For beam-sensitive or non-conducting NMs, they generally need a coating (platinum, gold, or graphite) or staining (especially TEM) before imaging. Coatings enhance brightness and contrast at the expense of changes in shape, size, and surface texture. One more limitation of these techniques relates to the single-particle evaluation in a very small sample quantity, which makes questionable the representativeness of the data and its statistical relevance in the evaluation of batch homogeneity. Besides coating and staining downsides, images must be carefully interpreted since artefacts could modify the imaging of the NPs, such as crystals related to buffer drying [8].

Nevertheless, electron microscopy evolved considerably. As an example, SEM can be configured with an ultrahigh resolution field emission setup (field emission SEM) that can drastically reduce the accelerating voltages and increase spatial resolution. This feature reduces charge accumulation in the sample, but may still need coating and dehydration. As most nanosized medicines are vehicled as suspensions, vitrification of samples in amorphous ice by cryogenic techniques became a great choice: samples freeze very quickly and resemble the liquid spatial distribution. The coating over the frozen sample gives a more accurate shape description. Several drug products are evaluated by cryo-EM, specially liposomes [9]. Of note, the cryogenic setup is more expensive and still scarce in analytical laboratories.

AFM gives 3D analysis of NMs with a nanometric topographic resolution and also some mechanical properties. It is a good tool to directly image NMs and works also on samples rich in water [3]. On the other hand, AFM has a few contrast materials and lack other options offered by SEM. It can also be difficult to perform AFM for samples that are not well attached to a surface and can be displaced by the AFM tip [10].

8.3 Size average, distribution, and nanomaterial concentration

Size can be measured in the nano range through equipment and methods based mainly on laser-light scattering/diffraction, EM, and physical separation, followed by detection of an NM property. Microscopy methods allow for particle visualization and consequent shape assessment with absolute number description, whereas laser-based methods depend on mathematical models related to the particle shape for size determination. Physical separation happens mainly through analytical ultracentrifugation, field flow fractionation, and gel permeation, with the former also relying on shape models ('perfect sphere') and the latter on comparison with model particles.

The analytical choice comes from equipment availability, capability to detect and characterize the NM in the specific size range, sample characteristics (amount, composition, and physical state), and intended use of data (formulation characterization, production in-line, at-line, and offline control). It should also be accounted that a method may impose drying, dilution, and other sample modifications that might alter the NP original attributes

[3]. For example, organic NM may be subjected to substantial changes in size in the wet and dry states, leading to minor dimensions measured by EM in dry matter than the ones measured in liquid state by dynamic light scattering (DLS) [7]. For this reason, it is important to report the "type" of size measured (e.g., hydrodynamic versus projected particle radius and ensemble versus single particle analysis) and the NP state (dry or wet). The USP chapter also recommends the use of complementary methods when the measured attribute is critical (e.g., performing DLS and EM analyses) [3].

The same microscopy methods used for shape determination apply to size evaluation, but they require higher training/cost/time requirements than scattering techniques and may take several samples to determine a reliable size distribution. In particular, AFM precisely gives the particle size and shape, even in a polydisperse sample. The disadvantage of AFM is that the number of NMs analyzed is smaller than that from DLS, and it is important to critically evaluate the results to avoid under/overestimation of the total sample size distribution [11].

Light scattering techniques [DLS and nano tracking analysis (NTA)] are low/medium cost techniques and easy to manipulate, require little sample preparation, and provide screening analysis with a fast check of the sample, but with low-resolution results. DLS helps especially when biological interactions are pursued (e.g., protein corona), and it is the first choice for quality control (QC) for most nanostructured drug products [8,12]. DLS can measure the hydrodynamic size and distribution of NM based on intensity, determining the fluctuations in the intensity of light scattering from NMs in Brownian motion. For that, the software assumes that NM has a spherical shape, and the sample viscosity and refractive index is known. Since scattering intensity is much higher for bigger particles, polydisperse samples can present higher size averages. One more concern is with particle aggregation state: the method does not distinguish between larger particles and small aggregates. However, in purified samples with a known particle individual, such as protein solutions, DLS does provide aggregation kinetic profiles [3,8].

NTA has a number-based measurements of size, which allows to distinguish different populations in a polydisperse sample and gives a more reliable size distribution than DLS. It also complements DLS measuring by giving the NM concentration in the sample (number of particles per mL) [12]. Since NTA requires lower NM density (10^8 to 10^{12} particles/mL and 10^7 to 10^9 particles/mL, respectively), it has better resolution than DLS, being less susceptible to the influences of high intensity scattering from bigger NMs. However, it is more expensive than DLS equipment and may require extensive sample dilution, together with a more complicated sample insertion in the equipment [11].

Part of the uncertainty brought in DLS measurements of polydispersed samples comes from the high sensitivity to bigger nanoparticles. Data acquisition in multiangle DLS (MADLS) counterbalance this phenomena, bringing a better correlation of size and scattering and consequently better size determination of distinct particle populations [13]. So far, due to the novelty, this methodology is not standardized and fewer publications use it for drug product analysis.

Laser diffraction (LD) differs from dynamic measurements because it looks at diffraction or scattered laser intensity vs diffraction angle pattern to determine particle size; therefore, movement of particles is not considered as a size parameter. DLS is more suitable for NMs ≤ 50 nm, while LD provides better results for bigger particles (starting from 50–100 nm, depending on the equipment) [11]. Due to the low limit of detection of size, this technique is not standardized for NM material characterization.

Another multiangle option refers to the static light scattering, a standardized technique that can determine the size of undiluted samples and follow aggregation/agglomeration kinetics [3,10]. Small angle X-ray scattering (SAXS) can also be used to obtain NM morphological and heterogeneity/aggregation information, despite providing less detail than EM/AFM and requiring dilution of monodisperse populations.

All these techniques perform measurements under a liquid or powder condition, in a static or flow mode. However, to monitor nanoaerosols produced in manufacturing or NM distribution after aerolization (inhalation products), an impactor equipment is required to separate particles between its stages according to their aerodynamic particle size distribution [14,15]. Some of these techniques give a concentration data (e.g., NTA and MADLS) based on direct nanoparticle properties; fluorescence also relates to NM concentration, allowing for direct determination or indirect quantification by fluorescent probes. Fluorescence principles are better explored in the API content section.

8.4 Nanomaterial surface properties

NMs have a high surface area to volume ratio, which gives them a huge reactive interface with the local environment. This means that the same material can change its properties depending on how it is used—as bulk or NM, together with the chemical composition, charge, and reactivity [3]. The charge of an NM suspension interferes with the toxicity, environmental impact, and physiological fate. Hence, the knowledge of NM surface properties enables us to predict, establish, and optimize formulations [16].

Surface charge assessment relies on acoustic, electric, and optical properties, with emphasis on zeta potential determination by electrokinetic potential of colloidal suspensions. A nonstandardized method that is worth mentioning is the sensitive tunable resistive pulse sensing, which is capable of solving charge and size of individual particles. However, polydisperse populations require change of the conical pore to accommodate different size ranges and make absolute measurements more difficult [7,10].

ZP measurement is helpful to predict whether NP will be favored to aggregate or agglomerate or will remain in suspension as discrete particles. High ZP values ($|\zeta| \geq$ 15 mV) indicate high repulsion among NMs, and low ZP values indicate that NMs are prone to aggregate from an electrostatic point of view [3]. However, NMs that have steric stabilization could have low ZP values and maintain discrete particles [6]. It is important to consider several details of ZP measurement because it depends on the local environment, solvents, pH, and background electrolyte concentration [7,10,11].

NM surface reactivity and loading may depend on porosity and surface area. Pores interfere drastically in the NM surface-to-volume ratio, which can increase API loading, decrease NM sealing, interfere in targeting and cell uptake, and so forth. Porosity needs to be characterized according to the size, dimensions, and volume of the pore cavity. Along with direct pore visualization by EM, dry samples of NMs absorb nitrogen or expand helium according to its surface area and porosity, which is the reason why analytical techniques based on these phenomena are frequent and standardized.

Of note, samples need to be frozen at very low temperatures, a step that may change surface area or pore density [17].

Dynamic vapor sorption (DVS) also evaluates pore distribution and surface area in dried particles, with the advantage of working at room temperature. As a downside, DVS analysis follows water sorption and desorption profiles on the NM surface, which could lead to hydrolysis degradation or solid-state transformations [verifiable by powder X-ray diffraction (XRD) after DVS]. Nevertheless, the transformations upon water uptake are useful to determine sample stability under humidity, crystal changes, and other properties, which are relevant for formulation design and optimization. Some experiments show octanol as an alternative vapor to sorption experiments [18,19].

Both gravimetric and gas adsorption analyses rely on the application of mathematical equations to model the NM behavior, with the Brunauer–Emmett–Teller theory for surface area calculation [19]. Other models can be fit to isotherms to represent different aspects of the NM, such as hydrophilic layers and hydrophobic cores [20].

8.5 Nanomaterial-active pharmaceutical ingredient structure, composition, and crystal form

Structure, composition, and crystal form compose a set of features one should know for practically all medicines. Therefore, most techniques are not built up for NMs, so that data should be carefully interpreted to take this into account. The most common properties measured are thermal behavior, crystal profile, and chemical composition.

Differential scanning calorimetry (DSC) and thermal gravimetric analysis (TGA) are usual techniques to understand the thermal behavior of NMs, APIs, and their interactions. Besides the final product, thermal analysis aid in process development, since one can mimic thermal conditions of real unit operations and follow their consequences in physical and chemical states. TGA detects mass variation derived from a change in physical state and/or chemical composition of samples upon controlled heating. So, a TG curve may contain different weight loss processes such as dehydration, decomposition, oxidation, and loss of volatiles [21]. Dehydration mass loss correlates with residual moisture, a property directly related with dry product stability and drying process efficiency. There are five main factors to consider to obtain good and reproducible TGA results: sample purity and particle size; heating rate; atmosphere (static or dynamic and type of gas); and crucible and sample weight (higher weight increases sensitivity and decreases resolution) [22]. It is interesting to consider this fast and user-friendly technique when analyzing API-NM interactions, since NM could protect the API from degradation but could also accelerate this process. It is also possible to analyze gas products from TGA (TGA-FTIR, TGA-MS, and TGA-GC/MS) [23]. In particular cases, such as inorganic nanoparticles coated with organic substances, it is possible to determine coating mass proportion due to mass loss of the organic material. For the same reason, the API encapsulation rate can be determined by TGA if the NM is inorganic and the loading relates to organic material. Both assay types need more samples and a highly sensible TGA [24].

If TGA associates the weight loss to the temperature increments (up to 1500°C), then DSC gives information of thermal events (crystallization, melting, and glass transition).

Phase changes are recorded according to the heat flow of the sample compared to the reference crucible at a certain temperature treatment [25]. These characterizations bring information upon compatibility between NM-API and further formulation stability. A DSC analyzer submits the sample to controlled cooling, heating, temperature holding, and combination of thermal steps. These treatments provoke endothermic and exothermic events including melting of crystals, glass transitions, and thermal degradation. Therefore, thermal shifts can be related with API or NM crystal form and the purity of that physical species.

DSC allows to identify whether an API-NM incorporation changed the original API crystalline state to an amorphous compound or to a different polymorph (if it has a different melting point). It also predicts original crystalline API internalization into the nanocarrier due to the lack of its crystalline melting peak. The dislocation of melting peaks of NM and API indicates their interaction, which can be further investigated by complementary techniques [25]. Temperature and the velocity it changes in DSC direct influence property measurement. For example, slow heating rates can increase the resolution of peaks, whereas faster rates increase sensitivity with the possible cost of slowing down crystallization events or causing peak dislocations [25,26]. Generally, it is not necessary to prepare a sample for analysis and the measurements are straightforward, but in the characterization phase, several temperatures and rates must be tested to evaluate time-related transitions [25].

XRD also detects the presence of polymorphs, solvates, or cocrystals that can be created due to formulation manufacturing or excipient interaction. XRD is more precise than DSC in this matter because different crystals diffract the laser in a different way, but not necessarily have different melting points. In addition, it verifies the degree of crystallinity of the API and API-NM formulation [27]. Powder XRD is a nondestructive and most common technique applied to pharmaceutical NMs, but higher sensitivity comes with the use of SAXS. SAXS can elucidate particle size, polydispersity, and NM morphology [28]. Since crystalline material has a diffraction signature, NM composition can be elucidated when comparing diffractograms of samples with databases. However, most drug-related compounds have amorphous content that does not diffract light significantly, so excipients may be disregarded in this analysis.

One of the spectroscopic techniques most applied to study API-NM interactions and surface composition is the Fourier transform infrared spectroscopy (FTIR). It evaluates the absorption of infrared electromagnetic radiation by the molecules in the sample and gives spectra that comprises the fingerprint of pure molecules and their binding modifications and changes in the functional groups binding due to the presence of other compounds. The interpretation of the spectra provides information upon molecule structures and interactions, and it is recommended by health agencies and pharmacopeias as substance identification [28]. UV, fluorescence, and mass spectrometry also give NM information, but will be discussed in the API section.

Nuclear magnetic resonance (NMR) also applies for quantitation and structure determination of NMs, besides morphology in situ in solid phase or solution. It is often applied to analyze interactions or coordination between the surface of a certain NM and the ligand. Ligand density, atomic composition, and its influence on NM shape and size are also characterizations provided by the NMR technique [28].

It is pertinent to consider the NM-API characterization by different analytical techniques, since they are often complementary. For example, despite DSC being a rapid, user-friendly technique that does not require sample preparations, it does not provide structural information and its information would be enriched if combined with a spectroscopic technique. Evidently, it is of major importance to verify the particularities and limitations of both the sample and the technique. The overview of techniques presented here is not exhaustive due to the large amount of alternatives in chemical analysis.

8.6 Active pharmaceutical ingredient content

The NM-based delivery system can be associated with the total or partial API content from the formulation. Therefore, characterization must include the API-NM-associated amount, assurance of API content integrity postproduction, and detection of impurities and degradation products [20].

The API-NM association can be measured related with the percentage of API incorporated in the carrier, generally called encapsulation efficiency, regardless of where the carried substance is located within the carrier. Drug loading, in turn, is concerned with the carrying weight capacity of the carrier system. For both determinations, there is a need to separate the free from the carrier-associated API, for example, using centrifugal filter devices, size exclusion spin columns, or solid phase extraction columns [3].

Quantification of API relies mainly on UV-vis spectrophotometry. UV-vis determines API content by its discrete wavelength absorption, which is directly proportional to API concentration over a range that varies among the analytes in solution (Beer–Lambert law) [29]. The absorption of a specific wavelength of UV/Vis radiation occurs by one or more chromophores that are molecular groups with π bond and atoms with nonbonding orbitals. The spectrum of emission and detection goes from 185 nm up to 1000 nm, detected by an UV/Vis spectrophotometer [30]. Although this works well for pure substances, excipients for the formulation or API degradation products may also absorb on the same wavelength and bind to the API or alter pH, which can also cause change intensity and the maximum absorbance wavelength (λ) [20].

The intensity of fluorescence emitted by a sample upon light stimulation also relates to molecule concentration. Emission measurements implicate that the excited electrons from the API return to the relaxed state with photon emission [31]. Measuring the emission spectra with the fluorimeter brings high sensitivity and selectivity, which is especially useful when the API has low absorption of light in the UV region. A second useful situation concerns measurement of a highly diluted drug in biological fluids, a common need for pharmacokinetic studies [29].

Fluorescence or UV/vis detection gained a higher specificity when preceded by a column chromatographic step to separate samples into their constituents, especially high performance liquid chromatography (HPLC)-dominated API content protocols, since it separates excipients and degradation products and delivers them with high sensitivity, repeatability, and specificity [32,33]. However, at the cost of sensitivity, the UV/Vis detector can be replaced by multiple photodiode arrays that give information over several wavelengths at the same time [34].

HPLC separations rely mainly on differences of molecule partition between the mobile liquid phase and the column stationary phase, which makes analytes reaching detectors in different times [35]. The normal phase HPLC has stationary phases more polar than the mobile phase, and reversed phase (RP) has the opposite polarity mode. RP-HPLC is the method of choice for most APIs due to the stability and reproducibility of the stationary phases, together with the wide range of components for the mobile phase. Concerning mobile phase formulation, it is usually composed of water and buffered solutions, with methanol or acetonitrile to reduce the polarity; adjustments in these components provide adequate retentive characteristics for the compounds of interest. Other factors that affect the retention time of analysis include temperature, pH of the buffer and/or mobile phase, stationary phase properties, flow rate, and mobile phase composition [36,37].

The columns most used in RP-HPLC are silica-based, with C3, C4, C8, or C18 alkyl chains attached. They are compatible with aqueous and some organic mobile phases, since it does not react, dissolve, or swell in them [38]. High molecular weight substances, such as protein drugs, can benefit a size exclusion column that separates species by size, by HPLC or LC systems with lower pressure. Classical silica-based columns also do not perform well with highly polar drugs, and alternative ion-exchange chromatography is a compendial alternative. They can be based on modified silica to became anionic or cationic, besides other polymers and resins [39,40].

When the compounds are volatile, gas chromatography stands out. Substances separate between an inert gas flow and a liquid or solid stationary phase inside the column. Like HPLC, drug polarity influence interactions and consequent retention times in the column. Then, separated compounds pass generally through a flame ionization detector (FID) or a more expensive mass spectrometry (the last one especially useful for degradation products). The sample undergoes pyrolysis under the air-hydrogen flame in the FID, decomposing in ions and electrons that are detected by a high-impedance picoammeter.

Regardless of the method choice, they must be developed and validated during formulation development in order to assess the loading of the API as well as the possible interaction between the formulation components [41]. For that, it is necessary to comply with the criteria of specificity, linearity, precision, repeatability, determination of the analytical curve range, detection limit, and quantification limit [41].

8.7 Active pharmaceutical ingredient degradation products, other impurities, and stability assessment

API-NM association can protect the cargo from degradation, but manufacturing steps that require heating, high energy, or pH shifts may degrade molecules. The manufacturing stress can be summed up or even escalate API–excipient interactions, bringing unstable formulations after production or through storage time. For example, nanostructured lipid carriers require solid lipid melting to incorporate the API, but the heating can degrade it [20]. APIs also undergo chemical reactions depending on the pharmaceutical dosage form and environmental conditions, resulting in degradation products during storage or transportation. These products decrease the API content and have the potential to cause adverse effects in patients, so they need to be identified and kept under a threshold related with its biological safety and API daily dose. Recommendations on thresholds and analytical reporting can be found on ICH guideline Q3B and in ICH-M7 for mutagenic impurities [42,43].

Hydrolysis and oxidation are the main the causes of API instability. Hydrolysis is the most common pathway for API breakdown, in which the API molecule reacts with water, resulting in the cleavage of a chemical bond within that molecule. Esters and amides are the most common groups found in APIs prone to hydrolysis. Water reacts with esters more rapidly than with amides, and these reactions can be catalyzed by either acid or base. The rate depends on the pH of the aqueous solution. Degradation can happen during the process of API association to a NM, exposing the drug to severe conditions of high temperature or oxidant excipients/impurities, for example [20]. Likewise, metabolism of esters and amides in APIs happens through a hydrolysis mechanism catalyzed by hydrolytic enzymes from tissues and plasma [44,45].

Oxidation involves the removal of electrons from a molecule (or the addition of oxygen) and triggered by light, heat, or traces of certain metals. Oxidative degradation can often be reduced to acceptable levels by storing susceptible drugs in the absence of light (e.g., using amber vials) and oxygen (e.g., storing under nitrogen or argon), or by using formulation strategies like higher purity excipients, antioxidants, and protective coating [46].

A clear understanding of the organic chemistry of API degradation is essential to maintain the stability, efficacy, and safety of a drug product throughout its shelf-life. So, health agencies require forced degradation studies to assure that the API content analysis is specific to the API and that degradation can be detected. The stress conditions include temperature, humidity, light, and pH variation changes. The knowledge produced with this technique is important to know the unwanted products and thus understand and avoid potentially problematic stages of the production process [47].

HPLC coupled with a UV detector is the most used technique to monitor or detect API degradation, since degradation products usually appear as new peaks. However, identification of overlapping peaks is usually done with HPLC-DAD (photodiode array ultraviolet detector), which detects peak purity. The products that surpass the thresholds need a full identification by high resolution techniques, which mostly include separation through a column (HPLC; LC; gas chromatography) to isolate the substance, coupled or followed by a detector that produces a mass spectra (mass spectrometry), an UV spectra (DAD), proton NMR spectra, or a combination of detection modes [34].

Elemental impurities may cause adverse events to patients and instability to the formulation during its shelf-life. Residual solvents, although generally not related with API degradation, may bring toxicological hazards. As a consequence, they have to be below limits, indicated by health agencies and organization as the ICH documents of the Q3 series (Q3A to Q3E).

Degradation products, as the API content, must be followed during product storage, which is called long-term stability. Before this, products are tested in accelerated conditions (variations in temperature, humidity, and UV radiation) to predict their behavior in the long run. ICH QA series (QA1 to Q1F) indicates general stress conditions to submit product samples and, depending on drug degradation mechanisms, to extrapolate stability data to the shelf life in ambient conditions.

8.8 Active pharmaceutical ingredient release assay

API release is the process by which the API molecules dissociate from nanostructures and migrate to the external environment. The local mode of in vivo release will depend on the administration route, API physicochemical properties, mechanism of release from the carrier, and targeting abilities of the formulation. It is an essential property to know as release kinetics correlates with targeting and plasma profile. In a research laboratory environment, the in vitro drug release kinetics can be measured through the dispersion of the product into a dissolution media inside a dissolution apparatus, measuring the released API over time with a suitable sensitive analytical technique. Whenever possible, the in vitro release method should reflect the route of administration of the drug product.

This API release test comprises the essential toolbox to assess safety, efficacy, and quality profile of any NM-based drug delivery system, ensuring that these attributes are maintained throughout the lifecycle of a given medicine. From an industry perspective, an in vitro profile that correlates with the in vivo release kinetics (IVIVC) would have a long-term advantage as a surrogate for in vivo bioequivalence testing required to qualify higher level scale-up and post-approval changes for modified release. Also, an IVIVC method helps in screening candidate formulations due to release properties. However, the testing strategy can vary between the development and QC stages, whereas the former can focus on the establishment of an IVIVC; the QC method conditions focus on faster and simpler conditions, which may include higher temperatures or surfactants to expedite drug dissociation.

IVIVC also complies with rational use of animals in research. Determination of pharmacokinetic parameters requires drug content measurements in the plasma or blood fluid (e.g., aqueous humor), which demands frequent sampling, complex drug extraction from biological samples, highly sensitive analytical instruments, as well as extensive animal/human experiments. The animal studies, such as with rabbits and other mammals, together with instrumentation evolution to characterize NMs, enabled an extensive understanding of the in vivo drug release process [48]. Based on these data, it is possible to obtain an IVIVC to establish "a predictive mathematical model describing the relationship between an in vitro property and a relevant in vivo response" by the U.S. FDA [49].

In general, the methods for the establishment of an IVIVC include biorelevant concentrations of fluid components (plasma, saliva, and gastrointestinal fluid), specific proteins for protein–drug interactions, synthetic/biorelevant surfactants, enzymes, and cosolvents [50]. So far, the elucidation of the bionanointerface shows its importance in determining the biological fate of nanostructures. If the carrier design aims local API release for regional action or absorption, the fluid simulation correlates well with API fate, when the API pharmacokinetics is already known. However, when the carrier is absorbed or administered parenterally to reach the blood stream, the API content still bound to the carrier can extravasate from blood circulation, causing differences between the pharmacological or toxicological effects of nanomedicines when compared to a solution of the free drug [51]. Considering this, a recent published USP general chapter <1001> states that *"although desirable, in vitro and in vivo correlations may not be possible for modified-release parenteral dosage forms due to the complexity of the release mechanisms and the lack of knowledge about in vivo release conditions"* [52].

Testing dissolution precludes equipment selection. The most suitable apparatus and/or method configuration will rely on the product characteristics and its administration route. When NMs are associated with the API, there are different drug release setups and no standard in vitro dissolution method. As an example, an expert panel joined by the United States Pharmacopoeia has published a stimuli article showing the recent trends and developments in the area of in vitro performance of NM-based drug products. A thorough discussion is made on the methods used in the detection of the free and particle-bound fractions of the drug in the dissolution media, recommendations for the development and validation of the release assay, and the key parameters that should be documented to enable method reproducibility and results consistency within different laboratories [53].

Basically, the current in vitro dissolution methods for assessing the drug release from NMs have to be able to distinguish bound and nonbound API. Therefore, the assay has to be based on membrane diffusion methods, also called dialysis methods, or sample and separate methods, which include NM separation after sample collection. Both separation modes can be done on traditional or continuous flow (CF) methods [54]. Each of these techniques has its own particularities, advantages, and drawbacks that will be briefly discussed in this chapter.

The membrane methods are the most versatile and popular among the researchers for assessing the in vitro dissolution/release testing from NMs; they can be adapted in practically all available apparatus for dissolution testing (USP I, II, IV, shake-flask, Franz-Cells). The rationale is that diffusion happens through a dialysis membrane that separates the carrier from the released drug and acceptor media. Therefore, the membrane should be permeable to the free dissolved API but not to the NM. In addition, API or NM must not adsorb on the membrane because it would decrease exchange membrane area and influence results [55].

In the sample and separate methods, the nanostructured drug delivery systems are directly dispersed into the release medium, which is maintained under constant agitation to prevent NM aggregation. Drug release is then monitored over time by quantification after the physical separation from NM using techniques such as filtration, ultracentrifugation, and centrifugal ultrafiltration. Of note, this step can cause filter clogging or API absorption to filters or to NM. Equipment USP apparatuses I and II predominate, although other methods of separation and apparatuses are reported in the literature like the NanoDis system [56].

In the CF methods, drug release from the nanostructured drug delivery system is measured in a dissolution media, which is constantly circulating throughout a device containing the drug product. The amount of the drug released from the carrier is determined by collecting the eluent at periodic intervals. The most common apparatus used in CF methods is the Apparatus IV (Flow-Through Cells), with closed or open circuits. In the closed configuration, the dissolution media circulates in a loop, whereas the open option brings continuously fresh media. Due to dilution, the open configuration requires analytical methods with higher sensitivity. The CF methods are often associated with a sample and separate and/or a dialysis technique, by using either a filter with a reduced pore size or a dialysis-based device. The main issues related to the CF methods are the difficult equipment setup prior to the analysis, membrane or filter clogging due to their reduced porosity associated with the polymeric NMs, which can cause variations in the analysis flow rate, and API adsorption to the filters and/or glass beads (used to enable the laminar flow, disperse/hold the NM, and prevent NM aggregation) [57].

Although not currently applied for commercial APIs, some published methods rely on direct measurements, such as ion- or drug-selective electrodes. Direct measurements based on spectroscopic in line analyzers can also be efficient if the drug and NM carrier possess vibrational signatures that do not overlap.

References

[1] Dave VS. Chapter 4 - QbD considerations for excipient manufacturing. In: Beg S, Hasnain MS, editors. Pharmaceutical Quality by Design. Academic Press; 2019. p. 65–76. Available from: https://doi.org/10.1016/B978-0-12-815799-2.00004-6.

[2] Halwani AA. Development of pharmaceutical nanomedicines: from the bench to the market. Pharmaceutics 2022;14:106.

[3] USP. ⟨1153⟩ *Drug Products Containing Nanomaterials*. https://doi.usp.org/USPNF/USPNF_M13775_02_01.html; 2022. Available from: https://doi.org/10.31003/USPNF_M13775_02_01.

[4] FDA/CDER/"Yeaton, A. Drug products, including biological products, that contain nanomaterials - guidance for industry. 29 (2017).

[5] Hoshyar N, Gray S, Han H, Bao G. The effect of nanoparticle size on in vivo pharmacokinetics and cellular interaction. Nanomed (London) 2016;11:673–92.

[6] Pettitt ME, Lead JR. Minimum physicochemical characterisation requirements for nanomaterial regulation. Environ Int 2013;52:41–50.

[7] Faria M, et al. Minimum information reporting in bio–nano experimental literature. Nat Nanotech 2018;13:777–85.

[8] Caputo F, Clogston J, Calzolai L, Rösslein M, Prina-Mello A. Measuring particle size distribution of nanoparticle enabled medicinal products, the joint view of EUNCL and NCI-NCL. A step by step approach combining orthogonal measurements with increasing complexity. J Control Rel 2019;299:31–43.

[9] Standard Practice for Performing Cryo-Transmission Electron Microscopy of Liposomes. https://www.astm.org/e3143-18b.html.

[10] Modena MM, Rühle B, Burg TP, Wuttke S. Nanoparticle characterization: what to measure? Adv Mater 2019;31:1901556.

[11] Bhattacharjee S. DLS and zeta potential – what they are and what they are not? J Contr Rel 2016;235:337–51.

[12] Maguire CM, Rösslein M, Wick P, Prina-Mello A. Characterisation of particles in solution – a perspective on light scattering and comparative technologies. Sci Technol Adv Mater 2018;19:732–45.

[13] Austin J, Minelli C, Hamilton D, Wywijas M, Jones HJ. Nanoparticle number concentration measurements by multi-angle dynamic light scattering. J Nanopart Res 2020;22:108.

[14] United States Pharmacopeia. General Chapter, ⟨1603⟩ Good Cascade Impactor Practices. USP-NF. Rockville, MD: United States Pharmacopeia. https://doi.usp.org/USPNF/USPNF_M13055_03_01.html; 2022. Available from: https://doi.org/10.31003/USPNF_M13055_03_01.

[15] ISO/TR 27628:2007(en), Workplace atmospheres—Ultrafine, nanoparticle and nano-structured aerosols—Inhalation exposure characterization and assessment. https://www.iso.org/obp/ui/#iso:std:iso:tr:27628:ed-1:v1:en.

[16] Bantz C, et al. The surface properties of nanoparticles determine the agglomeration state and the size of the particles under physiological conditions. Beilstein J Nanotechnol 2014;5:1774–86.

[17] Kéri A, et al. Porosity determination of nano- and sub-micron particles by single particle inductively coupled plasma mass spectrometry. J Anal Spectrom 2020;35:1139–47.

[18] Mesallati H, Umerska A, Tajber L. Fluoroquinolone amorphous polymeric salts and dispersions for veterinary uses. Pharmaceutics 2019;11.

[19] Kondor A, et al. On the BET surface area of nanocellulose determined using volumetric, gravimetric and chromatographic adsorption methods. Front Chem Eng 2021;3.

[20] Beraldo-Araújo VL, et al. Levofloxacin in nanostructured lipid carriers: preformulation and critical process parameters for a highly incorporated formulation. Int J Pharm 2022;626:122193.

[21] Nasrollahzadeh M, Atarod M, Sajjadi M, Sajadi SM, Issaabadi Z. Chapter 6 - Plant-mediated green synthesis of nanostructures: mechanisms, characterization, and applications. In: Nasrollahzadeh M, Sajadi SM, Sajjadi M, Issaabadi Z, Atarod M, editors. Interface Science and Technology, Vol. 28. Elsevier; 2019.
[22] Heal G.R. Thermogravimetry and derivative thermogravimetry. In: *Principles of Thermal Analysis and Calorimetry*; 2002, pp. 10–54. Available from: https://doi.org/10.1039/9781847551764-00010.
[23] Mansfield E, Banash M. Thermal Analysis of Nanoparticles: Methods, Kinetics, and Recent Advances. *NIST*; 2021.
[24] Dongargaonkar AA, Clogston JD. Quantitation of surface coating on nanoparticles using thermogravimetric analysis. In: McNeil SE, editor. Characterization of Nanoparticles Intended for Drug Delivery. Springer; 2018. p. 57–63. Available from: https://doi.org/10.1007/978-1-4939-7352-1_6.
[25] Gabbott P. A practical introduction to differential scanning calorimetry. Principles and Applications of Thermal Analysis. John Wiley & Sons, Ltd.; 2008. p. 1–50. Available from: https://doi.org/10.1002/9780470697702.ch1.
[26] Gabbott P. Fast scanning DSC. Principles and Applications of Thermal Analysis. John Wiley & Sons, Ltd.; 2008. p. 51–86. Available from: https://doi.org/10.1002/9780470697702.ch2.
[27] Holder CF, Schaak RE. Tutorial on powder X-ray diffraction for characterizing nanoscale materials. ACS Nano 2019;13:7359–65.
[28] Mourdikoudis S, Pallares RM, Thanh NTK. Characterization techniques for nanoparticles: comparison and complementarity upon studying nanoparticle properties. Nanoscale 2018;10:12871–934.
[29] Siddiqui MR, AlOthman ZA, Rahman N. Analytical techniques in pharmaceutical analysis: a review. Arab J Chem 2017;10:S1409–21.
[30] What Causes Molecules to Absorb UV and Visible Light. *Chemistry LibreTexts* https://chem.libretexts.org/Bookshelves/Physical_and_Theoretical_Chemistry_Textbook_Maps/Supplemental_Modules_(Physical_and_Theoretical_Chemistry)/Spectroscopy/Electronic_Spectroscopy/Electronic_Spectroscopy_Basics/What_Causes_Molecules_to_Absorb_UV_and_Visible_Light; 2013.
[31] 15.1: Theory of Fluorescence and Phosphorescence. *Chemistry LibreTexts* https://chem.libretexts.org/Bookshelves/Analytical_Chemistry/Instrumental_Analysis_(LibreTexts)/15%3A_Molecular_Luminescence/15.01%3A_Theory_of_Fluorescence_and_Phosphorescence; 2022.
[32] Weich A, de OLIVEIRA DC, de MELO J, Goebel K, Rolim CMB. Validation of UV spectrophotometric and HPLC methods for quantitative determination of atenolol in pharmaceutical preparations. Lat Am J Pharm 2007;6.
[33] Rahman H, Manirul Haque S. Development and validation of chromatographic and spectrophotometric methods for the quantitation of rufinamide in pharmaceutical preparations. TJPS 2021;0:0.
[34] Singh, R. Current trends in forced degradation study for pharmaceutical product development. in; 2012.
[35] Raghavan R, Joseph JC. Chromatographic methods of analysis: high-performance liquid chromatography. Encyclopedia of Pharmaceutical Science and Technology, Fourth Edition. CRC Press; 2015.
[36] Martin PD, Jones GR, Stringer F, Wilson ID. Comparison of normal and reversed-phase solid phase extraction methods for extraction of β-blockers from plasma using molecularly imprinted polymers. Analyst 2003;128:345–50.
[37] de Villiers A, et al. Evaluation of ultra performance liquid chromatography: Part I. Possibilities and limitations. J Chromatogr A 2006;1127:60–9.
[38] Vervoort RJM, Debets AJJ, Claessens HA, Cramers CA, de Jong GJ. Optimisation and characterisation of silica-based reversed-phase liquid chromatographic systems for the analysis of basic pharmaceuticals. J Chromatogr A 2000;897:1–22.
[39] Derayea SM, Ahmed HM. Applications of ion-exchange chromatography in pharmaceutical analysis. In: Inamuddin, editor. Applications of Ion Exchange Materials in Biomedical Industries. Springer International Publishing; 2019. p. 119–38. Available from: https://doi.org/10.1007/978-3-030-06082-4_5.
[40] United States Pharmacopeia Vol 31, National Formulary 26, General Chapter: <621> Chromatography. http://www.uspbpep.com/usp31/v31261/usp31nf26s1_c621.asp.
[41] ICH. Validation of analytical procedures: text and methodology Q2 (R1); 2005.
[42] EMA. ICH Q3A (R2) Impurities in new drug substances - Scientific guideline. *European Medicines Agency*. https://www.ema.europa.eu/en/ich-q3a-r2-impurities-new-drug-substances-scientific-guideline; 2018.

[43] EMA. ICH M7 Assessment and control of DNA reactive (mutagenic) impurities in pharmaceuticals to limit potential carcinogenic risk - Scientific guideline. *European Medicines Agency*. https://www.ema.europa.eu/en/ich-m7-assessment-control-dna-reactive-mutagenic-impurities-pharmaceuticals-limit-potential; 2018.
[44] Melo SR, de O, Homem-de-Mello M, Silveira D, Simeoni LA. Advice on degradation products in pharmaceuticals: a toxicological evaluation. PDA J Pharm Sci Technol 2014;68:221–38.
[45] Snape T.J., Astles A., Davies J. Understanding the chemical basis of drug stability and degradation. *Pharm J.* https://pharmaceutical-journal.com/article/ld/understanding-the-chemical-basis-of-drug-stability-and-degradation.
[46] Gabrič A, Hodnik Ž, Pajk S. Oxidation of drugs during drug product development: problems and solutions. Pharmaceutics 2022;14:325.
[47] Peltonen L. Practical guidelines for the characterization and quality control of pure drug nanoparticles and nano-cocrystals in the pharmaceutical industry. Adv Drug Deliv Rev 2018;131:101–15.
[48] Shen J, Burgess DJ. In vitro–in vivo correlation for complex non-oral drug products: where do we stand? J Contr Rel 2015;219:644–51.
[49] FDA Guidance for industry: extended release oral dosage forms: development, evaluation and application of in vitro/in vivo correlation (issued 9/1997, Posted 9/26/1997) - ECA Academy. https://www.gmp-compliance.org/guidelines/gmp-guideline/fda-guidance-for-industry-extended-release-oral-dosage-forms-development-evaluation-and-application-of-in-vitro-in-vivo-correlat.
[50] Gupta R, Chen Y, Xie H. In vitro dissolution considerations associated with nano drug delivery systems (NDDS). Wiley Interdiscip Rev Nanomed Nanobiotechnol 2021;13:e1732.
[51] Mast M-P, et al. Nanomedicine at the crossroads – a quick guide for IVIVC. Adv Drug Deliv Rev 2021;179:113829.
[52] United States Pharmacopeia. General Chapter, ⟨1001⟩ In Vitro Release Test Methods for Parenteral Drug Preparations. USP-NF. Rockville, MD: United States Pharmacopeia. https://doi.usp.org/USPNF/USPNF_M5433_02_01.html; 2022. Available from: https://doi.org/10.31003/USPNF_M5433_02_01.
[53] Wacker MG, Lu X, Burke M, Nir L, Fahmy R. Testing the in-vitro product performance of nanomaterial-based drug products: view of the USP expert panel. Dissol. Technol 2022;29:6–20.
[54] D'Souza S. A review of *in vitro* drug release test methods for nano-sized dosage forms. Adv Pharm 2014;2014:e304757.
[55] Nothnagel L, Wacker MG. How to measure release from nanosized carriers? Eur J Pharm Sci 2018;120:199–211.
[56] Lombardo SM, Günday Türeli N, Koch M, Schneider M, Türeli AE. Reliable release testing for nanoparticles with the NanoDis system, an innovative sample and separate technique. Int J Pharm 2021;609:121215.
[57] Shen J, Burgess DJ. In vitro dissolution testing strategies for nanoparticulate drug delivery systems: recent developments and challenges. Drug Deliv Transl Res 2013;3:409–15.

CHAPTER

9

Inorganic and metal-based nanoparticles

Gajanan Paul, Ujjwal Gupta*, Hinal Shah*, Farhan Mazahir and A.K. Yadav*

Department of Pharmaceutics, National Institute of Pharmaceutical Education and Research, Raebareli, Uttar Pradesh, India

9.1 Introduction

In the past two or three decades, the medical field has witnessed great progress in the field of the drug delivery system, from conventional methods to the advanced nanodelivery system to the various new techniques, and these have proved to be effective therapies and safer to the mankind. Even the smallest molecules like peptides and nucleic acids are easily delivered to the target site. Nanotechnology-based techniques are widely used to diagnose and treat various malignant, neurodegenerative, and respiratory diseases. The use of Au, Ag, Fe, and Gd has gained a lot of focus because of their less radioactivity and robust shape and size. Nanoparticles are used in the gene delivery systems, effective in replacing the gene involved in causing cancer and other genetic disorders [1]. Polymeric nanoparticles (NPs) are used widely in the controlled and sustained release formulations polylactic glycolic acid, and chitosan is a widely used polymer, as it is highly biocompatible and biodegradable and approved by FDA. Various metallic NPs, that is, iron oxide, gold, and silver, have shown promising results for the diagnosis of cancer and radiotherapy and less toxicity as compared to other NPs. Fig. 9.3 shows various metallic NPs which, by the enhanced permeability and retention (EPR) effect, help in the diagnosis of cancer. Further, in various scientific studies, it is shown that the iron oxide NPs have unique optical properties that allow them to act as biosensors for living cells, whereas the various scientific literature has shown that silver NPs have wide use in electronic devices, textiles, wound dressing, antimicrobial coatings, and biomedical devices [2]. There are also carbon-

* Authors Gajanan Paul, Ujjwal Gupta, and Hinal Shah contributed equally to this chapter.

Molecular Pharmaceutics and Nano Drug Delivery
DOI: https://doi.org/10.1016/B978-0-323-91924-1.00006-X

based and lipid-based NPs and nanoemulsions used in the bioimaging application. Liposomes which are used commonly for the delivery of nutraceuticals and biologics have high encapsulation efficiency and extended circulation time. As with the increase in demand, carbon NPs are used in gene therapy and imaging. The various literature also suggests that the nanoemulsion can be administered by parental, transdermal, and ocular routes, as they have the property to protect the encapsulated drug from enzymatic degradation and hydrolysis and they have shown the increased uptake of drug in the cancer cells, leading to the reduction of tumor growth [3].

9.2 Enhanced permeability and retention effect

In the tumor tissues, the absence of the vasculature supportive tissues initiates the leaky vessels, pores, and poor lymphatic system formation, which offers a great advantage to treat cancer. This process is called the unchanged EPR effect. Generally, the treatment of cancer by the EPR mechanism is growing day to day and helping in many ways to design the novel therapies. In the abnormal and leaky vasculature system and EPR effect in the tumor tissues, NPs tend to accumulate higher than in other tissues, so the NP system also enhances the half-life of the drug because it protects it from renal clearance. There are various factors, protein binding and NP aggregation, which affect the EPR effect because of the increase in the size of the NP system due to complex formation [4,5]. According to various scientific studies, it has also been observed that the EPR effect is abolished by the reticuloendothelial system present in the liver and spleen; to overcome this problem, surface modification can be done, and hence the EPR effect can be enhanced. EPR effects have other factors like Bradykinin, cyclooxygenases, heme oxygenase, carbon monoxide, and so forth [5]. Nanomedicines nowadays are having an effect worldwide by varying their biopharmaceutical properties and increasing patient compliance. Nanomedicines can be formulated like liposomes, micelles, microbubbles, and magnetic NPs. Moreover, these formulations are very effective and can penetrate cancer cells in the future; biological molecules like monoclonal antibodies and aptamers can be improved by the EPR effect.

9.3 Blood–brain barrier

All of the tissues and organs in the body rely on blood arteries to provide oxygen and nutrients. The blood–brain barrier (BBB), which allows blood vessels to vascularize the central nervous system (CNS) and has unique features. Ions, chemicals, and cells are tightly regulated between the blood and the brain. This fine management of CNS homeostasis enables normal neuronal activity and survival. It is also protects neuronal tissue from poison and infections. A series of physical, transport, and regulatory factors work together to maintain the physiological barrier [6]. Capillaries are divided into three structural groups. The epidermis and lung have continuous nonfenestrated capillaries that are connected by cellular connections and have a complete basement. There is no fenestra (pores) in the basal membrane. The plasma membrane of their cells continually fenestrated intestinal villi and endocrine vessels. The structure of glands is similar to that of a continuous structure but possesses diaphragmed fenestra all over their body membrane. Discontinuous capillaries in the liver exhibit wide gaps throughout the cell and are characterized by a lack of continuity [7]. Because the BBB's restrictive nature makes drug delivery to the CNS difficult, significant efforts have been made. To develop modulation or bypassing methods, the BBB is used for therapeutic delivery, and loss of some, or all, of these barriers is observed. In neurological diseases such as stroke, multiple sclerosis (MS), brain damage and neurodegenerative disorders, characteristics are the most important factor in the pathogenesis and progression of these disorders. Ion dysregulation, altered signaling homeostasis, and BBB dysfunction can all result from BBB failure in immunological cells and chemicals entering the body [6,7].

9.3.1 History of blood–brain barrier

Ehrlich and his colleague Goldmann performed experimental work supporting a BBB over 100 years ago within in vivo vital staining of organs following systemic infusion of dyes. While Ehrlich and Goldman's contributions are frequently mentioned in the literature, other authors produced key work that pre-and post-dated Goldmann in studies of the BBB. According to Ehrlich, acidic vital dyes are used to stain the peripheral organs of animals. Following systemic injection, the entire body is affected, except the brain and spinal cord. Although, Ehrlich was not one of them in the context of a BBB, who explain this observation. On the other hand, in the CNS, it was thought that the drug receptors expressed in peripheral tissues bind the important organs. In the year 1913, it was thought that the flow of nutrients from the blood to the brain required a mandatory passage via an intermediary CSF compartment of the BBB's anatomical location to the CSF production, which takes place in the choroid plexus (ChPs) [8].

9.3.2 Cells of the blood–brain barrier

Endothelial cells (ECs), which form the walls of blood vessels, and mural cells, which exist on the abluminal surface of blood arteries, are the two basic cell types that make up blood vessels. The BBB's features are mostly exhibited within the ECs, although they are also induced and are sustained by crucial contacts with others. Immune cells, glial cells, and brain cells are all examples of mural cells in the neurovascular unit that interact [9].

9.3.2.1 Endothelial cells

ECs are modified simple squamous epithelial cells that form the walls of blood arteries and are derived from mesoderm. Large arteries and veins can have lots of ECs in their diameter, whereas the smallest capillary has only a few. It is made up of a single EC folding in itself to form and create the vessel's lumen. These microvascular ECs in the CNS are extremely rare. Thin cells have a thickness 39% less than muscles. With a distance of less than a quarter of a mile between them, ECs and the luminal and parenchymal surfaces are separated by a micron [10].

9.3.2.2 Pericytes

Pericytes are brain capillary constituents that occur at various frequencies in distinct vascular beds. They are most common in the CNS, especially the retina, and are connected by a basement membrane. ECs form a peg-socket-like direct synaptic connection. N-cadherin forms focal interactions with the endothelium as well as connexins. Their tight interaction with ECs permits ions, metabolites, second messengers, ribonucleic acids, and different amino acids to be exchanged between the cell. Pericytes also have a role to perform important responsibilities in preserving BBB integrity and assisting in microvascular stability and angiogenesis. Pericytes, which have contractile properties comparable to smooth muscle cells, can regulate the flow of blood (to some extent), the diameter of capillaries, and cerebral blood flow [11].

9.3.2.3 Astrocytes

Astrocytes are a type of glial cell that has polarized cellular processes that surround either neuronal processes or blood vessels. Astrocytes provide a cellular interface between the CNS and the rest of the body. Several grafting and cell culture investigations have indicated the role of various neurovascular unit (NVU) cells in the development and maintenance of the BBB. When a 3-day-old quail's avascular tissue brain graft was put into the ECs in chick embryos' coelomic cavity, the graft was vascularized, resulting in a functional BBB [12].

9.3.2.4 Tight junctions

Tight junctions (TJs) are cell adhesions connecting the membrane of two cells, and they are made up of numerous transmembrane proteins that interact directly via extracellular components. TJs in the CNS are specialized in their molecular and structural composition to create a high-resistance electrical barrier, and the paracellular permeability of the BBB is determined by the unique mix of TJ proteins at the BBB [12,13].

TJs are derived from between the ECs, and it was found that cellular adhesions are produced on the apical region of the lateral membrane by homotypic and heterotypic contacts of transmembrane molecules related to the cytoskeleton via interactions with cytoplasmic protein adapters [13].

9.3.2.5 Mural cells

Mural cells include vascular smooth muscle cells that surround major vessels and pericytes, which only partially cover the microvasculature's endothelial walls. Pericytes are special cells, and do not express specific/single marker which makes their study difficult. These cells are frequently mixed up with other cells that are found in the perivascular area. The most widely accepted method is currently positive reactivity to both PDGFR-b and NG2, which is a molecular identifier of CNS pericytes; however, alternative markers exist [14].

9.3.3 Regulation of the blood–brain barrier

ECs in mammals are known to undergo dynamic alterations in response to various stimuli. The dynamic alterations of ECs are influenced by ceratin activities such as cellular, physical, and chemical stimuli. Chemical signaling appears to have a crucial function in various kinds of physiology of cells. Shear stress, for example, is a type of physical stimulation that is one of the most significant but underappreciated physiological stimuli, which contributed to the differentiation and maturation of vascular ECs as well as other cellular and molecular processes. Several variables peculiar to the microniche of the NVU maintain and regulate the persistence of a functional BBB throughout adulthood. The interactions between astrocytes and ECs are complex and known to alter the phenotype of the barrier via regulating EC morphology and angiogenesis. The morphology of ECs are affected by the normal or pathological conditions, and influnce the integrity of BBB (i.e. leakiness). The appropriate preservation environment for synaptic and neuronal activity is provided by certain ion channels and transporters at the BBB. The abluminal sodium is a good example of a pump that (Na^+, K^+-ATPase) transports Na^+ into the brain and K^+ out of the brain to maintain a high concentration of Na^+ and low levels of K^+ in the interstitial fluid. The luminal Na^+, K^+, and Cl^- cotransporters, that is, Na^+, K^+, and Cl^- and Na^+, K^+, and $2Cl^-$ are transferred from the blood to the endothelium. Calcium transporters (Na^+–Ca^{2+} exchanger) and voltage-gated K^+ channel are regulated to transport the ion across the BBB [7,10,12].

9.3.4 Disturbance of the blood–brain barrier in the central nervous system disorder

The BBB is disrupted in a variety of neurological illnesses, including stroke, Alzheimer's disease (AD), epilepsy, and others. Traumatic brain injury imaging is used to determine the functional aspects of human patients and for postmortem examination. The diseased state of the brain is discovered using brain samples. Different neurological illnesses cause to break down the BBB. The various neurological disorders are represented in Fig. 9.3. Working with animals is also an option for disease models and cell cultures of the BBB. The use of models has allowed for the discovery of certain interesting facts. TJs, transporters, transcytosis, and LAM expression are just some of the features of the BBB that can be affected by the malfunction. This can result in breakdown edema, ionic homeostasis disturbance, altered ionic homeostasis immunological infiltration, and signaling eventually, leading to neuronal dysfunction and degeneration. Even though BBB malfunction is common, it has been considered, in some cases, as a continuation of the original insult in some disorders including MS, epilepsy, and AD. The BBB is damaged in most CNS disorders as a result of the pathology's inflammation, injury, or degenerative processes. The BBB, on the other hand, is only targeted by the pathogenic process in a few disorders by the factors of disease. These disorders include neuromyclitis optica and MS. In MS, astrocytes are not typically thought to be a key target of the immune system. Even though BBB rupture and astrocyte physiological changes are hallmarks of MS pathogenesis [14,15].

Fig. 9.1 shows the various pathways of the BBB, which is further described below.

9.3.4.1 *Paracellular pathway*

Lipophilic or low molecular weight solutes are transmitted through the BBB via the paracellular route by the passive diffusion activity, and then they affect the electrochemical, hydrostatic, and osmotic factors' gradient. In this system, TJ has a structural role and is influenced by the solute concentration when it comes to functionality; the junctional complex's permeability is controlled by the endothelial cytoskeleton's contractility and sticky forces. One of the most important blood–brain exchange systems has been identified. Paracellular diffusion, on the other hand, is a minor element in the development of brain-targeted drugs [7].

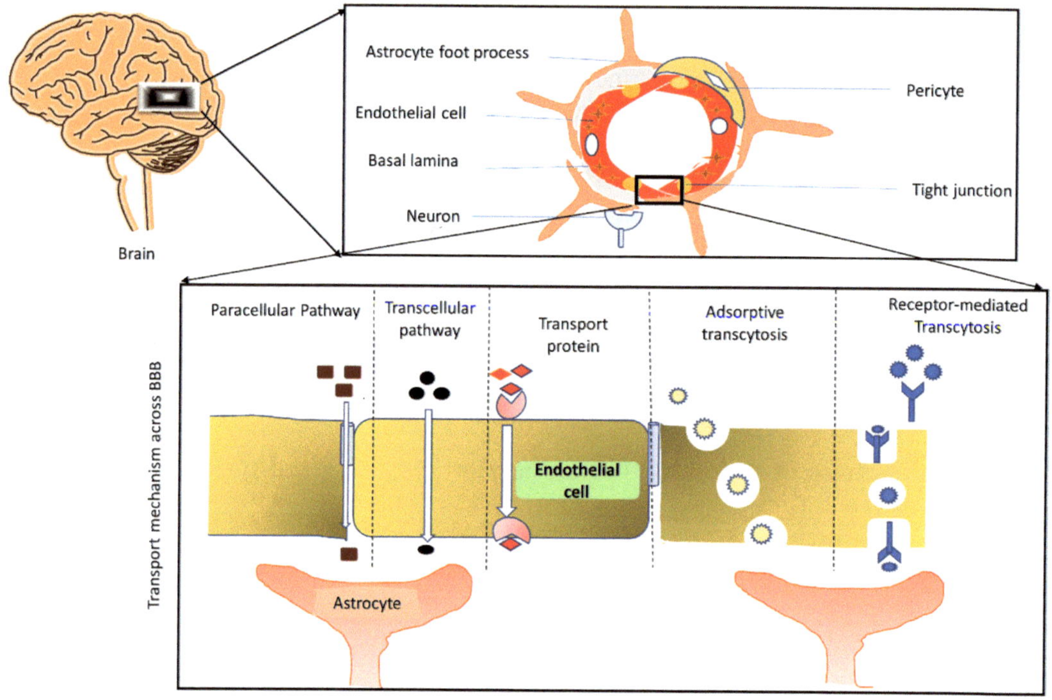

FIGURE 9.1 Pathways of blood–brain barriers.

9.3.4.2 *Transcellular pathway*

This type of pathway is either energy-dependent or energy-independent, and the diffusion occurs via luminal and abluminal membrane of the capillary endothelium, receptor-mediated transcytosis (RMT), efflux transport system, endocytosis of positively charged molecules, and carrier-mediated transport [8].

9..3.4.3 *Passive diffusion*

A wide range of lipid-soluble substances can flow through the BBB and passively reach the brain. Calculating a drug's logo (octanol/water) partition coefficient at room temperature determines its lipid solubility. The rate of change in pH is related to the rate of change at which a substance penetrates the CNS, as well as its lipid solubility, which contains both unionized and ionized species in solution; unionized species cross the BBB. Another important aspect in calculating the molecular weight is the size of the molecule. Small compounds can freely pass through the BBB. Once the drug's MW is greater than 400 Dais, it is difficult to permeate the BBB.

Only lipid-soluble molecules with less than 10 hydrogen bonds and a diameter of roughly 180 Da can diffuse across brain endothelia passively. Different BBB transcellular transport mechanisms are used instead to carefully regulate the entry and departure of chemicals into and out of the CNS. The "carrier-mediated transport" refers to the transfer of essential nutrients like glucose in hydrophilic substances, which is assisted by the principal transport channel. To get to the other side, fatty acids and amino acids must cross the BBB [10,11].

9.3.4.4 *Active efflux*

The BBB's luminal, blood-facing endothelial plasma membrane expresses many ATP-binding cassette proteins. They are ATP-dependent efflux pumps. Xenobiotic and endogenous metabolite pumps reduce the permeability of a variety of poisons, including pharmaceuticals. P-glycoprotein (Pgp—multidrug resistance protein ABCB) is the major efflux transporter in the BBB, and P-gp is a common efflux transporter in the BBB. On the other side, MRP isoforms appear to be expressed in both luminal and abluminal membranes, and they seem to prefer water-soluble conjugates as a substrate. Because the medications will be conjugated by drug converting enzymes, bi-directional efflux from the endothelium is anticipated to render them cytotoxic-free [12]

9.3.4.5 *Receptor-mediated transcytosis*

It is a process employed by the BBB for the uptake of compounds like hormones, insulins, leptin, and low-density lipoproteins. There are two types of vesicular transport systems: RMT and adsorptive-mediated transcytosis. RMT is a pathway where macromolecules orligands bind to specific receptors present on the cell surface, and promp the cells to uptake macromolecules or ligands. The receptors and ligand are joined together to create a cluster. A caveola is formed, which pinches off and becomes a vesicle. Both the ligand and the receptors are internalized by ECS. When a cell is directed across the cytoplasm to the cell's opposing side, exocytosis happens. It is the principal way for brain ECs to take in chemicals like hormones or high-molecular-mass proteins like insulin and leptin. IGF, transferrin, and density lipoproteins cross the BBB. This route is a type of active transport system that relies on temperature and has the potential to get saturated. Recognition of receptor ligands increases the production of the development of covered pits that finally envelop the ligand. An endocytic vesicle is a type of endocytic vesicle. The second phase entails an examination. The endosomal fusion separates the ligand from the receptor. Not all vesicles can get across the BBB because some lysosomes fuse with others, losing their content [6,16].

9.3.4.6 *Carrier-mediated transport*

The BBB separates the brain from the rest of the body, preventing the flow of numerous critical polar chemicals required for metabolisms, such as glucose and amino acids. As a result, other pathways for vital nutrients to reach the body are required. It is vital to have a brain. CMTs are genes that are encoded within a cell. The solute carrier transporter gene family is a group of genes that transports solutes. More than 300 transporter genes are encoded by this gene membrane-bound protein that aids in transportation through biological membranes of a diverse range of substrates. To achieve intact protein or peptide transcytosis, the lysosomal compartment within the cell must be avoided. This is achieved by directing the major source of energy. The endosome and its contents are removed from the lysosomal compartment when degradation ensues [11,13].

9.3.4.7 Charged compound interaction

The carrier-mediated pathway is a saturable transfer system that allows substances to flow from the systemic circulation to the brain parenchyma. It can either be energy-dependent or self-contained. These carriers are normally polarized. The luminal and the abluminal membranes are both affected. There are a variety of carrier systems expressed in brain ECs that may selectively transport a broad range of chemicals, including glucose, which is passively transported by the glucose transporter protein type-1 (GLUT-1) transporter. There are many different amino acids to choose from. There are many different energy-dependent carrier proteins, each with its n function that is defined by the physico-chemical qualities of each individual. Neutral, and aromatic amino acids are taranfered by the N- or L- transporters [6].

9.4 Neurological disease

9.4.1 Alzheimer's disease

AD is a well-known protein conformational disease and a chronic neurodegenerative disease. Dementia affects 47 million people worldwide, with the number expected to double (to 131 million) by 2050 [17]. Two prototypical lesions of AD are senile plaques, which are extracellular lesions composed of a nucleus of β-amyloid protein accumulation (Aβ42), and neurofibrillary tangles, which are intraneuronal findings composed of phosphorylated and microtubule-associated tau protein (P-tau) [18,19]. Amyloid pathology causes β-secretases (BACE1) and γ-secretases to cleave amyloid precursor protein (APP), an integral protein on the plasma membrane, to produce insoluble Aβ fibrils. After then, the Aβ oligomer diffuses into synaptic clefts and obstructs synaptic signaling. PSEN1 and PSEN2 mutations result in greater A42/A40 ratios, and mutations in one of three genes (APP, PSEN1, and PSEN2) are apparent [20] (Fig. 9.2).

9.4.1.1 Iron oxide nanoparticles

To develop noninvasive magnetic resonance imaging (MRI) techniques for the diagnosis of AD, we produced antibody-conjugated superparamagnetic iron oxide NPs (SPIONs) for use as an in vivo agent for MRI detection of amyloid plaques in AD. We now provide results from trials performed in APP/PS1 transgenic mice, revealing the ability of novel anti-APP-conjugated SPIONs to traverse the BBB and act as a contrast agent for plaque MRI. Plaque complicity increased from 5.10.5 to 8.30.2 when the plaque contrast to noise ratio was identical in control AD mice and AD animals treated with SPIONs. In the SPION-treated AD mice, the number of MRI-detectable plaques per brain increased from 347 ± 45 in the control AD mice and 668 ± 86 in the SPION-treated AD animals. These findings reveal that in transgenic mice, our SPION-enhanced amyloid-detection approach provides an effective, noninvasive MRI detection tool [21].

9.4.1.2 Gadolinium nanoparticles

Oligomers are more pathogenic and neurotoxic; they have been a popular AD biomarker. Using oligomers is a reliable and useful technique for detection and tomography

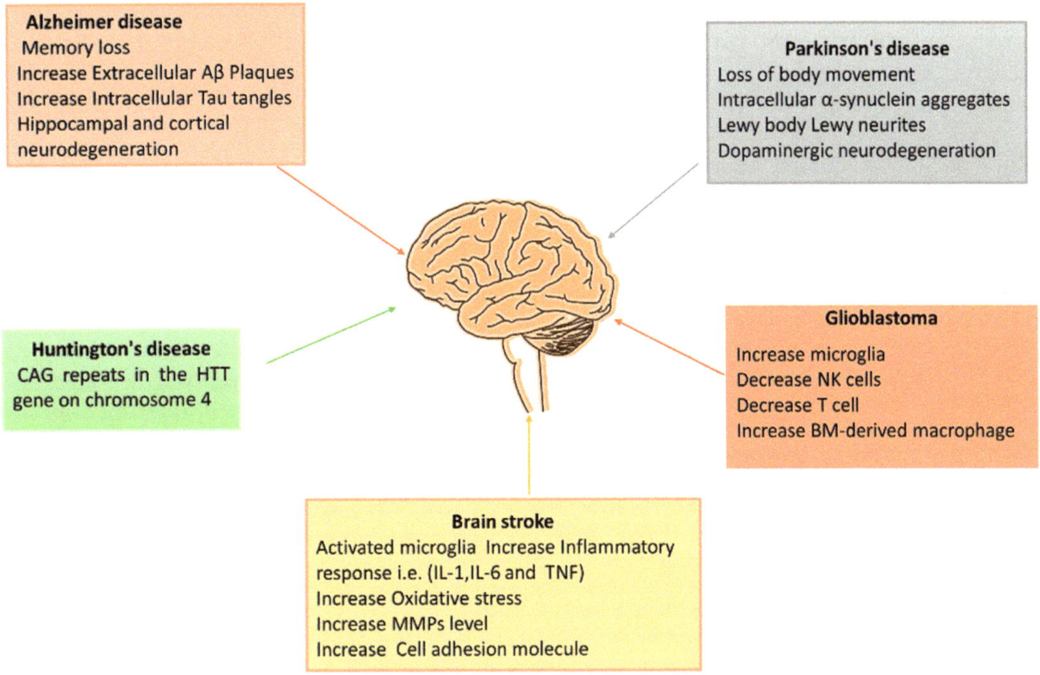

FIGURE 9.2 Representation of various neurological disorders.

for the early identification of AD, assessing disease progression, and evaluating the efficacy of possible AD treatments. For the real-time model of content in an AD mouse model, the first oligomer-specific Gd^{3+}-based NPs were synthesized using NP@SiO_2@F-SLOH as multimodal near-infrared imaging (NIRI)/T1-weighted MRI contrast agents, in vivo and ex vivo NIRI agents with high sensitivity and selectivity to A oligomers, as well as MRI agents with beneficial resolution in various age groups for the AD mouse model; the NP@SiO_2@F-SLOH was successful. The NP probe, meanwhile, prevents A fibrillation and protects neurons from A-induced damage, suggesting that it could be utilized as treatment for AD. All of these findings indicate that this effective and sensitive nanomaterial (NM) has a lot of promise for application as a valuable theranostics MRI nanoprobe. While the common use of MRI is as a clinical diagnostic tool, no clinically derecognized contrast agents for cerebral AD biomarker imaging are now available. We describe the design and development of the first BBB penetrable theranostics that target amyloid (A). Gadolinium and tetraactic acid based cyanine dye diaplyed multifunctional properties as a multimodal probe, including good biocompatibility, low cytotoxicity, high Aβ selectivity, strong fluorescence augmentation upon binding with Aβ species, paramagnetic properties, high stability, good BBB penetrability, and quick removal from the mouse. The dyad's longitudinal relaxivity (r^1) was found to be 4.42 m/Ms at 3 Tesla(T), indicating that it might be used as a T1-weighted (one of the basic pulse sequences in MRI that shows differences in tissue T1 relaxation periods) MRI contrast agent. In transgenic mouse models of AD, the probe had been successfully assessed for one- and two-photon stimulated fluorescence and MRI of A. It can also prevent A aggregation, protect against A-induced toxicity, and promote the production of reactive oxygen species (ROS). Our findings show the dyad's remarkable theranostics power for AD diagnosis and therapy, as well as the tremendous potential for MRI in humans [22].

9.4.2 Parkinson's disease

In 1817, James Parkinson published the first report on Parkinson's disease (PD), describing it as "paralysis agitans." PD is a chronic, progressive neurological condition that affects 1%–2% of the world's population over 65 and 4%–5% of those over 85. Every year, 60,000 people in the United States are diagnosed with PD, resulting in a significant socioeconomic cost of $20 billion each year [23]. Tremors, slower movements, and rigidity are all motor symptoms and alterations in taste and smell perception, gastrointestinal dysfunction, and sleep disturbances are nonmotor symptoms of PD [24]. Degeneration of dopaminergic neurons in the SN as well as intraneuronal protein clumps known as Lewy bodies (LB) is observed, and Lewy neurites are neuropathologic markers of PD. It was long considered that 50% to 70% of substantia nigra (SN) dopaminergic neurons die by the time clinical motor symptoms become evident [25]. α-synuclein, a tiny (140 amino acid) protein found mostly in the neocortex, hippocampus, SN, thalamus, and cerebellum, is the most important component of LB. The SN and the cornu ammonis (CA2/3) region of the hippocampus have the most Lewy neurites, which are nerve cell terminals that contain an aggregation synuclein [15]. Alterations in the seven genes α-synuclein (SNCA), parkin (PARK2), UCH-L1 (PARK5), DJ1 (PARK7), LRRK2 (PARK8), ATP13A2 (PARK9), and PINK (PARK6) have been shown to produce familial parkinsonism definitively [26]. It has long been assumed that by the time clinical motor symptoms appear, 50% to 70% of SN dopaminergic neurons die [25]. The parkin gene has the most mutations, ranging from 1.96% to 39.1% in the Indian case series. SNCA has no mutations, while DJ1, PINK1, and LRRK2 have mutations [27].

9.4.2.1 Iron oxide

The progressive loss of dopaminergic neurons in the midbrain is a hallmark of PD, and stem cell transplantation is a viable treatment option. In these studies, tracking the biological properties of the transplanted cells in vivo is crucial for gaining a fundamental understanding of stem cell function and determining clinical success. To make unique ultrasmall SPIONs coated with polyacrylic acid (PAA) and methoxy polyethylene glycol (PEG) amine, we employed a thermal breakdown technique and a two-step modification. According to TEM and FTIR, USPIO-PAA/PEG NPs have a uniform diameter of 10.070.55 nm and an absorption peak of the conforming ligands. MTT revealed that cells incubated with USPIO-PAA/PEG NPs survived for more than 96% of the time. The synthesized USPIO-PAA/PEG exhibited an excellent relaxation rate of $84.65\,s^{-1}\,Mm^{-1}$, and the effective uptake was tracked using MRI. HADSCs were also identified and labeled with USPIO-PAA/PEG before being transplanted into the striatum of 6-hydroxydopamine-induced PD rat models. Transplantation with tagged HADSCs significantly reduced apomorphine-induced rotations in PD mice and increased the number of dopaminergic neurons in SN, according to MRI findings. Overall, the development of USPIO-PAA/PEG NPs provides a useful tool for in vivo cell therapy tracing as well as a novel method for tracking stem cells with therapeutic potential in PD [28].

9.4.3 Brain stroke

A stroke is a neurological condition in which blood arteries get blocked [29]. Clots occur in the brain, disrupting blood flow by blocking arteries and rupturing blood vessels, resulting in bleeding. A brain stroke occurs when an artery ruptures, resulting in the unexpected death of brain cells owing to a lack of oxygen. Dementia and depression are common side effects of stroke [30]. There are two types of strokes: ischemic and hemorrhagic. Around 85% of stroke people die as a result of cerebral ischemic occlusions. Cerebral hemorrhagic stroke accounts for 10%–15% of all strokes [31]. Stroke affects 13.7 million people worldwide each year and is the second foremost cause of death, accounting for 5.5 million deaths. The risk of stroke in those aged 75–84 is 25 times that in people aged 45–54. Stroke affects one out of every four persons in their lifetime, and there are more than 80 million stroke survivors worldwide. When compared to Caucasians, women are at the same or higher risk of stroke than men, and Hispanic/Latino Americans have a higher prevalence of all forms of strokes. According to studies, black people have roughly twice as many strokes as white people. Ischemic and hemorrhagic strokes account for the majority of strokes. An ischemic thrombotic stroke is the most prevalent type of stroke; nevertheless, low oxygen partial pressures, hypotension, and reduced oxygen consumption are also extra physiologic conditions that can cause ischemia and neuronal death or dysfunction [32].

9.4.3.1 Gold nanoparticles

Exosomes are proving to be effective therapeutic options for a variety of illnesses. Extracellular vesicles can overcome biological barriers, such as the BBB and act as effective drug and gene therapy transporters. However, a paucity of data on exosome trafficking, biodistribution, and challenges in imaging in deep brain locations in vivo are all hurdles to therapeutic development. We recognize noninvasive in vivo neuroimaging and exosome tracking approaches based on glucose-coated gold NP (GNP) labeling and computed tomography (CT) imaging. Instead of the usual and less efficient indirect labeling through parent cells, exosomes were directly labeled with GNPs. On a mechanical level, we discovered that glucose-coated GNPs were uptaken into mesenchymal stem cell (MSC) exosomes via an active energy-dependent mechanism driven by the GLUT-1 and requiring endocytic proteins. Next, we determined the best size and administration route for exosome labeling; we found that 5 nm GNPs enabled better exosome labeling and that intranasal administration resulted in superior brain accumulation and, as a result, improved in vivo neuroimaging. When compared to intravenous administration, we also used a mouse model of localized brain ischemia to track intranasally given GNP-labeled exosomes, which demonstrated increased accumulation at the lesion site over 24 hours, in contrast to nonspecific migration and clearance from control brains. As a result, this exosome labeling technology has the potential to be employed as a powerful diagnostic tool for several brain disorders as well as potentially improving exosome-based neuronal recovery therapy [33].

The primary goal is to create a CT-based approach for detecting thrombi in the brain and guiding thrombolytic therapy. In vitro and in vivo images of fib-GC-GNPs and a non-targeted control agent in C57Bl/6 mice ($n = 107$) with FeCl3-induced carotid thrombosis and/or embolic ischemic stroke were displayed in C57Bl/6 mice ($n = 107$) with FeCl3-induced carotid thrombosis and/or embolic ischemic stroke. Fibrin-binding ability was higher with fib-GC-GNPs than with GC-GNPs, with thrombi visible on micro-CT (MCT) with high density. CT imaging with fib-GC-GNP is recommended for the initial detection and quantification of cerebral thrombi and monitoring of the tPA-mediated thrombolytic effect, which reveals the histological stroke response. MCT might also detect chronic thrombosis for up to 3 weeks without the need for extra NP delivery. Fib-GC-GNP-based direct cerebral thrombus imaging greatly improves the value and information obtainable by regular CT, has multiple uses in basic/translational research, and will be viable to allow for modified thrombolytic therapy in clothing by (1) optimizing tPA dosing to match thrombus burden and (2) enabling the rational triage [34].

9.4.3.2 Iron oxide nanoparticles

Because the early inflammatory response of immune cells within the ChPs in response to neuroinflammation is unknown in vivo in many brain disorders, there is a significant need to develop imaging tools that would allow for noninvasive monitoring of ChP involvement in these disorders. MRI coupled with SPIO particles is a minimally invasive technique for tracking phagocytic cells in inflammatory diseases (SPIO). In a mouse model of neuroinflammation generated by intraperitoneal lipopolysaccharide administration, we wanted to see if USPIO-enhanced MRI might be utilized to detect ChP participation in vivo. We detected significant USPIO-related signal decreases in the ChPs of animals with neuroinflammation compared to controls using high-resolution MRI. To statistically analyze their findings, they used a four-point grading system. Ex vivo investigations indicated USPIO build up as well as immune cell absorption in the ChP stroma. We confirmed the translational potential of our technique using the therapeutically relevant USPIO ferumoxytol. USPIO accumulation in the chips might be used as an imaging biomarker to look for ChP involvement in neuroinflammatory diseases, and it could be used swiftly in clinical practice [35].

Human MSCs (hMSCs) were labeled using silica-coated magnetite composite NPs ($Fe_3O_4@SiO_2$) and core-shell NPs for in vitro and in vivo MRI studies. The NPs are 24–30 nm in diameter, with an 8 nm Fe_3O_4 core and an 8 nm SiO_2 shell. The NPs distributed in water have a transverse relaxivity of $\sim$106 m/Ms, according to the researchers. After a 12-hour incubation period with hMSCs at a concentration of 100 mg Fe/mL, cellular absorption of $Fe_3O_4@SiO_2$ is 20–100 pg Fe/cell, with the majority of the $Fe_3O_4@SiO_2$ found in the cytoplasm. The viability and differentiation of human bone marrow-derived stromal stem cells (hMSCs) are unaffected by this degree of absorption. Single-cell sensitivity is achieved in vitro using $Fe_3O_4@SiO_2$-labeled hMSCs equally distributed in an agarose gel at 11.7 T. $Fe_3O_4@SiO_2$-labeled hMSCs injected into the left hemisphere of nude mice produce imaging sensitivity comparable to $\sim$130 hMSCs [36]

9.4.3.3 *Gd nanoparticles*

Identifying the dynamics of BBB disruption in an acute ischemic stroke is critical for preventing symptomatic hemorrhagic change. Current approaches for assessing BBB permeability, on either side, are not quantitative and are only used in the context of acute reperfusion therapy. Nanoparticles, whether healthy or not, use a combination of passive and active activities to cross the BBB. Imaging and measuring their transfer rate capacity can help researchers better understand how the BBB degrades and how to best administer neuroprotective drugs. Researchers developed a unique endovascular stroke model of acute ischemic stroke treated with mechanical thrombectomy and monitored by positron emission tomography (PET)-MRI before creating an endovascular stroke model of acute ischemic stroke treated with mechanical thrombectomy and monitored by PET-MRI. Small clinical gadolinium Gd-DOTA (1 nm) and AGuIXVR NPs (5 nm) utilized for brain theranostics were employed to measure cerebral capillary permeability [37].

9.4.4 Huntington's disease

In 1872, an American family doctor named George Huntington coined the term "Huntington's disease" (HD) [38]. HD is an autosomal dominant neurological disorder that is rare, deadly, and progressive. In the Caucasian population of the United States and most of Europe, the majority rate of HD is 5–10 per 100,000 [39]. This sickness lasts between 17 and 20 years. Psychiatric symptoms (such as depression, suicidal ideation, mania, apathy, and schizophrenia-like symptoms), cognitive defects (such as interpersonal deficits, lack of attention, and motor skill learning deficits), motor impairment (such as chorea, rigidity, gait abnormalities, and bradykinesia), sleep disturbances, and weight loss are all caused by HD. HD is caused by a CAG trinucleotide repeat expansion in the huntingtin (HTT) gene on chromosome 4 that is autosomal and dominantly inherited on chromosome 4; a mutation in the exon-1 region of the HTT gene has been discovered, leading to the expansion of a CAG repeat region in this exon. The polyglutamine (poly Q) domain at the N-terminus of the HTT protein is increased in HD patients. The typical HTT gene has around 35 CAG repeats; mutations that increase this to around 40 CAGs induce HD to occur with full incidence, and people with 36–39 CAG repeats in HTT show a variety of HD symptoms [40,41].

9.4.4.1 *Iron oxide nanoparticles*

We observed the properties of SPIONs conjugated with an amyloid oligomer-specific scFv antibody (W20) attached to PEGylated SPIONs. The findings revealed that W20-SPIONs, which have a diameter of roughly 11.8 nm and an appropriate relaxation capacity for use as an MRI contrast agent, were stable and nontoxic. W20-SPIONs penetrated the BBB and were precisely bound to the oligomer region in transgenic mouse models of PD and HD, resulting in MRI signals that distinguished PD and HD from healthy controls. These findings demonstrated W20-SPIONs' promise in early-stage PD and HD diagnosis, as well as a new method for evaluating the efficacy of new medications [42].

9.4.5 Glioblastoma

Glioblastoma (GBM) is an extremely prevalent malignant primary brain tumor, accounting for around 57% of all gliomas and 48% of all primary malignant CNS tumors [43]. GBMs can form anywhere in the brain, including the brain stem, cerebellum, and spinal cord. The four lobes of the brain account for 61% of all primary gliomas: frontal (25%), temporal (20%), parietal (13%), and occipital (3%) [44]. The putative cell of origin is used to classify GBM. Astrocytic tumors (astrocytoma, anaplastic astrocytoma, and GBM), oligodendrogliomas, ependymomas, and mixed gliomas are all examples of these [45]. GBM is a rare tumor that affects less than 10 persons per 100,000 worldwide. It can occur at any age, with the greatest incidence occurring between the ages of 55 and 60. It is responsible for 2.5% of cancer-related deaths and is the third foremost cause of cancer-related death in people aged 15 to 34 [43]. The ratio of GBM prevalence is higher in men as compared to women. GBM is 1.58 times more familiar in males compared with females [45–47]. In terms of ethnicity, non-Hispanic whites have the highest incidence, followed by American Indians and Alaska Natives, who have a 40% lower incidence. GBM is becoming more common in North America, Australia, and Northern and Western Europe on a global scale [47]. GBM patients have a poor prognosis, with a 1-year life expectancy of 37.2% and a 5-year survival rate of 5.1% [47], and a median survival of $\sim$10 months [46].

9.4.5.1 *Gold nanoparticles*

Nanoparticles can be utilized to deliver targeted drugs, which are very useful in the treatment of brain tumors. Then, because of the great spatial resolution required, a thorough evaluation of NPs from the tumor's neighboring microvasculature is necessary. The purpose of this study is to use whole-organ imaging in vivo and post-mortem, as well as nanoscale three-dimensional (3D) X-ray microscopy, to develop an experimental solution to this problem. A 3D X-ray and fluorescence imaging examination of the link between xenografted glioma cells and tumor-induced angiogenic microvasculature was possible, thanks to the use of GNPs as contrast agents. The pictures of the angiogenic microvessels revealed NP leaking. Complementary investigations revealed that fluorescent GNPs allow for visible-light identification of cells following endocytotic internalization [48].

It is critical to use PET imaging to monitor and quantitatively evaluate the transport and localization of Au NPs to optimize operations and minimize undesirable effects (NMs), a photothermal agent that is often utilized. Two of the challenges in coupling radiometals to Au NMs via a chelator are radiometal detachment and NM surface property changes. This study established a simple and general chelator-free Copper-64 (64Cu) radiolabeling method by chemically reducing 64Cu on the surface of PEG-stabilized Au NMs, regardless of their shape and size, or 64Cu-integrated NMs, which are radiochemically stable and can provide accurate and sensitive NM localization over noninvasive PET imaging. We helped with the integration of 64Cu onto RGD peptide-modified Au nanorods (NRs) for tumor theranostics [49].

9.4.5.2 *Gadolinium nanoparticles*

Activation and Guidance of Irradiation by X-ray (AGuIX) NPs are made of a polysiloxane network enclosed by gadolinium chelates. They have a variety of traits. They are simple to make, have tiny hydrodynamic diameters (5 nm), and are biodegradable due to siloxane bond hydrolysis. Dynamic light scattering and relaxometry were used to quantify deterioration in diluted circumstances at physiological pH. Positive contrast agents and efficient radiosensitizers are other names for AGuIX NPs. The efficacy of their MRI and radiosensitization with DOTAREM, a feasible gadolinium-based molecular medication, is compared in this research. In an investigation with healthy animals, we observed that AGuIX had a higher contrast in MRI pictures than DOTAREM for the same number of injected gadolinium animals. AGuIX delivers superior contrast upon injection than DOTAREM because it has a stronger longitudinal relaxivity and a twofold longer residence duration in the blood circulation. MRI identifies a rapid and significant rise in contrast after intravenous injection of the AGuIX in 9 L gliosarcoma-bearing rats, which reaches a plateau 7 minutes later. After being injected with a precise amount of gadolinium, we agreed to a treatment plan that included 20 minutes of microbeam radiation therapy. There was no significant change in median survival time after microbeam radiation therapy in the presence or absence of gadolinium chelates (38 and 44 days, respectively). The median survival period has been improved to 102.5 days, thanks to AGuIX particles showing interest in this nanomedicine treatment. This remarkable radio sensitizing observation could be explained by the particles' long-term tumor absorption, which results in a large nanoscale build up under irradiation [50].

9.4.5.3 *Iron oxide nanoparticle*

SPIONs have shown multifunctional benefits in cancer theranostics as a result of their systemic diffusion. Nanoparticles administered intratumorally can boost the therapeutic potential of local treatment (including localized hyperthermia). As a result, it is critical to create a realistic pharmacokinetic model for predicting NP distribution for both clinically relevant routes of delivery. In C57/Bl6 mice with subcutaneous GL261 GBMs, the biodistribution of SPIONs (of two diameters, i.e., 130 and 60 nm) radiolabeled with zirconium-89 or technetium-99 and intratumoral or intravenous administration were studied. A novel pharmacokinetic model was developed based on PET/CT biodistribution data to well understand the pharmacokinetics of SPIONs following both delivery methods. The occurrence of radiolabeled NPs within the glioma site (with low levels in the liver and spleen) was recognized by PET imaging analysis of the NPs (confirmed by histology) at all studied time points following intratumoral injection (with low amounts in the liver and spleen). The mathematical model demonstrated the dynamic redistribution of NPs in the organism for 72 hours, with a 100-hour equilibrium. When NPs were given intravenously, they revealed a specific distribution pattern, with rapid particle retention in all organs (particularly the liver and spleen) and, as a result, a sluggish release rate [51]. Individuals with brain tumors require a special contrast agent for MRI during surgical operations or postoperative radiography. Lactoferrin-conjugated SPIONs (Lf-SPIONs) were used to identify brain gliomas in vivo in this investigation. The Lf-SPIONs were preferred for MRI because of their hydrodynamic diameter of roughly 5 nm, the saturation magnetization of 51 emu/g Fe, and T2 relaxivity of 75.6 m/Ms. Lf-SPIONs had a superior image or sensitivity to display brain glioma on MR images compared to SPIONs in a rat model of C6 glioma. Lf-SPIONs significantly improved T2-weighted imaging of brain glioma in vivo till 48 hours after injection. After 48 hours, Lf-SPIONs were found surrounding the vascular area of tumor slices. When reverse transcription polymerase chain reaction (RT-PCR) and Western blot were used to compare brain tumor tissues to normal brain tissues, high-level expression of Lf receptors was found. According to these findings, Lf-SPIONs could be used as a sensitive and specific MRI contrast agent in the diagnosis of brain glioma [42].

9.4.6 Breast cancer

9.4.6.1 Silver nanoparticles

Silver NPs have played a crucial role in the identification and treatment of breast cancer. The immobilized gemcitabine present on the NP surface makes a covalent bond to thiol linkers through the sensitive amide bond; various scientific studies showed that the amide bond prevents the breakage of NPs under physiological pH and remains under breast cancer cells. The various scientific literature studies have shown that 14 nm GNPs eliminate breast cancer cells and show a synergistic effect [52].

9.4.6.2 Gold nanoparticles

GNPs have shown a very promising result in the visualization and bioimaging of breast cancer. Imaging of tumors is done by GNPs for in vivo photoacoustic tomography. When the gold nanocages conjugated with monoclonal antibodies are used to target breast cancer cells, the overall studies show that these nanocages have good therapeutic activity for breast cancer cells. The cell proliferation is also inhibited by regulating the c-mica gene by loading the GNPs by oligonucleotides sequence (POY2T). Mortality in the case of breast cancer has been reduced by mammographic screening, but radiological imaging is specific to 71%, as reported in the literature [53].

9.4.6.3 Gadolinium nanoparticles

Molecular imaging of cancer can be done by using tri-gadolinium nitride metallofullerene. MRI provides high-resolution 3D images of soft tissues. Various researches are ongoing to develop safe MRI contrast agents, which may have high sensitivity to molecular bioimaging [54]

9.4.6.4 Iron nanoparticles

Variations in miRNA levels play a function in carcinogenesis. Dextran-coated iron oxide NPs have been utilized in the treatment of breast cancer in several studies and have shown to be effective. Because the hydroxyl group is present on the surface of the dextran-coated NPs, the NPs bind to the anticancer cells via a linker or direct conjugation [55].

9.4.7 Prostate cancer

9.4.7.1 Silver nanoparticles

There are very vital nanocarriers used in nanomedicines having antibacterial, antiviral, and antifungal activities. Cisplatin loaded in GNPs, which is used to treat prostate cancer, is usually the leading cause of death in men all over the world. The uptake of cisplatin by PC-3 cells is improved by cisplatin-loaded GNPs, resulting in increased cisplatin absorption and decreased cisplatin cytotoxicity [56].

9.4.7.2 *Gold nanoparticles*

These NPs of different shapes and sizes are synthesized by the various physical, chemical, and biological methods, which are used in the diagnosis and treatment of prostate cancer. Mostly, the biologically synthesized GNPs act as a potential tool for biosensors, immunoassays, photoimaging, photothermal therapy, and targeted drug delivery system [13,56] These NPs show their action either by local heating to destroy the cells or for the drug release, giving it a therapeutic effect. There is a great possibility of conjugating the NPs by various biologically active moieties such as amines and thiol groups to make them productive for use in biosensing, bioimaging, and sensing for electron microscopy markers. In the imaging of focal ablation of the prostate tissues, AuroLase is under active clinical trials, which use NP-directed laser irradiation, as it targets the external site and it does not show any toxicity for the normal cells [57].

9.4.7.3 *Gadolinium nanoparticles*

These NPs are used in MRI, which has a high potential for the diagnosis of prostate cancer due to its soft tissue resolution, but in some cases, MRI and CT are less sensitive, so there is a need to develop a better imaging system; after various studies, it was found that multimodal molecular imaging has complementary advantages. Among them, the fluorescence bimodal imaging probes are a point of interest, as shown in various scientific literature studies. Usually, in this imaging, gadolinium NPs are used with the fluorescent dye, as the dye used is highly sensitive in the infrared region. The NPs are conjugated with the monoclonal antibodies against prostate-specific membrane antigen [55].

9.4.7.4 *Iron nanoparticles*

The chemical coprecipitation method is used for the preparation of the iron-based NPs. DNA nanocomposites are used to treat prostate cancer cells in vitro and in vivo. They have a strong inhibitory effect and are used as a potential method of treatment [58]

9.4.8 Lung cancer

9.4.8.1 *Silver nanoparticles*

The common lung cancer cell line to be introduced toward the various silver NPs is A-549. In various studies, the NPs carrying doxorubicin are targeted to the overexpressed transferrin receptor in the A549 and HCC827 human cancer cell lines. The studies have further identified and are still working on the invention of new technologies and methods for the treatment of lung cancer. Though the silver nanosphere is prepared by reducing hydrazine monohydrates and using BSA as a stabilizing agent, these nanospheres are evaluated for cancer cell lines and found to be therapeutically active [53]

9.4.8.2 *Gold nanoparticles*

Among the various NMs, gold nanoclusters (NCs) have applications in drug delivery, biosensing, biolabeling, and other vaccine delivery system because of their biocompatible, optical, and physicochemical properties and fluorescent properties. Gold is chemically inactive, which has high compatibility in the human body. Nanosized gold materials offer several advantages due to their less toxicity, spectroscopic properties, and negligible quenching. The gold NMs help in multiple imaging and provide precise information about the monitoring of LC. The dendrimer GNPs offer the best tissue resolution and increase therapeutic efficacy. Their effect is very much superior when compared with gadolinium chelates [59].

9.4.8.3 *Gadolinium nanoparticles*

Ln-containing compounds have the potential for bioimaging applications and are used as biomarkers. Gadolinium oxide NRs doped with luminescent rare earth metal compounds are excellent MRI contrast agents and can be used as a bifunctional biomarker because of their magnetism and luminescence [60].

9.4.8.4 *Iron nanoparticles*

In the past few decades, the magnetic nanostructure has become the focus of study in chemistry and biology due to its biomedical application such as magnetic bioseparation, MRI, and magnetoreception. Recently, the fluorescent dye body has received attention in lung cancer treatment. Bodipy dyes have a potential for bioimaging in the lung cancer lead sensor-based bodily receptor attached covalently to the surface of the iron oxide NPs. Similarly, these NPs can accumulate in the cancer cell, making them a good contrasting agent for the MRI [61].

9.4.9 Ovary cancer

9.4.9.1 *Silver nanoparticles*

Ovarian cancer is the sixth most common malignancy around the world; the standard management involves surgical tumor debulking and chemotherapy. Silver NPs with graphene have gained a lot of attention, as they can be used for surface-enhanced Raman scattering (SERS) because their particle shape and size can be altered, as these NPs can be synthesized by green methods like microwave radiation and methods which involve biomolecules like gelatin, bacteria, and plant extracts. Silver has a high therapeutic effect but is more toxic at less concentration than compared to other NPs due to its small size, as the average size is around 10 nm over the surface of graphene sheets [62].

9.4.9.2 *Gold nanoparticles*

In this content, multifunctional GNPs are established as a potential theranostics agent for cancer diagnosis and therapy, as they can successfully carry an increasing amount of the drug molecule to the disease site [63].

9.4.9.3 *Gadolinium nanoparticles*

Gadolinium is used for MRI and cancer therapy because of its ability to create auger electrons and cause DNA damage. Various scientific literature studies show that gadolinium NPs loaded with silica are used for cancer and tumor spheroid. Further, through irradiation with monochromatic X-rays, complete eradication of tumor can be done, but this effect requires accurate energy just above the K-edge energy of gadolinium. The NPs are prepared by using the sol-gel method by utilizing CTAB as a templating agent; using these NPs, destruction of the tumor is observed when brought under monochromatic X-rays of 50.25 Kev. However, this effect is time-dependent and depends upon the amount of gadolinium [64].

9.4.9.4 Iron nanoparticles

SPIONs have shown promising results in imaging, drug delivery, surgery, and hormonal therapy. SPOIN size plays an important role in the targeting of the tumor site by using EPR effect. Folic acid incorporated in the iron oxide NPs is a user agent in the MRI for the detection of ovarian cancer tissues. The NP with the size of 9.2 nm does not show any toxicity for the human skov-3 cell lines, and this indicates that it is a potential area for the treatment of ovarian cancer [65].

9.4.9.5 Advancements in delivering the nanoparticles to the lungs

Lungs offer a great total area to NPs to show enhanced effectiveness, help to prevent first-pass metabolism, and give better local and systemic action. According to Mansour et al. and Sung et al., NPs for localized noninvasive pulmonary delivery enable even distribution of drugs throughout the tissues of the lungs, improve pharmacokinetics of drugs, allow for sustained drug release, reduce undesirable systemic effects, and induce cellular uptake. Nanoparticles can be specifically targeted to desired components of the lungs like within the small airways and alveoli. The absorption of NPs is mainly reliant on the interaction between lung clearance mechanisms and molecular properties of airborne particles. Sung et al. proposed that the size, shape, and biodistribution of NPs within the lungs direct how they interact with lung tissue and the surface composition of NPs regulates the subsequent response. Delivery of NPs to lungs is dependent on both NP internal environments. According to Mahajan et al., physiological barriers to the delivery of NPs include mucosal fluid and alveolar fluid [66] (Fig. 9.3).

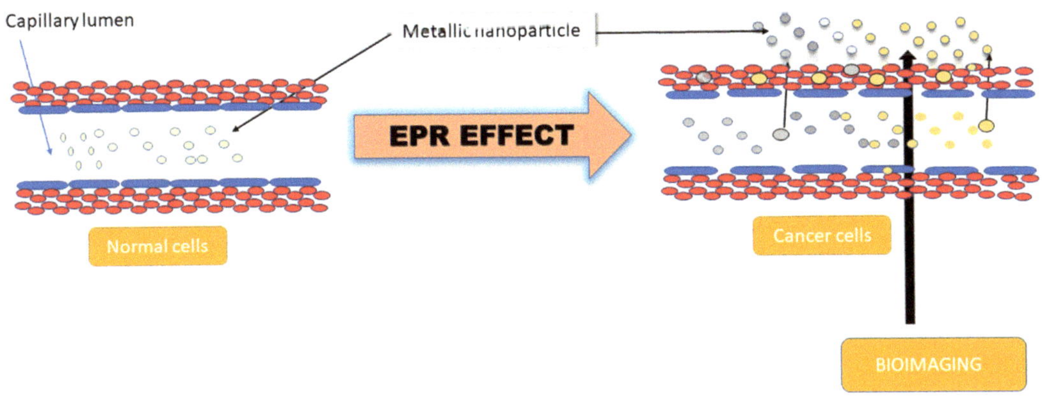

FIGURE 9.3 Cancer bioimaging by metallic nanoparticles.

9.4.9.6 *Targeting and performance of nanoparticles in the body*

The overall diameter of NPs lies between the ranges of submicron sizes. A large number of NPs have been discovered and developed as transporters of different molecules including drugs for various clinical uses. Different constituents are utilized because of the fabricating property that they possess. They usually exhibit their distinctive physical properties because of the submicron sizes; hence such properties are used in delivering the desired drugs according to the disease. They possess a great total area on their surface as compared to micromaterials ($>1\ \mu m$) with comparable total mass. This feature makes NPs deliver the drugs with enhanced efficacy to cells/tissues. After administration, the NPs tend to accumulate at the neoplasm, injury bleeding sites, and other inflammation associated ailments. Thus, they possess appropriate characteristics for utilization in transporters in targeted delivery of drug molecules and bioimaging.

9.4.9.7 *Route of administration and in vivo behavior of nanoparticles*

Various routes of administration can be exploited for the delivery of NPs like intravenous/intraperitoneal injection, oral route, and pulmonary inhalation. The most widely exploited route is intravenous injection. Because of the small molecular size of NPs, they can easily depart away from the damaged vessels of neoplasm, injury, sites of bleeding, and persistent infection without any difficulty. In such conditions, the enhanced blood flow and endothelial permeability lead to the disease-specific accumulation of NPs. Considering EPR phenomena, the most prominent disorder for targeting by NPs administered by the IV route is cancer. There are still certain confines of NPs via the intravenous route for treating disorders like chronic obstructive pulmonary disease (COPD), such as asthma and tuberculosis. Diseases like COPD, idiopathic pulmonary fibrosis, and CF possibly might not form very pervious vasculature inside pathologic wound/injury; therefore, it is a task to attain effective delivery of NPs aimed at such pathological conditions. Rapidly dividing cells can lead to lesser penetration of NPs, which inhibits NPs to get to the desired site of action. Biodistribution of NPs in the body is studied widely to understand nontargeted delivery to the lungs. In a recent study, larger-sized NPs (100–300 nm) which were labeled with ^{14}C were given in the form of an injection to mice and rats. Majorly, they showed accumulation in the reticuloendothelial system, but somewhat lesser accumulation was also observed in the lungs. Properly designed NPs that are specially designed for delivery to the lungs can lead to improvements in the pharmacokinetics of drugs. Methotrexate-loaded albumin NP and doxorubicin-loaded solid lipid NPs were found to have an extensive distribution within the lungs. Hence, NPs should be designed and developed considering their type and properties, which greatly influence their biological behavior. Pulmonary inhalation as a route of administration of NPs is of high importance in the case of chronic lung diseases. It then has the advantage of providing greater lung distribution (>3 times higher) when compared with intravenous or oral delivery. During inhalation, NPs are dispersed within a gas-type system. Dosage forms like powders, as well as suspensions in fluid form, have been made available, and further instruments specially designed to disperse a substance and for inhalation have been very essential. The spray-drying process helps to formulate inhalational powder containing NPs, to which lactose can be added as a carrier matrix to improve aerosolization. Nebulizers are utilized for delivering NP suspensions to the pulmonary system via the inhalation process. Liposomes and solid lipid NPs are extensively utilized for inhalation to the lungs because of their property to preserve their size, without forming aggregates. The phenomena of surface modification of NPs with the help of hydrophilic polymers are also widely used to inhibit aggregation and opsonization of NPs in vivo [67].

9.4.9.8 Advances in inorganic nanoparticles

Inorganic NPs have progressed for biomedical uses in current years due to their brilliant optical as well as magnetic attributes. Widespread research is being performed to synthesize inorganic NPs. Noble metal, metal oxide, as well as semiconductor NPs in the size range between 1 and 100 nm possess exclusive characteristics related to their size, which encouraged scholars to examine NPs for different bioimaging purposes. These uses would give rise to a huge range of vital elements for diagnosis in the biomedical field. Fluorescent semiconductor nanocrystals and quantum dots like cadmium selenide-zinc sulfide are being developed for serving as a possible fluorescence marker, because of their excellent optical characteristics. Latest developments for the manufacture of organometallic compounds supported the synthesis of magnetic NPs (like ferric oxide and ferrous oxide) based on their shape and size and synthesis of QDs (like cadmium sulfide and cadmium telluride). Different types of contrast agents, as well as optical markers, proved to be necessary for various kinds of bioimaging and diagnostic techniques like fluorescent imaging, optical coherence tomography, MRI, and position emission tomography. MRI and PET are one of the best techniques to perform bioimaging inside the body, while imaging based on fluorescence is best performed outside the body. Au as well as Ag NPs have been the ideal materials and are in the developing stage as substitutes for semiconductor NCs. Noble metallic nanocrystals exhibit surface plasmon resonance, which brings very strong improvement in the ability to absorb as well as scatter. These have been utilized for optical imaging-based contrast agents to detect proteins as well as DNA. Even if single particles of nanometer size can be imaged with the help of scattered light or photothermal technique, their use in bioimaging is still restricted because other components of cells also scatter the light. The latest research focused on synthesis facilitated the discovery of various metal NPs for use as contrast agents. Magnetic iron oxide (γ-Fe_2O_3 or Fe_3O_4) NPs are studied for their bioimaging property as T2 (negative) contrast agents for clinical diagnosis purpose. The use of contrast agents is done to enhance the tissue contrast in this technique. Contrast agents are of the following types: positive and negative. Positive contrast agents have the property to shorten longitudinal relaxation time (T1), leading to brightening (hyperintense) of MR images, while negative contrast agents have the property to transverse relaxation time (T2), leading to darkening (hypointense) of MR images. For medical bioimaging, gadolinium-based paramagnetic chelates (such as Gd-DTPA [diethylene triamine pentaacetic acid]) have functioned as T1 contrast agents. Iron oxide-based magnetic NPs can be certainly modified to acquire various biological and pharmacological targeting entities. Magnetic NPs (MNPs) (Fe_2O_3, Fe_3O_4) have been functionalized as negative T2 contrast agents for MRI in recent studies. Luminescent gadolinium oxide (Gd_2O_3) hybrid magnetic NPs are utilized as T1 contrast agents in MRI. Nanoshells made of Au_3Cu_1 have also been utilized to serve as MR contrast agents [68]. Various inorganic elements such as gold, silver, iron oxide, and silica are extensively used for making NPs. Because of the presence of their plasmonic and magnetic properties, they produce imaging contrast by CT, MR, as well as PET. They are being widely utilized in disease identification and imaging. They are cationic and hence can easily bind to negatively charged DNA and RNA and can be used for gene delivery, although the success rate of inorganic NPs for the treatment of chronic lung disorders is low. However, GNPs were effectively targeted toward cells of the epithelium of alveoli of mice affected by COPD. Because of their cationic nature, they tend to bind to negatively charged serum proteins, which causes aggregation on intravenous administration. A recent study proposed that this can be prevented by using a surface modification of GNPs with PEG. Lower excretion rates of GNPs still obstruct their clinical uses and long-term studies. Also, they are not capable of carrying large quantities of drug substances; hence, these points should be considered before the beginning of clinical trials of inorganic NPs [67].

9.4.9.9 *Surface modifications and bioconjugation of nanoparticles*

The original synthesized form of NPs is not suitable for biological use due to its surface characteristics. A phenomenon called surface modification is needed for enhancing the aqueous dispersibility and biocompatibility of NPs and also to obtain suitable functional groups for bioconjugation purposes, as represented in Fig. 9.4. The addition of biomolecules like proteins, antibodies, RNA, and so forth to the surface of NPs is performed by conventional bioconjugate chemistry. These molecules can be attached either via physical adsorption or via covalent coupling to the NP surface. In direct attachment by surface assimilation, the electrostatic and hydrophobic interaction among biologic molecules plus

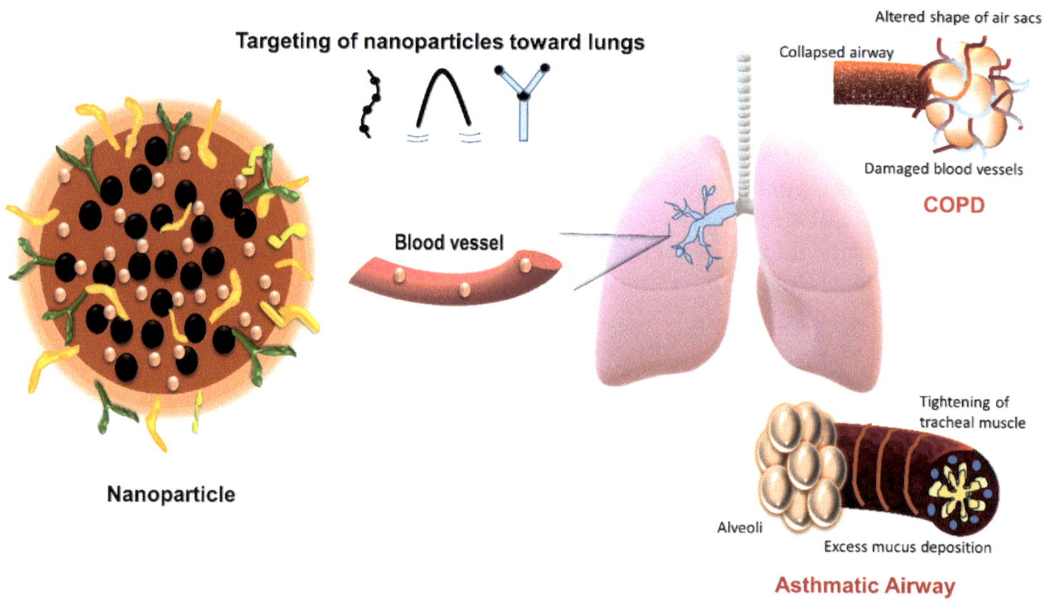

FIGURE 9.4 Bioimaging of respiratory disorders by surface modification of nanoparticles.

the surface of NPs prevail as compared to the interaction between NPs themselves. There are certain demerits of physical adsorption like:

1. Smaller amount of control for the regulation of several biomolecules being attached on the surface of NPs.
2. Alignment and positioning of biomolecules.
3. Desorption of biomolecules from the surface of NPs.

To overcome these limitations of physical adsorption, the covalent coupling is given more preference. Usually, first, the surface of NPs is modified by the addition of different functional groups before covalent coupling. Examples of such functional groups include sulfide, amine, and carboxyl groups. These functional groups have importance in supplying suitable sites for conjugation of biomolecule and regulating the colloidal stability of NPs [69].

9.4.10 Tuberculosis

9.4.10.1 Gold nanoparticles

9.4.10.1.1 Diagnosis of tuberculosis using gold nanoparticles

GNPs possess exclusive physiochemical as well as optical properties to best suit medical imaging and treatment together with integrative analysis. Their optical characteristics along with antigen/antibody as well as certain biological molecules allow them for bioimaging of infectious agents. Choi and Frangioni et al. and Sonawane and Nimse et al. proposed that GNPs do not cause any alteration to the functional activity even after antigen immobilization. Kim et al. proposed that functionalization of GNPs at the surface leads to increment of antigen–antibody reaction, hence enhancing the intensity of immunoassay signals, which finally causes the sensitivity of the assay to rise. The assay was highly precise together with generated consistent outcomes using small quantities of mycobacterium DNA. Chandra et al. and Cordeiro et al. proposed that the calorimetry of a specific gene or sequence present in samples through GNP probes provided an affordable technique of diagnosis. Baptista et al. reported GNPs for bioimaging of tuberculosis, in which they used DNA probes alongside gold NPs intended for colorimetric assay of mycobacterium. Essentially, on 526 nm wavelength, if there is the occurrence of complementary DNA, then the solution containing nanoprobe does not show any color change and retains pink color, while it becomes purple if complementary DNA is absent (due to the formation of nanoprobe aggregates). Baptista et al. said that the abovementioned method proved to be more precise than other techniques like InnoLiPA-Rif-TB. The instance of contamination was found to be very low, and the method was found to take only 15 minutes per sample. Tsai et al. proposed the insertion sequence (IS6110) of mycobacterium for enhancement of assay sensitivity together with microfluidics technology, a method that used calorimetric identification of these NPs, in addition to the IS6110 sequence. Khan et al. proposed that SPR is of high importance and was found to give red color to GNP colloid. The method observes changes in the surface refractive index, made due to coupling or decoupling of NPs. Masson, Nguyen, Wang, and Fan proposed that SPR technology offers high optical sensor sensitivity, which allows for the identification of small quantities of disease-specific analyte without many specifications to be followed. Hsieh et al. proposed designing the SPR-based CFP-10CFP-10 antigen detection technique by Yang et al., which provided high utility in the diagnosis of mycobacterium. Scientists proposed GNP-modified indium tin oxide electrodes for indirectly identifying *Mycobacterium tuberculosis* using genomic DNA obtained from samples.

9.4.10.1.2 Gold nanoparticle-mediated dipstick assay

Stephen et al. developed a method in which colloidal GNPs were taken and coating of *M. tuberculosis* antigen was done on them with the help of alkanethiol derivatives and anti-MTB rabbit antibodies. These gold NPs containing antigen coating perform the task of the detector in this assay. Binding occurs between these antigen-coated gold NPs and the serum samples or antibodies, which are immobilized on the nitrocellulose membrane. The formation of red color occurs as a result of this binding of gold NPs on the nitrocellulose membrane, which can be visualized easily [70].

9.4.10.1.3 UV Spectroscopy-based detection using gold nanoparticles

Gold NPs were used for the detection of *M. tuberculosis* with the help of UV-Vis spectroscopy visually. It was based on the recognition of oligonucleotide.

9.4.10.1.4 A calorimetric assay using gold nanoparticles for diagnosis of *Mycobacterium tuberculosis*

A calorimetric assay using GNPs has been described in easy as well as quick diagnosis of Mycobacterium DNA. Firstly, PCR was performed for the amplification of the DNA sample. Conjugation between gold NPs and thiolated oligonucleotide particular to bacterium was done. This included combining nanoprobes along with the test DNA. The solution containing nanoprobes had been observed to have red color because of surface plasmon resonance phenomena. When the amount of sodium chloride is high, it leads to an accumulation of nanoprobes when complementary DNA is not present in the sample. This leads to a color change of the solution from red to purple. When nanoprobes go through cross-linking by complementary DNA of mycobacterium, accumulation does not occur and no color change is observed and the solution retains its red color [69].

9.4.10.1.5 Gold nanoparticle-based conjugate for detection of tuberculosis

Given the high efficacy of nanotechnology, some researchers refined high-throughput techniques on the principle of nanotechnology in the detection of TB, which is nanodisk mass spectroscopy. Culture filtrate protein 10 kDa (CFP-10) and 6 kDa early secretory target (ESAT-6) serve as TB markers. By conjugating ESAT-6 and CFP-10 antibodies to the surface of silica NPs, this assay facilitated a sensitive investigation of both antibodies present in the disease state. The prime requirement for the identification of active Mtb is clinical sensitivity and specificity. Both the markers of tuberculosis can be measured at small concentrations also. Researchers evolved the Au-Cu nanoshell dot-blot immunoassay in identifying culture filtrate protein 10. The assay included reducing Cu ions on GBP-CFP10G2-Au NPs compound (GBP is a gold binding peptide and G2 represents Group 2 antibody genes). It possesses binding capabilities for Au as well as an antigen that is responsible for the production of red spots, which can be easily visualized. The amount of the TB antigen is proportional to the intensity of the color produced, with a limit of detection of 7.6 μpg/mL. This technique may identify culture filtrate protein 10 antigen in TB patients from their samples of urine and can be performed for real-time detection of CFP-10 antibody with large sensitivity and precision for rapid diagnosis of tuberculosis [70].

9.4.10.2 *Silver nanoparticles*

9.4.10.2.1 Silver nanoparticles-based noncross-linking assay for detection of *Mycobacterium tuberculosis*

In such an assay, NPs get accumulated or stable along with molecular recognition elements. These elements assimilate on top of NPs by taking the help of electrostatic force. When a sample is added to the abovementioned complex, a color change is produced because of disruption or stabilization of the NP. To support this, Teengam et al. developed a noncross-linking assay implementing silver NPs by which the presence of *M. tuberculosis* and MERS coronavirus could be observed in the microfluidic paper analytical instrument. It was less responsive toward identifying the DNA/RNA of the infectious agent; hence amplification techniques like PCR need to be incorporated. However, this assay allowed three nucleic acid biomarkers to be detected visually. Various NP probes comprising metals have been designed for the identification of DNA/RNA sequences associated with disease-causing organisms. As SPR is dependent on the size of metallic NPs in aggregation assay, many disease-causing pathogens like the Middle East Respiratory Syndrome Coronavirus, *M. tuberculosis*, and HPV can be identified. Silver NPs are highly conductive and therefore utilized in electrochemically identifying HIV and *M. tuberculosis* [70].

9.4.10.3 *Silica nanoparticles*

9.4.10.3.1 Silica nanoparticle-based imaging

Sun et al. reported that mesoporous silica NPs can be used in imaging, drug delivery, and biosensing. Qin et al. combined silica NPs with fluorescent dye in indirect immunofluorescence microscopy. It contains an SYBR Green I mediated assay, which leads to staining of only bioconjugated fluorescent silica NPs. Fluorescent signals were fivefold intense compared to the old fluorescence isothiocyanate build identification technique. This gave accurate outcomes in 2 hours and hence was a good technique for identifying mycobacterium [71].

9.4.10.3.2 Silica nanoparticle-based fluorescent microscopy

Dye-doped silica NPs were used for the detection of *M. tuberculosis* with the help of fluorescence microscopy as a detection technique, and the signal was amplified within 4 hours as its detection limit. It was based on the recognition of antibodies.

9.4.10.3.3 Silica nanoparticles for rapid diagnosis of *Mycobacterium tuberculosis*

Tan group used silica NPs for the rapid identification of *M. tuberculosis*. In that method, they used anti-mycobacterium antibody for detecting *M. tuberculosis* together with an antibody binding protein, which was labeled with RuBpy-doped Si-NPs for the production of a fluorescent signal for analysis. Fluorescent-based indirect immunofluorescence microscopy was used as a detection technique that proved successful in detecting *M. tuberculosis* in both the bacterial mixture and spiked sputum. The assay was completed in 4 hours, including sample pretreatment [69].

9.4.10.4 Iron oxide nanoparticles

9.4.10.4.1 Superparamagnetic iron oxide nanoparticles for bioimaging of tuberculosis

Akbarzadeh et al. proposed that magnetic NPs have optimum properties for them to be used in nanomedicine, especially imaging therapy. Their surface can be modified with antibodies, antibiotics, and carbohydrates for the detection of bacteria. Cristea et al. and Sabale et al. proposed the use of SPIONs (iron oxide NPs). It is primarily utilized for the treatment and delivery of drug molecules through MRI. IgG-coupled IONPs have facilitated improving the limit of detection (104 CFU/mL) with the help of nano-MALDI techniques. Kaittanis et al. and Vallabani and Singh reported utilizing diagnostic magnetic resonance along with Fe oxide NPs in detecting Mycobacterium DNA. Engstrom and coworkers invented a method in which they labeled streptavidin-tagged magnetic nanobeads with biotin and used the same for detecting rpoB gene mutation in *M. tuberculosis*.

9.4.10.4.2 Iron oxide nanoparticles in magnetic resonance imaging of tuberculosis

Engstrom et al. proposed a method for the detection of *M. tuberculosis*. It comprised an assay containing 11 padlock probes, which are used for targeting the 23 S ITS region of the bacterium. Out of the total probes, one probe was utilized for detecting MTBC, the second probe was utilized for detecting wild-type, and the rest of the probes were for detecting mutation in the RRDR-rpoB gene. The Brownian relaxation principle guides this detection system, and the signal is identified by AC susceptometry. Sable et al. checked the potential of SPIONs for enhancement of sensitivity and specificity of MRI for detection of tuberculosis. It is helpful for the study of antibody–antigen and parasite–host interactions. Activation of SPIO NPs was done by making conjugates with anti-MTB surface antibodies. Inoculation of this conjugate with the bacterium was done, and MRI was performed, which gives specific target recognition by decreasing signal intensity. Skoura et al. stated that the following technique proved to be accurate in identifying extrapulmonary tuberculosis [70].

9.4.11 Asthma

9.4.11.1 Gold nanoparticles

9.4.11.1.1 Cyclodextrin-stabilized gold nanoclusters for bioimaging

Gold NCs have extensive applications and are developing materials, as they are highly fluorescent and possess optimum magnetic properties. They lie within different ranges of the size of subnanometer to about 2 nm. They are decently water-soluble, ultrasmall in size, photoluminescent, and highly photostable, have high emission rates, possess large Stokes shift, and are highly biocompatible. All these characteristics of gold NCs make them an ideal candidate for biosensing, biological labeling, and bioimaging. A recent study focused on synthesizing Au NCs by using a stabilizer and pointed out toward increasing its water solubility and fluorescence and utilized them in identifying copper ions. Cyclodextrin is an oligosaccharide containing (α-1,4)-linked α-D glucopyranose unit. An important feature of cyclodextrin is it combines with a different group of atoms to make conjugates having the host and the guest, which is formed because molecules and cyclodextrin interact with each other hydrophobically. This leads to an increase in solubility and activity of the molecule, which forms a bond with cyclodextrin, protects it from degradation, assists the immobilization of proteins on metallic surfaces, regulates the amount of aggregation, and, when this complex gets attached to NPs, increases controlled delivery of drugs. A cyclodextrin-functionalized gold NC had been utilized in identifying metal ions along with biomacromolecules. Heavy metal ions are highly toxic to humans. Co^{2+} ion concentration, when not regulated, becomes toxic to cells. Its toxicity can occur by the creation of ROS, which is associated with many disorders including interstitial lung diseases, cancer, asthma, and pneumonia. Until now, only limited probes without labels in fluorescent as well as calorimetric identification are developed for copper ions. In addition, these methods have not been effectively used for the identification of these redox-active transition metals in living cells. A study proposed an easy and effective method for preparing Au NCs capped with cyclodextrin, where glutathione was made available during the process as it functions as an antioxidant required to enhance photoluminescence. These Au NCs displayed red-fluorescence emitting optical and sufficiently stable fluorescence as that of different red-luminescent NMs and were utilized for the imaging of cells or other biological moieties. They also had large biocompatibility and exhibited no damaging effect on normal cells. Because of such optical characteristics, it was possible to make an effective fluorescent probe. These sensing probes containing Au NCs possess the deep penetrating ability, and therefore a faster detection of Co^{2+} ions was made possible in biomedical devices [72].

9.4.11.2 *Magnetic nanoparticles*

9.4.11.2.1 Magnetic nanoparticle-based bioimaging

An electronic nose based on nanosensors was invented. It was able to identify specific volatile organic compounds in exhaled gas in a noninvasive way. Past clinical research showed that this technique can differentiate between the breaths exhaled by asthmatic individuals as well as nonasthmatic individuals, in addition to predicting the degree of disease. It is also possible to detect the asthma type using this technique, whether it is neutrophilic, eosinophilic, mixed granulocytic, or paucigranulocytic. This method has been utilized to carry out precise and noninvasive evaluations to differentiate asthmatic patients with eosinophils, neutrophils, and polynuclear granulocyte phenotypes. The efficiency of this method was assessed by a clinical trial (NCT02026336), and it was found that asthma type can be certainly differentiated using this method [70].

9.4.11.3 *Polystyrene nanoparticles*

9.4.11.3.1 Loaded inhaled polystyrene nanoparticles with innate immune cells for bioimaging

Molecular imaging of inflammatory lung diseases like asthma is restricted till now. The eployment of innate immunity cells in the lungs protects from antimicrobial infection. Innate immune cells were utilized in the bioimaging of pulmonary tissue, with the help of loaded inhaled polystyrene NPs along with fluorescent dye Itrybe. With the help of fluorescence reflectance imaging of ovalbumin-based allergic airway inflammation in SKH-1 mice, inside as well as outside the body, the results reported after the administration of these NPs inside the nose and lungs of infected ones show the expressively larger intensity of fluorescence as compared to the noninfected ones up to 1 day. Immunofluorescence was performed outside the animal body, which showed that CD68 + CD11c + ECF-L + MHCIIlow cells had taken up these NPs, detecting those in the form of M2 macrophages of alveoli in peribranchial and regions of alveoli. Analysis inside the animal body was confirmed using flow cytometry methods, overlapping tile analysis, and confocal microscopy, demonstrating an expressively larger amount of these NPs consisting of macrophages in infected animal's lungs as compared with controls. Some of the cells having these NPs were detected to be accessory cells. Flow cytometry of tracheobronchial lymph nodes displayed that I try be NPs were found to be a minor amount in infected ones 1-day past inhalation. The following method can improve the pre-symptomatic diagnosis of inflammation inside the body and facilitate the tracking of inhaled NPs [72].

9.4.12 Chronic obstructive pulmonary disease

9.4.12.1 Iron oxide nanoparticles

9.4.12.1.1 Conjugated supermagnetic iron oxide nanoparticles for imaging lungs

Aillon et al. reported that iodine NCs could as used as another alternative as contrast agents for visualizing lungs. PET and MRI have been the widely used techniques for lung imaging using NPs. Through MR dual simultaneous 19F/1H neovascular molecular imaging, the study of targeted micelles expressed on lung ECs was conducted. The influence of supermagnetic iron oxide NPs conjugated with a biocompatible antibody was studied for its in vivo effect after administration to the lungs. It enabled precise targeting and imaging of a macrophage subpopulation in lipopolysaccharide-induced COPD in a mice model [73].

9.4.12.2 Selenium nanoparticles

9.4.12.2.1 Detection of a diagnostic marker of chronic obstructive pulmonary disease using selenium nanoparticles

An important diagnostic marker of oxidative stress produced in COPD or asthma is hydrogen peroxide. Wang et al. developed a hydrogen peroxide sensor. It was built from biosynthesized selenium NPs made using the bacterial strain Bacillus subtilis. The resultant selenium NPs were spherical and could be transformed into 1D trigonal wires. A carbon electrode was prepared with selenium NPs colloidal suspension and a drop containing an enzyme called horseradish peroxidase. Cyclic voltammetry studies affirmed that selenium NPs increased the detection of hydrogen peroxide in the detection limit of 80 nM. This material can be utilized for detecting hydrogen peroxide in COPD patients' breaths that they exhale [74].

9.4.13 Influenza

9.4.13.1 Gold nanoparticles

9.4.13.1.1 Gold nanoparticle-based bioassay for targeting and bioimaging

Various kinds of NPs like gold, platinum, hybrid particles, and metal–organic frameworks are being used as enzyme mimics in bioassays for targeting diseases caused by a respiratory syncytial virus, avian influenza, and salmonella. Various bioassays utilizing enzymes for the function of catalytic turnover agents in identification have been designed in the same way as immunoassays on the surface of well plates. It was observed that conversion of this technology to the lateral flow format resulted in a 100-fold increase in detection limits by enzyme detection element as compared to the old GNP-based lateral flow stripes.

9.4.13.1.2 Reductive nanoparticle enlargement for increased sensitivity of assays for detecting influenza

GNPs are abundantly used to serve as detection elements in commercial lateral flow assays. The size of particles is usually from 15 to 50 nm; further, they could be identified both by visual means and by employing simple hand-held readers. However, the detection limits for such assays are low enough for the detection of low-intensity infections. To increase the sensitivity of these assays, one can chemically increase the size of particles, which enables them to become visually intense. A lateral flow assay works in such a way that there is the formation of NP-rich composite in the presence of disease-causing allergen. Then, in the consecutive step, a mixture of the molecular precursor as well as a reducing agent is poured into the test. The GNPs present at both portions perform the function of nucleation sites for the accumulation of metal. Silver enhancement is one of the most widely used techniques to increase the size of NPs and involves reducing ions into the parent metal of silver. This is done on the GNPs in the existence of an acid buffer. The technique can lead to producing action of particles of a huge variety of size range. Horton et al. in 1991 reported for the first time the use of silver enhancement in paper diagnostics in which an assay was designed to identify immunoglobulin G in mice as well as confirmed a 100-fold enhancement in detection limits. Since then, it is widely used for the diagnosis of many infectious diseases such as influenza, HIV, malaria, *Y. pestis*, and *E. coli* [75].

9.4.13.1.3 Calorimetric immunoassay based on Au nanoparticles

Calorimetric immunoassay based on GNPs is one of the most efficient methods of imaging. The staining of GNPs with silver may enhance the responsiveness of the method. On its own, it may be employed to test the device built upon lateral flow assay. Such a method is reasonably possible under controlled environmental conditions. However, more research is needed in the area of GNPs-based immunoassay for increasing sensitivity and specificity of detection.

9.4.13.2 *Magnetic nanoparticles*

9.4.13.2.1 Superconducting quantum interference device containing magnetic nanoparticles for detection of influenza virus

For the detection of the avian influenza H5N1 virus, the concept of clustering of virus target-induced magnetic NPs was implemented at a concentration of approximately 5 pg/mL of viral load using superconducting quantum interference device (SQUID). MNPs undergo cluster formation due to interaction between viruses and antibodies developed on the surface of NPs. However, their reaction toward external AC magnetic field is considerably less as compared to the single, distinct MNPs. Thus, engineered MNPs were developed to produce a quick, efficacious, and easy technique for parting as well as detecting smaller amounts of microbes. They exhibit great detection efficacics because they possess a large surface-to-volume ratio and quick reaction kinetics. Therefore, these days MNP-based diagnosis is preferred over PCR. The most obvious limitation of using equipment like SQUID is its cost, due to which it is difficult to put into practice in developing countries.

9.4.14 Pneumonia

9.4.14.1 Silver nanoparticles

9.4.14.1.1 Silver nanoparticle-based surface-enhanced Raman scattering for imaging of pneumonia

Ag NPs have been successfully employed for SERS based on identifying specific determinants. This method can also be utilized for single-molecule determination because of the sensitivity of SERS. The sensitivity of SERS for detection is dependent on the proximity between analytes and the surface of NPs. Scientists reported SERS-active Ag NR assay for identification as well as for distinguishing molecular fingerprints of different disease-causing organisms like *M. pneumonia* and respiratory syncytial virus. Also, this technique can categorize viruses at the strain level.

9.4.15 Anthracis

9.4.15.1 Europium nanoparticles

9.4.15.1.1 Europium (Eu III)-based fluorescence nanoparticle sensor for diagnosis of B. anthracis

Lu et al. proposed the use of Europium (Eu III)-based fluorescence NP sensor in the early diagnosis of diseased spores present in the form of a water-based fluid mixture. Calcium dipicolinate (CaDPA) serves as a marker for bacillus spores. By detecting CaDPA, these spores can be identified. Conjugation between Eu III-complex (sensing moiety) and dye-doped silica NPs was done, which detects CaDPA. Hence, an NP sensor with ideal dimensions was developed, leading to the maximum possible surface area for detecting B. anthracis spores. It offered a detection limit of 0.2 nM CaDPA within only 2 minutes.

9.4.15.2 Silica nanoparticles

9.4.15.2.1 Bioimaging of infectious diseases via silica nanoparticles

It was observed that luminescent silica NPs show merits of multiplexing capability, higher sensitivity, photostability, and ease of functionalization, as compared to conventional fluorescent dyes. Every silica NP is capable of encapsulating tens to thousands of fluorescent dye molecules, leading to the production of highly accurate and consistent signals. Such optical characteristics of silica NPs make them highly suitable for bioimaging and real-time tracking [69].

Acknowledgment

The authors are thankful to National Institute of Pharmaceutical Education and Research-Raebareli, (NIPER-R) and Ministry of Chemicals and Fertilizers, Department of Pharmaceuticals, Govt. of India, for all kind support. The communication number for this manuscript has been provided by NIPER-R, and the communication number is NIPER-R/Communication/306.

References

[1] Bahadar H, Maqbool F, Niaz K, Abdollahi M. Toxicity of nanoparticles and an overview of current experimental models. Iran Biomed J 2016;20(1):1–11.

[2] Tan P, Li H, Wang J, Gopinath SCB. Silver nanoparticle in biosensor and bioimaging: clinical perspectives. Biotechnol Appl Biochem 2021;68(6):1236–42.

[3] Aslan N, Ceylan B, Koç MM, Findik F. Metallic nanoparticles as X-Ray computed tomography (CT) contrast agents: a review. J Mol Struct 2020;1219:128599.

[4] Subhan MA, Yalamarty SSK, Filipczak N, Parveen F, Torchilin VP. Recent advances in tumor targeting via EPR effect for cancer treatment. J Pers Med 2021;11(6):571.

[5] Wu J. The enhanced permeability and retention (EPR) effect: the significance of the concept and methods to enhance its application. J Pers Med 2021;11(8):771.

[6] Kadry H, Noorani B, Cucullo L. A blood-brain barrier overview on structure, function, impairment, and biomarkers of integrity. Fluids Barriers CNS 2020;17(1):69.

[7] Tajes M, Ramos-Fernández E, Weng-Jiang X, et al. The blood-brain barrier: structure, function, and therapeutic approaches to cross it. Mol Membr Biol 2014;31(5):152–67.

[8] Banks WA. The blood-brain barrier in neuroimmunology: tales of separation and assimilation. Brain Behav Immun 2015;44:1–8.

[9] Profaci CP, Munji RN, Pulido RS, Daneman R. The blood-brain barrier in health and disease: important unanswered questions. J Exp Med 2020;217(4):e20190062.

[10] Keaney J, Campbell M. The dynamic blood-brain barrier. FEBS J 2015;282(21):4067–79.

[11] Pardridge WM. CSF, blood-brain barrier, and brain drug delivery. Expert Opin Drug Deliv 2016;13 (7):963–75.

[12] Krasemann S, Haferkamp U, Pfefferle S, et al. The blood-brain barrier is dysregulated in COVID-19 and serves as a CNS entry route for SARS-CoV-2. Stem Cell Rep 2022;17(2):307–20.

[13] Andreone BJ, Chow BW, Tata A, et al. Blood-brain barrier permeability is regulated by lipid transport-dependent suppression of caveolae-mediated transcytosis. Neuron. 2017;94(3):581–94.

[14] Pollak TA, Drndarski S, Stone JM, David AS, McGuire P, Abbott NJ. The blood-brain barrier in psychosis. Lancet Psychiatry 2018;5(1):79–92.

[15] Fu BM. Transport across the blood-brain barrier. Adv Exp Med Biol 2018;1097:235–59.

[16] Huang X, Hussain B, Chang J. Peripheral inflammation and blood-brain barrier disruption: effects and mechanisms. CNS Neurosci Ther 2021;27(1):36 4.

[17] Tiwari S, Atluri V, Kaushik A, Yndart A, Nair M. Alzheimer's disease: pathogenesis, diagnostics, and therapeutics. Int J Nanomed 2019;14:5541–54.

[18] Silva MVF, Loures CMG, Alves LCV, de Souza LC, Borges KBG, Carvalho MDG. Alzheimer's disease: risk factors and potentially protective measures. J Biomed Sci 2019;26(1):33.

[19] Haque RU, Levey AI. Alzheimer's disease: a clinical perspective and future nonhuman primate research opportunities. Proc Natl Acad Sci U S A 2019;116(52):26224–9.

[20] Masters CL, Bateman R, Blennow K, Rowe CC, Sperling RA, Cummings JL. Alzheimer's disease. Nat Rev Dis Prim 2015;1:15056.

[21] Sillerud LO, Solberg NO, Chamberlain R, et al. SPION-enhanced magnetic resonance imaging of Alzheimer's disease plaques in AβPP/PS-1 transgenic mouse brain. J Alzheimers Dis 2013;34(2):349–65.

[22] Wang X, Chan HN, Desbois N, et al. Multimodal theranostic cyanine-conjugated gadolinium(III) complex for *in vivo* imaging of amyloid-β in an Alzheimer's disease mouse model. ACS Appl Mater Interfaces 2021;13(16):18525–32.

[23] Georgiopoulos C, Witt ST, Haller S, et al. A study of neural activity and functional connectivity within the olfactory brain network in Parkinson's disease. Neuroimage Clin 2019;23:101946.

[24] Gaba A. Recent studies on nutrition and Parkinson's disease prevention: a systematic review. Open J Prev Med 2015;05(05):197–205.

[25] Simon DK, Tanner CM, Brundin P. Parkinson disease epidemiology, pathology, genetics, and pathophysiology. Clin Geriatr Med 2020;36(1):1–12.

[26] Cherian A, Divya KP. Genetics of Parkinson's disease. Acta Neurol Belg 2020;120(6):1297–305.

[27] Nuytemans K, Theuns J, Cruts M, Van Broeckhoven C. Genetic etiology of Parkinson disease associated with mutations in the SNCA, PARK2, PINK1, PARK7, and LRRK2 genes: a mutation update. Hum Mutat 2010;31 (7):763–80.

[28] An L, Tao Q, Wu Y, et al. Synthesis of SPIO nanoparticles and the subsequent applications in stem cell labeling for Parkinson's disease. Nanoscale Res Lett 2021;16(1):107.
[29] Kuriakose D, Xiao Z. Pathophysiology and treatment of stroke: present status and future perspectives. Int J Mol Sci 2020;21(20):7609.
[30] Bivard A, Lin L, Parsonsb MW. Review of stroke thrombolytics. J Stroke 2013;15(2):90–8.
[31] Pare JR, Kahn JH. Basic neuroanatomy and stroke syndromes. Emerg Med Clin North Am 2012;30(3):601–15.
[32] Janardhan V, Qureshi AI. Mechanisms of ischemic brain injury. Curr Cardiol Rep 2004;6(2):117–23.
[33] Betzer O, Perets N, Angel A, et al. In vivo neuroimaging of exosomes using gold nanoparticles. ACS Nano 2017;11(11):10883–93.
[34] Kim JY, Ryu JH, Schellingerhout D, et al. Direct imaging of cerebral thromboemboli using computed tomography and fibrin-targeted gold nanoparticles. Theranostics. 2015;5(10):1098–114.
[35] Hubert V, Dumot C, Ong E, et al. MRI coupled with clinically-applicable iron oxide nanoparticles reveals choroid plexus involvement in a murine model of neuroinflammation. Sci Rep 2019;9(1):10046.
[36] Yi P, Chen G, Zhang H, et al. Magnetic resonance imaging of $Fe_3O_4@SiO_2$-labeled human mesenchymal stem cells in mice at 11.7 T. Biomaterials. 2013;34(12):3010–19.
[37] Debatisse J, Eker OF, Wateau O, et al. PET-MRI nanoparticles imaging of blood-brain barrier damage and modulation after stroke reperfusion. Brain Commun 2020;2(2):fcaa193.
[38] Bates GP, Dorsey R, Gusella JF, et al. Huntington disease. Nat Rev Dis Prim 2015;1:15005.
[39] McColgan P, Tabrizi SJ. Huntington's disease: a clinical review. Eur J Neurol 2018;25(1):24–34.
[40] Roos RA. Huntington's disease: a clinical review. Orphanet J Rare Dis 2010;5:40.
[41] Margolis RL, Ross CA. Diagnosis of Huntington's disease. Clin Chem 2003;49(10):1726–32.
[42] Liu XG, Lu S, Liu DQ, et al. ScFv-conjugated superparamagnetic iron oxide nanoparticles for MRI-based diagnosis in transgenic mouse models of Parkinson's and Huntington's diseases. Brain Res 2019;1707:141–53.
[43] Taylor OG, Brzozowski JS, Skelding KA. Glioblastoma multiforme: an overview of emerging therapeutic targets. Front Oncol 2019;9:963.
[44] Al-Shaya HM, Li H, Beg OU, et al. Phytochemical profile and antioxidation activity of Annona fruit and its effect on lymphoma cell proliferation. Food Sci Nutr 2019;8(1):58–68.
[45] Hanif F, Muzaffar K, Perveen K, Malhi SM, Simjee ShU. Simjee ShU. Glioblastoma multiforme: a review of its epidemiology and pathogenesis through clinical presentation and treatment. Asian Pac J Cancer Prev 2017;18(1):3–9.
[46] Tan AC, Ashley DM, López GY, Malinzak M, Friedman HS, Khasraw M. Management of glioblastoma: state of the art and future directions. CA Cancer J Clin 2020;70(4):299–312.
[47] Omuro A, DeAngelis LM. Glioblastoma and other malignant gliomas: a clinical review. JAMA. 2013;310(17):1842–50.
[48] Lai SF, Ko BH, Chien CC, et al. Gold nanoparticles as multimodality imaging agents for brain gliomas. J Nanobiotechnol 2015;13:85.
[49] Sun X, Huang X, Yan X, et al. Chelator-free (64)Cu-integrated gold nanomaterials for positron emission tomography imaging-guided photothermal cancer therapy. ACS Nano 2014;8(8):8438–46.
[50] Chen D, Zhou Y, Yang D, et al. Positron emission tomography/magnetic resonance imaging of glioblastoma using a functionalized gadofullerene nanoparticle. ACS Appl Mater Interfaces 2019;11(24):21343–52.
[51] Klapproth AP, Shevtsov M, Stangl S, Li WB, Multhoff G. A new pharmacokinetic model describing the biodistribution of intravenously and intratumorally administered superparamagnetic iron oxide nanoparticles (SPIONs) in a GL261 xenograft glioblastoma model. Int J Nanomed 2020;15:4677–89.
[52] Hepokur C, Kariper İA, Mısır S, et al. Silver nanoparticle/capecitabine for breast cancer cell treatment. Toxicol Vitro 2019;61:104600.
[53] Malik P, Mukherjee TK. Recent advances in gold and silver nanoparticle-based therapies for lung and breast cancers. Int J Pharm 2018;553(1–2):483–509.
[54] Ayat NR, Vaidya A, Yeung GA, et al. Effective MR molecular imaging of triple negative breast cancer with an EDB-fibronectin-specific contrast agent at reduced doses. Front Oncol 2019;9:1351.
[55] Yalcin S. Dextran-coated iron oxide nanoparticle for delivery of miR-29a to breast cancer cell line. Pharm Dev Technol 2019;24(8):1032–7.
[56] El-Sheikh SMA, Edrees N, El-Sayed H, et al. Could cisplatin loading on biosynthesized silver nanoparticles improve its therapeutic efficacy on human prostate cancer cell line and reduce it's in vivo nephrotoxic effects? Biol Trace Elem Res 2022;200(2):582–90.

[57] Singh P, Pandit S, Mokkapati VRSS, Garg A, Ravikumar V, Mijakovic I. Gold nanoparticles in diagnostics and therapeutics for human cancer. Int J Mol Sci 2018;19(7):1979.
[58] Xiao F, Liu J, Zheng Y, et al. The targeted inhibition of prostate cancer by iron-based nanoparticles based on bioinformatics. J Biomater Appl 2021;36(1):3–14.
[59] Lakshmi BA, Kim S. Quercetin mediated gold nanoclusters explored as a dual functional nanomaterial in anticancer and bio-imaging disciplines. Colloids Surf B Biointerfaces 2019;178:230–7.
[60] Hemmer E, Takeshita H, Yamano T, et al. In vitro and in vivo investigations of upconversion and NIR emitting $Gd_2O_3:Er^{3+}$, Yb^{3+} nanostructures for biomedical applications. J Mater Sci Mater Med 2012;23(10):2399–412.
[61] Topel SD, Topel Ö, Bostancıoğlu RB, Koparal AT. Synthesis and characterization of Bodipy functionalized magnetic iron oxide nanoparticles for potential bioimaging applications. Colloids Surf B Biointerfaces 2015;128:245–53.
[62] Choi YJ, Gurunathan S, Kim JH. Graphene oxide-silver nanocomposite enhances cytotoxic and apoptotic potential of salinomycin in human ovarian cancer stem cells (OvCSCs): a novel approach for cancer therapy. Int J Mol Sci 2018;19(3):710.
[63] Maity R, Chatterjee M, Banerjee A, et al. Gold nanoparticle-assisted enhancement in the anti-cancer properties of theaflavin against human ovarian cancer cells. Mater Sci Eng C Mater Biol Appl 2019;104:109909.
[64] Matsumoto K, Saitoh H, Doan TLH, et al. Destruction of tumor mass by gadolinium-loaded nanoparticles irradiated with monochromatic X-rays: implications for the Auger therapy. Sci Rep 2019;9(1):13275.
[65] Talluri S, Malla RR. Superparamagnetic iron oxide nanoparticles (SPIONs) for diagnosis and treatment of breast, ovaria,n and cervical cancers. Curr Drug Metab 2019;20(12):942–5.
[66] Wang L, Feng M, Li Q, Qiu C, Chen R. Advances in nanotechnology and asthma. Ann Transl Med 2019;7 (8):180.
[67] Yhee JY, I'm J, Nho RS. Advanced therapeutic strategies for chronic lung disease using nanoparticle-based drug delivery. J Clin Med 2016;5(9):82.
[68] Nam J, Won N, Bang J, et al. Surface engineering of inorganic nanoparticles for imaging and therapy. Adv Drug Deliv Rev 2013;65(5):622–48.
[69] Tallury P, Malhotra A, Byrne LM, Santra S. Nanobioimaging and sensing of infectious diseases. Adv Drug Deliv Rev 2010;62(4–5):424–37.
[70] Zhong W, Zhang X, Zeng Y, Lin D, Wu J. Recent applications and strategies in nanotechnology for lung diseases. Nano Res 2021;14(7):2067–89.
[71] Gupta AK, Singh A, Singh S. Diagnosis of tuberculosis: nanodiagnostics approaches. Nano Biomed 2019;261–83.
[72] Markus MA, Napp J, Behnke T, et al. Tracking of inhaled near-infrared fluorescent nanoparticles in lungs of SKH-1 mice with allergic airway inflammation. ACS Nano 2015;9(12):11642–57.
[73] Siafaka PI, Okur NÜ, Karantas ID, Okur ME, Gündoğdu EA. Current update on nanoplatforms as therapeutic and diagnostic tools: a review for the materials used as nanotheranostics and imaging modalities. Asian J Pharm Sci 2021;16(1):24–46.
[74] Schröfel A, Kratošová G, Šafařík I, Šafaříková M, Raška I, Shor LM. Applications of biosynthesized metallic nanoparticles - a review. Acta Biomater 2014;10(10):4023–42.
[75] Markwalter CF, Kantor AG, Moore CP, Richardson KA, Wright DW. Inorganic complexes and metal-based nanomaterials for infectious disease diagnostics. Chem Rev 2019;119(2):1456–518.

CHAPTER

10

Dendrimers: promises and challenges in drug delivery

Aadil Sk Khatik, Satish Kurdhane, Sanya Batheja and Umesh Gupta

Nanopolymeric Drug Delivery Lab, Department of Pharmacy, School of Chemical Sciences and Pharmacy, Central University of Rajasthan, Ajmer, Rajasthan, India

10.1 Introduction

Nanotechnology is a concept used to monitor, repair, build, and regulate biological systems at a scale of 100 nm or less. Nanomedicine includes the use of nanoparticles, nanofibers, nonporous membranes, nanochips, nanotubes, and nanosensors among many more artificial nanodevices and nanostructures. The development of nanotechnology was greatly aided by the unique class of macromolecules known as dendrimers. The dendrimers are well-crafted synthetic polymeric structures with low polydispersity and curved surface functions. Initially, these polymeric hyperbranched molecules were discovered by Fritz Vogtle in 1978, Donald Tomalia, and associates in the early 1980s and George R. Newkome simultaneously, but separately. The synthesized macromolecules were referred to as "arborols" by the researchers, which is Latin for "trees." Dendrimers may alternatively be referred to as "cascade molecules." However, this word is less popular. In the beginning of the dendritic era, Tomalia's poly (amidoamine) (PAMAM) dendrimer [1], Newkome arborols (unimolecular micelles) [2], and Meijer's (polypropylene imine) (PPI) dendrimer [3] established the characteristic features of the respective dendrimers for their commercial use [4,5]. Dendronized polymers are those that have a dendron-like bond, and Flory is responsible for the creation of branched or hyperbranched polymers. Both the polymers were comprised of similar functional characteristics [6,7]. Various types of linear polymers such as polyethylene glycol (PEG), polyglutamic acid, polysaccharide, poly(allylamine hydrochloride), and N-(2 hydroxypropyl)methyl acrylamide were employed for the approval of highly branched polymer formation *via* clinical evaluation. It resulted in the formation of a well-structured, highly branched, and clearly defined polymeric

Molecular Pharmaceutics and Nano Drug Delivery
DOI: https://doi.org/10.1016/B978-0-323-91924-1.00010-1

architecture [8]. The creation of hyperbranched polymers involves continually adding monomer units, much like the branches of a tree [9]. One of the most promising nanocarrier platforms can be seen in the architecture of dendrimer, which are in the range of 1 to 100 nm in diameter [10]. Due of their widespread commercial availability, PAMAM and PPI dendrimers are the two most frequently researched dendrimers. Apart from them, poly (L-lysine) dendrimer [11], phosphorous dendrimer (P-dendrimer) [12], PEGylated dendrimer [13], carbosilane dendrimer [14], and peptide dendrimer [15] are also thoroughly investigated [16].

10.2 Structural architecture and properties

Dendrimers are globular and spherical nanovehicles with a specific architecture made up of three elements: (1) core (central structure having functional moieties), (2) branching units (extension of the core moiety which helps in depiction of the dendritic generation), and (3) surface functional groups (functional moieties present at the terminals of the structure). These functional groups play a key role in determining dendrimer functionality. Dendrimers set themselves apart from linear polymers due to their high symmetry, monodispersity, and surface polyvalency. The generation reaction that takes place and results in higher generation and degree of branching creates a three-dimensional spherical structure. A well-defined core shell architecture having low polydispersity was created by distinct synthetic approaches [17]. One of the most important aspects of architecture is the systematic construction of monomeric units into branch cells. The dendron clump resembles a tree. The structure of a starburst dendrimer resulted from the union of tree-like dendrons to the core having varied sizes and morphologies [18]. In comparison to the organic dendrimer, a heteroatom-based dendrimer holds a comparatively minor position. Yet, there is already a wide variety of topologies available, especially for silicon and phosphorous-based dendrimer [18].

Many significant dendrimer classes, including poly(2,2-bis(hydroxymethyl)propionic acid), poly(ether hydroxylamine), poly(ester amine), polyglycerol, poly-L-lysine, melamine, aminobis-(methylene phosphonic acid) scaffold dendrimer, and so forth. were created as the potential nanovehicles [19]. The developmental stage of a dendrimer from a dendron indicates increased molecular weight along with the number of their surface groups doubled at each generation development stage. For instance, G3 dendrimer has 32 functional groups and G7 dendrimer has potentially 512 surface groups. When the G2 PAMAM dendrimer with an ethylene diamine core was synthesized, it was in the range of 5 to 10 nm, and it exhibits a high surface area-to-volume ratio. They are exceedingly flexible at first and amorphous in smaller generation before becoming spherical, globular confirmation [20]. Materials with a smaller size, such as a G5 PAMAM dendrimer, resemble the hemoglobin protein in terms of their forms and sizes. Growing generations of the dendrimer, such as G7 PAMAM, have larger internal-to-external surface area ratios and are destined for rigorous confirmation [21]. The flow characteristics of the dendrimer are one of the distinctive features. Due to their chain entanglement, certain linear polymers exhibit high viscosity at higher concentrations; nevertheless, a globular dendrimer has less chain entanglement, so it exhibits low viscosity even at a higher concentration [22]. For greater reactivity, the surface groups of the dendrimer control the solubility and miscibility. Dendrimers with hydrophilic groups were soluble in polar solvents, while those with hydrophobic groups are soluble in nonpolar solvents. In comparison to the equivalent properties of linear polyester, dendritic polyester has a greater solubility in the solvents like tetrahydrofuran [9].

The charge of a dendrimer has an impact on toxicities and interactions with cellular membranes. Cationic dendrimer interacts strongly and nonspecifically with an anionic lipoidal cellular membrane. A surface group with more charges has a faster production rate and a stronger interaction with lipoidal layers. More toxicities are seen in a higher generation dendrimer than lower generations [23]. The surface of the dendrimer is changed with amine functional groups to lessen various sorts of toxicities. Modification of the PAMAM dendrimer lowers these kinds of harmful electrostatic interactions by adding neutral (hydroxyl or acetyl) or negatively charged (carboxyl) groups. Consequently, a changed surface charge on the dendrimer is required for the specificity of target cells and tissues whether it is ligand- or protein-targeted [24]. Interest in employing dendrimer in biomedical applications is greatly influenced by its biological characteristics. When the generation and concentration of PAMAM dendrimers (G2, G3, G3, and G4) increase, they are reacted with erythrocyte and alteration in protein confirmation. The 2.5 and 3.5 generations of the PAMAM dendrimer only weakly interact with proteins. With an anionic charge and a carboxylate surface, dendrimer are noncytotoxic over a wide concentration range [25].

10.3 Nomenclature

The generation of a dendrimer is radial growth of a dendritic molecule. The famous de Gennes compact packing model has had the most attention for about 20 years. It determines that peripheral gathering found at the surface of a dendrimer after some generation, as shown in Fig. 10.1. The surface area A_z is determined by Eq. (10.1), where Z represents the total number of functional groups at the terminal, A_D depicts the total surface of the dendrimer, N_Z represents the number of surface moieties per generation, r depicts the radius of dendrimer, N_c illustrates the number of branches from the core, N_b illustrates the number of branches at each generation, and G represents the number of generations.

$$A_z = A_D N_Z (r^2 / N_C \cdot N_b \cdot G) \tag{10.1}$$

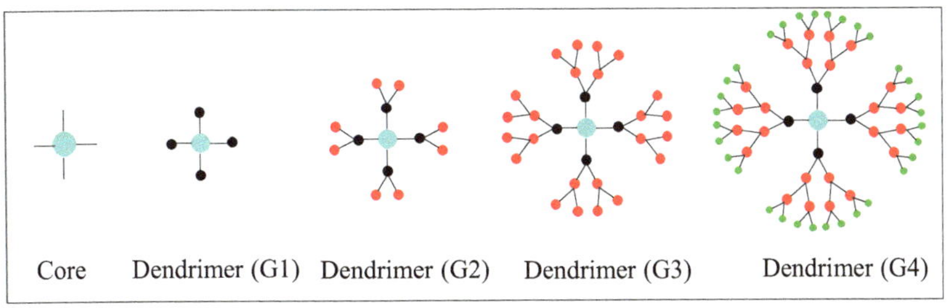

FIGURE 10.1 Representation of core and different generations of the dendrimer.

It indicates that lowering of a high generation number is due to A_z. The compactly packed generation G1 is achieved when A_z is similar to the van der Waals radii. A simple equation was provided for a PAMAM dendrimer having a branch cell segment, P:

$$G_1 = 2.88(\ln P + 1.5) \tag{10.2}$$

According to this equation, the compact packed generation is arrived between 10 and 11 [26].

10.4 Synthesis of dendrimer

10.4.1 Divergent method

This is the first proposed method for the preparation of the dendrimer [27]. This method rose from the seminal work of Tomalia and Newkome. In this method, firstly, the multifunctional core is formed as a result of self-assembly of a dendrimer. Then, the outer extension of the core is formed by the addition of the sequences using the Michael addition reaction. The ethylenediamine (EDA) is used as an initiator for the formation of multifunctional core. It contains the four-armed form of nitrogen which helps in increasing the extensions through amidation reaction. The two abovementioned steps were repeated continuously to yield a different generation of the dendrimer. In this method, the formation of the dendrimer happens in a stepwise manner. The core formation is considered to be the first one followed by the building a molecule toward the periphery by monomer coupling and transforming the monomer group to produce a reactive surface for coupling. After the formation of the first-generation dendrimer (G1), in the next step, the (G1) activated or unprotected reacted with the other monomer to form second generation (G2). The process continues till the desired generation is obtained (as shown in Fig. 10.2A) [27]. The reaction of the generation should be complete, and it should avoid the ununiformly formed branches (inequality in the branch length). This problem can affect the functionality and symmetry of the dendrimer. Hence, it could be an intractable challenge to determine the variation between perfect and imperfect dendrimers. The divergent method is widely commercialized for the development of highly symmetric dendrimers. The peculiarity of this method is that it obtains a higher yield but with less purity, or in other words, purity is compromised to obtain a higher yield. The imperfect dendrimer formation can be avoided by taking the surplus quantity of the reagent.

10.4.2 Convergent method

This method was developed by the Fréchet and Hawker in 1989–90 [27]. It is an alternative to the divergent method, which usually produces a purer form of dendrimer. Unlike the divergent method, this method involves the dendrimer synthesis, which starts from the exterior of the structure (surface) to the multifunctional core (interior). A wide range of dendrimers with different functionalities is the product of this reaction. This approach of synthesis overcomes the issues of the divergent approach like purity and

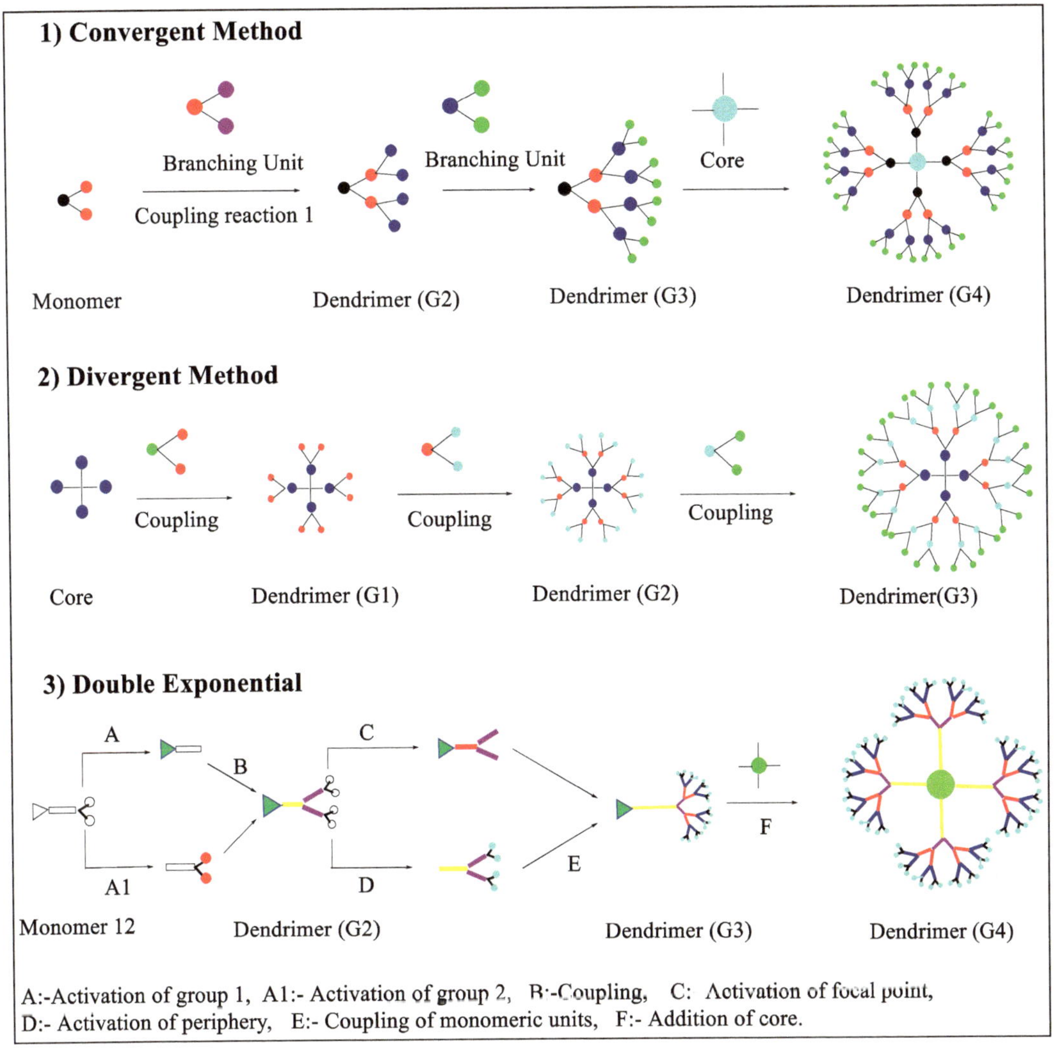

FIGURE 10.2 Synthesis of dendrimer *via* different methods; (A) convergent method, (B) divergent method, and (C) double exponential method.

structural defects. The yield is compromised for the purity and symmetry. So, unlike the divergent method, it is used at the laboratory scale only. However, for commercial scale, the divergent method is the favored option. Dendrimers synthesized using this method have mixed structural features, as different parts are conjugated to generate dendrimers, which contain heteromorphologies. This functionality becomes the reason for development of multifunctional designs.

It is a two-step method which includes activation of the monomer, followed by their coupling to the core. Firstly, the surface groups are coupled to the monomer to form a dendritic segment, for example, zero generation (G0). Secondly, activation of (G0) is done in order to couple with another monomer, and the resultant moiety is called as the G1 or dendritic wedge. These two steps are repeated to get the desired dendrimer by reacting different functionality monomers. Finally, to obtain a whole dendrimer, this formed exterior was coupled with the multifunctional core (as shown in Fig. 10.2B). By using the convergent method, only a small-sized dendrimer can be synthesized due to generation of stearic hindrance between dendron while attaching to core [27] Stearic hindrance occurs as result of the coupling of the multiple dendron focal point of core, leading to the smallest size (not more than 6th gen) with limited yield.

10.4.3 Click chemistry

The principle of click chemistry was firstly described by Barry Sharpless in 2001. The unmet needs of drug discovery and chemistry were involved in it [28]. This principle of click chemistry has been applied for the preparation of dendrimers. In click chemistry, functional groups were modified to rapidly synthesize higher generation of dendrimers. The click chemistry includes various reactions such as Diel-alder, thiol-yene, azide-alkyne, TAD-click/ trans click, sulfur fluoride exchange, and so forth [29]. By using this reaction, a wide range of high chemical yield, stereospecific, and stable products with harmless byproducts were obtained. All generations (G2 and G3) were isolated directly as pure solids, and sodium chloride is the only major byproduct of this reaction [29].

Click reactions applied to the dendrimer are as follows:

- Azide-alkyne reaction
  - CuAAC (copper-catalyzed azide-alkyne cycloaddition)
  - SPAAC (strain-promoted alkyne-azide cycloaddition)
- Thiol-yne reaction
- Diel-alder reaction
- TAD-click/ trans-click chemistry

10.4.4 Lego chemistry

Lego chemistry is a method that involves the core and branched monomer. The monomer and core used consists of highly functional groups. The terminal groups are made up of hydrazine and phosphine [30]. After some variation in synthetic preparation scheme, the established scheme permits proliferation of the surface groups of dendrimers from 50 to 250 groups in one step. Advantages include requirement of least solvent and easy purification with environment friendly byproducts (water and nitrogen) [31].

10.4.5 Double exponential method

This method was firstly studied by Shinkai, Franchet, and Roy [30]. This method resembles a rapid growth technique of linear polymer preparation. This method works by producing monomers from both convergent and divergent methods using a single initiator. Further, orthogonally protected trimer is prepared by reacting the resultant. The produced trimer is then used for further growth of the dendrimer by using it as a repeating unit (as shown in Fig. 10.2C) [31]. The strength of this approach is rapid synthesis, and it can be easily combined with convergent and divergent methods [32].

10.5 Types of dendrimers

Current synthetic chemistry led to the development of several dendritic polymers. Dendritic polymers are created using a dendritic scaffold that is comparable to the ideal dendrimer. Yet, by altering certain functional group modifications on the surface, new functional characteristics can be obtained. Several generations of dendrimers are created, depending upon the target, which tends to increase solubility and decrease dendritic toxicity. The structural architectures of different types of dendrimers such as PAMAM dendrimer, poly (propylene imine) dendrimer, poly (L-lysine) dendrimer, poly (ethylene imine) dendrimer, peptide dendrimer, glycodendrimer, and other recently created types are mentioned in Fig. 10.3 [33].

10.5.1 Poly (amidoamine) dendrimer

PAMAM was the first dendrimer developed by the Tomalia's group using a divergent technique. It differs from other dendrimers; amidoamine grows from the central functional group, whereas amine does not [1]. PAMAM, which is employed in biomedical applications, is first created and marketed. The unaltered PAMAM surface is positively charged, interacting with red blood cells (RBCs) and other cells exhibiting cytotoxicity or hemolytic toxicity. PAMAM dendrimer's cytotoxicity and hemolytic toxicity are dependent on their charge, concentration, and production. In comparison to higher generation (G2–G4), G0, and G1, which have reduced toxicity. PAMAM dendrimer with the same charge anionic and neutral toxicity exhibits decreased toxicity. Fatty acids, such as lauric acid ($nC_{11}H_{23}COOH$), changed the surface of the dendrimer to increase their permeability. Surface modification of the PAMAM dendrimer *via* PEGylation or lauryl moiety was said to reduce cytotoxicity and increase permeability. The terminal amine group of PAMAM dendrimer is linked to several functional groups, such as hydroxyl (-OH), carboxylic acid (–COOH), or PEG [34]. Steric branching of the G7–10 generation makes PAMAM dendrimer's drug or guest loading less effective. PAMAM and tris-(hydroxymethyl) amino methane have been combined to carry several antibacterial compounds [35].

In 1993, Haensler and Szoka [36] showed that the DNA-PAMAM dendrimers have a high capacity for transfection in mammalian cells. A better compound is formed by the lower generation of the amino functional dendrimer, which also improves the endocytosis of DNA into the nucleus. The complexation of dendrimers with DNA is supported by the electrostatic interaction between the positive end amino group of PAMAM and negative phosphate group of DNA. It has been discovered that improving the dendrimer surface by combining a hydrophobic dye molecule (Oregon green448) and a sugar molecule (cyclodextrin) enhances transfection ability. From generation G0 through G10, the size range is consistently between 1 and 14 nm. PAMAM displays a $pK_a = 6.85$ with primary amine at

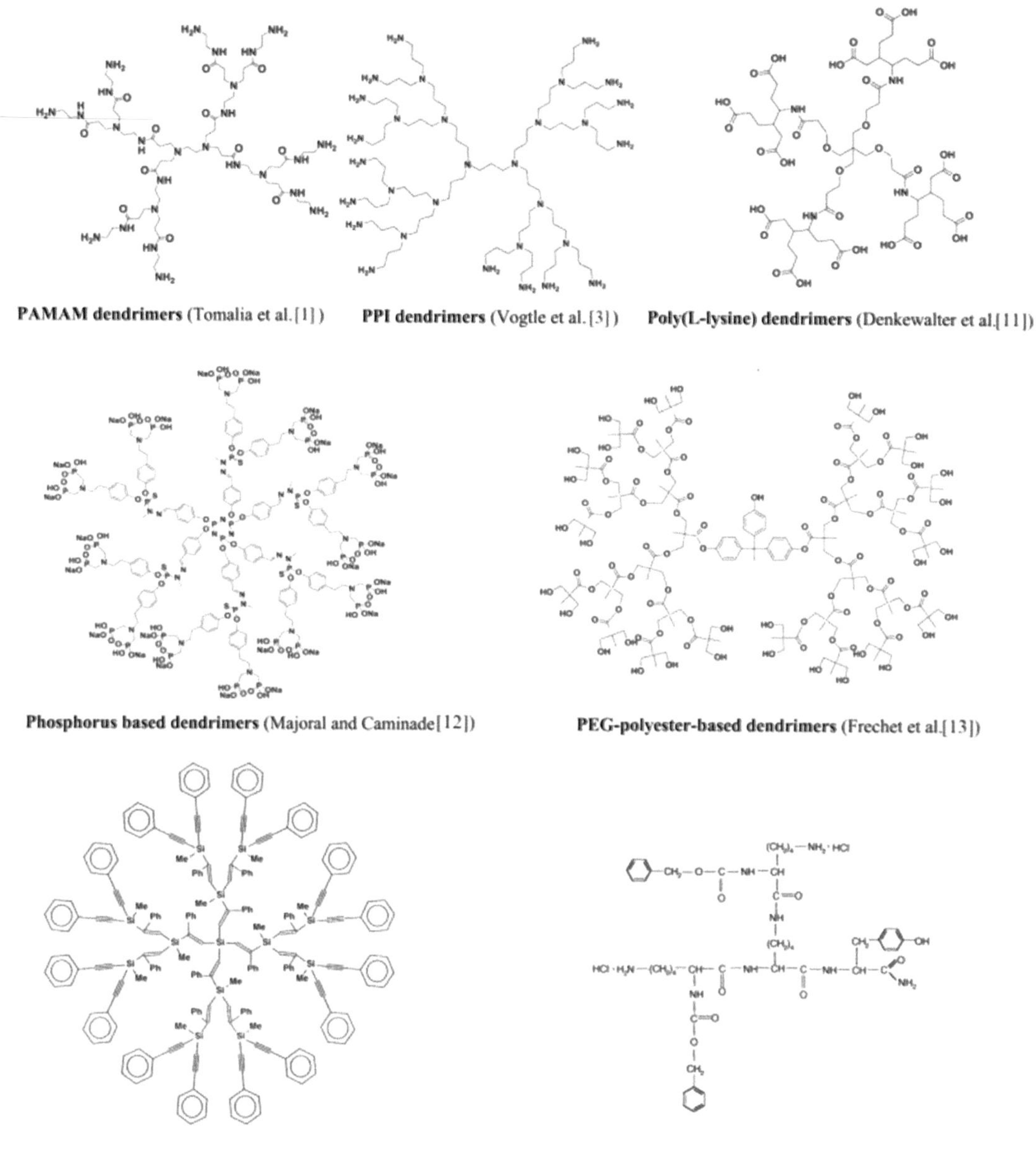

FIGURE 10.3 Chemical structure of the selected type of dendrimer. *Source: Extracted from Janaszewska A, Lazniewska J, Trzepí Nski P, Marcinkowska M, Klajnert-Maculewicz B. Cytotoxicity of dendrimers. Biomolecules 9(8) (2019) 330 [16].*

the surface and a $pK_a = 3.86$ with tertiary amine in the core. Both the kinds of a particular generation also transport to the epithelial layer of the gastrointestinal wall, indicating the benefits of oral distribution [37]. In the study, the release rate and encapsulation of doxorubicin (DOX) were affected by various groups, including acetyl (PAMAM-G5-NHAc), glycidol hydroxyl (PAMAM-G5-NGlyOH), and carboxyl (PAMAM-G5-SAH), and the rate increased under an acidic (PH5.5) condition, rising by 39.5%, 60.9%, and 68.6%, respectively, in comparison to 5.5%, a multidrug resistance issue. Dual medication delivery is done using PAMAM and carbon dots (CDs). Covalent connections between blue-emitting CDs and DOX and PAMAM dendrimers, which include the efflux inhibitor D-tocopheryl PEG 1000 succinate and the target ligand peptide arginine-glycine-aspartic acid (RGD) peptide, are prepared (TGPS). The PAMAM dendrimer/CD nanohybrid system as a whole thus have the potential in therapeutic applications [38]. PAMAM dendrimers are also hypothesized to serve as a framework for contrast agents for magnetic resonance imaging (MRI), improving contrast and lowering dose requirements [39].

10.5.2 Polypropylene imine dendrimer

PPI dendrimers are highly branching, amine-functionalized macromolecules that are mostly made by divergent synthesis. 1,4-diaminobutane (DAB) serves as the basis for the synthesis of the PPI dendrimer, also known as the DAB dendrimer. The twofold Michael addition of acrylonitrile to primary amine, followed by reduction of the nitrile to produce surface primary amines, regulates the terminal synthesis. PPI dendrimers are similar to PAMAM dendrimers, in that they both include tertiary amines within and primary amines on the outside [40]. Functional group modification of the PPI dendrimer is necessary for effective DNA and RNA transport. PPI dendrimers vary from PAMAM dendrimers in terms of size and polarity in their inner branching area. Alkyl and tertiary amine groups are present in the PPI interior area, although amide is also present in PAMAM and can bring more polarity to the inner region [41].

The various internal functional groups result in various behaviors of the drug molecule when they are encapsulated. The many amines functional groups on the surface of PPI dendrimers enable them to bind with additional targeted ligands such as Tf, folate, arginine, antibodies, peptides, and carbohydrates, among others [42]. In another study, the delivery of hydrophobic anticancer drugs and PEGylated diaminobutane PPI (G4) dendrimer was fabricated with folate. The development of formulation improves site-specific targeting with reduced toxicity and sustained release of etoposide at the tumor site [43]. In another study, transferrin (Tf) containing G3-PPI dendrimer successfully delivered the plasmid DNA across the blood–brain barrier by targeting the transferrin receptor in the brain. Fifth-generation PPI dendrimer also shows the potential ability to deliver various antitumor agents to brain tumor and gliomas [44].

10.5.3 Glycodendrimer

The term "glycodendrimer" refers to the dendrimer composed of a sugar moiety. The relationship between the different sugar molecules, including glucose, mannose, galactose, and disaccharide, is established for the synthesis of dendrimers. Also, glycodendrimer can be classified on the basis of placement of the sugar molecule at the core or branches. Glycodendrimer can be carbohydrate coated, carbohydrate centered, or carbohydrate based entirely. It can be synthesized using both divergent and convergent methods. Yet, the outcome of the convergent approach is additional branches that have been brought together from various sites where the core was attached. Several common structures of multifunctional glycodendrimer can be identified: fan, comb-like, and ellipsoidal shapes [45].

10.5.4 Liquid crystalline dendrimer

A liquid crystalline dendrimer is primarily composed of a mesogenic group, an aliphatic spacer, and a polymer chain. Mesogens that resemble rigid rods and are capable of producing mesophases are seen in LC dendrimers. LC mesophase formation largely depends on the spacers. Liquid crystals have a strong polymer bonding arrangement and are shaped like cylindrical rods. Mesogenic group, carbon chain spacer, and polymer chain make up the LIC dendrimer. For the dendrimer's cylindrical (rod-like) shape, spacers are crucial [32]. Dendrimers synthesized by the convergent method are reported by Percec and coworkers for the preparation of racemic AB2 cylindrical mesogenic monomers exhibiting conformational isomerism [46].

10.5.5 Core-shell dendrimer

These are superstructure dendritic assemblage, in which one dendrimer unit serves as the core and is affixed firmly to another dendrimer unit shell. The architecture of the core shell is developed with the repetitive fixing of shells around the core till the generation number of the core becomes higher than the shell [32]. The connection of additional shells is maintained by synthetic processes, which assist in the development of nanoparticles in the 1−100 nm range. Making a PAMAM dendrimer core with additional PAMAM dendrimers covalently linked as a shell is an essential technique that may be utilized to make larger dendritic molecules without adding more steps to the process [30].

10.5.6 Hybrid dendrimer

The hybrid dendrimer combines linear and hyperbranched polymer in the form of mixed-breed or surface conjugate copolymers. Round structures and a greater number of end functional groups of dendrimers are better prepared *via* dendritic fusion. The dendritic components' interconnection with various reactive terminals serves additional functions, such as stabilizers, surfactants, or adhesives [32]. To better understand the dendrimer performance, the two dendrimers can be arranged in various combinations, such as a flexible core with a rigid shell or a flexible shell with a rigid core. Hybrid dendrimers also have the benefit of being produced by merely covalently joining two dendrimers that have already been generated [30].

10.5.7 Chiral dendrimer

The chiral dendrimer are prepared by utilizing essentially different branches but which are chemically similar to the chiral core [32]. The chiral dendrimer contains three main components, such as chiral centers in the core of the dendrimer and a branching unit consisting of chiral centers, which joins the chiral molecules to the surface. In the wider area, these are utilized as a catalyst in the isolation of two enantiomers and identification of molecules [47]. Chiral dendrimers with a binaphthyl core are also employed for fluorescence-based selective enantiomer identification of chiral substances. Fluorescence has some benefits, including improved sensitivity, the ability to record responses in real time, and the capacity to detect multiple modes. Three sequences of zeroth- to second-generation chiral dendrimer were synthesized by the convergent method using chiral and nonracemic AB2 monomers [48].

10.5.8 Peptide dendrimer

The peptide dendrimer composed of amino acids that are in the core or branching unit is linked *via* peptide linkage. Recently, the peptide dendrimer has gained considerable attention in the field of nanotechnology. Several researchers have reported that peptide dendrimers have a pivotal role to play in delivery of viral vaccines, protein replication, and development of immunogenic or diagnostic agents [49]. The peptide dendrimer has a molecular weight ranging from 2 from 100 kDa, and it carries big protein molecules. It includes three main classes: grafted peptide, natural amino acids, and conventional peptide dendrimers. Peptide dendrimers are employed in the delivery of a gene as a nonviral vector [50]. The transfection ability is increased with the increase of generation of the dendrimer. It may cause steric hinderance, which leads to the difficulty in synthesis of the peptide dendrimer. To overcome this limitation, it is suggested to utilize the click chemistry for the synthesis of the peptide dendrimer [51].

10.5.9 Polyamidoamine organosilicon dendrimer

PAMAM organosilicon (PAMAMOS) is the class of linear copolymer dendrimers that includes PAMAM components as the hydrophilic core and organosilicon as a surface functionality. PAMAMOS is constructed by Michael addition reaction. The organosilicon unit is attached to the core of dendrimer (PAMAM) with free amino terminals. They are also called as reversed micelles type, which may include largely branched amphiphilic components. PAMAMOS can be prepared by a unreactive surface group, mainly trimethylsilane and trimethsiloxysilyl moieties, which may produce vinylsilyl, vinylsiloxysilyl, and alkoxysilyl [52]. The distinctive feature of PAMAMOS compared to the PAMAM dendrimer is solubility. The hydrophilic PAMAM dendrimer is soluble in water, methanol, and insoluble hydrocarbon, while hydrophobic trimethylsilane changes to the PAMAMOS dendrimer. They are observed to be insoluble in water and soluble in toluene. The solubilizing property of PAMAMOS makes it have an identical shape to the dendrimer [52].

10.5.10 Polylysine dendrimer

The characteristic feature of the polylysine dendrimer is biodegradability. It is metabolized by several enzymes available in the system and easily excreted due to its low molecular weight. The extent of biodegradability can be predicted by the peripheral amino groups and detaching of capping groups. These are employed in the pH-dependent drug delivery system [53].

10.5.11 Phosphorous dendrimer

The phosphorous dendrimers are thermodynamically stable. The construction of phosphorus dendrimers involves repetitive units of hydroxyl-benzaldehyde as the base medium with the polymeric core (PCl), followed by its condensation using phosphorhydrazide. The conformational changes could be observed with the increase in generation of dendrimers (G3 to G5). It tends to exhibit a highly rigid structure. Phosphorous dendrimers have been employed in different arenas of chemistry, material science, and biologicals [12].

10.5.12 Triazine dendrimer

1,3,5-Triazine is an essential molecule for the synthesis of dendrimers. The characteristic features of the triazine dendrimer include bioactive nature, better stability, controlled generation size, and greater production. These dendrimers exhibit enhanced antibacterial activity to the skin with increased stability and reduced toxicity [54]. Melamine-derived dendrimer has been explored for functionalization of carbon fiber. In the recent studies, triazine dendrimers were grafted onto the mesoporous materials (MCM-41 and SBA-15) to enhance loading of the support for high-throughput synthesis application [55].

10.6 Challenges of dendrimer in drug delivery

A dendrimer is a potential nanocarrier, having seen significant advancement in the field of medicine. However, notable shortcomings in the designing and applicability of the dendrimer have been observed, such as size limitation, stability issues, high cost, approval challenges, and so forth. Some of them are briefly discussed below.

10.6.1 Cationic toxicities

Among several limitations, ***dendritic toxicity*** is predominant. The dendritic toxicity is significantly related to the structure and architecture of the respective dendrimer. Dendrimers are cationic in nature and thus cause impairment of the biological membrane, resulting in apoptotic activity. Substantially, the cationic macromolecules have the tendency to interact with anionic cellular components such as plasma membrane, organelles (endosomes, mitochondria, and nuclei), and proteins [56]. The interaction of cationic macromolecules with the biological membrane results in the destabilization of the nanosystem, causing membrane rupture, which may lead to the production of reactive oxygen species (ROS) responsible for the cell death [57]. Several research groups have also reported the concentration- and generation-dependent toxicity of amine-terminated dendrimers, as discussed in Table 10.1.

TABLE 10.1 Different types of toxicities of dendrimer.

Type of dendrimer	Disease	Cell lines	Description	Toxicity	References
PPI (G3 and G4)	–	–	PPI G3 exhibits 4% hemolysis, while PPI G4 folate-modified dendrimer exhibits twofold higher hemolysis (8%) due to increased polycationic charge on the surface.	Hemolytic toxicity	[58]
PPI (G4)	Ovarian Cancer	CHO	PPI G4 dendrimers are highly cytotoxic to the CHO line but maltotriose-modified dendrimer reduces cytotoxicity up to 30%.	Cytotoxicity	[59]
PPI (G5)	Cancer	HUVEC	PPI dendrimers (G5) exhibits 65% cytotoxicity against HUVEC cell lines. Masking or PEGylation of the surface charge assists in the minimization of the induced cytotoxicity.	Cytotoxicity	[60]
PPI (G4 and G5)	Neuroblastoma	Neuro-2a	Piperazine-modified PAMAM dendrimers exhibit enhanced transfection efficiency among PAMAM-based vectors with 80% cytotoxicity	Cytotoxicity	[59]
PPI (G5)	Hepatocellular carcinoma	Hep G2	Concentration- and time-dependent cell viability, hemolysis, and hematological parameters were observed with significant results. It was concluded that the PPI G5 modification with amino acid could result in newer biocompatible nanovehicles	Cytotoxicity and hemolytic toxicity	[61]
PPI (G5)			Free-amine terminal of PPI G5 potentiates hemolysis of 2% RBC suspension from 14% to 34% at the concentration of 0.001 mg/mL and 1 mg/mL, respectively	Hemolytic toxicity	[38]
PAMAM	Reticular cell carcinoma	J774A.1	The cytotoxic response of J774A.1 cells to the PAMAM dendrimers, with varying generations (G-4, G-5, and G-6), were evaluated using the Alamar blue (AB) and MTT assays. The generation-dependent effect was highly observed on increased intracellular ROS, inflammatory mediators (MIP-2, IL-1, TNF-α), cytotoxicity. The author demonstrated the generation-dependent cytotoxic trend as follows: G6 > G5 > G4 Due to the increased free-amine terminals leading to cationic toxicity.	Cytotoxicity	[62]
PAMAM	Colorectal adenocarcinoma	Caco-2	Carboxy-PAMAM G3.5 and 4.5 are cytotoxic at conc. of 10.0 mM compared to G3 and G4, which are toxic at 1 mM.	Cytotoxicity	[37]

(Continued)

TABLE 10.1 (Continued)

Type of dendrimer	Disease	Cell lines	Description	Toxicity	References
PAMAM $G4\text{-}NH_2$	Colorectal adenocarcinoma	Caco-2	Cytotoxicity is dependent on the dendrimer generation, probably due to the intrinsic toxicity associated with the higher generation dendrimer.	Cytotoxicity	[63]
PAMAM (All Gen.)		RBC suspension	PEGylated dendrimer reduced 13.3–15.3 hemolysis due to less interaction with ammonium ions.	Hemolytic toxicity	[64]
PAMAM (G5)	Melanoma	SK-Mel-28	PAMAM (G5) dendrimer shows toxicity on SK-Mel-28 cells at minimum conc of 7.5 μM.	Cytotoxicity	[65]
PAMAM (G4)		HEK293	The author employed PAMAM G4 modification with PEG and folic acid (FA) to obtain partially substituted PAMAM dendrimers with different sizes, charges, and surface functionalities.As a result, it was observed that incorporation of FA and PEG increases cell viability of the PAMAM-based nanoformulation.Also, the pharmacokinetic profile of PEG-PAMAM illustrates the extended circulation time in the blood, exhibiting sustained drug release (71.1 min).	Cytotoxicity	[66]
PAMAM	Neurodegenerative disorders	mHippoE-18	Pyrrolidone-modified dendrimer exhibits 70% of cell viability, while unmodified PAMAM dendrimers exerts 20% cell viability. Thus, it was concluded that the reduction of free-amine terminal tends to potentiate the cell viability rate.	Cytotoxicity	[44]
PAMAM	Zebrafish embryo	100% mortality of zebrafish embryo	In-vivo toxicity of PAMAM dendrimers like G3, G4, and G5 have a 100% toxicity compared to G6-amonoethanol and anionic dendrimer.	Cytotoxicity	[67]
PAMAM G7		Fibrinogen aggregation	Cationic dendrimers induce coagulopathies through their ability to aggregate negatively charged blood proteins, including fibrinogen and albumin	Hematological toxicity	[68]

10.6.2 Obstacles in synthesis

10.6.2.1 Purification of dendrimer

The synthesis of dendrimers involves undesired side reactions, which could make the dendrimer impure. These impurities may be due to many functionalities like arm, dimers, or trailing generations. Many research groups have explored the obstacles faced during the purification of dendrimers, but yet not a single potential and easy method has been established with 99% purity of the dendrimer. Thus, purification of dendrimer is essential along with its accurate characterization to estimate the purity and reproducibility of the specific generation. Purification of the dendrimer also potentiates its biological activity.

In 2003, Rether et al. developed a technique for the separation and recovery of heavy metal ions using the N-benzoyl thiourea modified-PAMAM dendrimer. The purification process was performed by the polymer-supported ultrafiltration technique. In this study, the authors utilized PAMAM G2.5 dendrimer as a base polymer. The results exhibited that modified PAMAM dendrimer retained almost all metal ions at pH 9. The separation of heavy metal ions was achieved in the presence of aqueous solutions containing high concentrations of competing complexing agents such as triethanolamine or sodium nitrate [69].

In 2010, Balieu et al. prepared modified-PPI G1 dendrimer with glyceryl moiety by one step reaction, that is, surface decoration. The prepared glycerol-decorated PPI dendrimers were purified by solubilizing them in minimum quantity of methanol, followed by the addition of pentane/ethyl acetate to precipitate modified-PPI G1 dendrimer as a pure product with 78% yield [70]. In 2012, Mullen et al. purified the PAMAM G5 dendrimer simply by using the membrane dialysis method. After the purification process, the dendrimers were analyzed by gel-permeation chromatography, potentiometric titration, and reverse phase chromatography [71]. Recently, Kharwade et al. described the method for purification of PAMAM dendrimers by *azeotropic distillation*. The solvent system of toluene: methanol (9:1) was utilized for the solubilization and purification of PAMAM dendrimer [72]. Still, 100% purity cannot be achieved by any of the protocol mentioned above. Hence, purification of the dendrimer is still a major research area which needs to be explored.

10.6.2.2 Generation-dependent obstacles

Many research groups have reported the generation-dependent obstacles such as synthetic procedures, steric hindrance, membrane disruption, and so forth. With the increase in generation of dendrimer, the steric hindrance increases. Thus, it potentiates the need to understand the concept of the generation-dependent effect. In 1998, Pollak et al. determined the generation-dependent effect on the metalloporphyrin core dendrimer by using electrochemical and fluorescence quenching studies. In this study, the authors established that the metalloporphyrin core with higher generation dendron increases the distance between the porphyrin core and the electrode surface. However, high-generation dendrimers have the tendency to isolate a peripheral site without any restrictions [73].

In 2004, Devarakonda et al. investigated the effect of PAMAM dendrimer generation size and surface functional group on aqueous solubility of nifedipine. The aqueous solubility of nifedipine was measured at 30°C in Tris buffer at varied pH (pH 4, 7, and 10) by using the traditional rotary bottle method. The authors studied that the lower generation PAMAM dendrimers (<G3) exhibit more potential to significantly increase the solubility of poorly water-soluble drugs than the higher generation dendrimers (>G3) [74].

In 2010, Kojima et al. demonstrated the influence of generation of dendrimer and length of the PEG chain on biodistribution of the PEGylated dendrimer. The authors studied PEGylated l-lysine-bearing PAMAM dendrimers and non-PEGylated PAMAM dendrimers, among which the biodistribution of PEGylated dendrimers was found to be different from the non-PEGylated dendrimers. PEGylation induces prolonged blood circulation of dendrimers, which may assist in targeting of effected tissues. Therefore, the PEGylated dendrimers can be a potential drug carrier for cancer chemotherapy [75].

In 2014, Kesharwani et al. elaborated the generation dependent potential of PPI dendrimer on cancer targeting. The PPI dendrimer of different generation were synthesized and loaded with melphalan as a drug moiety. The in-vitro studies resulted into increased drug loading with the increased generation of dendrimers; from G4 to G5. It also exhibits a significant increase in generation-associated toxicity. Thus, the authors concluded that G4 dendrimer is superior to the G3 as well as G5 dendrimers due to their drug delivery applicability [76].

10.6.2.3 Uneconomical in nature

The production of dendrimer needs a high degree of precision; hence it is preferable for each generation to have a single size and molecular weight rather than the wide molecular weight dispersion found in most polymers. The synthesis of dendrimers could be done *via* different methods using proper equipment. The cost of reactors, purification assembly, azeotropic distillation, gel permeation chromatography, high-performance liquid chromatography, and so forth make it uneconomical in nature. The multistep synthesis of higher generation of dendrimer also illustrates the cost-excessiveness. The complex ligands and metal catalyst used in the synthesis are very expensive, for example, rhodium (Rh) and palladium(pd) [77].

In laboratories, the solid phase synthesis of dendrimer is still limited at milligram to gram scale. Due to the small-scale reactions, it is hard to ensure the completion of reaction and removal of the product from solid support. Huang et al. elaborated the Mitsunobu reaction for the synthesis of polyether dendrimer using expensive reagents with limited shelf life [78].

10.6.3 Drug leakage

Drug leakage is one of the most common issues being faced by the nanocarriers. The drug leakage or morphological change of the dendrimers can be estimated by the stability studies. Many researchers have observed the leakage of the drug from the dendritic core. For instance, in 2009, Parimi et al. developed a new insight regarding interaction of the lipid bilayer with the PAMAM dendrimer. The intrinsic activity of PAMAM may cause phospholipid bilayer disruption. Thus, it may lead to leakage of the drug from the core of the dendrimer [79].

Leakage of the drug from the PPI dendrimer may take place in varied temperatures (0,25 ± 2, 60°C ± 2°C) and light conditions [80]. In glycodendrimers, leakage of drug molecules is lower at room temperature because of hypothetical shrinkage of the dendrimer structure due to decrease in energy levels that molecules have to reduce in energy for efficient interaction with drug molecules. At higher temperatures, the uniform ring-like structure becomes unstable because the molecules have more free energy and the carbohydrate linkages could break. As a result, the structures become more brittle, and the drug is released to a greater extent than at ambient temperature. Also, it was discovered that formulations stored in light experienced greater drug leakage than those stored in darkness. They could be explained by cleavage at higher temperatures and in light, which causes bond breaking due to increased molecular kinetics [81].

10.6.4 Regulatory challenges

Commercialization of dendrimers was undertaken because of their unique features, and they were sent to FDA for clinical approval. During all stages of drug discovery and commercialization process, it is important to file patents to protect the intellectual properties of inventors and companies and also save money and time from being wasted in lawsuits or even losing legal cases. Nevertheless, considering the long time it takes to gain regulatory approval of a drug, passing the required clinical trials, and finally introducing a new pharmaceutical to the market, the allowed 20-year period (depending on the country) of patent protection diminishes the period of commercial exclusivity to 12 years or less [82]. Dendrimers are currently used in preclinical in vivo effectiveness trials (as mentioned in Table 10.2) [83].

10.7 Biomedical applications of dendrimer

10.7.1 Drug delivery

Multifaceted properties like multifunctional core, variability of surface, monodispersity, surface conjugation, branched structure, high solubility, low viscosity, and so forth make dendrimers a perfect candidate as a drug delivery vehicle. The internal multifunctional core assists in the encapsulation and targeting of a drug at specific sites with the aimed ligand. The high local density of ligand and flexibility and deformability of a dendrimer are some add-on characteristics responsible for it. Since the last few decades, the evolution of a novel drug delivery system has gained immerse attention. The NDDS has showcased its potential in the treatment and management of several disease such as skin disease, neurodegenerative disease cancer, and so forth [105]. Cancer is one of the leading causes of mortality worldwide. Various research groups have utilized dendrimers as a potential nanocarrier for the targeting of carcinoma cells.

In 1970, the primary dendrimer-based nanoformulation was commercialized by Starpharma Ltd., Australia, for the prevention and treatment of genital herpes (HSV-2) HIV and other sexually transmitted infections. The first dendrimer-based nanotherapeutic agent was launched in 1970, for example, VivaGel [19]. Many researchers have utilized dendrimers as a potent drug delivery system by mainly two approaches: (1) by drug encapsulation and (2) drug dendrimer conjugation core of dendrimers. The drug encapsulation helps in providing sustained drug release at a site of action, whereas drug dendrimer conjugation potentiates rapid drug release at the site of action for instance.

TABLE 10.2 Preclinical studies using dendrimers-based nanomedicine for in-vivo therapy.

Application	Platform	Active agent	Remark/clinical status	References
Inflammation				
Drug delivery	PAMAM (G5)	Methotrexate	Collagen-induced arthritis	[83]
	PAMAM(G4)	Naked dendrimers	Chlamydia-induced reactive arthritis	[84]
	Phosphorous ABC terminated	Naked dendrimers	Rheumatoid arthritis	[85]
	PAMAM (G4)	Naked indomethacin	Improved drug solubility and increased accumulation in inflammatory regions in arthritic rats	[86]
	PAMAM	Methyl prednisolone	Allergen-induced lung inflammation	[87];
	Mannose	Mannose-grafted dendrimers	Acute lung inflammation prevention	[88]
	PAMAM (G4)	Fluocinolone acetonide	Retinal degradation model	[89]
Cancer				
Drug delivery or intrinsic dendrimers surface chemistry	PAMAM (G3.5)	Cisplatin	Increased MTD and bioavailability of cisplatin, prolonged survival of mice with melanoma	[90]
	PEG-PLL	Doxorubicin	Greater antitumor activity in breast cancer compared to liposomal formulation	[91]
	PEG_PAMAM	Methotrexate	Greater antitumor activity compared to non-PEG dendrimers	[92]
	PEG-PAMAM	Doxorubicin	RGD-conjugated PAMAM dendrimers showed greater tumor accumulation with PEG than without, and improved survival in animals with gliomas	[93]
	PPI	Surfactant	Greater antitumor activity in brain tumors	[94]
Gene delivery				
	PAMAM	Oligo-DNA	Dendrimers could effectively deliver 111In-labeled oligo-DNAs to tumor	[95]
	PAMAM	*Angiostatin gene*	Intratumoral administration of dendrimers with the angiostatin gene effectively inhibited tumor growth	[96]
	PPI	DNA	Intravenous administration of transferrin-bearing PPI dendrimers led to rapid and sustained tumor regression	[97]

(Continued)

TABLE 10.2 (Continued)

Application	Platform	Active agent	Remark/clinical status	References
Infectious disease				
Drug delivery or intrinsic dendrimers surface chemistry	PAMAM	N-acetyl-neuraminic acid	Inhibition of HA-mediated adhesion in the influenza model	[98]
	PEG-PPI	RIF	Tuberculosis treatment	[99]
Gene delivery	PAMAM	Si RNA	Suppressed HIV infection in the humanized mouse model	[100]
Diagnostic				
Mr contrast	PAMAM G4, G6	Gd	Enhanced retention, reduced renal clearance	[101]
CT/SPECT	PAMAM G4	Tri-iodinated and chelated ^{99}Tc	Increases blood circulation time and provides effective simultaneous contrast enhancement in both CT and SPECT	[102]
PET	Peptide dendrimers conjugated	Cyclic 9-amino acid peptide (LyP-1)	Ability to detect atherosclerotic plaques using in vivo PET imaging	[103]
CEST	PPI, PAMAM G2, G5	DOTAM, MRI contrast agents	Used for pH mapping, to detect gliomas at very low agent concentrations	[104]

PAMAM, poly(amido amine); *ABP*, azabisphosphonate; *G*, generation; *MTD*, maximum tolerated dose; *PPI*, polypropylenimine; *RGD*, arginine-glycine-aspartic acid; *PEG*, poly(ethylene glycol); *PLL*, poly-l-lysine; *PETIM*, poly(propyl ether imine); *DG*, dendrimers glucosamine; *HA*, hemagglutinin; *RIF*, rifampicin; *HIV*, human immunodeficiency virus; *HSV*, herpes simplex virus; *siRNA*, short interfering ribonucleic acid, *CT*, computed tomography; *SPECT*, single-photon emission computed tomography; *Mr*, magnetic resonance; *MRI*, magnetic resonance imaging; *LyP-1*, cyclic 9-amino acid peptide; *PET*, tetracarboxy amide; *CEST*, chemical exchange saturation transfer. positron emission tomography; *DOTAM*, 2,2′,2,″2‴-(1,4,7,10-tetraazacyclododecane-1,4,7,10-tetrayl) tetraacetic acid.

10.7.2 Gene delivery

To exterminate genetic morbidities, gene delivery is functioning as a novel platform. This new technology for the DNA transfection works by expressing aimed protein or antisense oligonucleotide to deactivate or silence the targeted gene with siRNA, which is responsible for pairing and subsequent cleavage of corresponding mRNA. Hence, the selection of the appropriate gene delivery vector (viral or nonviral) plays a significant role in gene delivery [106]. For gene delivery, viruses are the primary and most favored vector. Along with this, the viral vector has some disadvantages like scarce specificity, poor transfection rate, being prone to various enzymatic ruin, for example, nuclease, poor cellular intake, high toxicity (naked siRNA), and low stability, which limit the use of viruses in gene therapy. In addition to this, negative charge and strong hydrophilic nature prevent it from crossing the cell membrane easily. As a result, the use of a viral vector was hampered [107]. Hence, nonviral vectors are getting more attention because of their low cytotoxicity, high immunogenicity, and high compaction capacity. Nonviral vectors like cationic polymers, lipids, liposomes, exosomes, peptide, proteins, and so forth can be a better replacement for viral vectors because of their properties like flexibility, safety, facile synthesis, and easy modification with ligand [108]. The negatively charged genetic material can be complexed with a positively charged carrier, and so, endocytosis can be improved [109]. Cationic-amine terminated dendrimer (PAMAM and PPI) can be complexed with nucleic acid through electrostatic interactions, which lead to the generation of a stable compact complex called dendriplexes. The transfection efficiency is usually calculated by the amine-phosphate ratio. The excess amine groups on dendriplexes are responsible for promoting cellular interactions, which may lead to severe toxicity and low transfection efficiency. Thus, it is essential to optimize every parameter of the complex. PAMAM dendrimer was firstly proposed by Haenslernad Szoka in 1993 as a nonviral dendrimer carrier. PAMAM [110], PPI [111], triazine, viologen dendrimer [112], carbosilane [113], phosphorous dendrimer [114], and PLL dendrimer [115] are utilized as the nonviral dendritic nanocarriers [108]. Different research groups have worked on different dendrimers, as specified in Table 10.3.

10.7.3 Surface-engineered dendrimer

Normal cell toxicity, retroendothelial system, immunogenicity, drug stability, drug hydrophobicity, leakage of drug, and so forth are some of the major limitations faced during the dendritic formulation. The nanosized cationic nature of the dendrimer is also responsible for the interaction with the cell membrane and cell organelles, proteins, enzymes, and so forth [19]. The commonly used dendrimers like PAMAM, PPI, and PLL all induce significant cytotoxicity because of cationic charge rendering on their edge. To circumvent these stumbling blocks, surface modification of dendrimers needs to be performed in order to reduce free terminal cationic groups. For handling this issue, neutral and anionic molecules are used, which prevent interaction with the cell membrane. This surface modification technique enables improved solubility and enhanced drug encapsulation efficiency with improved pharmacokinetic and bio-distribution profile. In addition, the site-specific activity assists in better transfection efficiency and stability enhancement [27]. Several research groups have developed novel surface-modified strategies for circumventing the toxicity-associated or generation-based hurdles, as shown in Table 10.4. Some of the surface-modified strategies are as follows:

1. Lipid-modified dendrimer
2. Fluorinated dendrimer
3. Amino acid-modified dendrimer
4. Saccharide-modified dendrimer
5. Protein- and peptide-modified dendrimer
6. Polymer-modified dendrimer
7. Nanoparticle-modified dendrimer
8. Cationic moiety-modified dendrimer
9. Ligand-modified dendrimer (photosensitizer, fluorophore, hormone, folic acid, and aminoglycoside-modified dendrimer) [108].

TABLE 10.3 Summary table of dendrimer-mediated gene delivery.

S. No.	Type of dendrimer	Generation	Ligand	Result	References
1	PAMAM	1	EpDT3 aptamer	Enhanced endocytosis by EpDt3 aptamer. In-vivo studies depict a significant anticancer activity of PAMAM-PEG-EpDT3/ pMEG3 NPs against castration-resistant prostate cancer.	[116]
		2	Hyaluronic acid	HA lowers cytotoxicity of the polymer and increases GTE. DNA delivery capacity of PAMAM G4 3850%−5% and PAMAM G5%−5% improved.	[117]
		3	4,4′-Dithio-dibutryic acid and pDNA	The prepared NCs/pDNA polyplexes have higher GTE than single G3 and G5 PAMAM.	[118]
		5	Cholesteryl chloroformate, alkyl-PEG and DOX.	Better antitumor effect than individual gene and drug delivery for colon cancer cell line C26.	[119]
		6	Histidine and Arginine and pDNA	G2-HAR dendrimers have high GTE than G2 and G3 and less cytotoxicity than G6. used for gene delivery in ID.	[120]
2	PPI	5	siRNA, DTBP PEGylation and LHRH	The dendrimer is stable in serum for 48 h and against nuclease. Enhanced cell specific delivery	[121]
		3	Transferrin and pDNA	In vitro studies of dendriplexes exhibit higher cellular uptake in murine brain endothelioma. In vivo administration of dendriplexes exhibits threefold higher gene expression in the brain.	[44]

DTBP, Dimethyl-3–3′-dithiobispropionimidate; *LHRH*, luteinizing hormone releasing hormone; *pDNA*, plasmid DNA; *DOX*: doxorubicin; *PEG*, polyethylene glycol; *GTE*, gene transfection efficiency; *HAR*, Histidine-Arginine, *CRPC*, castration-resistant prostate cancer; *ID*, inflammatory disorder.

10.8 Diagnostic applications

Molecular imaging has been widely explored, and there has been remarkable progress in nanomedicine. It allows for real-time visualization of the cellular function of an organism and also its molecular interactions. Modern imaging technology has been evolved for the diagnosis and recognition of disease. This technique includes (1) fluorescence imaging, computed tomography (CT scan), MRI, positron emission tomography, and single photon emission tomography. To meet the challenges required for precise diagnosis of morbidity and for improved specificity, various contrast agents were prepared in the laboratory [128]. The ability of the dendritic surface to attach various groups like solubility enhancer, cell-specific targeting moieties, highly branched structure, and 3D architecture makes dendrimers a peculiar carrier

TABLE 10.4 Summary of surface-engineered dendrimers in gene and drug delivery.

Tech	Conjugated molecule	Results	References
PEGylated dendrimer	PEG	Improved drug loading, decreased hemolytic toxicity of the PAMAM dendrimer.	[122]
FA-conjugated dendrimer	FA-PEG	Folic acid–PEG-PAMAM has low hemolytic toxicity compared to PEG-PAMAM and the PAMAM dendrimer.	[123]
Antibody-conjugated Dendrimer	Anti-HER2-mAb	Low systemic toxicity and rapid internalization.	[124]
Lipid-conjugated PAA dendrimer	Lauric acid, myristic acid, palmitic acid	Increased gene transfection efficiency on stem cells. Increase cellular uptake of DNA as increase chain length. (Lauric acid <myristic acid < palmitic acid)	[125]
Fluorinated dendrimer	PAMAM-fluorinated dendrimer	Heptafluorobutyric acid-modified G-5 PAMAM dendrimers (G5-F768) show highest TE (>90%) as compared to the lipofectamine. Fluorination of PPI dendrimer also enhances transfection efficiency.	[126]
Peptide-conjugated dendrimer	Arg-Gly-Asp, LHRH (QHWSYKCLRP)	Minimization of cytotoxicity as a result of tripeptide PAMAM dendrimer.	[127]
Drug and drug-antibody conjugated dendrimer	Flurbiprofen	Less hemolytic cytotoxicity compared to the PAMAM dendrimer.	[121]

FA, folic acid; *Dox*, doxorubicin; *Arg-Gly-As*, arginine-glycine-aspartate; *PPI*, poly(propylimine); *LHRH*, luteinizing hormone releasing hormone; *PEG*, polyethylene glycol; *PAMAM*, poly(amidoamine); *PAA*, polyacrylic acid; *HER*, human epidermal growth factor receptor.

for contrasting agents compared to other nanomedicines. The bioactive agents can be encapsulated, adsorbed, or chemically conjugated on the dendritic surface to provide diagnostic or therapeutic applications. As per the literature, first in vivo applications of diagnostic agents with the dendrimer were revealed by Weiner and his colleagues in 1996. The authors developed an ion-chelate complex of the PAMAM derivative. The study demonstrates an increase in rotational correlation time of the ion-chelate complex with the increased molecular weight. Also, it suggested that a low molecular weight derivative cascade polymer with a rigid side chain could be a potential MRI contrasting agent [129].

Weiner et al. have also demonstrated a PAMAM-complexed diagnostic agent using gadolinium as a complexing agent. A dendrimer-based reagent exhibits blood pool properties and excellent relaxivity values when gadolinium is complexed with the PAMAM surface, compared with small diagnostic agents such as Magnevist, Schering, and AG [129]. Paramagnetic metal chelates such as Gd (III)-DOTA, Gd (III)-DTPA, and their derivatives are utilized as a diagnostic agent due to an increase in the relaxation rate of the surrounding water protons. Gadolinium is an FDA-approved diagnostic agent used in MRI, which has a greater contrast between normal and abnormal tissue in the body. It is safer than iodine and rapidly cleared by the kidney [130].

A series of Gd (III)DTPA-functionalized PPI dendrimer was reported by Kobayashi et al.; the authors demonstrated that r_1 almost linearly increased with the molecular weight of the dendrimer without reaching a plateau value, eventually resulting in an r_1 value of 29 mM/s for the fifth generation of dendritic contrast agent [131]. To further improve the Gd (III)-labeling efficiency for enhanced MRI applications, Cheng et al. developed a new platform of dendrimer nanoclusters (DNCs) via crosslinking of G5 PAMAM dendrimer with a bifunctional amine-reactive cross-linker. The formed DNCs can be linked with DTPA for Gd (III) chelating, targeting ligand FA, and the FI dye for in vitro and in vivo targeted optical and MRI of cancer cells overexpressing the folic acid receptors [132]. However, properties like low molecular weight, rapid renal clearance, and sometimes gadolinium ion release from Gd chelate (which cause inhibition of the calcium channel and nephrogenic and skin fibrosis) limit the use of this agents. Currently, scientists are focusing on high molecular weight macromolecules of gadolinium. Still, release of GD ions is a critical concern. To solve this, the nanoparticle of Gd is prepared with inorganic agents, which exhibits higher reflexivity and excellent Gd 3 + ion-retaining ability. Gd_2O_3-incorporated mesoporous silica NP(Gd_2O_3-SBA-15a) and bovine serum albumin (Gd_2O_3-BSA with AuNPs) have been shown to be efficient contrasting agents in MRI [133]. Recently, Fan et al. reported hypoxia due to targeted delivery of PAMAM G5 dendrimer (Gd-Au DENPs-Nit)-entrapped gold nanoparticles. The prepared nanohybrid with a 3.2 nm diameter core exhibits excellent X-ray attenuation ($r_1$relaxivity of 1.32 mM/S) along with good cellular uptake in the cancer cell, exhibiting dual activity [134]. To overcome the small molecular weight shortcoming of iodine, dendrimers have been exploited by covalently linking with small iodine on the surface of dendrimers [135].

In 2006, Fu et al. developed modified dendrimers by using t-Boc lysine (G3-G5) as an amplifier and PEG (3–12 kDa) as a core. The study resulted in an array containing multiple free amino terminal groups being conjugated to stable and highly soluble triiodopthalamide. Among different modifications, PEG (12 kDa) exhibits a strong and persistent intravascular enhancement with prolonged blood half-life (approx. 35 minutes), analyzed by dynamic CT imaging [136]. In another study, Guo et al. first synthesized the gold-DNEP NPs using G5 amine terminated dendrimers as a template. Further, this template complexed with an iodine-based CT contrast agent di-trizoic acid (DTA). The result demonstrated that the NPs were able to complex 59 DTA molecules per particle and exhibited a significantly enhanced X-ray attenuation property in comparison to a single element-based contrast agent [137].

10.9 Conclusion

In this chapter, we briefly reviewed the history of dendrimers, generations of dendrimers, and their characteristic features. Dendrimers have been widely utilized as a potential nanovehicle in distinct forms, for example, antibody-conjugated dendrimer, dendrimer-drug conjugates, dendrimer-gene complexes, and many more. The chapter summarizes epitome of dendrimers being utilized in the diagnosis, treatment, and management of different diseases/disorders. The challenges of the dendritic approach are due to the several reasons, among which inherently associated toxicity, generation-dependent obstacles, expensive nature, drug leakage, and regulatory challenges are major challenges being faced. As per the findings of distinct research groups, the challenges of dendrimers are cross-linked to one another. The cationic nature of dendrimers potentiates their inherent toxicity, which increases with the increase in generation size. It results in different types of toxicities such as hemolytic toxicity, cytotoxicity, and hematological toxicity. Thus, there is an unmet need to devise new strategies to overcome these challenges. In recent studies, the surface modifications have been an asset in overcoming the toxic effects of dendrimers. Being a potent nanocarrier, the surface-engineered dendrimers exhibited a remarkable impact in site-specific targeting, enhanced therapeutic efficacy, enhanced biocompatibility, and reduced side effects. Thus, the recent advancements may lead to the generation of new dendrimer-associated therapeutics that may enable the development of novel therapeutics.

References

[1] Tomalia DA, Baker H, Dewald J, Hall M, Kallos G, Martin S, et al. A new class of polymers: starburst-dendritic macromolecules. Polym J 1985;17(1):117–32. Available from: https://doi.org/10.1295/polymj.17.117.

[2] Newkome GR, Yao ZQ, Baker GR, Gupta VK. Cascade molecules: a new approach to micelles. 1aA [27]-arborol. J Org Chem 1985;50(11):2003–4. Available from: https://doi.org/10.1021/JO00211A052/SUPPL_FILE/JO00211A052_SI_001.PDF.

[3] Buhleier E, Wehner W, Voegtle F. 'Cascade'- and 'nonskid-chain-like' syntheses of molecular cavity topologies. Chem Inform 1978;9(25). Available from: https://doi.org/10.1002/CHIN.197825228.

[4] Yang H, Kao WJ. Dendrimers for pharmaceutical and biomedical applications. Biomater Sci 2012;17(1):3–19. Available from: https://doi.org/10.1163/156856206774879171.

[5] Tomalia DA, Naylor AM, Goddard WA. Starburst dendrimers: molecular-level control of size, shape, surface chemistry, topology, and flexibility from atoms to macroscopic. Matter Angew Chem Int Ed Engl 1990;29(2):138–75. Available from: https://doi.org/10.1002/ANIE.199001381.

[6] Flory PJ. Principles of Polymer Chemistry. 1st Ed. London, U.S.A: Cornell University Press; 1953. Available from: https://doi.org/10.1126/science.119.3095.555.b.

[7] Klajnert B, Bryszewska M. Dendrimers: properties and applications. Acta Biochim Pol 2001;48(1):199–208. Available from: https://doi.org/10.18388/abp.2001_5127.

[8] Madaan K, Kumar S, Poonia N, Lather V, Pandita D. Dendrimers in drug delivery and targeting: drug-dendrimer interactions and toxicity issues. J Pharm Bioallied Sci 2014;6(3):139–50. Available from: https://doi.org/10.4103/0975-7406.130965.

[9] Fréchet JMJ. Functional polymers and dendrimers: reactivity, molecular architecture, and interfacial energy. Science 1994;263(5154):1710–15. Available from: https://doi.org/10.1126/SCIENCE.8134834.

[10] Duncan R. Polymer conjugates as anticancer nanomedicines. Nat Rev Cancer 2006;6(9):688–701. Available from: https://doi.org/10.1038/nrc1958.

[11] Denkewalter R., Kolc J., Lukasavage,W. Macromolecular highly branched homogeneous compound based on lysine units, April 6, 1979.

[12] Launay N, Caminade AM, Majoral JP. Synthesis and reactivity of unusual phosphorus dendrimers. A useful divergent growth approach up to the seventh generation. J Am Chem Soc 1995;117(11):3282–3. Available from: https://doi.org/10.1021/JA00116A037/SUPPL_FILE/JA3282.PDF.

[13] Ihre H, Padilla De Jesús OL, Fréchet JMJ. Fast and convenient divergent synthesis of aliphatic ester dendrimers by anhydride coupling. J Am Chem Soc 2001;123(25):5908–17. Available from: https://doi.org/10.1021/JA010524E.

[14] Schlenk C, Frey H. Carbosilane dendrimers- synthesis, functionalization, application. Silicon Chemistry. Vienna: Springer; 1999. p. 3–14. Available from: https://doi.org/10.1007/978-3-7091-6357-3_1.

[15] Klajnert B, Janiszewska J, Urbanczyk-Lipkowska Z, Bryszewska M, Shcharbin D, Labieniec M. Biological properties of low molecular mass peptide dendrimers. Int J Pharm 2006;309(1–2):208–17. Available from: https://doi.org/10.1016/J.IJPHARM.2005.10.039.

[16] Janaszewska A, Lazniewska J, Trzepí Nski P, Marcinkowska M, Klajnert-Maculewicz B. Cytotoxicity of dendrimers. Biomolecules 2019;9(8):330. Available from: https://doi.org/10.3390/BIOM9080330.

[17] Abbasi E, Aval SF, Akbarzadeh A, Milani M, Nasrabadi HT, Joo SW, et al. Dendrimers: synthesis, applications, and properties. Nanoscale Res Lett 2014;9(1):1–10. Available from: https://doi.org/10.1186/1556-276X-9-247/FIGURES/8.

[18] Tomalia DA, Hedstrand DM, Ferritto MS. Comb-burst dendrimer topology: new macromolecular architecture derived from dendritic grafting. Macromolecules 2002;. Available from: https://doi.org/10.1021/MA00006A039.

[19] Kesharwani P, Jain K, Jain NK. Dendrimer as nanocarrier for drug delivery. Prog Polym Sci 2014;39 (2):268–307. Available from: https://doi.org/10.1016/J.PROGPOLYMSCI.2013.07.005.

[20] Percec V, Cho WD, Mosier PE, Ungar G, Yeardley DJP. Structural analysis of cylindrical and spherical supramolecular dendrimers quantifies the concept of monodendron shape control by generation number. J Am Chem Soc 1998;120(43):11061–70. Available from: https://doi.org/10.1021/JA9819007.

[21] Maiti PK, Çağin T, Wang G, Goddard WA. Structure of PAMAM dendrimers: generations 1 through 11. Macromolecules 2004;37(16):6236–54. Available from: https://doi.org/10.1021/MA035629B/SUPPL_FILE/MA035629BSI20040618_125851.

[22] Hawker CJ, Farrington PJ, Mackay ME, Wooley KL, Fréchet JMJ. Molecular ball bearings: the unusual melt viscosity behavior of dendritic macromolecules. J Am Chem Soc 1995;117(15):4409–10. Available from: https://doi.org/10.1021/JA00120A028/ASSET/JA00120A028.FP.PNG_V03.

[23] Hong S, Bielinska AU, Mecke A, Keszler B, Beals JL, Shi X, et al. Interaction of poly(amidoamine) dendrimers with supported lipid bilayers and cells: hole formation and the relation to transport. Bioconjug Chem 2004;15(4):774–82. Available from: https://doi.org/10.1021/BC049962B.

[24] Hong S, Leroueil PR, Majoros IJ, Orr BG, Baker JR, Banaszak Holl MM. The binding avidity of a nanoparticle-based multivalent targeted drug delivery platform. Chem Biol 2007;14(1):107–15. Available from: https://doi.org/10.1016/J.CHEMBIOL.2006.11.015.

[25] Malik N, Wiwattanapatapee R, Klopsch R, Lorenz K, Frey H, Weener JW, et al. Dendrimers: relationship between structure and biocompatibility in vitro, and preliminary studies on the biodistribution of 125I-labelled polyamidoamine dendrimers in vivo. J Control Rel 2000;65(1–2):133–48. Available from: https://doi.org/10.1016/S0168-3659(99)00246-1.

[26] Astruc D, Boisselier E, Ornelas C. Dendrimers designed for functions: from physical, photophysical, and supramolecular properties to applications in sensing, catalysis, molecular electronics, photonics, and nanomedicine. Chem Rev 2010;110(4):1857–959. Available from: https://doi.org/10.1021/CR900327D/SUPPL_FILE/CR900327D_SI_001.PDF.

[27] Santos A, Veiga F, Figueiras A. Dendrimers as pharmaceutical excipients: synthesis, properties, toxicity and biomedical applications. Materials. 2019;13(1):65. Available from: https://doi.org/10.3390/MA13010065.

[28] Geng Z, Shin JJ, Xi Y, Hawker CJ. Click chemistry strategies for the accelerated synthesis of functional macromolecules. J Polym Sci 2021;59(11):963–1042. Available from: https://doi.org/10.1002/POL.20210126.

[29] Svenson S, Tomalia DA. Dendrimers in biomedical applications-reflections on the field. Adv Drug Deliv Rev 2005;57(15):2106–29. Available from: https://doi.org/10.1016/J.ADDR.2005.09.018.

[30] Patel V, Rajani C, Paul D, Borisa P, Rajpoot K, Youngren-Ortiz SR, et al. Dendrimers as novel drug-delivery system and its applications. Drug Delivery Systems. U.S.A: Academic Press Ed., Elsevier; 2020. p. 333–92.

[31] Nanjwade BK, Bechra HM, Derkar GK, Manvi FV, Nanjwade VK. Dendrimers: emerging polymers for drug-delivery systems. Eur J Pharm Sci 2009;38(3):185–96. Available from: https://doi.org/10.1016/J.EJPS.2009.07.008.

[32] Sherje AP, Jadhav M, Dravyakar BR, Kadam D. Dendrimers: a versatile nanocarrier for drug delivery and targeting. Int J Pharm 2018;548(1):707–20. Available from: https://doi.org/10.1016/J.IJPHARM.2018.07.030.

[33] Bugno J, Hsu HJ, Hong S. Tweaking dendrimers and dendritic nanoparticles for controlled nano-bio interactions: potential nanocarriers for improved cancer targeting. J Drug Target 2015;23(7–8):642–50. Available from: https://doi.org/10.3109/1061186X.2015.1052077.

[34] Luong D, Kesharwani P, Deshmukh R, Mohd Amin MCI, Gupta U, Greish K, et al. PEGylated PAMAM dendrimers: enhancing efficacy and mitigating toxicity for effective anticancer drug and gene delivery. Acta Biomater 2016;43:14–29. Available from: https://doi.org/10.1016/J.ACTBIO.2016.07.015.

[35] Pilkington GA, Pedersen JS, Briscoe WH. Dendrimer nanofluids in the concentrated regime: from polymer melts to soft spheres. Langmuir 2015;31(11):3333–42. Available from: https://doi.org/10.1021/LA504870F/ASSET/IMAGES/MEDIUM/LA-2014-04870F_0010.GIF.

[36] Haensler J, Szoka FC. Polyamidoamine cascade polymers mediate efficient transfection of cells in culture. Bioconjug Chem 1993;4(5):372–9. Available from: https://doi.org/10.1021/BC00023A012/ASSET/BC00023A012.FP.PNG_V03.
[37] Sadekar S, Ghandehari H. Transepithelial transport and toxicity of PAMAM dendrimers: implications for oral drug delivery. Adv Drug Deliv Rev 2012;64(6):571–88. Available from: https://doi.org/10.1016/J.ADDR.2011.09.010.
[38] Li D, Fan Y, Shen M, Bányai I, Shi X. Design of dual drug-loaded dendrimer/carbon dot nanohybrids for fluorescence imaging and enhanced chemotherapy of cancer cells. J Mater Chem B 2019;7(2):277–85. Available from: https://doi.org/10.1039/C8TB02723D.
[39] Longmire M, Choyke P, Kobayashi H. Dendrimer-based contrast agents for molecular imaging. Curr Top Med Chem 2008;8(14):1180–6. Available from: https://doi.org/10.2174/156802608785849021.
[40] Boas U, Christensen JB, Heegaard PMH. Dendrimers: design, synthesis and chemical properties. J Mater Chem 2006;16(38):3785–98. Available from: https://doi.org/10.1039/B611813P.
[41] Shao N, Su Y, Hu J, Zhang J, Zhang H, Cheng Y. Comparison of generation 3 polyamidoamine dendrimer and generation 4 polypropylenimine dendrimer on drug loading, complex structure, release behavior, and cytotoxicity. Int J Nanomed 2011;6:3361–72. Available from: https://doi.org/10.2147/IJN.S27028.
[42] Kesharwani P, Tekade RK, Gajbhiye V, Jain K, Jain NK. Cancer targeting potential of some ligand-anchored poly(propylene imine) dendrimers: a comparison. Nanomed Nanotechnol Biol Med 2011;7(3):295–304. Available from: https://doi.org/10.1016/J.NANO.2010.10.010.
[43] Sideratou Z, Kontoyianni C, Drossopoulou GI, Paleos CM. Synthesis of a folate functionalized PEGylated poly(propylene imine) dendrimer as prospective targeted drug delivery system. Bioorg Med Chem Lett 2010;20(22):6513–17. Available from: https://doi.org/10.1016/J.BMCL.2010.09.058.
[44] Somani S, Blatchford DR, Millington O, Stevenson ML, Dufès C. Transferrin-bearing polypropylenimine dendrimer for targeted gene delivery to the brain. J Control Rel 2014;188:78–86. Available from: https://doi.org/10.1016/J.JCONREL.2014.06.006.
[45] Roy R, Baek MG. Glycodendrimers: novel glycotope isosteres unmasking sugar coding. Case study with T-antigen markers from breast cancer MUC1 glycoprotein. Rev Mol Biotechnol 2002;90(3–4):291–309. Available from: https://doi.org/10.1016/S1389-0352(01)00065-4.
[46] Percec V, Chu P, Ungar G, Zhou J. Rational design of the first nonspherical dendrimer which displays calamitic nematic and smectic thermotropic liquid crystalline phases. J Am Chem Soc 1995;117(46):11441–54. Available from: https://doi.org/10.1021/JA00151A008/SUPPL_FILE/JA11441.PDF.
[47] Quintana S, García MÁ, Marina ML, Gómez R, de la Mata FJ, Ortega P. Synthesis of chiral carbosilane dendrimers with L-cysteine and N-acetyl-l-cysteine on their surface and their application as chiral selectors for enantiomer separation by capillary electrophoresis. Tetrahedron: Asymmet. 2017;28(12):1797–802. Available from: https://doi.org/10.1016/J.TETASY.2017.10.028.
[48] McElhanon JR, McGrath DV. Constitution, configuration, and the optical activity of chiral dendrimers. J Am Chem Soc 1998;120(8):1647–56. Available from: https://doi.org/10.1021/JA970150I.
[49] Manikkath J, Hegde AR, Kalthur G, Parekh HS, Mutalik S. Influence of peptide dendrimers and sonophoresis on the transdermal delivery of ketoprofen. Int J Pharm 2017;521(1–2):110–19. Available from: https://doi.org/10.1016/J.IJPHARM.2017.02.002.
[50] Sadler K, Tam JP. Peptide dendrimers: applications and synthesis. Rev Mol Biotechnol 2002;90(3–4):195–229. Available from: https://doi.org/10.1016/S1389-0352(01)00061-7.
[51] Luo K, Li C, Li L, She W, Wang G, Gu Z. Arginine functionalized peptide dendrimers as potential gene delivery vehicles. Biomaterials 2012;33(19):4917–27. Available from: https://doi.org/10.1016/J.BIOMATERIALS.2012.03.030.
[52] Dvornic PR. PAMAMOS: The first commercial silicon-containing dendrimers and their applications. J Polym Sci, Part A-1 Polym Chem 2006;44(9):2755–73. Available from: https://doi.org/10.1002/POLA.21368.
[53] Mehta D, Leong N, McLeod VM, Kelly BD, Pathak R, Owen DJ, et al. Reducing dendrimer generation and PEG chain length increases drug release and promotes anticancer activity of PEGylated polylysine dendrimers conjugated with doxorubicin via a cathepsin-cleavable peptide linker. Mol Pharm 2018;15(10):4568–76. Available from: https://doi.org/10.1021/ACS.MOLPHARMACEUT.8B00581/SUPPL_FILE/MP8B00581_SI_001.PDF.
[54] Vembu S, Pazhamalai S, Gopalakrishnan M. Potential antibacterial activity of triazine dendrimer: synthesis and controllable drug release properties. Bioorg Med Chem 2015;23(15):4561–6. Available from: https://doi.org/10.1016/J.BMC.2015.06.009.

[55] Zhao M, Meng L, Ma L, Wu G, Xie F, Ma L, et al. Stepwise growth of melamine-based dendrimers onto carbon fibers and the effects on interfacial properties of epoxy composites. Compos Sci Technol 2017;138:144–50. Available from: https://doi.org/10.1016/J.COMPSCITECH.2016.11.013.
[56] Mecke A, Majoros IJ, Patri AK, Baker J, Banaszak Holl M, Orr B. Lipid bilayer disruption by polycationic polymers: the roles of size and chemical functional group. Langmuir 2005;21(23):10348–54. Available from: https://doi.org/10.1021/LA050629L.
[57] Jain K, Kesharwani P, Gupta U, Jain NK. Dendrimer toxicity: let's meet the challenge. Int J Pharm 2010;394 (1–2):122–42. Available from: https://doi.org/10.1016/J.IJPHARM.2010.04.027.
[58] Kesharwani P, Mishra V, Jain NK. Generation dependent hemolytic profile of folate engineered poly(propyleneimine) dendrimer. J Drug Deliv Sci Technol 2015;28:1–6. Available from: https://doi.org/10.1016/J.JDDST.2015.04.006.
[59] Hashemi M, Tabatabai SM, Parhiz H, Milanizadeh S, Amel Farzad S, Abnous K, et al. Gene delivery efficiency and cytotoxicity of heterocyclic amine-modified PAMAM and PPI dendrimers. Mater Sci Eng C 2016;61:791–800. Available from: https://doi.org/10.1016/J.MSEC.2016.01.023.
[60] Stasko NA, Johnson CB, Schoenfisch MH, Johnson TA, Holmuhamedov EL. Cytotoxicity of polypropylenimine dendrimer conjugates on cultured endothelial cells. Biomacromolecules 2007;8(12):3853–9. Available from: https://doi.org/10.1021/bm7008203.
[61] Agashe HB, Dutta T, Garg M, Jain NK. Investigations on the toxicological profile of functionalized fifth-generation poly(propylene imine) dendrimer. J Pharm Pharmacol 2010;58(11):1491–8. Available from: https://doi.org/10.1211/JPP.58.11.0010.
[62] Naha PC, Davoren M, Lyng FM, Byrne HJ. Reactive oxygen species (ROS) induced cytokine production and cytotoxicity of PAMAM dendrimers in J774A.1 cells. Toxicol Appl Pharmacol 2010;246(1–2):91–9. Available from: https://doi.org/10.1016/J.TAAP.2010.04.014.
[63] Kolhatkar RB, Kitchens KM, Swaan PW, Ghandehari H. Surface acetylation of polyamidoamine (PAMAM) dendrimers decreases cytotoxicity while maintaining membrane permeability. Bioconjug Chem 2007;18 (6):2054–60. Available from: https://doi.org/10.1021/BC0603889.
[64] Bhadra D, Bhadra S, Jain S, Jain NK. A PEGylated dendritic nanoparticulate carrier of fluorouracil. Int J Pharm 2003;257(1–2):111–24. Available from: https://doi.org/10.1016/S0378-5173(03)00132-7.
[65] Schilrreff P, Mundiña-Weilenmann C, Romero E, Morilla M. Selective cytotoxicity of PAMAM G5 core–PAMAM G2. 5 Shell tecto-dendrimers on melanoma cells. Int J Nanomed 2012;7:4121–33. Available from: https://doi.org/10.2147/IJN.S32785.
[66] Diaz C, Benitez C, Vidal F, Barraza LF, Jiménez VA, Guzman L, et al. Cytotoxicity and in vivo plasma kinetic behavior of surface-functionalized PAMAM dendrimers. Nanomed Nanotechnol Biol Med 2018;14 (7):2227–34. Available from: https://doi.org/10.1016/J.NANO.2018.07.005.
[67] Pryor JB, Harper BJ, Harper SL. Comparative toxicological assessment of PAMAM and thiophosphoryl dendrimers using embryonic zebrafish. Int J Nanomed 2014;9(1):1947–56. Available from: https://doi.org/10.2147/IJN.S60220.
[68] Jones CF, Campbell RA, Brooks AE, Assemi S, Tadjiki S, Thiagarajan G, et al. Cationic PAMAM dendrimers aggressively initiate blood clot formation. ACS Nano 2012;6(11):9900–10. Available from: https://doi.org/10.1021/NN303472R/SUPPL_FILE/NN303472R_SI_007.MP4.
[69] Rether A, Schuster M. Selective separation and recovery of heavy metal ions using water-soluble N-benzoylthiourea modified PAMAM polymers. React Funct Polym 2003;57(1):13–21. Available from: https://doi.org/10.1016/J.REACTFUNCTPOLYM.2003.06.002.
[70] Balieu S, Zein AE, De Sousa R, Jérôme F, Tatibouët A, et al. One-step surface decoration of poly(propyleneimines) (PPIs) with the glyceryl moiety: new way for recycling homogeneous dendrimer-based catalysts. Adv Synth Catal 2010;352(11–12):1826–33. Available from: https://doi.org/10.1002/ADSC.201000229.
[71] Desai PP, Date AA, Patravale VB. Overcoming poor oral bioavailability using nanoparticle formulations – opportunities and limitations. Drug Discov Today Technol 2012;9(2):e87–95. Available from: https://doi.org/10.1016/J.DDTEC.2011.12.001.
[72] Kharwade R, More S, Warokar A, Agrawal P, Mahajan N. Starburst pamam dendrimers: synthetic approaches, surface modifications, and biomedical applications. Arab J Chem 2020;13(7):6009–39. Available from: https://doi.org/10.1016/J.ARABJC.2020.05.002.

[73] Pollak KW, Leon JW, Fréchet JMJ, Maskus M, Abruña HD. Effects of dendrimer generation on site isolation of core moieties: electrochemical and fluorescence quenching studies with metalloporphyrin core dendrimers. Chem Mater 1998;10(1):30–8. Available from: https://doi.org/10.1021/cm970312+.
[74] Devarakonda B, Hill RA, De Villiers MM. The effect of PAMAM dendrimer generation size and surface functional group on the aqueous solubility of nifedipine. Int J Pharm 2004;284(1–2):133–40. Available from: https://doi.org/10.1016/J.IJPHARM.2004.07.006.
[75] Kojima C, Regino C, Umeda Y, Kobayashi H, Kono K. Influence of dendrimer generation and polyethylene glycol length on the biodistribution of PEGylated dendrimers. Int J Pharm 2010;383(1–2):293–6. Available from: https://doi.org/10.1016/J.IJPHARM.2009.09.015.
[76] Kesharwani P, Tekade RK, Jain NK. Generation dependent cancer targeting potential of poly(propyleneimine) dendrimer. Biomaterials 2014;35(21):5539–48. Available from: https://doi.org/10.1016/J.BIOMATERIALS.2014.03.064.
[77] Liu S, Chang CH, Paul BK, Remcho VT. Convergent synthesis of polyamide dendrimer using a continuous flow microreactor. Chem Eng J 2008;135(SUPPL. 1):S333–7. Available from: https://doi.org/10.1016/J.CEJ.2007.07.022.
[78] Ya-Ting Huang A, Kao CL, Selvaraj A, Peng L. Solid-phase dendrimer synthesis: a promising approach to transform dendrimer construction. Mater Today Chem 2023;27:101285. Available from: https://doi.org/10.1016/J.MTCHEM.2022.101285.
[79] Parimi S, Barnes TJ, Prestidge CA. PAMAM dendrimer interactions with supported lipid bilayers: a kinetic and mechanistic investigation. Langmuir 2008;24(23):13532–9. Available from: https://doi.org/10.1021/LA8022858/ASSET/IMAGES/MEDIUM/LA-2008-022858_0008.GIF.
[80] Kesharwani P, Tekade RK, Jain NK. Formulation development and in vitro–in vivo assessment of the fourth-generation PPI dendrimer as a cancer-targeting vector. Futur Med 2014;9(15):2291–308. Available from: https://doi.org/10.2217/NNM.13.210.
[81] Bhadra D, Yadav AK, Bhadra S, Jain NK. Glycodendrimeric nanoparticulate carriers of primaquine phosphate for liver targeting. Int J Pharm 2005;295(1–2):221–33. Available from: https://doi.org/10.1016/J.IJPHARM.2005.01.026.
[82] Chauhan A, Patil C, Jain P, Kulhari H. Dendrimer-based marketed formulations and miscellaneous applications in cosmetics, veterinary, and agriculture. Pharmaceutical Applications of Dendrimers Elsevier 2020;325–34. Available from: https://doi.org/10.1016/B978-0-12-814527-2.00014-7.
[83] Kannan RM, Nance E, Kannan S, Tomalia DA. Emerging concepts in dendrimer-based nanomedicine: from design principles to clinical applications. J Intern Med 2014;276(6):579–617. Available from: https://doi.org/10.1111/JOIM.12280.
[84] Thomas TP, Goonewardena SN, Majoros IJ, Kotlyar A, Cao Z, Leroueil PR, et al. Folate-targeted nanoparticles show efficacy in the treatment of inflammatory arthritis. Arthritis Rheum 2011;63(9):2671–80. Available from: https://doi.org/10.1002/ART.30459.
[85] Gérard HC, Mishra MK, Mao G, Wang S, Hali M, Whittum-Hudson JA, et al. Dendrimer-enabled DNA delivery and transformation of chlamydia pneumoniae. Nanomed Nanotechnol Biol Med 2013;9(7):996–1008. Available from: https://doi.org/10.1016/J.NANO.2013.04.004.
[86] Hayder M, Poupot M, Baron M, Nigon D, Turrin CO, Caminade AM, et al. A Phosphorus-based dendrimer targets inflammation and osteoclastogenesis in experimental arthritis. Sci Transl Med 2011;3(81). Available from: https://doi.org/10.1126/SCITRANSLMED.3002212/SUPPL_FILE/3-81RA35_SM.PDF.
[87] Inapagolla R, Guru BR, Kurtoglu YE, Gao X, Lieh-Lai M, Bassett DJP, et al. In vivo efficacy of dendrimer–methylprednisolone conjugate formulation for the treatment of lung inflammation. Int J Pharm 2010;399(1–2):140–7. Available from: https://doi.org/10.1016/J.IJPHARM.2010.07.030.
[88] Blattes E, Vercellone A, Eutamène H, Turrin CO, Théodorou V, Majoral JP, et al. Mannodendrimers prevent acute lung inflammation by inhibiting neutrophil recruitment. Proc Natl Acad Sci U S A 2013;110(22):8795–800. Available from: https://doi.org/10.1073/PNAS.1221708110/SUPPL_FILE/PNAS.201221708SI.PDF.
[89] Iezzi R, Guru BR, Glybina IV, Mishra MK, Kennedy A, Kannan RM. Dendrimer-based targeted intravitreal therapy for sustained attenuation of neuroinflammation in retinal degeneration. Biomaterials 2012;33(3):979–88. Available from: https://doi.org/10.1016/J.BIOMATERIALS.2011.10.010.
[90] Malik N, Evagorou EG, Duncan R. Dendrimer-platinate: a novel approach to cancer chemotherapy: anticancer drugs. Anticancer Drugs 1999;10(8):767–76.

[91] Kaminskas LM, McLeod VM, Kelly BD, Cullinane C, Sberna G, Williamson M, et al. Doxorubicin-conjugated PEGylated dendrimers show similar tumoricidal activity but lower systemic toxicity when compared to PEGylated liposome and solution formulations in mouse and rat tumor models. Mol Pharm 2012;9(3):422–32. Available from: https://doi.org/10.1021/MP200522D/SUPPL_FILE/MP200522D_SI_001.PDF.

[92] Jiang YY, Tang GT, Zhang LH, Kong SY, Zhu SJ, Pei YY. PEGylated PAMAM dendrimers as a potential drug delivery carrier: in vitro and in vivo comparative evaluation of covalently conjugated drug and noncovalent drug inclusion complex. J Drug Target 2010;18(5):389–403. Available from: https://doi.org/10.3109/10611860903494203.

[93] Zhang L, Zhu S, Qian L, Pei Y, Qiu Y, Jiang Y. RGD-modified PEG–PAMAM–DOX conjugates: in vitro and in vivo studies for glioma. Eur J Pharm Biopharm 2011;79(2):232–40. Available from: https://doi.org/10.1016/J.EJPB.2011.03.025.

[94] Gajbhiye V, Jain NK. The treatment of glioblastoma xenografts by surfactant conjugated dendritic nanoconjugates. Biomaterials 2011;32(26):6213–25. Available from: https://doi.org/10.1016/J.BIOMATERIALS.2011.04.057.

[95] Sato N, Kobayashi H, Saga H, Nakamota Y, Ishimori T, Togashi K, et al. Tumor targeting and imaging of intraperitoneal tumors by use of antisense oligo-DNA complexed with dendrimers and/or avidin in mice1 | Clinical Cancer Research | American Association for Cancer Research. Clin Cancer Res 2001;7(11):3606–12.

[96] Vincent L, Varet J, Pille JY, Bompais H, Opolon P, Maksimenko A, et al. Efficacy of dendrimer-mediated angiostatin and TIMP-2 gene delivery on inhibition of tumor growth and angiogenesis: in vitro and in vivo studies. Int J Cancer 2003;105(3):419–29. Available from: https://doi.org/10.1002/IJC.11105.

[97] Koppu S, Oh YJ, Edrada-Ebel RA, Blatchford DR, Tetley L, Tate RJ, et al. Tumor regression after systemic administration of a novel tumor-targeted gene delivery system carrying a therapeutic plasmid DNA. J Control Rel 2010;143(2):215–21. Available from: https://doi.org/10.1016/J.JCONREL.2009.11.015.

[98] Landers JJ, Cao Z, Lee I, Piehler LT, Myc PP, Myc A, et al. Prevention of influenza pneumonitis by sialic acid–conjugated dendritic polymers. J Infect Dis 2002;186(9):1222–30. Available from: https://doi.org/10.1086/344316.

[99] Vijayaraj Kumar P, Agashe H, Dutta T, Jain N. PEGylated dendritic architecture for development of a prolonged drug delivery system for an antitubercular drug. Curr Drug Deliv 2006;4(1):11–19. Available from: https://doi.org/10.2174/156720107779314794.

[100] Price CF, Tyssen D, Sonza S, Davie A, Evans S, Lewis GR, et al. SPL7013 gel (VivaGel®) retains potent HIV-1 and HSV-2 inhibitory activity following vaginal administration in humans. PLoS One 2011;6(9):e24095. Available from: https://doi.org/10.1371/JOURNAL.PONE.0024095.

[101] Kobayashi H, Sato N, Kawamoto S, Saga T, Hiraga A, Laz Haque T, et al. Comparison of the macromolecular MR contrast agents with ethylenediamine-core versus ammonia-core generation-6 polyamidoamine dendrimer. Bioconjug Chem 2000;12(1):100–7. Available from: https://doi.org/10.1021/BC000075S.

[102] Criscione JM, Dobrucki LW, Zhuang ZW, Papademetris X, Simons M, Sinusas AJ, et al. Development and application of a multimodal contrast agent for SPECT/CT hybrid imaging. Bioconjug Chem 2011;22(9):1784–92. Available from: https://doi.org/10.1021/BC200162R/SUPPL_FILE/BC200162R_SI_001.PDF.

[103] Seo JW, Baek H, Mahakian LM, Kusunose J, Hamzah J, Ruoslahti E, et al. 64Cu-labeled LyP-1-dendrimer for PET-CT imaging of atherosclerotic plaque. Bioconjug Chem 2014;25(2):231–9. Available from: https://doi.org/10.1021/BC400347S/SUPPL_FILE/BC400347S_SI_002.PDF.

[104] Castelli DD, Terreno E, Longo D, Aime S. Nanoparticle-based chemical exchange saturation transfer (CEST) agents. NMR Biomed 2013;26(7):839–49. Available from: https://doi.org/10.1002/NBM.2974.

[105] Gupta U, Perumal O. Chapter 15 - Dendrimers and its biomedical applications | request PDF. In: Kumbar SG, editor. Natural and Synthetic Biomedical Polymers. Elsevier; 2014. p. 243–57. Available from: https://doi.org/10.1016/B978-0-12-396983-5.00016-8.

[106] Farzaneh F, Trefzer U, Sterry W, Walden P. Gene therapy of cancer. Immunol Today 1998;19(7):294–6. Available from: https://doi.org/10.1016/S0167-5699(98)01280-8.

[107] Thomas CE, Ehrhardt A, Kay MA. Progress and problems with the use of viral vectors for gene therapy. Nat Rev Genet 2003;4(5):346–58. Available from: https://doi.org/10.1038/NRG1066.

[108] Yang J, Zhang Q, Chang H, Cheng Y. Surface-engineered dendrimers in gene delivery. Chem Rev 2015;115(11):5274–300. Available from: https://doi.org/10.1021/CR500542T.

[109] Gupta U, Perumal O. Dendrimers and its biomedical applications. Nat Synth Biomed Polym 2014;243–57. Available from: https://doi.org/10.1016/B978-0-12-396983-5.00016-8.

[110] Conti DS, Brewer D, Grashik J, Avasarala S, Da Rocha SRP. Poly(amidoamine) dendrimer nanocarriers and their aerosol formulations for SiRNA delivery to the lung epithelium. Mol Pharm 2014;11(6):1808–22. Available from: https://doi.org/10.1021/MP4006358.

[111] Kullberg M, McCarthy R, Anchordoquy TJ. Systemic tumor-specific gene delivery. J Control Rel 2013;172 (3):730–6. Available from: https://doi.org/10.1016/J.JCONREL.2013.08.300.

[112] Merkel OM, Mintzer MA, Librizzi D, Samsonova O, Dicke T, Sproat B, et al. Triazine dendrimers as nonviral vectors for in vitro and in vivo RNAi: the effects of peripheral groups and core structure on biological activity. Mol Pharm 2010;7(4):969–83. Available from: https://doi.org/10.1021/MP100101S.

[113] Perisé-Barrios AJ, Jiménez JL, D'Omínguez-Soto A, De La Mata FJ, Corbí AL, Gomez R, et al. Carbosilane dendrimers as gene delivery agents for the treatment of HIV infection. J Control Rel 2014;184(1):51–7. Available from: https://doi.org/10.1016/J.JCONREL.2014.03.048.

[114] Ferenc M, Pedziwiatr-Werbicka E, Nowak KE, Klajnert B, Majoral JP, Bryszewska M. Phosphorus dendrimers as carriers of SiRNA–characterisation of dendriplexes. Molecules 2013;18(4):4451–66. Available from: https://doi.org/10.3390/MOLECULES18044451.

[115] Inoue Y, Kurihara R, Tsuchida A, Hasegawa M, Nagashima T, Mori T, et al. Efficient delivery of SiRNA using dendritic poly(L-Lysine) for loss-of-function analysis. J Control Rel 2008;126(1):59–66. Available from: https://doi.org/10.1016/J.JCONREL.2007.10.022.

[116] Tai Z, Ma J, Ding J, Pan H, Chai R, Zhu C, et al. Aptamer-functionalized dendrimer delivery of plasmid-encoding LncRNA MEG3 enhances gene therapy in castration-resistant prostate cancer. Int J Nanomed 2020;15:10305–20. Available from: https://doi.org/10.2147/IJN.S282107.

[117] Hu H, Wang H, Liang S, Li X, Wang D. Synthesis and characterization of a PAMAM dendrimer nanocarrier functionalized by HA for targeted gene delivery systems and evaluation in vitro. J Biomater Sci Polym Ed 2021;32(2):205–28. Available from: https://doi.org/10.1080/09205063.2020.1827921.

[118] Mekuria SL, Li J, Song C, Gao Y, Ouyang Z, Shen M, et al. Facile formation of PAMAM dendrimer nanoclusters for enhanced gene delivery and cancer gene therapy. ACS Appl Bio Mater 2021;4(9):7168–75. Available from: https://doi.org/10.1021/ACSABM.1C00743.

[119] Pishavar E, Ramezani M, Hashemi M. Co-delivery of doxorubicin and TRAIL plasmid by modified PAMAM dendrimer in colon cancer cells, in vitro and in vivo evaluation. Drug Dev Ind Pharm 2019;45 (12):1931–9. Available from: https://doi.org/10.1080/03639045.2019.1680995.

[120] Lee Y, Lee J, Kim M, Kim GY, Choi JS, Lee M. Brain gene delivery using histidine and arginine-modified dendrimers for ischemic stroke therapy. J Control Rel 2021;330:907–19. Available from: https://doi.org/10.1016/J.JCONREL.2020.10.064.

[121] Taratula O, Garbuzenko OB, Kirkpatrick P, Pandya I, Savla R, Pozharov VP, et al. Surface-engineered targeted PPI dendrimer for efficient intracellular and intratumoral SiRNA delivery. J Control Rel 2009;140 (3):284–93. Available from: https://doi.org/10.1016/J.JCONREL.2009.06.019.

[122] Qi R, Gao Y, Tang Y, He RR, Liu TL, He Y, et al. PEG-conjugated PAMAM dendrimers mediate efficient intramuscular gene expression. AAPS J 2009;11(3):395–405. Available from: https://doi.org/10.1208/S12248-009-9116-1.

[123] Singh P, Gupta U, Asthana A, Jain NK. Folate and folate-PEG-PAMAM dendrimers: synthesis, characterization, and targeted anticancer drug delivery potential in tumor bearing mice. Bioconjug Chem 2008;19 (11):2239–52. Available from: https://doi.org/10.1021/BC800125U.

[124] Shukla R, Thomas TP, Peters JL, Desai AM, Kukowska-Latallo J, Patri AK, et al. HER2 specific tumor targeting with dendrimer conjugated anti-HER2 MAb. Bioconjug Chem 2006;17(5):1109–15. Available from: https://doi.org/10.1021/BC050348P.

[125] Santos JL, Oliveira H, Pandita D, Rodrigues J, Pêgo AP, Granja PL, et al. Functionalization of poly(amidoamine) dendrimers with hydrophobic chains for improved gene delivery in mesenchymal stem cells. J Control Rel 2010;144(1):55–64. Available from: https://doi.org/10.1016/J.JCONREL.2010.01.034.

[126] Wang M, Liu H, Li L, Cheng Y. A fluorinated dendrimer achieves excellent gene transfection efficacy at extremely low nitrogen to phosphorus ratios. Nat Commun 2014;5. Available from: https://doi.org/10.1038/NCOMMS4053.

[127] Asthana A, Chauhan AS, Diwan PV, Jain NK. Poly(amidoamine) (PAMAM) dendritic nanostructures for controlled site-specific delivery of acidic anti-inflammatory active ingredient. AAPS PharmSciTech 2005;6 (3). Available from: https://doi.org/10.1208/PT060367.

[128] Tomalia DA, Reyna LA, Svenson S. Dendrimers as multi-purpose nanodevices for oncology drug delivery and diagnostic imaging. Biochem Soc Trans 2007;35(Pt 1):61–7. Available from: https://doi.org/10.1042/BST0350061.

[129] Werner EJ, Avedano S, Botta M, Hay BP, Moore EG, Aime S, et al. Highly soluble tris-hydroxypyridonate Gd(III) complexes with increased hydration number, fast water exchange, slow electronic relaxation, and high relaxivity. J Am Chem Soc 2007;129(7):1870–1. Available from: https://doi.org/10.1021/JA068026Z.

[130] Patri AK, Majoros IJ, Baker JR. Dendritic polymer macromolecular carriers for drug delivery. Curr Opin Chem Biol 2002;6(4):466–71. Available from: https://doi.org/10.1016/S1367-5931(02)00347-2.

[131] Langereis S, Dirksen A, Hackeng TM, Van Genderen MHP, Meijer EW. Dendrimers and magnetic resonance imaging. N J Chem 2007;31(7):1152–60. Available from: https://doi.org/10.1039/B616960K.

[132] Cheng Z, Thorek DLJ, Tsourkas A. Gadolinium-conjugated dendrimer nanoclusters as a tumor-targeted T1 magnetic resonance imaging contrast agent. Angew Chem Int Ed Engl 2010;49(2):346–50. Available from: https://doi.org/10.1002/ANIE.200905133.

[133] Mekuria SL, Debele TA, Tsai HC. Encapsulation of gadolinium oxide nanoparticle (Gd_2O_3) contrasting agents in PAMAM dendrimer templates for enhanced magnetic resonance imaging in vivo. ACS Appl Mater Interfaces 2017;9(8):6782–95. Available from: https://doi.org/10.1021/ACSAMI.6B14075.

[134] Fu Y, Nitecki DE, Maltby D, Simon GH, Berejnoi K, Raatschen HJ, et al. Dendritic iodinated contrast agents with PEG-cores for CT imaging: synthesis and preliminary characterization. Bioconjug Chem 2006;17(4):1043–56. Available from: https://doi.org/10.1021/BC060019C.

[135] Qiao Z, Shi X. Dendrimer-based molecular imaging contrast agents. Prog Polym Sci 2015;44:1–27. Available from: https://doi.org/10.1016/J.PROGPOLYMSCI.2014.08.002.

[136] Kojima C, Turkbey B, Ogawa M, Bernardo M, Regino CAS, Bryant LH, et al. Dendrimer-based MRI contrast agents: the effects of PEGylation on relaxivity and pharmacokinetics. Nanomedicine 2011;7(6):1001–8. Available from: https://doi.org/10.1016/J.NANO.2011.03.007.

[137] Guo R, Wang H, Peng C, Shen M, Zheng L, Zhang G, et al. Enhanced X-ray attenuation property of dendrimer-entrapped gold nanoparticles complexed with diatrizoic acid. J Mater Chem 2011;21(13):5120–7. Available from: https://doi.org/10.1039/C0JM04094K.

CHAPTER

11

Development of advanced diagnostic platform for detection of infectious diseases

Deepshikha Shahdeo, Drishya Prakashan and Sonu Gandhi

DBT-National Institute of Animal Biotechnology (DBT-NIAB), Hyderabad, Telangana, India

11.1 Introduction

Diagnostics plays an important part in health care industry, as the demand for a more powerful and efficient diagnostic device is increasing rapidly all over the world [1–3]. Advanced and high-end diagnostics has exceptionally changed the present scenario and replaced the conventional methods of diagnostics with more efficient ones. The advancement in technology and expertise has made it possible to provide rapid results in the identification of different pathogens [4]. New inventions in this area are feasible and have reduced the gap between laboratory testing and delivery of the results. Moreover, these rapid tests are easy, simple, and accurate for the detection of the pathogens with improved clinical outcomes in the diagnostic industry. One can easily and quickly identify the desired targets in a variety of samples with these devices because they convert the presence of particular biological analytes into recognized signals [5,6]. Apart from the conventional methods, modern diagnostics methods created a revolution in the health care industry [7–9]. Development of the point-of-care strategy helps in controlling the spread of disease as well as reducing the cost in health care, as it does not require trained operators and high-cost resources.

One of the major causes of death worldwide is infectious disease. They are caused by microbes like bacteria, virus, fungus, and so forth [10]. Despite the present advances in diagnosis and treatment, the spread of disease is still not under control. Recently, the pandemic of novel coronavirus 2019 has affected a large number of people across the globe [11]. The rapid growth in the infection rate makes it extremely difficult to reduce the spread of disease, leading to huge loss in economic and health care sectors

Molecular Pharmaceutics and Nano Drug Delivery
DOI: https://doi.org/10.1016/B978-0-323-91924-1.00008-3

of the global community. Hence, a better diagnostic platform for the early detection of the microbes in the shortest possible time and at low cost is important to prevent the spread of the disease [12,13].

Traditionally, pathogens were detected by microscopic examination, staining, or culturing of the organisms, which were based on their phenotypic characters. However, these methods are not reliable, as they are time-consuming and less sensitive. Moreover, many microbes cannot be identified by phenotypic characters. In order to overcome the constraints associated with the conventional diagnostics methods, modern diagnostics methods were developed. Other conventional techniques include genotype-based assays such as quantitative real-time polymerase chain reaction (PCR) [14–16].

Point-of-care testing (POCT) is necessary for early diagnosis and the improvement of patient health outcomes [17–19]. POCT allows people to self-test, without going to hospitals, thus reducing health care time, cost, and also the chances of infection from contagious disease. Hence, they facilitate better monitoring and management of disease. The POCT devices are sensitive, specific, accurate, user-friendly, rapid, and cost-effective. In addition, they provide a platform to screen a large number of samples with high efficiency in a short time [18,20,21].

Nanotechnology has tremendous applications in disease diagnosis and its treatment. The application of nanomaterials has been increased rapidly in recent years. Nanomedicine is a new branch where nanomaterials are used for medical applications. Nanoparticles are extremely small particles with a size range of 0.1 to 100 nm [22]. Due to this small size, the optical and magnetic properties of nanomaterials can be easily manipulated to generate a detectable signal [23–25]. The use of nanoparticles can improve the pharmaceutical medication release at the target site, thereby reducing the chance of their localization in healthy tissues and hence side effects [26]. Nanomaterials are used for surgery [27], cancer diagnostics and its therapy [28,29], detecting indicators of diseases like antibodies, specific proteins, viruses, drug delivery, and implant technology [14]. Most biological molecules and structures have a size similar to that of nanomaterials; hence, these materials can be used for biomedical applications and research both in vitro and in vivo. Nanomaterial-based methods have demonstrated high potential in health care, and it has raised high expectation to the patients as an affordable and excellent solution for treating different diseases. Despite these applications, to be clinically relevant, nanoparticle-based methods have to overcome many challenges, including their toxicity, delivery methods, and their therapeutic efficiency. Nanoparticles like quantum dots, gold nanoparticle (AuNP), magnetic nanoparticle, nanoshell, and nanotubes are promising candidates for diagnostics and therapeutic purposes.

11.2 Traditional laboratory techniques for the diagnosis and treatment of diseases

Some of the common traditional laboratory techniques for the detection of infection diseases are *electron microscopy* (EM) for viral and bacterial visualizations [30], *complement fixation test* (CFT) [31], *hemagglutination inhibition* test [32], *culture and drug susceptibility* test [33], *serologic test* (enzyme-linked immunosorbent assay, ELISA), and so forth [34,35].

Traditional approaches for detecting and identifying infectious disease rely mostly on specific microbiological and biochemical identification. Assay sensitivity and specificity are significant factors in clinical and diagnostic microbiology, and these are used to evaluate a newly designed test following comparison with a reference gold standard method.

In several developed countries, EM was used for the visualization and counting of the virus (Fig. 11.1A) [36,37]. However, the specimen preparation is required, which overall makes the analysis a tedious process. Other than that, EM requires the technical skills and expertise, which are not feasible for the developing countries like India and Bangladesh. Recently, a cell culture-based approach combined with EM has made a significant contribution to viral identification [38]. The only major drawback of the cell culture is that it takes a longer period of time for viral isolation, and experienced personnel are required

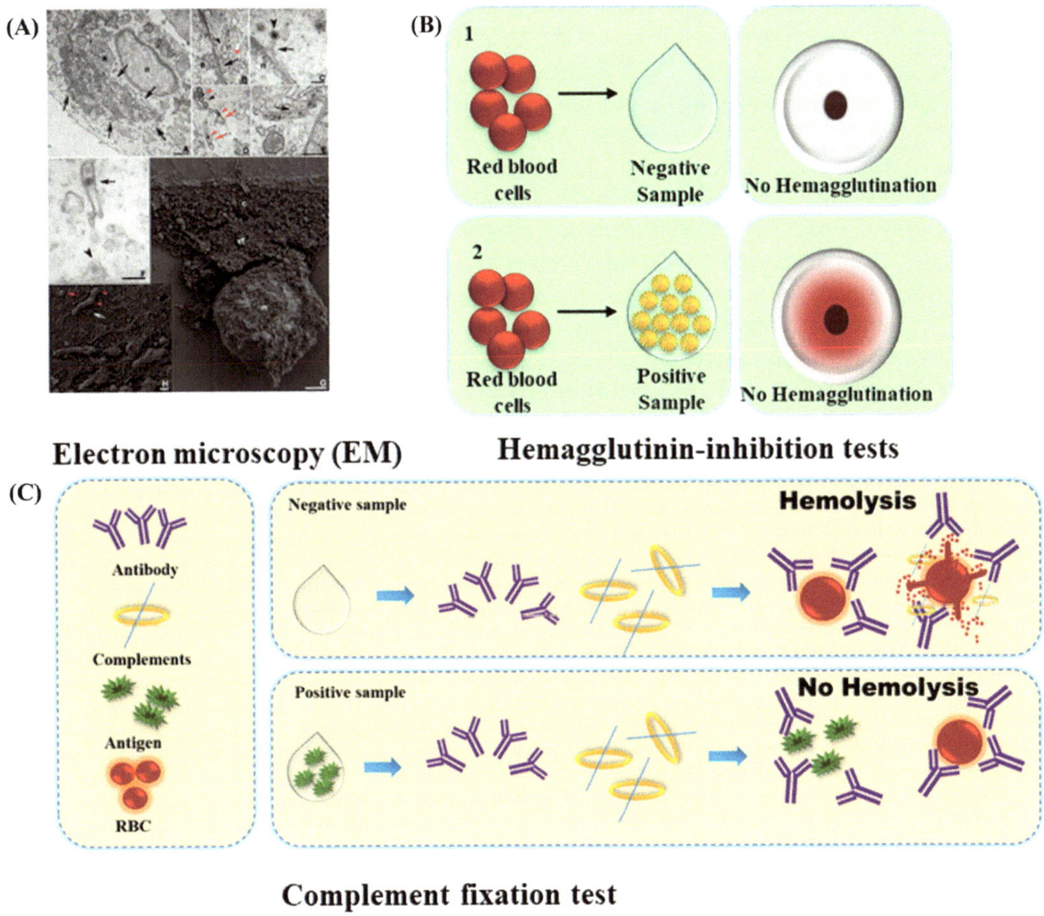

FIGURE 11.1 Different conventional techniques available for the detection of infectious diseases: (A) Different microcopy technique for the detection of Zika virus [36]; (B) hemagglutinin-inhibition test for detection malaria; and (C) complement fixation test used for screening of a specific antibody against a variety of possible pathogens. Source: *Open access.*

for handing of mammalian cell culture infected with viral load. The *shell vial technique* is the alternative the conventional cell culture technique for rapid detection of viral load [39]. In this technique, inoculated cells are centrifuged, incubated, and further stained with monoclonal antibodies. This is specific to the viruses that cause infection, to the respiratory systems, Herpes simplex virus, or Varicella zoster virus. The viral tier is detectable 1–5 days later.

Hemagglutinin-inhibition test is a process based on tendency of some viruses to cause blood agglutination (Fig. 11.1B). It is a simple, inexpensive, and rapid technique mainly used for the influenza virus. The principle of test is based on hemagglutinin (HA), an envelope protein that is capable of binding to red blood cells and forming a lattice fretwork known as "agglutination." Serial dilutions of the serum samples are mixed with the constant amount of erythrocyte and viral HA. In the presence of influenza antibodies, the process of clumping is inhibited. The rate of dilution is that at which complete agglutination is identified, recognized, and recorded. Agglutination assays have been carried out to diagnose a larger spectrum of viral illnesses other than influenza. However, the test is laborious and rigorous, especially in terms of quality control.

CFT is a immunological medical test and usually used for screening of a specific antibody against the varieties of possible pathogens. It is widely preferred for diagnosis of chronic brucella (Fig. 11.1C). Other than that, *microimmunofluorescence* test is the gold standard technique for the chlamydial antibody detection. CFT was shown to be simple, efficient, and required reasonable material. However, in comparison to gold standards, it is a time-consuming technique and has low sensitivity. Optimization via reactant titration and control preparation is critical for attaining efficient testing.

The list of conventional techniques listed is not comprehensive, and the only common techniques usually used are listed in Table 11.1.

11.3 Recent emerging technology for diagnosis of infectious diseases

Biosensors are devices that measure the amount of a biological analyte in a sample. It consists of mainly two parts: bioreceptor and transducer, which are integrated in one system [13,54–57]. The bioreceptor part contains a biomolecule that can specifically recognize the target analyte and transform it into a measurable signal via a transducer [58]. Nanoparticle-based biosensors are used in various fields including biomedical, environment, pharmaceutical, cosmetics, and food [59–62]. The presence of environmental pathogens, their toxins, organic pollutants, and heavy metals can be easily identified with the use of biosensors [63,64] (Fig. 11.2).

Different types of biosensors used are immunosensors, enzyme-based, cell-based, fluorescent, DNA biosensors, thermal, and piezoelectric biosensors [66]. Recently, label-free biosensors that do not use reporter molecules to identify the target species are widely used [67]. Label-free assays are very easy to prepare, are low-cost, and require less facilities and manpower. Among the different biosensors, electrochemical biosensors have been widely used for pathogen detection. Electrochemical biosensors utilize an electrode for target detection. Electrochemical biosensors are widely used for diagnostics, food quality analysis [68,69], and environmental monitoring [70,71]. Numerous electrochemical

TABLE 11.1 Different conventional diagnostic techniques and their advantages and disadvantages for detection of several infectious diseases.

S. No.	Diagnostic technique	Advantage	Disadvantage	References
1.	Immunological test—antibody test	Cost-effective	Least sensitive	[40,41]
2.	Microscopic examination	Low cost, easily accessible	Low sensitivity	[42–44]
3.	Polymerase chain reaction	Fast, accurate, high sensitivity and specificity	Standard lab settings, expertise required, costly	[14,45–48]
4.	Next generation sequencing	High sensitivity and identification accuracy	Costly, bioinformatic skills required	[49]
5.	Nucleic acid-based amplification techniques	Highly sensitive and specific	Long run time needed and specific primers required for the target	[50]
6.	DNA based test—microarray technique	Highly sensitive and specific	Not cost-effective, requires a standard lab setup	[51]
7.	Serologic test—ELISA	Rapid detection and highly sensitive	Lab setting required	[41,52]
8.	Immunofluorescence assay	Highly sensitive in comparison to microscopy	Time-consuming, standard lab setting required	[42]
9.	Hemagglutinin-inhibition tests	Quick, simple, and cost-effective	Laborious and rigorous	[32,53]
10.	Complement fixation test	Simple and cost-effective	Lacks sensitivity	[31]
11.	Mass spectrometry	Highly sensitive and great accuracy	Expensive and time-consuming	

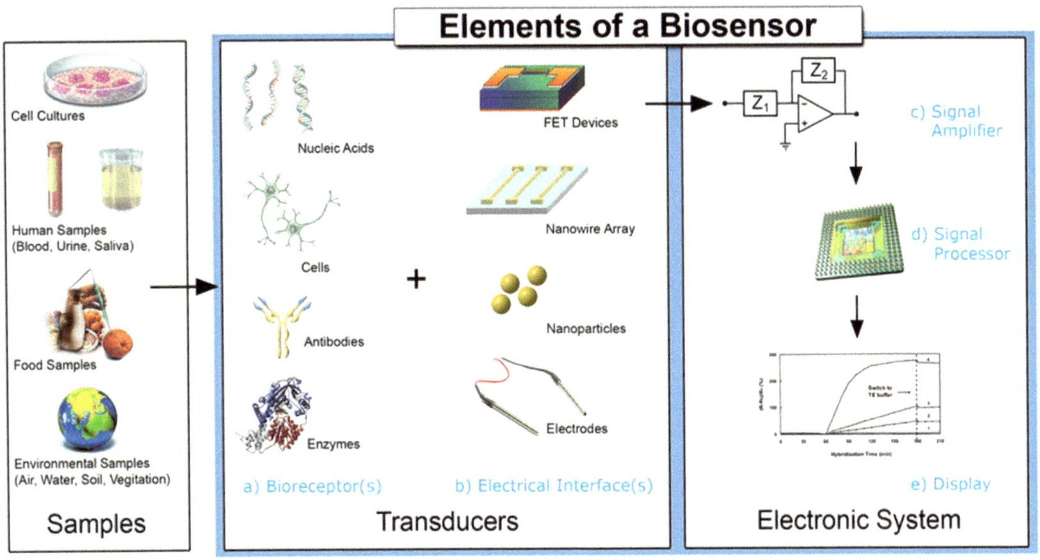

FIGURE 11.2 Schematic representation of the mechanism of action of a biosensor; as shown in the figure, a biosensor mainly consists of bioreceptors, transducer to convert the chemical signal to electrical signal, an amplifier to increase the signal/noise ratio, and display to observe the numerical values [65]. Source: *Open access.*

biosensors have been developed in order to detect various microorganisms such as *E. coli*, *Staphylococcus*, *Mycobacterium*, and so forth so far [71–73]. Furthermore, POC biosensors are developed for the recent pandemic COVID-19 [4,42].

11.3.1 Diagnostic techniques for COVID-19

Currently, advanced electrode materials such as carbon-based hybrids are gaining a lot of attention due to their biocompatibility and conductivity. Pencil graphite can be used as an alternative to its costly electrode counterpart [74]. Apart from the carbon-based electrode, boron-doped diamond is another material that is in great demand for its better electronic, mechanical, and chemical properties [75,76]. In addition to this, effective immobilization of the biosensing element on the electrode is highly significant for the development of an advanced biosensor [77–79].

COVID-19 is an airborne contagious viral disease, which was declared a pandemic in March 2020. Severe acute respiratory syndrome coronavirus 2 (SARS-CoV-2) resulted in the coronavirus disease 2019 [80,81]. Fever, cold, cough, body pain, and headaches are the common symptoms of the diseases; however, it might progress to a life-threatening respiratory syndrome and can affect the lung, kidney, and heart [81,82]. Currently, RT-PCR is the most reliable technique for the accurate diagnosis of SARS-CoV-2 [1,83]. However, several new technologies are emerging to the fill the void. In the recent days, POC devices mainly consist of nucleic acid or are antibody-based. Nucleic acid is usually detected in the sputum of the patient, while antibody is detected in their serum/blood. After 5 days of infection, IgM and IgG are produced against the viral antigen [84]. The antibodies produced can be then detected in the plasma of the patient. Moitra et al. demonstrated the development of a colorimetric assay that can be detected by the naked eye [85] (Fig. 11.3A). N-gene-specific thiolated antisense oligonucleotides are made to absorb onto AuNPs. Changes in surface plasmon resonance (SPR) can be identified in 15 minutes when the target RNA sequence (N-gene) is present. Furthermore, RNaseH was used to break RNA from the RNA–DNA complex, resulting in precipitation that could be seen due to AuNP aggregation. At 0.18 ng/L, our developed assay demonstrated low limit of detection (LOD) and very less cross-reactivity with MERS-CoV.

Another extensively used technique is the immunochromatography strip assay also called as lateral flow immunoassay (LFA). LFA is a cellulose-based technology that has grown in popularity as a POCT device for detecting Ab in the blood. It consists of a nitrocellulose membrane with a sample pad and a conjugate pad integrated in it. The sample (blood, cells, and antibodies) is put on the sample pad and permitted to migrate to the conjugate pad by capillary action, where the antibody forms complex with AuNPs-conjugated antigen (SARS-CoV-2 spike) and flows by capillary action to the test and control lines. In addition to this, colorimetric visualization also uses fluorophores, latex nanoparticles, and AuNPs. Surface-enhanced Raman spectroscopy (SERS)-based LFA with dual-layered 5,5′-dithiobis-dithiobis-dithiobis-dithiobis-dithiobis-dithiobis-dithiobis-dithiobis-dithiobis- (2-nitrobenzoic acid) SARS-CoV-2 and DTNB-modified SiO_2@Ag NPs were reported for the identification of SARS-CoV-2 (Fig. 11.3B) [86,87]. Meanwhile, various SPR-based sensors for detecting SARS-CoV-2-specific nucleocapsid (Nu) antibodies (Abs) are

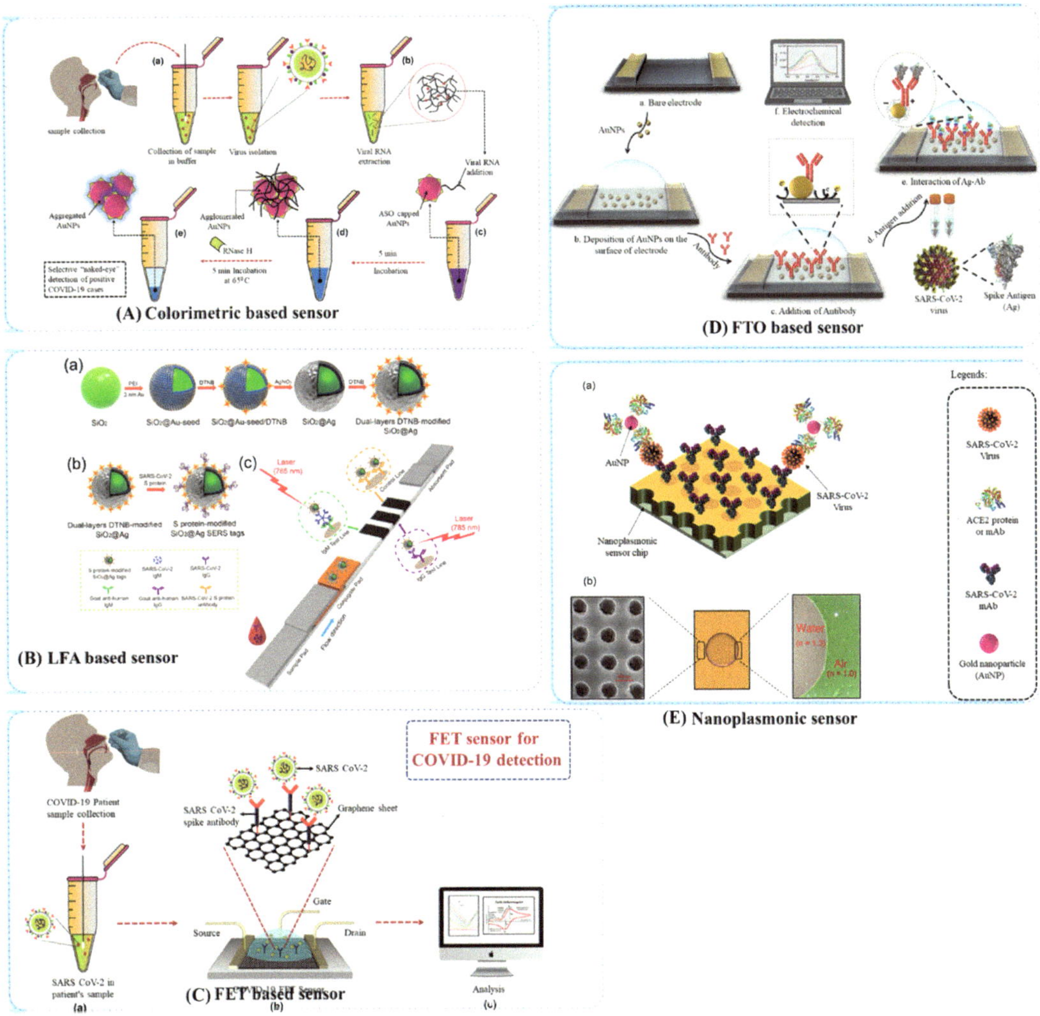

FIGURE 11.3 Different diagnostic platforms available for the diagnosis of SARS-CoV-2: (A) Colorimetric assay detectable with naked eyes [1,85]; (B) surface-enhanced Raman spectroscopy (SERS)-based lateral flow immunoassay (LFA) modified with DTNB-altered SiO2@Ag NPs for the detection of SARS-CoV-2 [86,87]; (C) graphene-modified field effect transistor (FET)-based electrochemical sensor for quick identification of SARS-CoV-2 in the real samples [88]; (D) AuNP-functionalized graphene-activated FTO-based electrochemical sensor for the recognition of Spike S1 antigen of SARS-CoV-2 [2]; (E) SARS-CoV-2 specific monoclonal antibody modified nanoplasmonic resonance sensors for detection of SARS-CoV-2 viral particles via optical detection technology [1,89]. Source: *(A, C, E) Open access; (B, D) Reprinted with copyright permission.*

being developed. Several SARS-CoV-2-infected people had antibodies developed against the nucleocapsid protein during infection, which can be used to promote vaccine research. The SPR sensor was covered with a peptide layer functionalized with recombinant Nu Ag, to detect SARS-CoV-2 Abs in nM concentration. The experiment was carried out on human serum that was undiluted, and the results were obtained in under 15 minutes using portable SPR equipment. This method enables more research into label-free, rapid POC Abs testing.

As discussed previously in this chapter, electrochemical biosensors are also playing a crucial role in the current scenario of pandemic. Scientists are working to develop numerous sensors in collaboration with different highly efficient conductive nanomaterials to fabricate advanced electrochemical biosensors. Seo et al. [88,90,91] developed an electrochemical sensor based on a field effect transistor for rapid detection of SARS-CoV-2. Graphene was employed as a conductive base, and Spike S1 Ag was detected when a particular antibody (Ab) was bound by 1-pyrenebutyric acid N-hydroxysuccinimide ester. The given experiment's LOD was determined to be 1 fg/mL in phosphate buffer saline and 100 fg/mL in clinical transport medium (Fig. 11.3C). Roberts et al. recently developed a label-free fluorine-doped tin oxide (FTO)-based electrochemical sensor for SARS-CoV-2 Spike S1 antigen detection. Differential pulse voltammetry and cyclic voltammetry were measured after interaction of Ag with FTO/ AuNPs complex coupled with in-housed generated Spike S1 antigen [2] (Fig. 11.3D).

Using nanoplasmonic sensors is another emerging technique, which is highly efficient in diagnosis. The nanoscale light used in this sensor is below the diffraction limit. It converts the free photons to localized charge-density oscillation. Nanoplasmonic resonance sensors were fabricated by coating SARS-CoV-2 monoclonal antibody (mAbs) for identification of SARS-CoV-2 virus particles via one-step optical detection technology. 370 vp/mL was found to be the LOD of the given technology. This approach can be measured in both the traditional ELISA reader and a mobile phone attached to the instrument [89] (Fig. 11.3E).

11.3.2 Diagnostic techniques for tuberculosis

Mycobacterium tuberculosis (M. tuberculosis) is a dangerous pathogenic bacterium that causes tuberculosis (TB), one of the leading causes of infectious disease-related death [92]. Approximately 1/3 of the world's population is infected with TB currently. TB infection is a big public health problem because it can develop as a result of an infection with acquired immune deficiency syndrome. For effective *M. tuberculosis* detection, clinical diagnosis, water and environmental analysis, food safety, and biodefense are all key topics [93]. The main concern in preventing efficient treatment to morbidity and mortality, notably in HIV-associated and drug-resistant TB cases, was a lack of adequate diagnostic methods for timely detection [93,94].

The gold standard method, for example, microbial culture-based assays, is currently the most widely utilized procedure. Cell culture, cell counts, and cell enrichment are typical techniques, but they are time-consuming and complex processes because bacteria grows slowly, such as *M. tuberculosis* [95,96]. TB poses a huge global public health threat, necessitating the development of more rapid and sensitive testing tools [97]. PCR, latex agglutination, ELISA, radiometric detection, and gene-probe amplified *M. tuberculosis* direct test are among the methods and techniques for quick detection of *M. tuberculosis* that have been developed to date. However, most of these approaches are not suitable for real-time detection and necessitate a normal laboratory setup that is not practical for TB testing in the field [98,99].

Biosensing technologies are particularly suited for this purpose because of the recent advancements in sensing technology research. Biosensors are used in a variety of applications, including clinical testing, disease diagnosis, food safety, bioprocessing, and environmental monitoring [7,9,21,100]. Biosensors are important because of their high accuracy and efficiency in detecting a wide range of analytes (saliva, blood, and urine).

To detect *M. tuberculosis* antigen, Daz-González et al. demonstrated a voltametric immunosensor based on enzymes [101]. A screen-printed carbon electrode altered with streptavidin was used for signal transduction. Biotinylated rabbit anti-*M. tuberculosis* antibodies were bonded onto the surface of the electrode using a streptavidin-biotin method. When *M. tuberculosis* antigens and monoclonal antibodies are used against *M. tuberculosis*, sandwich immunological complexes of rabbit anti-*M. tuberculosis*/*M. tuberculosis* antigens/monoclonal antibodies against *M. tuberculosis* could develop. The detector antibodies, which were rabbit IgG anti-mouse immunoglobulin G that had been alkaline phosphatase labeled, were then adsorbed onto the monoclonal antibodies. The enzymatic product produced when 3-indoxyl phosphate was used as a substrate for electrochemical analysis could cause an electrochemical change.

Danna et al. [102] developed a biomicrosystem for detection of ESTA-6. This biomicrosystem was made using physical vapor deposition of Au nanolayers on copper surfaces, as shown in Fig. 11.4A. The surface was thiolated using 20 mM 4-aminothiophenol and a polyclonal antibody (pAb) that was covalently attached. 40 independent replicas were used to characterize each step of the electroimmunosensor production procedure using impedance analysis. When ESAT-6 *M. tuberculosis* immunodominant protein samples were compared to negative controls, pure water, and 0.5 g/mL HSA, a maximum variation of 171% was achieved between each duplicate. As a result, this study demonstrates a noninvasive method for electrically monitoring the electroimmunosensor assembly process as well as a tool for its subsequent evaluation for antigen detection.

According to one study, scientists created a unique, highly accurate prototype bioelectronic TB antigen assay to identify TB-specific antigen, CFP10, in a small amount of serum and urine samples (39). It is the first developed bioelectronic immunoassay, which was utilized for identifying CFP-10 in clinical samples.

Recently, to monitor the response of antimycobacterial therapy, a rapid and quantitative blood-based assay was developed [103]. This newly developed blood-based assay is very sensitive and specific for TB infection. Nanodisk conjugated with antibodies was used to enrich the *M. tuberculosis*-specific peptides (CFP-10 and ESAT-6), as shown in Fig. 11.5. Recognition of *M. tuberculosis*-selective CFP-10 and ESAT-6 peptides, as well as the invention of antibody-conjugated nanodisks, considerably improve target peptide enrichment and MALDI of bound peptides, allowing for higher-throughput MALDI time-of-flight mass spectrometry detection. Additionally, trypsin digestion caused protein complexes to denaturate, allowing *M. tuberculosis* antigens to be liberated, which would otherwise go undetected in standard immunoassays. The NanoDisk-mass spectrometry method allows for fast determination of serum markers specific for active TB, overcoming obstacles associated with current methodologies, and it uses well-accepted clinical instrumentation to improve clinical translation potential.

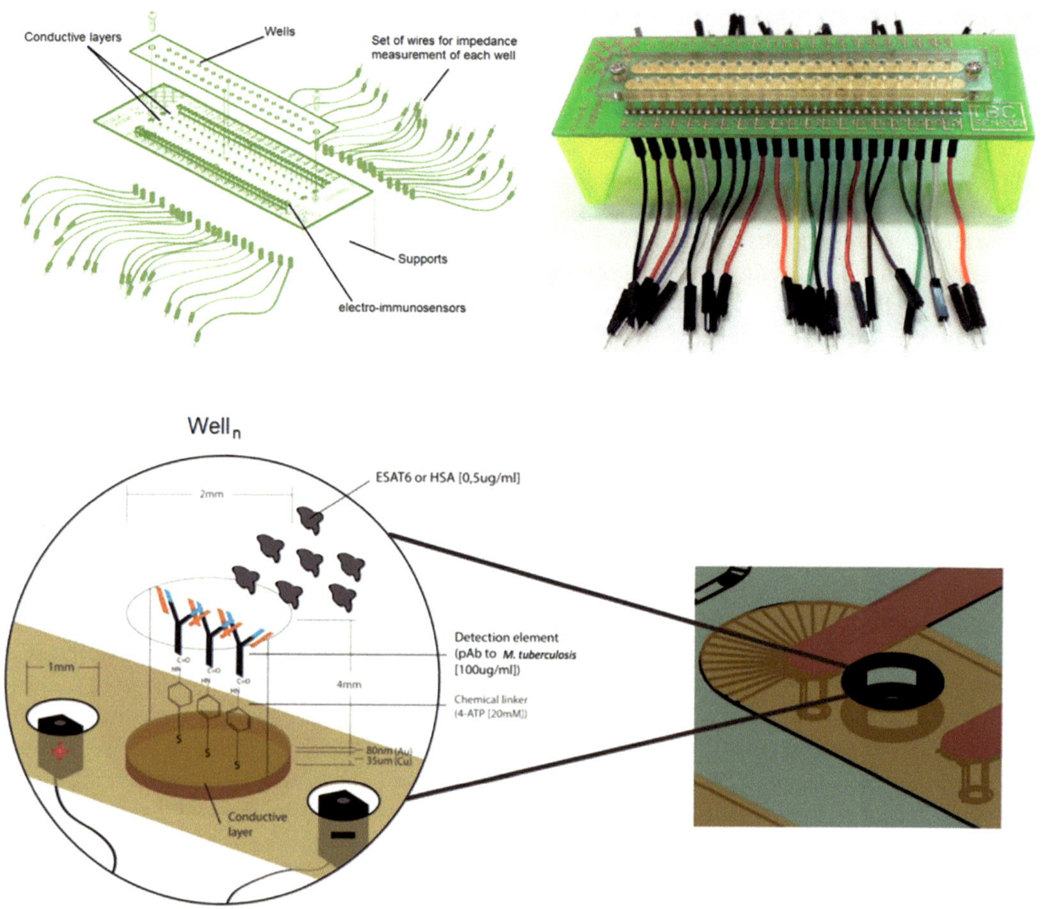

FIGURE 11.4 Schematic representation of the biomicrosystem. Image of a constructed biomicrosystem and illustration of an immunosensor well with reagent assembly and a capture probe layer are shown [102]. *Source: Open access.*

11.3.3 Diagnostic techniques available for malaria

Malaria is a major public health concern in densely populated, less developed tropical areas around the world [4]. Disease affects people and causes economic damage, and it can spread to new areas via visitors. Despite the fact that enough treatments exist for the successful treatment and cure of malaria, millions of people are infected each year, and thousands of people die. Early diagnosis of the infection has the potential to limit disease spread, save lives, and save money [104].

Nanoparticles are improving the sensitivity of the different electrochemical sensor. Magnetic nanoparticles were used to improve the sensitivity of the sensor. It is utilized to find Plasmodium falciparum's histidine-rich protein-2 (PfHRP-II). Monoclonal antibodies against these PfHRP-II were generated and functionalized with the magnetic nanoparticles

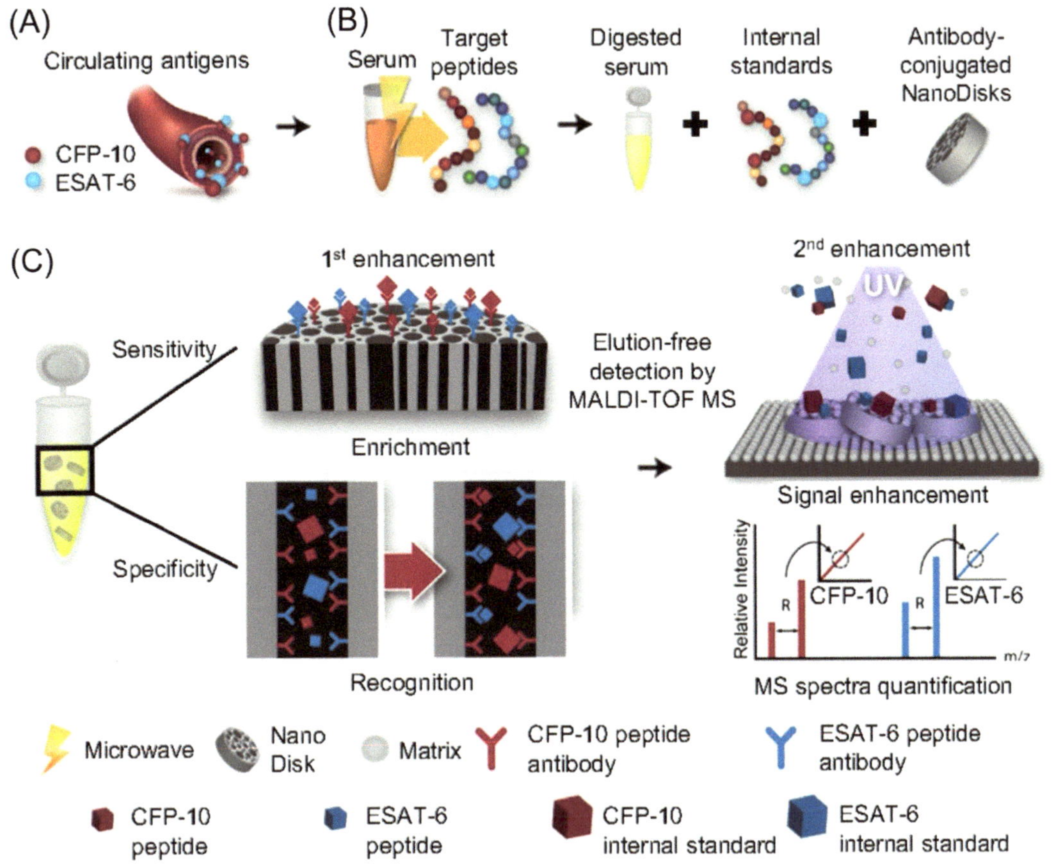

FIGURE 11.5 The NanoDisk-mass spectrometry platform is depicted schematically. (A) Active *M. tuberculosis* infections generate CFP-10 and ESAT-6 into the blood. (B) Microwave-assisted tryptic digestion is used on serum samples, which are then combined with functionalized nanodisks (C). Antibody-conjugated nanodisks recognize and enrich target peptides and boost the MALDI signal, and the target peptide can be quantified at low concentrations using the mass spectrometry intensity ratio of the target and isotope-labeled internal standard peptides [103]. Source: *Open access.*

and allowed to bind to the target analyte. Another secondary antibody against PfHRP-II-specific was labeled with the horseradish peroxide and used to develop the colorimetric and electrochemical sensor simultaneously. This technique yielded an LOD of 0.36 ng/mL in spiked serum samples, which is superior to traditional immunoassays (Fig. 11.6) [105,106].

11.3.4 Diagnostic techniques available for AIDS

Despite substantial efforts in HIV-1 early detection and its control and treatment, it still remains a major epidemic [12,107–109]. In 2014, there were 36.9 million HIV-positive persons globally, with 2.0 million new cases and 1.3 million fatalities. According to recent estimates, around 3,229,757 persons in Nigeria are infected with HIV, with approximately

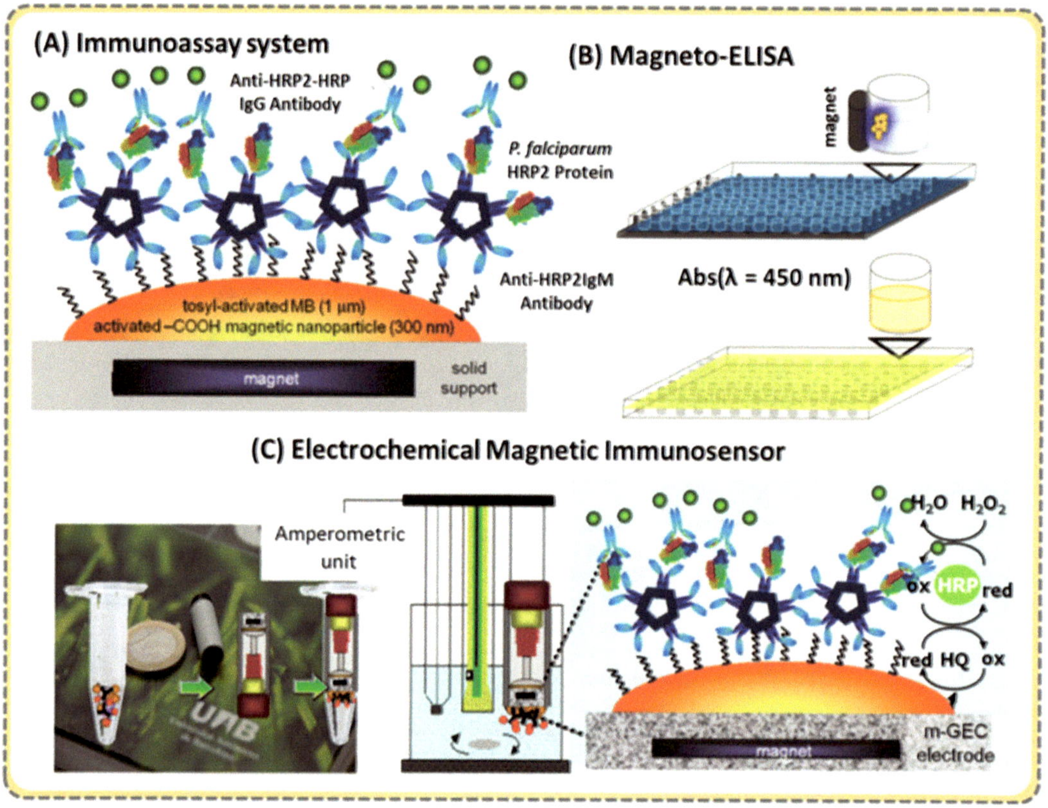

FIGURE 11.6 (A) IgM and IgG antibodies specific to PfHRP-II are used in a magnetic immunoassay format. (B) ELISA assay based on magnetic nanoparticles. (C) Electrochemical sensor based on magnetic nanoparticles and a catalytic reaction based on HRP for the creation of electrochemical signals [105]. Source: *Reprinted with Copyright permission.*

220,393 new HIV infections occurring in 2013 and 210,031 deaths from AIDS-related conditions. People who engage in low-risk groups are the main force behind the HIV epidemic in Nigeria, whereas high-risk groups such as female sex workers, homosexual men, and intravenous drug users contribute significantly to new infections [110]. Due to a multitude of aspects, such as suppressive antiretroviral treatment and syringe exchange programs, the overall occurrence of HIV-1 has declined in affluent countries [111]. Despite increased HIV testing availability, about half of all infected persons around the world are ignorant about their HIV status, and access to treatment is a major limitation. Recent quick tests of HIV are posing the risk of incorrect interpretation and necessitating complicated electronic data gathering, resulting in a poor connection to care and public health data loss. Mobile-phone-connected detection devices offer the possibility for easy testing and combining electronic data gathering with wireless networking.

Grey et al. created a portable smartphone-based digital diagnosis system based on shear horizontal surface acoustic wave (SH-SAW), which they tested with a sample of 133

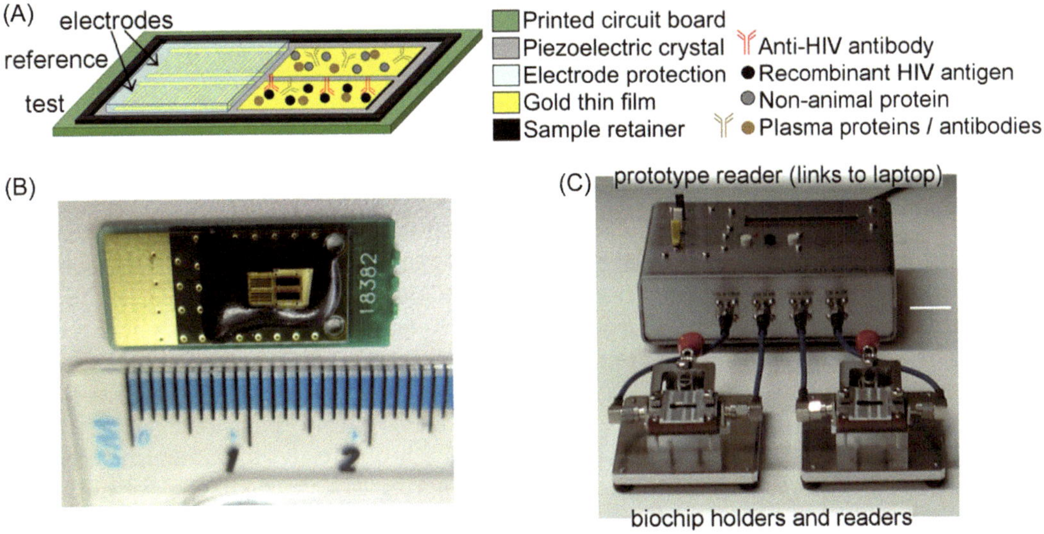

FIGURE 11.7 Biosensors and biochips based on SH-SAW; (A) important features of dual-channel biochips. (B) Dimensions of disposable laboratory biochips. The electrodes are shielded by glass, and the channels are encased in black resin. (C) Biochip holders and prototype readers in the laboratory [112]. Source: *Open access.*

HIV-positive patients [112]. They developed a small, portable laboratory prototype, as well as dual-channel biochips with in-situ reference control coating and a reduced configuration requiring only 6 μL of plasma. To detect anti-p24 or anti-gp41 antibodies, as well as a control, the dual-channel biochips were effectively produced using ink-jet printing with capture coatings. Plasma samples from 31 HIV patients and 102 healthy people were used to test biochips. In terms of sensitivity, specificity, low sample volume, and time to response, SH-SAW biosensors surpassed market rapid HIV tests. Within 5 minutes, individual biomarker testing indicated sensitivities of 100% (anti-gp41) and 64.5% (anti-p24) (combined sensitivity of 100%) and 100% specificity (Fig. 11.7).

11.4 Other diagnostic approaches and future perspective

Microfluidic technology has been positively known for the control of infectious diseases since it allows for timely therapy [18,111,113]. It offers a significant solution for distant areas and near-patient facilities by reducing patient turnaround trips between the clinic and the lab. When time is of the essence or physical space does not allow for the installation of traditional technology, they are widely useful. A lab-on-a-chip is a small device that combines lab processes [114–116]. To execute quick reactions in the chip or on a transportable device, it uses a very small sample volume. Microfluidic based diagnostics coupled with advanced equipment to carry out tests in lab at lower cost, with very less expenditure. The reactions span from nucleic acid amplification and detection to cell count and immunoassays. The WHO and nonprofit organizations like the Foundation for

Innovative New Diagnostics are collaborating to strengthen infectious disease surveillance and their control programs, establish new laws, and establish detection services that use less resources.

11.5 Conclusion

Diagnostic tools that have recently been created are transforming clinical practices and may assist in minimizing the occurrence of major infectious diseases. However, technical capabilities, on their own, are insufficient unless they are complemented by health promotion programs to raise awareness about the importance of early detection and routine screening of high-risk populations. Furthermore, diagnostics with high quality comes at the price that only wealthy countries can currently pay in routine practice, which is retarding the deployment of innovative procedures in the developing countries and native areas. Even so, efforts will still be continued to create new high-quality tests that are inexpensive in low-income nations, thereby significantly strengthening disease management measures for their people.

Acknowledgments

We are grateful for the research endowment under the Intensification of Research in High Priority Area (IRHPA) program from Science and Engineering Research Board (SERB), New Delhi (Grant Number IPA/2020/000069, CRG/2020/003014, and WEA/2020/000036) and Department of Biotechnology (DBT), New Delhi (Grant number BT/PR34216/AAQ/1/765/2019).

Conflicts of interest

The authors declare no conflict of interest.

References

[1] Roberts A, Chouhan RS, Shahdeo D, Shrikrishna NS, Kesarwani V, Horvat M, et al. A recent update on advanced molecular diagnostic techniques for COVID-19 pandemic: an overview. Front Immunol 2021;12. Available from: https://doi.org/10.3389/FIMMU.2021.732756.

[2] Roberts A, Mahari S, Shahdeo D, Gandhi S. Label-free detection of SARS-CoV-2 Spike S1 antigen triggered by electroactive gold nanoparticles on antibody coated fluorine-doped tin oxide (FTO) electrode. Anal Chim Acta 2021;1188:339207. Available from: https://doi.org/10.1016/J.ACA.2021.339207.

[3] Vidic J, Manzano M, Chang CM, Jaffrezic-Renault N. Advanced biosensors for detection of pathogens related to livestock and poultry Veterinary Res 2017;48(1):11BioMed Central Ltd. Available from: https://doi.org/10.1186/s13567-017-0418-5.

[4] Wang H, Naghavi M, Allen C, Barber RM, Carter A, Casey DC, et al. Global, regional, and national life expectancy, all-cause mortality, and cause-specific mortality for 249 causes of death, 1980–2015: a systematic analysis for the Global Burden of Disease Study 2015. Lancet 2016;388(10053):1459–544. Available from: https://doi.org/10.1016/S0140-6736(16)31012-1.

[5] Baek YH, Um J, Antigua KJC, Park JH, Kim Y, Oh S, et al. Development of a reverse transcription-loop-mediated isothermal amplification as a rapid early-detection method for novel SARS-CoV-2. Emerg Microbes Infect 2020;. Available from: https://doi.org/10.1080/22221751.2020.1756698.

[6] Yoo H, Jo H, Oh SS. Detection and beyond: challenges and advances in aptamer-based biosensors. Mater Adv 2020;1(8):2663–87. Available from: https://doi.org/10.1039/D0MA00639D.

[7] Banga I, Tyagi R, Shahdeo D, Gandhi S. Biosensors and their application for the detection of avian influenza virus. Nanotechnology in modern animal biotechnology. Elsevier; 2019. p. 1–16. Available from: https://doi.org/10.1016/b978-0-12-818823-1.00001-6.

[8] Kasoju A, Shrikrishna NS, Shahdeo D, Khan AA, Alanazi AM, Gandhi S. Microfluidic paper device for rapid detection of aflatoxin B1 using an aptamer based colorimetric assay. RSC Adv 2020;10(20):11843–50. Available from: https://doi.org/10.1039/d0ra00062k.

[9] Shahdeo D, Gandhi S. Next generation biosensors as a cancer diagnostic tool. Biosens Based Adv Cancer Diagn 2022;. Available from: https://doi.org/10.1016/b978-0-12-823424-2.00016-8.

[10] Rivera A, Messaoudi I. Pathophysiology of ebola virus infection: current challenges and future hopes. ACS Infect Dis 2015;1(5):186–97. Available from: https://doi.org/10.1021/ID5000426.

[11] Cui F, Zhou HS. Diagnostic methods and potential portable biosensors for coronavirus disease 2019. Biosens Bioelectron 2020;165:112349. Available from: https://doi.org/10.1016/J.BIOS.2020.112349.

[12] Nandi S, Mondal A, Roberts A, Gandhi S. Biosensor platforms for rapid HIV detection. Adv ClChem 2020;. Available from: https://doi.org/10.1016/bs.acc.2020.02.001.

[13] Roberts A, Chauhan N, Islam S, Mahari S, Ghawri B, Gandham RK, et al. Graphene functionalized field-effect transistors for ultrasensitive detection of Japanese encephalitis and Avian influenza virus. Sci Rep 2020;10(1):1–12. Available from: https://doi.org/10.1038/s41598-020-71591-w.

[14] Alharbi KK, Al-sheikh YA. Role and implications of nanodiagnostics in the changing trends of clinical diagnosis. Saudi J Biol Sci 2014;21(2):109–17. Available from: https://doi.org/10.1016/J.SJBS.2013.11.001.

[15] Debruyne EN, Delanghe JR. Diagnosing and monitoring hepatocellular carcinoma with alpha-fetoprotein: new aspects and applications. Clinica Chim Acta 2008;395(1–2):19–26. Available from: https://doi.org/10.1016/j.cca.2008.05.010.

[16] Kanji JN, Zelyas N, MacDonald C, Pabbaraju K, Khan MN, Prasad A, et al. False negative rate of COVID-19 PCR testing: a discordant testing analysis. Virol J 2021;18(1):1–6. Available from: https://doi.org/10.1186/S12985-021-01489-0.

[17] Mahari S, Prakashan D, Gandhi S, et al. Immunochromatographic assay for the point-of-care diagnosis of food borne Salmonella strains using smartphone application. Coll Surf B: Biointerfaces 2023;226:113319. Available from: https://doi.org/10.1016/j.colsurfb.2023.113319.

[18] Roberts A, Dhanaze H, Sharma GT, Gandhi S. Point-of-care detection of Japanese encephalitis virus biomarker in clinical samples using a portable smartphone-enabled electrochemical "Sensit" device. Bioeng Transl Med 2023;8:e10506. Available from: https://doi.org/10.1002/btm2.10506.

[19] Prakashan D, Narlawar SS, Byakodi M, Nagamani K, Gandhi S. Gold nanoparticle conjugate-based lateral flow immunoassay (LFIA) for rapid detection of RBD antigen of SARS-CoV-2 in clinical samples using a smartphone-based application. J Med Virol 2023;95:e28416. Available from: https://doi.org/10.1002/jmv.28416.

[20] Mohammadniaei M, Nguyen HV, Tieu MV, Lee MH. 2D materials in development of electrochemical point-of care cancer screening devices. Micromachines 2019;10(10). Available from: https://doi.org/10.3390/mi10100662 MDPI AG.

[21] Shahdeo D, Roberts A, Abbineni N, Gandhi S. Graphene based sensors. Compr Anal Chem 2020;91:175. Available from: https://doi.org/10.1016/BS.COAC.2020.08.007.

[22] Patil M, Mehta DS, Guvva S. Future impact of nanotechnology on medicine and dentistry. J Indian Soc Periodontol 2008;12(2):34. Available from: https://doi.org/10.4103/0972-124X.44088.

[23] Ashikbayeva Z, Tosi D, Balmassov D, Schena E, Saccomandi P, Inglezakis V. Application of nanoparticles and nanomaterials in thermal ablation therapy of cancer. Nanomaterials 2019 2019;9(9):1195. Available from: https://doi.org/10.3390/NANO9091195.

[24] Keshavarz M, Behpour M, Rafiee-Pour HA. Recent trends in electrochemical microRNA biosensors for early detection of cancer RSC Adv 2015;5(45):35651–60Royal Society of Chemistry. Available from: https://doi.org/10.1039/c5ra01726b.

[25] Mody VV, Siwale R, Singh A, Mody HR. Introduction to metallic nanoparticles. J Pharm Bioallied Sci 2010;2(4):282. Available from: https://doi.org/10.4103/0975-7406.72127.

[26] Baetke SC, Lammers T, Kiessling F. Applications of nanoparticles for diagnosis and therapy of cancer. Br J Radiol 2015;88(1054). Available from: https://doi.org/10.1259/BJR.20150207/ASSET/IMAGES/LARGE/BJR.20150207.G004.JPEG.
[27] Xiao L, Zhu A, Xu Q, Chen Y, Xu J, Weng J. Colorimetric biosensor for detection of cancer biomarker by Au nanoparticle-decorated Bi2Se3 nanosheets. ACS Appl Mater Interfaces 2017;9(8):6931–40. Available from: https://doi.org/10.1021/acsami.6b15750.
[28] Chen Y, Fu Y, Li X, Chen H, Wang Z, Zhang H. Peptide-functionalized NaGdF4 nanoparticles for tumor-targeted magnetic resonance imaging and effective therapy. RSC Adv 2019;9(30):17093–100. Available from: https://doi.org/10.1039/c9ra02135c.
[29] Gao J, Du B, Zhang X, Guo A, Zhang Y, Wu D, et al. Ultrasensitive enzyme-free immunoassay for squamous cell carcinoma antigen using carbon supported Pd-Au as electrocatalytic labels. Anal Chim Acta 2014;833:9–14. Available from: https://doi.org/10.1016/j.aca.2014.05.004.
[30] Goldsmith CS, Miller SE. Modern uses of electron microscopy for detection of viruses. Clin Microbiol Rev 2009;22(4):552. Available from: https://doi.org/10.1128/CMR.00027-09.
[31] Casals J, Palacios R. The complement fixation test in the diagnosis of virus infections of the central nervous system. J Exp Med 1941;74(5):409. Available from: https://doi.org/10.1084/JEM.74.5.409.
[32] Pedersen JC. Hemagglutination-inhibition assay for influenza virus subtype identification and the detection and quantitation of serum antibodies to influenza virus. Methods Mol Biol (Clifton, NJ) 2014;1161:11–25. Available from: https://doi.org/10.1007/978-1-4939-0758-8_2.
[33] Kim SJ. Drug-susceptibility testing in tuberculosis: methods and reliability of results. Eur Respir J 2005;25(3):564–9. Available from: https://doi.org/10.1183/09031936.05.00111304.
[34] Azri FA, Sukor R, Selamat J, Bakar FA, Yusof NA, Hajian R. Electrochemical immunosensor for detection of aflatoxin B 1 based on indirect competitive ELISA. Toxins 2018;10(5). Available from: https://doi.org/10.3390/toxins10050196.
[35] Souf S. Recent advances in diagnostic testing for viral infections. Biosci Horizons: Int J Stud Res 2016;9. Available from: https://doi.org/10.1093/BIOHORIZONS/HZW010.
[36] Caldas LA, Azevedo RC, da Silva JL, de Souza W. Microscopy analysis of Zika virus morphogenesis in mammalian cells. Sci Rep 2020;10(1):1–11. Available from: https://doi.org/10.1038/s41598-020-65409-y.
[37] Richert-Pöggeler KR, Franzke K, Hipp K, Kleespies RG. Electron microscopy methods for virus diagnosis and high resolution analysis of viruses. Front Microbiol 2019;10:3255. Available from: https://doi.org/10.3389/FMICB.2018.03255/BIBTEX.
[38] Leland DS, Ginocchio CC. Role of cell culture for virus detection in the age of technology. Clin Microbiol Rev 2007;20(1):49. Available from: https://doi.org/10.1128/CMR.00002-06.
[39] Jayakeerthi RS, Potula RV, Srinivasan S, Badrinath S. Shell vial culture assay for the rapid diagnosis of Japanese encephalitis, West Nile and Dengue-2 viral encephalitis. Virol J 2006;3(1):1–7. Available from: https://doi.org/10.1186/1743-422X-3-2/TABLES/2.
[40] Erlanger BF. Principles and methods for the preparation of drug protein conjugates for immunological studies. Pharmacol Rev 1973;25(2):271–80. Available from: http://www.ncbi.nlm.nih.gov/pubmed/4581044.
[41] Steingart KR, Flores LL, Dendukuri N, Schiller I, Laal S, Ramsay A, et al. Commercial serological tests for the diagnosis of active pulmonary and extrapulmonary tuberculosis: an updated systematic review and meta-analysis. PLoS Med 2011;8(8). Available from: https://doi.org/10.1371/JOURNAL.PMED.1001062.
[42] Srivastava S, Singh PK, Vatsalya V, Karch RC. Developments in the diagnostic techniques of infectious diseases: rural and urban prospective. Adv Infect Dis 2018;8(3):121–38. Available from: https://doi.org/10.4236/AID.2018.83012.
[43] Cattamanchi A, Huang L, Worodria W, Den Boon S, Kalema N, Katagira W, et al. Integrated strategies to optimize sputum smear microscopy: a prospective observational study. Am J Respir Crit Care Med 2011;183(4):547. Available from: https://doi.org/10.1164/RCCM.201008-1207OC.
[44] Cuevas LE, Al-Sonboli N, Lawson L, Yassin MA, Arbide I, Al-Aghbari N, et al. LED fluorescence microscopy for the diagnosis of pulmonary tuberculosis: a multi-country cross-sectional evaluation. PLoS Med 2011;8(7). Available from: https://doi.org/10.1371/JOURNAL.PMED.1001057.
[45] Helb D, Jones M, Story E, Boehme C, Wallace E, Ho K, et al. Rapid detection of Mycobacterium tuberculosis and rifampin resistance by use of on-demand, near-patient technology. J Clin Microbiol 2010;48(1):229–37. Available from: https://doi.org/10.1128/JCM.01463-09.

[46] Johnston SP, Pieniazek NJ, Xayavong MV, Slemenda SB, Wilkins PP, Da Silva AJ. PCR as a confirmatory technique for laboratory diagnosis of malaria. J Clin Microbiol 2006;44(3):1087. Available from: https://doi.org/10.1128/JCM.44.3.1087-1089.2006.

[47] Khairnar K, Martin D, Lau R, Ralevski F, Pillai DR. Multiplex real-time quantitative PCR, microscopy and rapid diagnostic immuno-chromatographic tests for the detection of Plasmodium spp: performance, limit of detection analysis and quality assurance. Malar J 2009;8(1). Available from: https://doi.org/10.1186/1475-2875-8-284.

[48] Lawn SD, Nicol MP. Xpert® MTB/RIF assay: development, evaluation and implementation of a new rapid molecular diagnostic for tuberculosis and rifampicin resistance. Fut Microbiol 2011;6(9):1067–82. Available from: https://doi.org/10.2217/FMB.11.84.

[49] Behjati S, Tarpey PS. What is next generation sequencing. Arch Dis Child Educ Pract Ed 2013;98(6):236. Available from: https://doi.org/10.1136/ARCHDISCHILD-2013-304340.

[50] Bremer JW, Lew JF, Cooper E, Hillyer GV, Pitt J, Handelsman E, et al. Diagnosis of infection with human immunodeficiency virus type 1 by a DNA polymerase chain reaction assay among infants enrolled in the Women and Infants' Transmission Study. J Pediatrics 1996;129(2):198–207. Available from: https://doi.org/10.1016/S0022-3476(96)70243-3.

[51] Maciej S. Synteza i aktywność biologiczna nowych analogów tiosemikarbazonowych chelatorów żelaza. Uniw Śląski 2013;343–54 https://doi.org/10.2/JQUERY.MIN.JS.

[52] Pottumarthy S, Wells VC, Morris AJ. A comparison of seven tests for serological diagnosis of tuberculosis. J Clin Microbiol 2000;38(6):2227. Available from: https://doi.org/10.1128/jcm.38.6.2227-2231.2000.

[53] Xiang DX, Chen Q, Pang L, Zheng CL. Inhibitory effects of silver nanoparticles on H1N1 influenza A virus in vitro. J Virol Methods 2011;178(1–2). Available from: https://doi.org/10.1016/j.jviromet.2011.09.003.

[54] Chou S-F, Hsu W-L, Hwang J-M, Chen C-Y. Development of an immunosensor for human ferritin, a nonspecific tumor marker, based on surface plasmon resonance. Biosens Bioelectron 2004;19(9):999–1005. Available from: https://doi.org/10.1016/j.bios.2003.09.004.

[55] Mahari S, Gandhi S. Electrochemical immunosensor for detection of avian Salmonellosis based on electroactive reduced graphene oxide (rGO) modified electrode. Bioelectrochemistry 2022;144:108036. Available from: https://doi.org/10.1016/J.BIOELECHEM.2021.108036.

[56] Roberts A, Gandhi S. Japanese encephalitis virus: a review on emerging diagnostic techniques. Front Biosci—Landmark 2020;. Available from: https://doi.org/10.2741/4882.

[57] Xu L, Li D, Ramadan S, Li Y, Klein N. Facile biosensors for rapid detection of COVID-19. Biosens Bioelectron 2020;170:112673. Available from: https://doi.org/10.1016/j.bios.2020.112673.

[58] Kawamura A, Miyata T. Biosensors. Biomaterials nanoarchitectonics 2016;157–76. Available from: https://doi.org/10.1016/B978-0-323-37127-8.00010-8.

[59] Krishnan D, Kim F, Luo J, Cruz-Silva R, Cote LJ, Jang HD, et al. Energetic graphene oxide: challenges and opportunities Nano Today 2012;7(2):137–52Elsevier. Available from: https://doi.org/10.1016/j.nantod.2012.02.003.

[60] Roberts A, Kesarwani V, Gupta R, Gandhi S. Electroactive reduced graphene oxide for highly sensitive detection of secretory non-structural 1 protein: a potential diagnostic biomarker for Japanese encephalitis virus. Biosens Bioelectron 2022;198:113837. Available from: https://doi.org/10.1016/J.BIOS.2021.113837.

[61] Singh L, Kruger HG, Maguire GEM, Govender T, Parboosing R. The role of nanotechnology in the treatment of viral infections. Ther Adv Infect Dis 2017;4(4):105. Available from: https://doi.org/10.1177/2049936117713593.

[62] Stephen Inbaraj B, Chen BH. Nanomaterial-based sensors for detection of foodborne bacterial pathogens and toxins as well as pork adulteration in meat products J. Food Drug Anal. 2016;24(1):15–28 Elsevier Taiwan LLC. Available from: https://doi.org/10.1016/j.jfda.2015.05.001.

[63] Koedrith P, Thasiphu T, Weon JI, Boonprasert R, Tuitemwong K, Tuitemwong P. Recent trends in rapid environmental monitoring of pathogens and toxicants: potential of nanoparticle-based biosensor and applications. Sci World J 2015;2015. Available from: https://doi.org/10.1155/2015/510982.

[64] Vigneshvar S, Sudhakumari CC, Senthilkumaran B, Prakash H. Recent advances in biosensor technology for potential applications—an overview. Front Bioeng Biotechnol 2016;4:11. Available from: https://doi.org/10.3389/FBIOE.2016.00011/BIBTEX.

[65] Grieshaber D, MacKenzie R, Vörös J, Reimhult E. Electrochemical biosensors - sensor principles and architectures. Sensors 2008;8(3):1400–58. Available from: https://doi.org/10.3390/S80314000.

[66] Mehrotra P. Biosensors and their applications—a review J Oral Biol Craniofacial Res 2016;6(2):153–9 Elsevier B.V. Available from: https://doi.org/10.1016/j.jobcr.2015.12.002.
[67] Peltomaa R, Glahn-Martínez B, Benito-Peña E, Moreno-Bondi MC. Optical biosensors for label-free detection of small molecules. Sensors (Basel, Switzerland) 2018;18(12). Available from: https://doi.org/10.3390/S18124126.
[68] Duffy M. The urokinase plasminogen activator system: role in malignancy. Curr Pharm Des 2004;10 (1):39–49. Available from: https://doi.org/10.2174/1381612043453559.
[69] Duffy MJ, McGowan PM, Harbeck N, Thomssen C, Schmitt M. UPA and PAI-1 as biomarkers in breast cancer: validated for clinical use in level-of-evidence-1 studies Breast Cancer Res 2014;16(4) BioMed Central Ltd. Available from: https://doi.org/10.1186/s13058-014-0428-4.
[70] Mishra GK, Sharma V, Mishra RK. Electrochemical aptasensors for food and environmental safeguarding: a review. Biosensors 2018;8(2):28. Available from: https://doi.org/10.3390/BIOS8020028.
[71] Talan A, Mishra A, Eremin SA, Narang J, Kumar A, Gandhi S. Ultrasensitive electrochemical immunosensing platform based on gold nanoparticles triggering chlorpyrifos detection in fruits and vegetables. Biosens Bioelectron 2018;105:14–21. Available from: https://doi.org/10.1016/j.bios.2018.01.013.
[72] Amiri M, Bezaatpour A, Jafari H, Boukherroub R, Szunerits S. Electrochemical methodologies for the detection of pathogens. ACS Sens 2018;3(6):1069–86. Available from: https://doi.org/10.1021/ACSSENSORS.8B00239.
[73] Furst AL, Francis MB. Impedance-based detection of bacteria. Chem Rev 2018;119(1):700–26. Available from: https://doi.org/10.1021/ACS.CHEMREV.8B00381.
[74] Yang C, Denno ME, Pyakurel P, Venton BJ. Recent trends in carbon nanomaterial-based electrochemical sensors for biomolecules: a review. Anal Chim Acta 2015;887:17–37. Available from: https://doi.org/10.1016/J.ACA.2015.05.049.
[75] Huang J, Harvey J, Fam D, Nimmo MA, Tok A. Novel biosensor for Interleukin-6 detection-review under responsibility of RMIT University. Procedia Eng 2013;60:195–200. Available from: https://doi.org/10.1016/j.proeng.2013.07.042.
[76] Baluchová S, Daňhel A, Dejmková H, Ostatná V, Fojta M, Schwarzová-Pecková K. Recent progress in the applications of boron doped diamond electrodes in electroanalysis of organic compounds and biomolecules – a review. Anal Chim Acta 2019;1077:30–66. Available from: https://doi.org/10.1016/J.ACA.2019.05.041.
[77] Bobrinetskiy II, Knezevic NZ. Graphene-based biosensors for on-site detection of contaminants in food Anal. Methods 2018;10(42):5061–70 Royal Society of Chemistry. Available from: https://doi.org/10.1039/c8ay01913d.
[78] Pumera M. Graphene in biosensing. Mater Today 2011;14(7–8):308–15. Available from: https://doi.org/10.1016/S1369-7021(11)70160-2.
[79] Raziq A, Kidakova A, Boroznjak R, Reut J, Öpik A, Syritski V. Development of a portable MIP-based electrochemical sensor for detection of SARS-CoV-2 antigen. Biosens Bioelectron 2021;178. Available from: https://doi.org/10.1016/J.BIOS.2021.113029.
[80] Djaileb A., Charron B., Jodaylami M.H., Thibault V., Coutu J., Stevenson K., et al. A rapid and quantitative serum test for SARS-CoV-2 antibodies with portable surface plasmon resonance sensing; 2020. https://doi.org/10.26434/CHEMRXIV.12118914.V1
[81] Wang N, Shang J, Jiang S, Du L. Subunit vaccines against emerging pathogenic human coronaviruses Front Microbiol 2020;11 Frontiers Media S.A. Available from: https://doi.org/10.3389/fmicb.2020.00298.
[82] Sheikhzadeh E, Eissa S, Ismail A, Zourob M. Diagnostic techniques for COVID-19 and new developments. Talanta, 220. Elsevier B.V; 2020. p. 121392. Available from: https://doi.org/10.1016/j.talanta.2020.121392.
[83] Torres MDT, de Araujo WR, de Lima LF, Ferreira AL, de la Fuente-Nunez C. Low-cost biosensor for rapid detection of SARS-CoV-2 at the point of care. Matter 2021;4(7):2403. Available from: https://doi.org/10.1016/J.MATT.2021.05.003.
[84] Liu J, Lian R, Zhang G, Hou B, Wang C, Dong J, et al. Changes in serum virus-specific IgM/IgG antibody in asymptomatic and discharged patients with reoccurring positive COVID-19 nucleic acid test (RPNAT. Ann Med 2021;53(1):34. Available from: https://doi.org/10.1080/07853890.2020.1811887.
[85] Moitra P, Alafeef M, Alafeef M, Alafeef M, Dighe K, Frieman MB, et al. Selective naked-eye detection of SARS-CoV-2 mediated by N gene targeted antisense oligonucleotide capped plasmonic nanoparticles. ACS Nano 2020;. Available from: https://doi.org/10.1021/acsnano.0c03822.

[86] Liu H, Dai E, Xiao R, Zhou Z, Zhang M, Bai Z, et al. Development of a SERS-based lateral flow immunoassay for rapid and ultra-sensitive detection of anti-SARS-CoV-2 IgM/IgG in clinical samples. Sens Actuators, B: Chem 2020;129196. Available from: https://doi.org/10.1016/j.snb.2020.129196.

[87] Yadav S, Sadique MA, Ranjan P, Kumar N, Singhal A, Srivastava AK, et al. SERS based lateral flow immunoassay for point-of-care detection of SARS-CoV-2 in clinical samples. ACS Appl Bio Mater 2021;4 (4):2974–95. Available from: https://doi.org/10.1021/ACSABM.1C00102.

[88] Seo G, Lee G, Kim MJ, Baek S-H, Choi M, Ku KB, et al. Rapid detection of COVID-19 causative virus (SARS-CoV-2) in human nasopharyngeal swab specimens using field-effect transistor-based biosensor. ACS Nano 2020;. Available from: https://doi.org/10.1021/acsnano.0c02823.

[89] Huang L, Ding L, Zhou J, Chen S, Chen F, Zhao C, et al. One-step rapid quantification of SARS-CoV-2 virus particles via low-cost nanoplasmonic sensors in generic microplate reader and point-of-care device. Biosens Bioelectron 2021;171:112685. Available from: https://doi.org/10.1016/J.BIOS.2020.112685.

[90] Narlawar S, Coudhury S, Gandhi S. Magnetic properties-based biosensors for early detection of cancer. Biosens Based Adv Cancer Diagn 2022;165–78. Available from: https://doi.org/10.1016/B978-0-12-823424-2.00010-7.

[91] Shahdeo D, Roberts A, Kesarwani V, Horvat M, Chouhan RS, Gandhi S. Polymeric biocompatible iron oxide nanoparticles labeled with peptides for imaging in ovarian cancer. Biosci Rep 2022;42(2):20212622. Available from: https://doi.org/10.1042/BSR20212622.

[92] Smith I. Mycobacterium tuberculosis pathogenesis and molecular determinants of virulence. Clin Microbiol Rev 2003;16(3):463. Available from: https://doi.org/10.1128/CMR.16.3.463-496.2003.

[93] Kyaw SP, Hanthamrongwit J, Jangpatarapongsa K, Khaenam P, Leepiyasakulchai C. Sensitive detection of the IS6110 sequence of Mycobacterium tuberculosis complex based on PCR-magnetic bead ELISA. RSC Adv 2018;8(59):33674–80. Available from: https://doi.org/10.1039/C8RA06599C.

[94] Seifert M, Vargas E, Ruiz-Valdepeñas Montiel V, Wang J, Rodwell TC, Catanzaro A. Detection and quantification of *Mycobacterium tuberculosis* antigen CFP10 in serum and urine for the rapid diagnosis of active tuberculosis disease. Sci Rep 2021;11(1):1–10. Available from: https://doi.org/10.1038/s41598-021-98471-1.

[95] Getahun H, Harrington M, O'Brien R, Nunn P. Diagnosis of smear-negative pulmonary tuberculosis in people with HIV infection or AIDS in resource-constrained settings: informing urgent policy changes. Lancet 2007;369(9578):2042–9. Available from: https://doi.org/10.1016/s0140-6736(07)60284-0.

[96] The Lancet Infectious Diseases. Tuberculosis and malaria in the age of COVID-19. Lancet Infect Dis 2021;21 (1):1. Available from: https://doi.org/10.1016/s1473-3099(20)30946-4.

[97] Sarro DSY, Kone B, Diarra B, Kumar A, Kodio O, Fofana B, et al. Simultaneous diagnosis of tuberculous and non-tuberculous mycobacterial diseases: time for a better patient management. Clin Microbiol Infect Dis 2018;3(3):1. Available from: https://doi.org/10.15761/cmid.1000144.

[98] He X, Zhou L, He D, Wang K, Qin D. Biosensing technologies for mycobacterium tuberculosis detection: status and new developments. Clin Dev Immunol 2011;2011. Available from: https://doi.org/10.1155/2011/193963.

[99] Pai M, Schito M. Tuberculosis diagnostics in 2015: landscape, priorities, needs, and prospects. J Infect Dis 2015;211:S21–8. Available from: https://doi.org/10.1093/infdis/jiu803.

[100] Chouhan RS, Horvat M, Ahmed J, Alhokbany N, Alshehri SM, Gandhi S. Magnetic nanoparticles—a multifunctional potential agent for diagnosis and therapy. Cancers 2021;13(9):2213. Available from: https://doi.org/10.3390/cancers13092213 MDPI AG.

[101] Díaz-González M, González-García MB, Costa-García A. Immunosensor for Mycobacterium tuberculosis on screen-printed carbon electrodes. Biosens Bioelectron 2005;20(10):2035–43. Available from: https://doi.org/10.1016/J.BIOS.2004.09.035.

[102] Sepulveda D, Aroca MA, Varela A, Portillo PD, Osma JF. Bioelectrochemical detection of Mycobacterium tuberculosis ESAT-6 in an antibody-based biomicrosystem. Sensors 2017;17(10):2178. Available from: https://doi.org/10.3390/S17102178.

[103] Liu C, Zhao Z, Fan J, Lyon CJ, Wu HJ, Nedelkov D, et al. Quantification of circulating Mycobacterium tuberculosis antigen peptides allows rapid diagnosis of active disease and treatment monitoring. Proc Natl Acad Sci U S A 2017;114(15):3969–74. Available from: https://doi.org/10.1073/PNAS.1621360114/-/DCSUPPLEMENTAL.

[104] Ragavan KV, Kumar S, Swaraj S, Neethirajan S. Advances in biosensors and optical assays for diagnosis and detection of malaria. Biosens Bioelectron 2018;105:188–210. Available from: https://doi.org/10.1016/J.BIOS.2018.01.037.

[105] De Souza Castilho M, Laube T, Yamanaka H, Alegret S, Pividori MI. Magneto immunoassays for plasmodium falciparum histidine-rich protein 2 related to malaria based on magnetic nanoparticles. Anal Chem 2011;83 (14):5570–7. Available from: https://doi.org/10.1021/AC200573S/SUPPL_FILE/AC200573S_SI_001.PDF.

[106] Álvarez DM, Castillo E, Duarte LF, Arriagada J, Corrales N, Farías MA, et al. Current antivirals and novel botanical molecules interfering with herpes simplex virus infection. Front Microbiol 2020;11. Available from: https://doi.org/10.3389/fmicb.2020.00139.

[107] Ding X, Yin K, Li Z, Liu C. All-in-one dual CRISPR-Cas12a (AIOD-CRISPR) assay: a case for rapid, ultrasensitive and visual detection of novel coronavirus SARS-CoV-2 and HIV virus. BioRxiv 2020;. Available from: https://doi.org/10.1101/2020.03.19.998724 2020.03.19.998724.

[108] Islam S, Shukla S, Bajpai VK, Han YK, Huh YS, Kumar A, et al. A smart nanosensor for the detection of human immunodeficiency virus and associated cardiovascular and arthritis diseases using functionalized graphene-based transistors. Biosens Bioelectron 2019;126:792–9. Available from: https://doi.org/10.1016/j.bios.2018.11.041.

[109] Ramana LN, Sharma S, Sethuraman S, Ranga U, Krishnan UM. Evaluation of chitosan nanoformulations as potent anti-HIV therapeutic systems. Biochim Biophys Acta—Gen Subj 2014;1840(1). Available from: https://doi.org/10.1016/j.bbagen.2013.10.002.

[110] Awofala AA, Ogundele OE. HIV epidemiology in Nigeria. Saudi J Biol Sci 2018;25(4):697–703. Available from: https://doi.org/10.1016/J.SJBS.2016.03.006.

[111] Lifson MA, Ozen MO, Inci F, Wang SQ, Inan H, Baday M, et al. Advances in biosensing strategies for HIV detection, diagnosis, and therapeutic monitoring. Adv Drug Deliv Rev 2016;103:90. Available from: https://doi.org/10.1016/J.ADDR.2016.05.018.

[112] Gray ER, Turbé V, Lawson VE, Page RH, Cook ZC, Ferns RB, et al. Ultra-rapid, sensitive and specific digital diagnosis of HIV with a dual-channel SAW biosensor in a pilot clinical study. NPJ Digital Med 2018;1 (1):1–8. Available from: https://doi.org/10.1038/s41746-018-0041-5.

[113] Huertas CS, Calvo-Lozano O, Mitchell A, Lechuga LM. Advanced evanescent-wave optical biosensors for the detection of nucleic acids: an analytic perspective Front Chem 2019;7:724 Frontiers Media S.A. Available from: https://doi.org/10.3389/fchem.2019.00724.

[114] Duffy GF, Moore EJ. Electrochemical immunosensors for food analysis: a review of recent developments. Anal Lett 2016;50(1):1–32. Available from: https://doi.org/10.1080/00032719.2016.1167900.

[115] Jugessur AS, Dou J, Aitchison JS, De La Rue RM, Gnan M. A photonic nano-Bragg grating device integrated with microfluidic channels for bio-sensing applications. Microelectr Eng 2009;86(4–6):1488–90. Available from: https://doi.org/10.1016/j.mee.2008.12.002.

[116] Mahendra Wijaya IP, Nie TJ, Gandhi S, Boro R, Palaniappan A, Hau GW, et al. Femtomolar detection of 2,4-dichlorophenoxyacetic acid herbicides via competitive immunoassays using microfluidic based carbon nanotube liquid gated transistor. Lab a Chip 2010;10(5):634–8. Available from: https://doi.org/10.1039/b918566f.

CHAPTER

12

Fundamentals of a targeted drug delivery system

Akash Chaurasiya[1], Sonali Singh[1], Kanan Panchal[1], Rishi Paliwal[2] and Akanksha Malaiya[2]

[1]Translational Pharmaceutics Research Laboratory, Department of Pharmacy, Birla Institute of Technology and Science, Pilani, Hyderabad, Telangana, India [2]Nanomedicine and Bioengineering Research Laboratory, Department of Pharmacy, Indira Gandhi National Tribal University, Amarkantak, Madhya Pradesh, India

Abbreviations

TDDS	Targeted drug delivery systems
DDS	Drug delivery systems
NP	Nanoparticle
PNP	Polymeric nanoparticles
NLC	Nanostructured lipid carriers
SLN	Solid lipid nanoparticles
RES	Reticuloendothelial system
USFDA	United States Food and Drug Administration
EPR	Enhanced permeability and retention

12.1 Introduction

Delivering drugs in a precise and accurate manner and the technology associated with them have always been cumbersome and challenging in the pharmaceutical research field. The idea of targeted drug delivery was first introduced by Paul Ehrlich, who termed it "magic bullet." It was conceptualized that the drug for the marked pharmacological action should be delivered at a specific site of action so as to minimize the undesirable toxicity and an optimal dose of the drug should be delivered, which cannot be achieved by using the traditional drug delivery systems (DDS). The most ideal condition is to deliver the drug directly to its target cell/tissue/organ in desired

Molecular Pharmaceutics and Nano Drug Delivery
DOI: https://doi.org/10.1016/B978-0-323-91924-1.00007-1

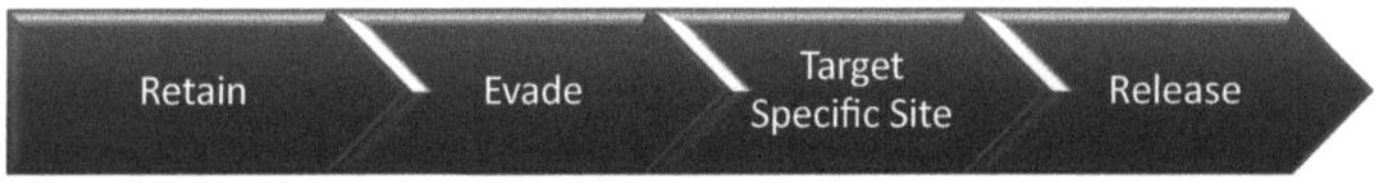

FIGURE 12.1 Mechanism of drug release.

concentrations. There are several pharmaceutical formulations employing the use of targeted DDS (TDDS) to deliver an accurate dose of a drug to the specific site to achieve a desirable pharmacological action [1].

The application of nanotechnology in DDS can improve drug solubility and distribution in various tissues and organs, obtain controlled or sustained release profiles, and promote the aggregation of drug molecules at a specific site of action [2]. There are several challenges while developing these targeted nano-sized DDS. After development, only a few enter the clinical trial, and a handful are approved. Also, the scale-up of such formulations is quite challenging. Despite these difficulties, there are several advantages of TDDS for better drug delivery, dose-effectiveness, and less toxic effects [3].

The overall function and performance of TDDS depend on four key requirements, viz, retain, evade, target, and release (Fig. 12.1). The challenging part while developing these DDS is to retain their contents (encapsulated/associated material) during preparation, processing, and final intended application. It should be able to evade the body's defense to reach the disease area. TDDS, either passively or actively through specific methods, provide high accumulation of drug substances at a specific target site, while avoiding healthy tissues and organs. Ultimately, the drug from the system must be released at the desired site of action and give a desirable and effective pharmacological action. There are different DDS intended for various sites of action as well as for differing therapeutic effects [4].

The need for targeted drug delivery over conventional DDS is because of the unsatisfactory performance of the drug concerning its pharmacodynamic, pharmacokinetic, pharmaceutical, and pharmacotherapeutic properties. Targeting drugs to a particular site of action through optimization of the DDS is not only important in enhancing the therapeutic efficacy but also in reducing toxicity and other side effects associated with the high doses and small therapeutic index. Thus, targeting is required to achieve solutions to these constraints and to overcome the innate disadvantages of conventional DDS [5]. Although parenteral drug delivery is highly invasive, oral delivery cannot be preferred to deliver pH-sensitive drugs and biologics like proteins, peptides, and other enzymes.

Supplying a high concentration of the medicine to the targeted site while bypassing the nontargeted area is the fundamental idea behind drug targeting. By reducing the side effects brought on by multiple site interactions, larger dosages, and nontarget concentrations, this approach helps to maximize the therapeutic effect of the medicines. Targeting also reduces drug interactions that are undesirable and affect the drug's ability to reach the targeted areas in the body [6]. Coordinated drug behavior, a targeted area, and a pharmaceutical carrier are key components of TDDS. The target is the particular organ, cell, or group of cells that the medicine will interact with when they are in a chronic or acute state [7]. The carrier is a carefully designed system that is necessary for the efficient delivery of the loaded medicine to the desired area. A drug-targeting complex should ideally be biochemically inert, biocompatible, nonimmunogenic, biodegradable, and physically and chemically stable both in vivo and in vitro. It should also be relatively easy to prepare, have a predictable and regulated pattern of drug release, be easy to eliminate from the body, and have little to no drug leakage while in transit [8].

12.2 Approaches for drug delivery

Drug delivery is a method to deliver the pharmaceutical dosage to the human body to achieve a certain desirable therapeutic effect. Various delivery system approaches are used to deliver the drug to the target site. By designing efficient dosage forms, one can deliver the drug to the human body and can minimize its toxic effects. Due to the versatility in the nature of the active molecules such as therapeutic enzymes, proteins, peptides, antibodies, and small molecules, optimization of these dosage forms is required. Innovative designs in drug delivery approaches improve the physical properties, therapeutic efficacy, and bioavailability of the drug molecule and reduce/mitigate the toxicity of these substances [1]. Table 12.1 describes different types of TDDS and their salient features.

12.3 Mechanism of drug targeting

There are many strategies by which drug molecules can be targeted to a certain site so that the toxic and other side effects can be mitigated (Fig. 12.2). Drug targeting can be further categorized into three orders of targeting. The drug carrier system's distribution to the target organ or tissue is constrained in first-order targeting. The second order is the selective targeting of a particular cell or cell type of a specific tissue or organ. Drugs that target macromolecules like DNA, proteins, and other intracellular components of the cell are designated under third-order targeting [18].

12.3.1 Passive targeting

In the passive targeting method, the body's natural reaction to the physicochemical properties of the drug or drug carrier system results in drug targeting. It relies on physiological body features such as the reticuloendothelial system (RES), monocyte–macrophage system, and the enhanced permeation and retention (EPR) effect [19]. In this method, nanocarriers are utilized to carry drugs and are designed meticulously to enter blood vessels at the disease area from the systemic circulation, creating the potential for large drug accumulation at the target site. The EPR effect, which causes sluggish lymphatic drainage, facilitates this procedure [20].

12.3.2 Active targeting

Active targeting is based on imposing targeting properties to the drug intrinsically (drug designed to target a specific molecule) and/or extrinsically (drug designed with certain targeting features, physical targeting programmed released at a certain temperature or pH,

TABLE 12.1 Different types of targeted drug delivery system, their components, uses, and special properties.

Types of TDDS	Components used	Uses	Special properties	References
Liposomes	Phospholipids dispersed in aqueous solution	Oral, topical and pulmonary targeted drug delivery	Unstable, requires special preparation and storage conditions	[9]
Niosomes	Cholesterol, charged substances, nonionic surfactants	Carrier for lipophilic and amphiphilic drugs	Stable, does not require special preparation and storage conditions	[10]
Transferosomes	Surfactants, alcohol, dye, phosphatidylcholine in buffer solution	Transdermal delivery for deeper penetration into epidermic layers	Ultraflexible and deformable vesicles	[11]
Polymeric nanoparticles	Polymer, drug, surfactant	Controlled release, improved in vivo and in vitro drug stability, enhanced therapeutic index and bioavailability	Facile synthesis, biocompatible, nontoxic, nonimmunogenic, biodegradable, inexpensive	[12]
Solid lipid nanoparticles	Lipid, surfactant, aqueous phase	Encapsulated drug, vitamins, xenobiotics	Nanosize, high drug loading, low toxicity and stability while production	[13]
Albumin nanoparticles	Albumin (protein), drug, surfactant	Drug delivery to different cancers	Biodegradability, biocompatibility, and favorable toxicological profiles	[14]
Nanocrystals	Lipid, polymer surfactant	Used to absorb poorly water-soluble drug quickly	Composed of 100% drug and no carrier material is used	[15]
Nanoemulsions	Oil phase, aqueous phase, surfactant	Used to deliver both hydrophilic as well as lipophilic drug for diseases like cancer	Greater surface area provides greater bioabsorption	[16]
Dendrimers	Drug, polymer	Used to deliver or carry drug molecules, peptides and genes	Higher branching and surface area, increased drug bioavailability	[17]

and ligand-based approach). Delivering drug molecules, theragnostic agents, and genes at the desired site of action while avoiding healthy tissues will reduce side effects and toxicity and will increase therapeutic effectiveness [21]. Comparing active targeting to passively targeted nanosystems, the amount of drug supplied to the target cell can be greatly increased. After aggregation in the tumor region, presumed active targeting can even boost the drug's effectiveness. This is accomplished by functionalizing the surfaces of the nanocarriers with ligands in order for them to bind to the receptors that are overexpressed on the tumor cells to achieve targeting. It is a specific ligand–receptor type interaction that happens following extravasation from the blood circulation [22]. This strategy increases the nanocarriers'

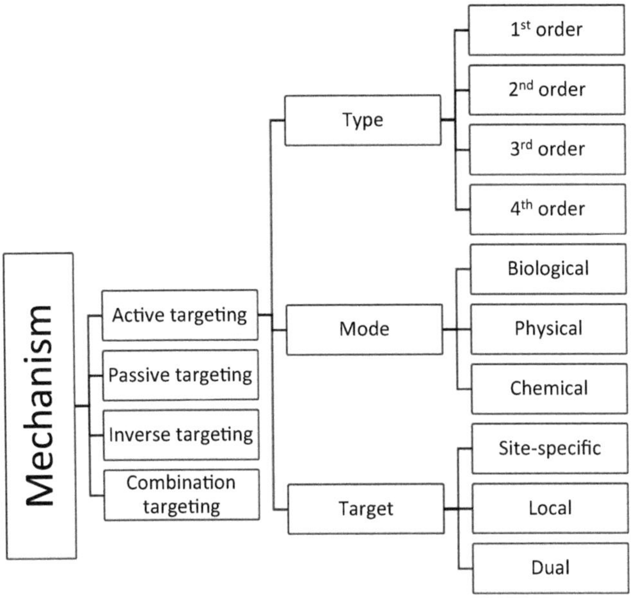

FIGURE 12.2 Mechanism of drug targeting.

affinity to the surface of cancer cells and hence increases drug penetration. Receptors like transferrin receptor and nicotinic acetylcholine receptor are examples of classical targets that enable the drug to reach the tumor microenvironment [23,24].

12.3.3 Inverse targeting

Inverse targeting can be achieved by blockage or saturation of passive targets or by blocking RES using sugar polymer or lipid micromolecules. Delivery of a carrier molecule having therapeutic activity itself is known as dual targeting, which synergistically enhances the efficacy of the drug. In the case of double targeting, geographical and temporal methodologies, viz, the placement of information in precise locations and the controlled delivery of time, are merged. Combination targeting is a method of directly approaching a target with drug-equipped polymers, carriers, and homing devices with molecular specificity [25].

12.4 Targeted drug delivery systems

Nanotechnology is a promising approach for drug delivery via different routes of administration. These are proven, reliable, and efficient systems for targeted drug delivery during many life-threatening diseases [26]. The application of nanotechnology as magic bullets in the delivery of actives to the brain, cancers, ocular sites, topical, transdermal, and so forth provides a new domain to the existing therapeutic regimen [27,28]. Table 12.2 enlists various nanostructured carrier systems used through different routes of

TABLE 12.2 Application of nanocarriers in targeted drug delivery.

Carrier	Therapeutic agent	Disease	Route	Application: Features/property	References
NLC	Meropenem	Soft tissue infection	Topical	Enhanced adhesion property, occlusion and sustained release	[31]
Hyaluronic acid NPs	Methotrexate	Breast cancer	Systemic delivery—IV	Sustained and prolonged release, reduced toxicity	[32]
Chitosan NPs	Doxorubicin	Breast cancer	Intracellular delivery	Increased potency of anticancer activity on MCF-cell lines	[33]
Nanogel	Diacerein	Arthritis	Topical	Overcomes drawback of the oral route, highly efficient, sustained and targeted release	[34]
Silver NPs	*Plectranthus barbatus*	Anti-oxidant activity	–	Free radical scavenging activity	[35]
NLC	Zopiclone	Insomnia	Nasal	Nose-to-brain delivery, faster and higher uptake	[36]
NLC	Docetaxel	Glioblastoma	Brain delivery	Sustained release, improved brain targeting action and potent anticancer activity	[37]
Chitosan NPs	Tedizolid Phosphate	Methicillin-resistant *Staphylococcus aureus* related ocular and orbital infection	Ocular	2.4-fold increase in trans corneal flux and apparent permeation, nonirritant properties	[38]
Micelles	Posaconazole	Ocular irritation and antifungal activity	Ocular delivery	Effective and safe delivery	[39]
PAMAM dendrimers	Docetaxel	Metastatic breast cancer	Cancer delivery	Sustained and controlled delivery, also used in chemophotothermal therapy	[40]
Nanoemulsion gel	Methotrexate	Local treatment for skin diseases	Topical	Higher penetration, optimum release and retention at the disease site	[41]
Microemulsions	Acemetacin	Analgesic and antiinflammatory	Transdermal	Higher penetration and significant analgesic and antiinflammatory effect	[42]
Liposomes containing in-Situ gel	Sumatriptan succinate	Migraine	Nasal	Nose-to-brain delivery, sustained impact on drug delivery, reduced toxicity	[43]

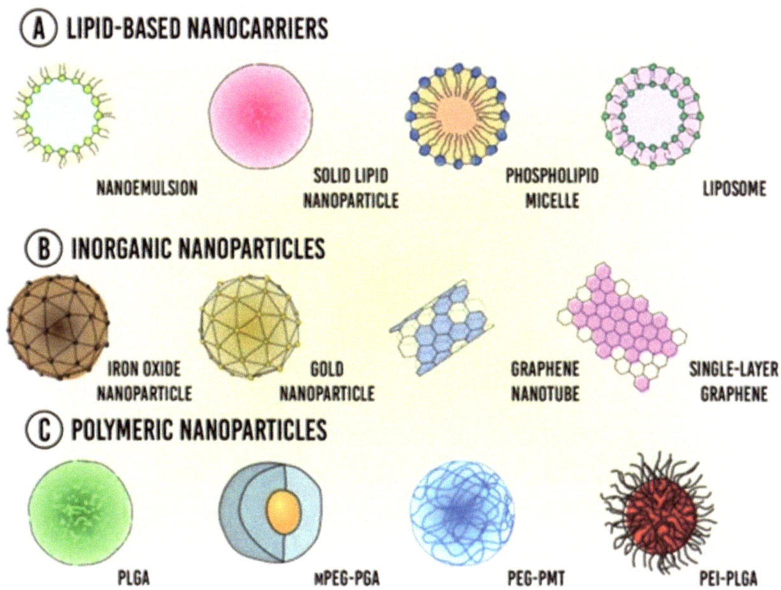

FIGURE 12.3 Different types of nanocarriers used for targeted drug delivery [44]. Source: *Reprinted from Lôbo GC, Paiva KL, Silva AL, Simões MM, Radicchi MA, Báo SN. Nanocarriers used in drug delivery to enhance immune system in cancer therapy. Pharmaceutics. 2021 Jul 28;13(8):1167. https://www.mdpi.com/1999-4923/13/8/1167. Copyright © 2021, The Author(s).*

administration for diverse therapeutic applications. Besides the ones enlisted, nanocarriers such as transferosomes, ethosomes, magnetic nanoparticles, carbon nanotubes, magnetic nanoparticles, and so on are also employed for biomedical applications [29]. Fig. 12.3 illustrates various nanocarrier systems employed for the purpose of targeted drug delivery. However, nanocarriers injected by these routes need to fulfill some primary requisites of being biodegradable, biocompatible, nonimmunogenic, as well as physically stable in vivo which is essential for it to be safe and efficacious. These must be developed in a way suitable for scaling-up and large-scale production, which makes the product useful for a clinical setup [3,30].

The drug can be loaded into polymeric nanoparticles (PNPs), which range in size from 1 to 1000 nm and can be made of natural or synthetic polymers. The drug may also be adsorbed or chemically attached to the surface of the PNP. The central matrix is made up of a variety of biodegradable polymers, including poly(lactic acid) (PLA), poly(lactic-coglycolic acid), poly(e-caprolactone) (PCL), chitosan, poly(alkyl cyanoacrylate), and poly (lysine). Typically, these are made from preformed polymers or by polymerizing monomers like alkyl cyanoacrylates and other similar substances. PNPs have drawn scientists to study drug compounds that target the brain [45,46]. Using biodegradable PNPs is one of the potential methods for delivering actives to the CNS, cancer, topical regions, and other areas. These are additionally being used as possible DDS because of their potential use throughout gene therapy, peptide, and protein delivery, as well as drug targeting to specific organs and tissues. In addition to recently created synthetic and semisynthetic polymers, natural polymers like chitosan, gelatin, sodium alginates, and others are still used in the development of novel DDS [45,46].

Advantages of PNPs

- Provide targeted and sustained drug delivery.
- Enhance the stability of any volatile pharmaceutical agents.
- Facile and economical large-scale fabrication by a multitude of methods.
- Significant improvement over traditional oral and intravenous methods of administration with respect to their efficiency and effectiveness.
- Ability to choose polymer and/or their combination to modify the release of drugs from PNPs to obtain a desirable pattern of drug release.
- Can be used for other activities related to drug delivery, such as tissue engineering.

12.4.1 Dendrimers

Nanomaterials called dendrimers are useful for therapeutic and diagnostic reasons. They have a peculiar tree-like structure and exhibit a variety of appealing qualities. They are especially appropriate for biomedical uses due to their monodispersity and tunable characteristics. The readily available polyamidoamine (PAMAM) dendrimers' properties, such as their surface charge or lipophilicity, could be simply tuned. The use of dendrimers is extensive in a variety of biological and diagnostic uses, including the delivery of drugs and genes, biosensing, the use of contrast agents, and so forth [47].

12.4.2 Liposomes

Amphipathic phospholipids are organized into circular bilayers called liposomes. Three distinct liposomal systems have been recognized by the New York Academy of Science since 1997: multilamellar (100 nm–20 mm), small unilamellar (10–50 nm), and large unilamellar (50–1000 nm) vesicles. The vesicles can contain various varieties of therapeutic molecules. The interior aqueous phase and lipid bilayer of liposomes, which are hydrophilic and hydrophobic substances, correspondingly [48,49].

12.4.3 Solid lipid nanoparticles

Solid lipid nanoparticles (SLNs), which are stabilized by different surfactants, are particles composed of highly purified solid lipids such as triglycerides, complex glyceride mixtures, or waxes. SLNs are made up of a solid hydrophobic lipid core that is comparatively rigid and solid at body and room temperatures. Physical stability, preserving incorporated drugs from deterioration, controlled drug release, and in vivo tolerability are the distinguishing features of SLNs. The low loading capacity, which is reliant on the drug's solubility in the lipid and the structure and polymorphic state of the lipid matrix, drug expulsion after crystallization, and comparatively high water content of the dispersion are other drawbacks that have been noted [50]. They are encircled by a phospholipid monolayer, which is further secured by the presence of significant amounts of surfactants. They are much less deleterious than polymer or ceramic nanoparticles due to their biodegradability. They can be produced with one of three hydrophobic core designs, a homogenous matrix, a drug-enriched shell, or a drug-enriched core, and have controllable pharmacokinetic characteristics. The shelf-life of SLN formulations is increased by the fact that they have been designed to be robust for a few years. Their tendency to be recognized by the RES still represents a significant limitation.

12.4.4 Nanostructured lipid carriers

Solid and liquid lipids are combined to create nanostructured lipid carriers (NLCs), a unique nanostructure with greater payload, smaller particle size, and resistance to drug expulsion. This process also creates a special nanostructure that is used to deliver drugs. They are reasonably simple to formulate and produce, and they can accommodate both hydrophilic and lipophilic pharmaceuticals. NLCs are second-generation lipid-based nanoparticles designed to overcome problems of entrapment efficiency and drug expulsion during storage encountered with SLNs [31]. NLCs possess greater flexibility for achieving the required release profiles and remain in an amorphous state even after solidification. These carrier systems are biocompatible, biodegradable, and employed for quick absorption [51,52].

12.4.5 Polymeric micelles

Polymeric micelles are formed by the spontaneous association of amphiphilic copolymers in an aqueous phase [53]. This property thus becomes an innovative tool to overcome various problems such as low water solubility and poor drug permeability. The key features of micelles such as size (diameter not exceeding 100 nm), size distribution, drug loading, and kinetics of drug release are critical for effective drug delivery [54]. The interaction between the hydrophobic and electrostatically neutral components of the commonly used copolymers, such as PLA, PCL, poly(L-amino acid):poly(aspartic acid) (PAsp), and phospholipids:phosphatidylethanolamine, results in the attractive force that causes micellization [55,56]. However, the compromised stability of the polymeric micelles compared to other lipidic and PNPs needs further developmental research [57].

12.5 Targeted drug delivery systems for the management of different disorders

Targeted drug delivery is described as a drug carrier complex/conjugate that delivers the drug exclusively to the preselected target cells in a specific manner. Drug targeting is the delivery of a drug to receptors or organs or any other specific part of the body, to which one aims to deliver the drug exclusively [2]. Over the years, there have been several medicines developed based on targeted nanotechnology that have been in clinical usage (Fig. 12.4). The drug's therapeutic index, as measured by its

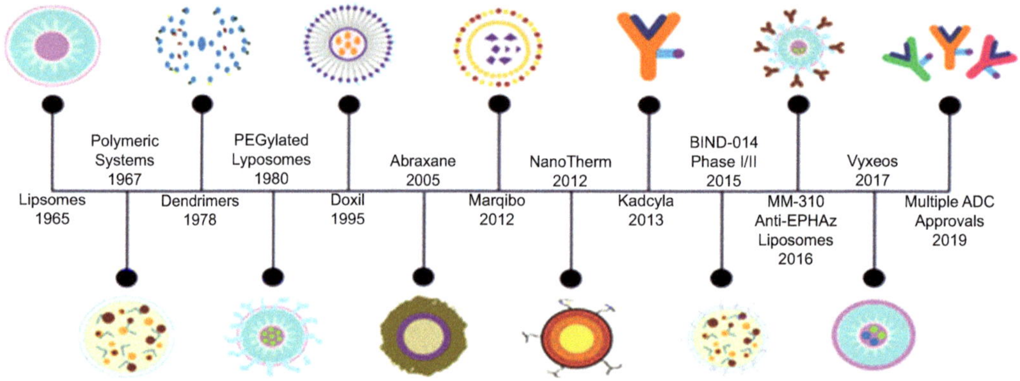

FIGURE 12.4 Timeline of the development of carrier-mediated agents [59]. Source: *Reprinted from Piscatelli JA, Ban J, Lucas AT, Zamboni WC. Complex factors and challenges that affect the pharmacology, safety and efficacy of nanocarrier drug delivery systems. Pharmaceutics. 2021;13(1):114. https://doi.org/10.3390/pharmaceutics13010114. (under the terms and conditions of the Creative Commons Attribution (CC BY) license).*

TABLE 12.3 Clinically approved nanotechnology-based product for targeted drug delivery application.

Trade name	Active drug/delivery system	Application
Invega Sustena®	Paliperidone palmitate/ nanocrystal	Schizophrenia
Diprivan®	Propofol/lipid emulsion	Anesthetic
Vyxeos®	Cytarabine and daeunorubicin/ liposomes	Acute myeloid leukemia
Doxil®/ Caelyx®	Doxorubicin/liposomes	Metastatic ovarian cancer and advanced Kaposi's sarcoma
Ambisome®	Amphotericin B/liposomes	Fungal infection
Onivyde®	Irinotecan/liposomes	Pancreatic cancer
Marqibo®	Vincristine sulfate/liposomes	Acute lymphoblastic leukemia
Abraxane®	Paclitaxel/nanosuspension	Metastatic breast cancer, non-small-cell lung cancer, pancreatic adenocarcinoma

pharmacological response and safety, relies upon the access and specific interaction of the drug with its corresponding receptor, while minimizing its interaction with nontarget tissue [58]. This targeted delivery would bypass the rest of the body, thus significantly reducing the overall toxicity while maintaining the therapeutic benefits of the drug. Table 12.3 enlists clinically approved nanotechnology based TDDS for the treatment of various diseases.

12.5.1 Brain delivery

Unlike other tissues, the blood–brain barrier (BBB) shields the brain from injuries. The BBB acts as the primary barrier to the entry of potentially harmful endogenous and exogenous molecules from the bloodstream, but it also creates an important challenge for the treatment of brain tumors. The BBB is composed of astrocytes' feet, pericytes, a basement membrane, and rigid junctions between endothelial cells [60]. The blood–cerebrospinal fluid barrier is the second barrier that hinders therapeutic drugs administered systemically from passing. Due to the BBB's complexity and structure, delivering drugs, diagnostic tools, and immunomodulators into the CNS and enabling them to pass through is not an easy task. Bevacizumab (for brain cancer) and natalizumab (for multiple sclerosis) failed clinical trials in people with acute dementia because of their inability to cross BBB. Therefore, the US Food and Drug Administration did not authorize biologicals for CNS disorders until 2019. A third obstacle to the delivery of therapeutic agents is the blood–tumor barrier within the tumor. The tight junctions of endothelial cells in the tumor are severely weakened, in contrast to normal brain capillaries. Drug penetration from the circulation into the tumor is constrained by the high intratumoral interstitial pressure produced by the leaky tumor vasculature. Additionally, the presence of various tumor microvessel populations and spatial variation in the capillary functions in the tumor region led to fluctuations in infiltration [26]. For instance, this might result in a heterogeneous distribution of drug molecules, which could potentially affect therapeutic outcomes. The BBB can be passed by passive diffusion for small molecules with a low molecular weight (less than 400–500 Da) and a high lipid partition coefficient. Consequently, it is crucial to obtain safe and efficient therapy through the delivery of pharmaceutically active compounds to specific sites in order to treat neurodegenerative diseases [61].

According to a published research, double emulsion solvent evaporation was used to create dopamine nanoparticles of borneol and lactoferrin for the treatment of Parkinson's disease. When compared to free dopamine, polymer-encapsulated dopamine formulation demonstrated less toxicity in an in vitro cytotoxicity study on SH-SY5Y and 16HBE cells [62]. In a related research, frovatriptan succinate polymeric NPs were developed for nasal delivery to the brain. Smooth NPs with a zeta potential of -35.17 ± 0.07 mV and a particle size of 264.4 ± 0.04 nm were produced using the double emulsification technique. An ex vivo diffusion investigation on goat nasal mucosa revealed that PNPs penetrated the mucosa about three times as quickly as pure drug solution. Fluorescence microscopy was used to show that PNPs were delivered to the brain in male Wistar rats after intranasal administration [63].

12.5.2 Cancer delivery

Cancer presents an imminent danger to life and has a poor prognosis. It is a pathophysiologically diverse disease that quickly progresses after onset into an uncontrollable stage [64]. For the majority of cancers, multimodality strategies like chemotherapy, radiotherapy, and surgical resection continue to be used as first-line treatment option. The two main types of chemotherapy used to treat various cancers are cytotoxic and cytostatic agents [65]. Direct tumor cell death, antiangiogenesis, prodifferentiation, disruption of growth factor pathways, and suppression of tumor invasion are all components of these drugs' mechanisms. Conventional chemotherapy is the major strategy causing undesirable side effects to the healthy tissue due to the nontargeting mechanism causing severe toxicity to normal cells. Additionally, because of their inherent properties like poor aqueous solubility, the requirement of high doses, inadequacy to attain desirable drug concentration in tumor or cancer cells, nonspecific biodistribution and development of multiple drug resistance make their use even more cumbersome [66]. Unconventional therapies such as photodynamic therapy, gene therapy, hormone therapy, and immunotherapy are potential adjuvant treatments that have shown promise in clinical trials for eradicating cancer [67]. The range of therapeutic agents including antibodies, genetic material, and photosensitizers, has been expanded by these additive treatments. Drug distribution is still a problem when treating cancer. In addition to complementing traditional chemotherapy and radiotherapy, the more recent methods of cancer treatment also avoid harming healthy tissues and preventing drug resistance. The use of nanotechnology for delivering these chemotherapeutics and other pharmaceutical actives to various cancers helps to improve their pharmacokinetic properties and solubility, reduce in vivo metabolism, prolong plasma half-life, and so on [64]. It also helps the drug to reach tumor tissue by passing through the discontinuous fenestrations in the endothelial layer and by evading circulation in the tumor microenvironment. In contrast to other normal tissue, which is surrounded by endothelial cells with tight junctions and functioning lymphatic drainage, they also primarily accumulate in the interstitial fluid of the tumor [68]. These properties act as a magic bullet to reduce the toxicity to the normal tissue compared to conventional drug treatment and provide beneficial effects to the patients by enhancing the permeability and retention effect [69].

In a research, an NLC gel of quercetin and resveratrol was produced with a particle size of 191 $\pm$5.20 nm, a zeta potential of -10.00 ± 0.30 mV, and an entrapment efficiency of 92.85% $\pm$ 0.25% to enhance their deposition in dermal and epidermal layers. NLC gel could be used as a potential carrier for the delivery of quercetin and resveratrol into the deeper layers of the skin as a result of a cytotoxicity research on human epidermoid carcinoma (A431) cell line by MTT assay. This would be a hopeful formulation for the treatment of skin cancer [70].

12.5.3 Ocular delivery

The limitations of traditional ocular therapy are overcome by nanocarriers, which also offer novel utility with increased therapeutic efficacy. Various nanocarriers have currently been designed for use in ocular applications. These extend ocular residence duration as well. Nanocarriers' surface charge and size are crucial for their fusion and retention at the target location [71].

Zeta potential is used to determine surface charge. The cornea and conjunctiva in ophthalmic delivery have a negative charge on their surfaces; as a result, the cationic NP is attracted to the anionic biomembrane through electrostatic interactions. This results in topical drug transport to the anterior segment of the eye and the retention of cationic NP on the negatively charged ocular tissues. The anionic NPs can diffuse into the retina, whereas the cationic NPs cause NPs to concentrate in different areas of the eye without doing so. These nanocarriers can transport therapeutics to the desired site despite ocular barriers, thanks to their nanosize and surface properties [72]. There are currently a few nanostructured ophthalmic products on the market, including Cyclokat® (a cationic nanoemulsion of cyclosporine A),

Cequa® (an ophthalmic nanomicellar solution of cyclosporine A), Visudyne® (a liposomal injection of verteporfin), and Artelac® Rebalance (Vitamin B12 liposomal eye drops). Due to the fact that they are biodegradable, biocompatible, safe, and efficient, these products are used to alleviate dry eye syndrome. Latanoprost and thymoquinone liposomes were prepared through studies using the thin film hydration technique to treat glaucoma. When compared to the test formulations, in vivo studies revealed that the drug-loaded liposomes substantially reduced intraocular pressure by up to 84 hours [73]. Another research developed betaxolol hydrochloride-loaded montmorillonite-chitosan nanoparticles with mean particle sizes of 460 nm and surface charges of 29 mV. This study showed that these chitosan NPs had a longer residence time and were more bioavailable on the corneal surface, suggesting that the current treatment method could be improved [74].

12.5.4 Transdermal delivery

One of the most appealing and cutting-edge methods for distributing medications through the epidermis is transdermal drug delivery. Compared to traditional dosage forms for the treatment of different illnesses, the transdermal route of drug administration offers a number of benefits. The epidermis serves as a reservoir and has the capacity to continuously and slowly release the drug that has penetrated it. Due to the existence of numerous absorption sites, it also reduces toxins and local irritability [27]. The present scenario demands a particular emphasis on the invention of safe medications with fewer side effects that support patient compliance, prevent hepatic first-pass metabolism, and so forth. However, due to the stratum corneum, which acts as an effective barrier to the penetration of drugs, and the highly organized structure of the skin, transdermal delivery is accompanied with some challenges [75]. Fortunately, it has been established that the use of nanocarriers significantly increases the penetration of drugs (both hydrophilic and lipophilic) through this barrier and offers the desired local or systemic effect [76].

In light of this, a microneedle patch containing nanoparticles loaded with capsaicin for transdermal drug administration was created. The zeta potential of the 106.8 nm-sized nanoparticles was −50.8 mV. When compared to native capsaicin, the plasma bioavailability of the capsaicin-loaded nanoparticles was higher in C57NL/6 mice. The dynamic release of MNPs in vitro and ex vivo peaked at 3 minutes [77]. In a different study, curcumin-loaded SLN microneedle patches were developed. The manufactured microneedles were also discovered to be nonirritating, demonstrating the improved efficacy of the novel formulations by reducing bradykinesia and increasing motor coordination and balance ability [78].

12.6 Characterization of targeted drug delivery systems

Characterizing the developed TDDS is a critical step, as it gives information about its physicochemical and functional properties. Different aspects of the DDS require to be characterized, which provides specific insights about the nature and behavior of the product. Also, the intended use such as the pattern of drug release, surface modification, and

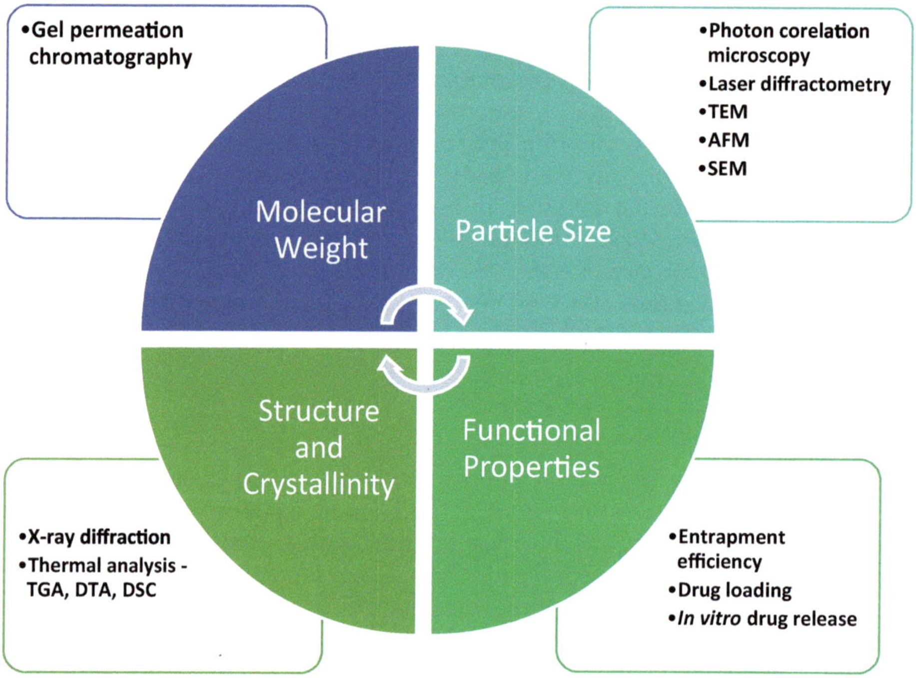

FIGURE 12.5 Characterization methods of targeted drug delivery system.

so on can be evaluated by certain in vitro tests [3]. Fig. 12.5 illustrates the different methods of characterizing these drug-loaded TDDS. The application of various characterization tools majorly depends on the intended application.

A critical aspect of the TDDS is its particle/globule size, as it helps it cross the biological membranes and barriers. The smaller the size of the drug carrier system, the greater will be its penetration through the fine fenestrations of the blood vasculature at the diseased site. Hence, it becomes important to determine the size of these nanocarriers to speculate their in vivo functionality. This diffusion is also affected by the morphology and the surface charge of the carrier system. Studying morphology not only provides information about its structural appearance but also helps in the developmental stage of certain nanostructures like nanoneedles, nanocapsules, and so on. On the other hand, the zeta potential, a reflection of the surface charge, indicates the stability of the formulation. The stability of the formulation will proportionally increase with the increase in the zeta potential as the charges on the surface of the carriers will cause their repulsion and thereby prevent aggregation. On the whole, size and zeta potential plays a vital role in determining the in vitro and in vivo stability of the drug formulation. Quasi-elastic light scattering, also known as dynamic light scattering, helps in the determination of particle/globule size as well as the surface charge by zeta potential measurement of TDDS [79]. Other techniques like atomic force microscopy, scanning electron microscopy, and transmission electron microscopy help to evaluate the particle size and the morphology of the developed nanocarrier systems [80,81].

In addition to the size, the molecular weight of the TDDS can be analyzed by gel permeation chromatography [82]. Accordingly, in the case of surface modification of the TDDS with ligands or other biochemical moieties characterization tests like infrared spectroscopy, nuclear magnetic resonance, and so on can be helpful. Structure and crystallinity as well are important parameters to be evaluated when it comes to delivering a drug molecule in the intact form to a specific site. This tells us about the nature, viz, crystalline or amorphous, of the drug loaded/encapsulated within the carrier system. Techniques like X-ray diffraction (XRD), small-angle XRD, and thermal analysis like differential scanning calorimetry, thermogravimetry, differential thermal analysis help in the analysis of the nature of the TDDS [83]. Understanding the nature of the drug and the glass transition temperature of the carrier system by thermal analysis also helps to anticipate the pattern of drug release in vitro and in vivo [84].

The abovementioned parameters directly or indirectly affect the drug loading and drug encapsulation efficiency. This majorly depends on the nature of the biomaterial, the size of the carrier system, the physicochemical property of the drug, and so on. The drug loading and entrapment efficiency are determined by quantification analysis using high-performance liquid chromatography methods, UV spectroscopy, or other spectral analysis [85]. The amount of drugs within the system correspondingly would determine the amount of drug released over time. The in vitro dissolution study is the most critical parameter to assess the drug release profile inside the body environment. In addition to the nature of the drug-loaded/encapsulated within the carrier system, the pattern of diffusion or erosion of the DDS governs the release mechanism [86].

12.7 Toxicology and regulatory aspect of targeted drug delivery systems

TDDS help in maximizing bioavailability, ameliorating pharmaceutical and pharmacodynamic profiles, and improving the biodistribution of drugs. These formulations enhance the solubility of drugs, and the targeting potential of the carrier systems facilitates site-specific delivery of entrapped therapeutics and longer circulation [87]. Although the TDDS have many advantages and exhibit positive usefulness, they possess challenges when it comes to their toxicity profiling and regulatory requirements. The formulation biomaterials of these nanocarriers comprise polymers, surfactants, organic solvents, and so on, which have in vivo toxicity issues. Thus, when it comes to formulating these systems, one must be careful about choosing the excipients for their safety and efficacy and compatibility with the drug, as their interaction can produce toxic substances, causing unwanted effects. Another possibility is the degradation of these components because of their mutual interaction, which can further produce other degradation products, which in turn can be harmful and can cause hazardous effects on the human body. Moreover, because of the nano size of these TDDS, they are capable of easily crossing biological barriers and accumulating in the specific organs of the body. So in the case of the generation of toxic or degraded components, they too accumulate within these tissues, leading to severe health hazards [88]. Therefore, identifying the potential risk of the drugs, excipients, and their interaction is crucial but challenging because it requires long-term studies and keen observations to generate adequate knowledge of their toxicological profile. Considering these factors, more stringent regulatory guidelines must be formulated to make their access more safe and efficacious accounting for their manufacturing process, storage conditions, dose and route of administration, and biological fate. Considering all these factors, DDS need to be evaluated at molecular, cellular, tissue, and organ level so that the toxic and hazardous effects related to these DDS can be minimized and effective therapy can be achieved [89].

12.8 Conclusion and future perspectives

Treatment of various human diseases, such as metabolic diseases, neurodegenerative diseases, cancers, and so on, depends on effective targeted delivery. Smart medication delivery systems and devices can be integrated with the human body for ideal drug delivery. Nanotechnology thus proves to be an important resolve in this sector. These nanosystems can be employed in the simplest forms such as tablets as well as complex injectable delivery platforms. They are also being used for theranostic purposes which can help in diagnosis and delivering therapy. Pharmaceutical companies are already working on developing clever TDDS employing nanotechnology by configuring the interface between a drug or other substance and the human body so that it only activates when the drug reaches its intended target.

TDDS are making significant advancements in the pharmaceutical domain. With the use of oral, transmucosal, transcutaneous, and needle-free immunization, global vaccine programs are very near to becoming a reality. Both gene therapy and protein therapeutic delivery have shown significant advancements. Novel medication delivery techniques have significantly improved cancer treatment. Drug distribution is being revolutionized by advancements in integrating microelectronics and nanotechnology, which ameliorate the therapeutic modalities.

However, the TDDS still faces some difficulties, which can be overcome with further research in that area. A major challenge is to develop these formulations at a lower cost and in a facile manner to ease their large-scale production and increase their availability to the patient masses. More fundamental research is needed to characterize these TDDS and accordingly formulate firm regulatory guidelines for streamlined approval and marketing of these products. Continuous updating of these regulatory guidelines is important as the new facets of this system are explored. A neat balance between the therapeutic dependence and safety profile of the TDDS needs to be identified so as to reap maximum benefits of these sophisticated drug delivery approaches. As new variations of diseases, particularly infections, may emerge, modifications and upgradation in the development of TDDS must be made. It must be realized that the science of drug delivery, especially targeting the delivery systems, is a continuous process that requires a multidimensional approach inclusive of biomaterial sciences, formulation expertise, scale-up and production techniques, and regulatory and quality stewardship.

References

[1] Liu G, et al. A review on drug delivery system for tumor therapy. Front Pharmacol 2021;12:735446. Available from: https://www.frontiersin.org/articles/10.3389/fphar.2021.735446/full (March 12, 2023).

[2] Tewabe A, et al. Targeted drug delivery—from magic bullet to nanomedicine: principles, challenges, and future perspectives. J Multidiscip Healthcare 2021;14:1711–24. Available from: https://www.dovepress.com/targeted-drug-delivery-from-magic-bullet-to-nanomedicine-principles-c-peer-reviewed-fulltext-article-JMDH (March 12, 2023).

[3] Panchal K, et al. An expanding horizon of complex injectable products: development and regulatory considerations. Drug Deliv Transl Res 2023;13(2):433–72. Available from: https://doi.org/10.1007/s13346-022-01223-5, https://link.springer.com/ (March 13, 2023).

[4] Ulbrich K, et al. Targeted drug delivery with polymers and magnetic nanoparticles: covalent and noncovalent approaches, release control, and clinical studies. Chem Rev 2016;116(9):5338–431. Available from: https://doi.org/10.1021/acs.chemrev.5b00589, https://pubs.acs.org/doi/ (March 12, 2023).

[5] Bae YH, Park K. Targeted drug delivery to tumors: myths, reality and possibility. J Contr Rel 2011;153 (3):198–205. Available from: https://linkinghub.elsevier.com/retrieve/pii/S0168365911003877 (March 12, 2023).

[6] Bruno BJ, Miller GD, Lim CS. Basics and recent advances in peptide and protein drug delivery. Ther Deliv 2013;4(11):1443–67. Available from: https://www.future-science.com/doi/10.4155/tde.13.104 (March 12, 2023).

[7] Panchal K, Sahoo RK, Gupta U, Chaurasiya A. Role of targeted immunotherapy for pancreatic ductal adenocarcinoma (PDAC) treatment: an overview. Int Immunopharmacol 2021;95:107508. Available from: https://linkinghub.elsevier.com/retrieve/pii/S1567576921001442 (May 14, 2022).

[8] D'Souza GGM, Weissig V. Subcellular targeting: a new frontier for drug-loaded pharmaceutical nanocarriers and the concept of the magic bullet. Expert Opinion Drug Deliv 2009;6(11):1135–48. Available from: http://www.tandfonline.com/doi/full/10.1517/17425240903236101 (March 12, 2023).

[9] Liu P, Chen G, Zhang J. A review of liposomes as a drug delivery system: current status of approved products, regulatory environments, and future perspectives. Molecules 2022;27(4):1372. Available from: https://www.mdpi.com/1420-3049/27/4/1372 (March 12, 2023).

[10] Kuotsu K, et al. Niosome: a future of targeted drug delivery systems. J Adv Pharm Technol Res 2010;1 (4):374. Available from: http://www.japtr.org/text.asp?2010/1/4/374/76435 (March 12, 2023).

[11] Rajan R, Vasudevan DT, Mukund VB, Jose S. Transferosomes - a vesicular transdermal delivery system for enhanced drug permeation. J Adv Pharm Technol Res 2011;2(3):138. Available from: http://www.japtr.org/text.asp?2011/2/3/138/85524 (March 12, 2023).

[12] Zielińska A, et al. Polymeric nanoparticles: production, characterization, toxicology and ecotoxicology. Molecules 2020;25(16):3731. Available from: https://www.mdpi.com/1420-3049/25/16/3731 (March 12, 2023).

[13] Westesen K, Bunjes H. Do nanoparticles prepared from lipids solid at room temperature always possess a solid lipid matrix? Int J Pharm 1995;115(1):129–31. Available from: https://linkinghub.elsevier.com/retrieve/pii/0378517394003478 (March 12, 2023).

[14] Satya Prakash S. Human serum albumin nanoparticles as an efficient noscapine drug delivery system for potential use in breast cancer: preparation and in vitro analysis. Int J Nanomed 2010;525. Available from: http://www.dovepress.com/human-serum-albumin-nanoparticles-as-an-efficient-noscapine-drug-deliv-peer-reviewed-article-IJN (March 12, 2023).

[15] Rao CNR, Thomas PJ, Kulkarni GU. 95 *Nanocrystals: synthesis, properties and applications*. Berlin, Heidelberg: Springer Berlin Heidelberg; 2007. Available from: http://link.springer.com/, 10.1007/978-3-540-68752-8 (March 13, 2023).

[16] Shah P, Bhalodia D, Shelat P. Nanoemulsion: a pharmaceutical review. Syst Rev Pharm 2010;1(1):24. Available from: http://www.sysrevpharm.org/text.asp?2010/1/1/24/59509 (March 12, 2023).

[17] Kesharwani P, Jain K, Jain NK. Dendrimer as nanocarrier for drug delivery. Prog Polym Sci 2014;39(2):268–307. Available from: https://linkinghub.elsevier.com/retrieve/pii/S0079670013000853 (March 12, 2023).

[18] Mahajan HS, Patil SB, Gattani SG, Kuchekar BS. Targeted drug delivery systems. Pharma Times 2007;39 (2):19–21.

[19] Bazak R, et al. Cancer active targeting by nanoparticles: a comprehensive review of literature. J Cancer Res Clin Oncol 2015;141(5):769–84. Available from: https://doi.org/10.1007/s00432-014-1767-3, http://link.springer.com/ (March 12, 2023).

[20] Torchilin VP. Passive and active drug targeting: drug delivery to tumors as an example. In: Schäfer-Korting M, editor. Drug delivery, handbook of experimental pharmacology. Berlin, Heidelberg: Springer Berlin Heidelberg; 2010. p. 3–53. Available from: http://link.springer.com/, 10.1007/978-3-642-00477-3_1 (March 12, 2023).
[21] Salahpour Anarjan F. Active targeting drug delivery nanocarriers: ligands. Nano-Struct Nano-Obj 2019;19:100370. Available from: https://linkinghub.elsevier.com/retrieve/pii/S2352507X19302926 (March 13, 2023).
[22] Dai L, et al. Tumor therapy: targeted drug delivery systems. J Mater Chem B 2016;4(42):6758–72. Available from: http://xlink.rsc.org/?DOI = C6TB01743F (March 13, 2023).
[23] Choudhury H, et al. Transferrin receptors-targeting nanocarriers for efficient targeted delivery and transcytosis of drugs into the brain tumors: a review of recent advancements and emerging trends. Drug Deliv Transl Res 2018;8(5):1545–63. Available from: https://doi.org/10.1007/s13346-018-0552-2, http://link.springer.com/ (March 13, 2023).
[24] Zhan C, Yan Z, Xie C, Lu W. Loop 2 of ophiophagus hannah toxin b binds with neuronal nicotinic acetylcholine receptors and enhances intracranial drug delivery. Mol Pharm 2010;7(6):1940–7. Available from: https://pubs.acs.org/doi/10.1021/mp100238j (March 13, 2023).
[25] Yadav KS, Mishra DK, Deshpande A, Pethe AM. Levels of drug targeting. Basic fundamentals of drug delivery. Elsevier; 2019. p. 269–305. Available from: https://linkinghub.elsevier.com/retrieve/pii/B9780128179093000078 (March 14, 2023).
[26] Unnisa A, Greig NH, Kamal MA. Nanotechnology: a promising targeted drug delivery system forbrain tumours and Alzheimer's disease. Current Med Chem 2023;30(3):255–70. Available from: https://www.eurekaselect.com/202689/article (March 13, 2023).
[27] Kurmi BD, Tekchandani P, Paliwal R, Paliwal SR. Transdermal drug delivery: opportunities and challenges for controlled delivery of therapeutic agents using nanocarriers. Current Drug Metabolism 2017;18 (5):481–95. Available from: http://www.eurekaselect.com/node/150362/article (March 13, 2023).
[28] Malaiya A, Singhai M, Paliwal SR, Paliwal R. Basics of targeted nanodrug delivery of chemotherapeutics for breast cancer therapy. Targeted nanomedicine for breast cancer therapy. Elsevier; 2022. p. 27–44. Available from: https://linkinghub.elsevier.com/retrieve/pii/B9780128244760000176 (March 13, 2023).
[29] Prajapati SK, et al. Biomedical applications and toxicities of carbon nanotubes. Drug Chem Toxicol 2022;45 (1):435–50. Available from: https://doi.org/10.1080/01480545.2019.1709492, https://www.tandfonline.com/doi/full/ (March 13, 2023).
[30] Paliwal R, Jayachandra Babu R, Palakurthi S. Nanomedicine scale-up technologies: feasibilities and challenges. AAPS PharmSciTech 2014;15(6):1527–34. Available from: https://doi.org/10.1208/s12249-014-0177-9, http://link.springer.com/ (March 13, 2023).
[31] Rajpoot K, et al. Meropenem-loaded nanostructured lipid carriers for skin and soft tissue infection caused by Staphylococcus aureus: formulation, design, and evaluation. AAPS PharmSciTech 2022;23(7):241. Available from: https://doi.org/10.1208/s12249-022-02381-y, https://link.springer.com/ (March 13, 2023).
[32] Malaiya A, Yadav AK. Hyaluronic acid anchored nanoparticulate carrier for delivery of methotrexate. Asian J Phar harmacol 2018;4(6):899–907. Available from: http://ajpp.in/uploaded/p227.pdf (March 13, 2023).
[33] Kurmi BD, Paliwal R, Paliwal SR. Dual cancer targeting using estrogen functionalized chitosan nanoparticles loaded with doxorubicin-estrone conjugate: a quality by design approach. Int J Biol Macromol 2020;164:2881–94. Available from: https://linkinghub.elsevier.com/retrieve/pii/S0141813020342641 (March 13, 2023).
[34] Kesharwani D, Paul SD, Paliwal R, Satapathy T. Exploring potential of diacerin nanogel for topical application in arthritis: formulation development, QbD based optimization and pre-clinical evaluation. Colloids Surfaces B Biointerfaces 2023;223:113160. Available from: https://linkinghub.elsevier.com/retrieve/pii/S0927776523000383 (March 13, 2023).
[35] Kumar Chandraker S, et al. Biofabrication of spherical silver nanoparticles using leaf extract of plectranthus barbatus andrews: characterization, free radical scavenging, and optical properties. Inorg Chem Commun 2022;142:109669. Available from: https://linkinghub.elsevier.com/retrieve/pii/S1387700322004774 (March 13, 2023).
[36] Taha E, et al. Cod liver oil nano-structured lipid carriers (Cod-NLCs) as a promising platform for nose to brain delivery: preparation, in vitro optimization, ex vivo cytotoxicity & in vivo biodistribution utilizing radioiodinated zopiclone. Int J Pharm: X 2023;5:100160. Available from: https://linkinghub.elsevier.com/retrieve/pii/S259015672300004X (March 13, 2023).

[37] Di Filippo LD, et al. Glioblastoma multiforme targeted delivery of docetaxel using bevacizumab-modified nanostructured lipid carriers impair in vitro cell growth and in vivo tumor progression. Int J Pharm 2022;618:121682. Available from: https://linkinghub.elsevier.com/retrieve/pii/S037851732200237X (March 13, 2023).
[38] Kalam MA, et al. Development and evaluation of chitosan nanoparticles for ocular delivery of tedizolid phosphate. Molecules 2022;27(7):2326. Available from: https://www.mdpi.com/1420-3049/27/7/2326 (March 13, 2023).
[39] Durgun ME, et al. Posaconazole micelles for ocular delivery: in vitro permeation, ocular irritation and antifungal activity studies. Drug Deliv Transl Res 2022;12(3):662–75. Available from: https://doi.org/10.1007/s13346-021-00974-x, https://link.springer.com/ (March 13, 2023).
[40] Mahdavijalal M, Panahi HA, Moniri E. Synthesis of PAMAM dendrimers anchored to WS2 nano-sheets for controlled delivery of docetaxel: design, characterization and in vitro drug release. J Drug Deliv Sci Technol 2023;79:104066. Available from: https://linkinghub.elsevier.com/retrieve/pii/S1773224722009777 (March 13, 2023).
[41] Latif MS, et al. Formulation development and in vitro/in vivo characterization of methotrexate-loaded nanoemulsion gel formulations for enhanced topical delivery. Gels 2022;9(1):3. Available from: https://www.mdpi.com/2310-2861/9/1/3 (March 13, 2023).
[42] Çağlar EŞ, Okur ME, Aksu B, Okur NÜ. Transdermal delivery of acemetacin loaded microemulsions: preparation, characterization, in vitro – ex vivo evaluation and in vivo analgesic and anti-inflammatory efficacy. J Disp Sci Technol 2023;1–11. Available from: https://doi.org/10.1080/01932691.2023.2175691, https://www.tandfonline.com/doi/full/ (March 13, 2023).
[43] Mathure D, et al. Preparation and optimization of liposome containing thermosensitive *in situ* nasal hydrogel system for brain delivery of sumatriptan succinate. ASSAY Drug Dev Technol 2023;21(1):3–16. Available from: https://doi.org/10.1089/adt.2022.088, https://www.liebertpub.com/ (March 13, 2023).
[44] Lôbo G.C., Paiva K.L., Silva A.L., Simões M.M., Radicchi M.A., Báo S.N. Nanocarriers used in drug delivery to enhance immune system in cancer therapy. Pharmaceutics. 13(8):1167. https://www.mdpi.com/1999-4923/13/8/1167
[45] Paliwal R, Sulakhiya K, et al. Role of nanoparticles in neurotoxicity. Nanomedical drug delivery for neurodegenerative diseases. Elsevier; 2022. p. 165–82. Available from: https://linkinghub.elsevier.com/retrieve/pii/B9780323855440000095 (March 13, 2023).
[46] Paliwal R, Kumar P, et al. Development of nanomedicines and nano-similars: recent advances in regulatory landscape. Current Pharm Design 2022;28(2):165–77. Available from: http://www.eurekaselect.com/197940/article (March 6, 2023).
[47] Shaikh A, Kesharwani P, Gajbhiye V. Dendrimer as a momentous tool in tissue engineering and regenerative medicine. J Contr Release 2022;346:328–54. Available from: https://linkinghub.elsevier.com/retrieve/pii/S0168365922002024 (March 13, 2023).
[48] Chaurasiya A, et al. A review on multivesicular liposomes for pharmaceutical applications: preparation, characterization, and translational challenges. Drug Deliv Transl Res 2022;12(7):1569–87. Available from: https://doi.org/10.1007/s13346-021-01060-y, https://link.springer.com/ (March 13, 2023).
[49] Paliwal SR, Paliwal R, Vyas SP. A review of mechanistic insight and application of PH-sensitive liposomes in drug delivery. Drug Deliv 2015;22(3):231–42. Available from: https://doi.org/10.3109/10717544.2014.882469, http://www.tandfonline.com/doi/full/ (May 18, 2022).
[50] Paliwal R, et al. Solid lipid nanoparticles: a review on recent perspectives and patents. Expert Opinion Ther Patents 2020;30(3):179–94. Available from: https://doi.org/10.1080/13543776.2020.1720649, https://www.tandfonline.com/doi/full/ (March 13, 2023).
[51] Akbari J, et al. Solid lipid nanoparticles and nanostructured lipid carriers: a review of the methods of manufacture and routes of administration. Pharm Dev Technol 2022;27(5):525–44. Available from: https://doi.org/10.1080/10837450.2022.2084554, https://www.tandfonline.com/doi/full/ (March 13, 2023).
[52] Gugleva V, Andonova V. Drug delivery to the brain – lipid nanoparticles-based approach. Pharmacia 2023;70(1):113–20. Available from: https://pharmacia.pensoft.net/article/98838/ (March 13, 2023).
[53] Kuperkar K, Patel D, Atanase LI, Bahadur P. Amphiphilic block copolymers: their structures, and self-assembly to polymeric micelles and polymersomes as drug delivery vehicles. Polymers 2022;14(21):4702. Available from: https://www.mdpi.com/2073-4360/14/21/4702 (March 13, 2023).
[54] Shalmani AA, et al. Effect of radical polymerization method on pharmaceutical properties of Π electron-stabilized HPMA-based polymeric micelles Biomacromolecules 2023;. Available from: https://doi.org/10.1021/acs.biomac.2c01261acs.biomac.2c01261, https://pubs.acs.org/doi/ (March 13, 2023)

[55] Guliy OI, et al. Polymeric micelles for targeted drug delivery systems. In *Pharmaceutical nanobiotechnology for targeted therapy*, Nanotechnology in the life sciencesIn: Barabadi H, Mostafavi E, Saravanan M, editors. Cham: Springer International Publishing; 2022. p. 521–59. Available from: https://link.springer.com/, 10.1007/978-3-031-12658-1_18 (March 13, 2023).
[56] Kotta S, et al. Progress in polymeric micelles for drug delivery applications. Pharmaceutics 2022;14(8):1636. Available from: https://www.mdpi.com/1999-4923/14/8/1636 (March 13, 2023).
[57] Ghezzi M, et al. Polymeric micelles in drug delivery: an insight of the techniques for their characterization and assessment in biorelevant conditions. J Contr Release 2021;332:312–36. Available from: https://linkinghub.elsevier.com/retrieve/pii/S0168365921001061 (March 13, 2023).
[58] Devarajan PV, Jain S, editors. Targeted drug delivery: concepts and design. Cham: Springer International Publishing; 2015. Available from: https://link.springer.com/, 10.1007/978-3-319-11355-5 (March 13, 2023).
[59] Piscatelli JA, Ban J, Lucas AT, Zamboni WC. Complex factors and challenges that affect the pharmacology, safety and efficacy of nanocarrier drug delivery systems. Pharmaceutics 2021;13(1):114. Available from: https://doi.org/10.3390/pharmaceutics13010114 (March 15 2023).
[60] Nance E, Pun SH, Saigal R, Sellers DL. Drug delivery to the central nervous system. Nature Rev Mater 2021;7(4):314–31. Available from: https://www.nature.com/articles/s41578-021-00394-w (March 13, 2023).
[61] Jamal A, et al. Insights into infusion-based targeted drug delivery in the brain: perspectives, challenges and opportunities. Int J Mol Sci 2022;23(6):3139. Available from: https://www.mdpi.com/1422-0067/23/6/3139 (March 13, 2023).
[62] Tang S, et al. Brain-targeted intranasal delivery of dopamine with borneol and lactoferrin co-modified nanoparticles for treating Parkinson's disease. Drug Deliv 2019;26(1):700–7. Available from: https://doi.org/10.1080/10717544.2019.1636420, https://www.tandfonline.com/doi/full/ (March 13, 2023).
[63] Deepika D, Dewangan HK, Maurya L, Singh S. Intranasal drug delivery of frovatriptan succinate–loaded polymeric nanoparticles for brain targeting. J Pharm Sci 2019;108(2):851–9. Available from: https://linkinghub.elsevier.com/retrieve/pii/S0022354918304489 (March 13, 2023).
[64] Khan MI, et al. Recent progress in nanostructured smart drug delivery systems for cancer therapy: a review. ACS Appl Bio Mater 2022;5(3):971–1012. Available from: https://doi.org/10.1021/acsabm.2c00002, https://pubs.acs.org/ (March 13, 2023).
[65] Shi Z, et al. Inorganic nano-carriers based smart drug delivery systems for tumor therapy. Smart Mater Med 2020;1:32–47. Available from: https://linkinghub.elsevier.com/retrieve/pii/S2590183420300065 (March 13, 2023).
[66] Lolage K.R., Wagh P.R. Nanocarriers for cancer-targeted drug delivery: review and challenges; 2020.
[67] Zeb A, et al. Potential and applications of nanocarriers for efficient delivery of biopharmaceuticals. Pharmaceutics 2020;12(12):1184. Available from: https://www.mdpi.com/1999-4923/12/12/1184 (March 13, 2023).
[68] Yu W, Liu R, Zhou Y, Gao H. Size-tunable strategies for a tumor targeted drug delivery system. ACS Central Sci 2020;6(2):100–16. Available from: https://doi.org/10.1021/acscentsci.9b01139, https://pubs.acs.org/doi/ (March 13, 2023).
[69] Dang Y, Guan J. Nanoparticle-based drug delivery systems for cancer therapy. Smart Mater Med 2020;1:10–19. Available from: https://linkinghub.elsevier.com/retrieve/pii/S2590183420300028 (March 13, 2023).
[70] Imran M, et al. Topical nanostructured lipid carrier gel of quercetin and resveratrol: formulation, optimization, in vitro and ex vivo study for the treatment of skin cancer. Int J Pharm 2020;587:119705. Available from: https://linkinghub.elsevier.com/retrieve/pii/S037851732030689X (March 13, 2023).
[71] Khiev D, et al. Emerging nano-formulations and nanomedicines applications for ocular drug delivery. Nanomaterials 2021;11(1):173. Available from: https://www.mdpi.com/2079-4991/11/1/173 (March 13, 2023).
[72] Gorantla S, et al. Nanocarriers for ocular drug delivery: current status and translational opportunity. RSC Adv 2020;10(46):27835–55. Available from: http://xlink.rsc.org/?DOI = D0RA04971A (March 13, 2023).
[73] Fahmy HM, et al. Treatment merits of latanoprost/thymoquinone – encapsulated liposome for glaucomatus rabbits. Int J Pharm 2018;548(1):597–608. Available from: https://linkinghub.elsevier.com/retrieve/pii/S0378517318304800 (March 13, 2023).
[74] Li J, et al. Montmorillonite/chitosan nanoparticles as a novel controlled-release topical ophthalmic delivery system for the treatment of glaucoma. Int J Nanomed 2018;13:3975–87. Available from: https://www.dovepress.com/montmorillonitechitosan-nanoparticles-as-a-novel-controlled-release-to-peer-reviewed-article-IJN (March 13, 2023).
[75] Babaie S, et al. Invasome: a novel nanocarrier for transdermal drug delivery. Nanomaterials 2020;10(2):341. Available from: https://www.mdpi.com/2079-4991/10/2/341 (March 13, 2023).

[76] Yu Y-Q, Yang X, Wu X-F, Fan Y-B. Enhancing permeation of drug molecules across the skin via delivery in nanocarriers: novel strategies for effective transdermal applications. Frontiers in Bioengineering and Biotechnology 2021;9:646554. Available from: https://doi.org/10.3389/fbioe.2021.646554/full, https://www.frontiersin.org/articles/ (March 13, 2023).

[77] Mudhol S, Peddha MS. Development of capsaicin loaded nanoparticles based microneedle patch for transdermal drug delivery. J Drug Deliv Sci Technol 2023;80:104120. Available from: https://linkinghub.elsevier.com/retrieve/pii/S1773224722010310 (March 13, 2023).

[78] Prabhu A, et al. Transdermal delivery of curcumin-loaded solid lipid nanoparticles as microneedle patch: an in vitro and in vivo study. AAPS PharmSciTech 2022;23(1):49. Available from: https://doi.org/10.1208/s12249-021-02186-5, https://link.springer.com/ (March 13, 2023).

[79] Ansari RR. Quasi-elastic light scattering in ophthalmology. In: Tuchin VV, editor. Handbook of coherent domain optical methods. New York, NY: Springer US; 2004. p. 437–64. Available from: http://link.springer.com/. doi: 10.1007/0-387-29989-0_11 (March 12, 2023).

[80] Hoo CM, Starostin N, West P, Mecartney ML. A comparison of atomic force microscopy (AFM) and dynamic light scattering (DLS) methods to characterize nanoparticle size distributions. J Nanoparticle Res 2008;10(S1):89–96. Available from: https://doi.org/10.1007/s11051-008-9435-7, http://link.springer.com/ (March 12, 2023).

[81] Brodusch N, et al. Scanning electron microscopy versus transmission electron microscopy for material characterization: a comparative study on high-strength steels. Scanning 2021;2021:1–19. Available from: https://www.hindawi.com/journals/scanning/2021/5511618/ (March 12, 2023).

[82] Shabir A, Alhusban F, Perrie Y, Mohammed AR. Effects of ball-milling on PLGA polymer and its implication on lansoprazole-loaded nanoparticles. J Basic Clinical Pharm 2011;2(2):71–82.

[83] Byrn SR, Zografi G, Chen XS. Differential scanning calorimetry and thermogravimetric analysis. Solid state properties of pharmaceutical materials. Hoboken: John Wiley & Sons, Inc.; 2017. p. 124–41. Available from: https://onlinelibrary.wiley.com/doi/10.1002/9781119264408.ch10 (March 12, 2023).

[84] Rieger J. The glass transition temperature tg of polymers—comparison of the values from differential thermal analysis (DTA, DSC) and dynamic mechanical measurements (Torsion Pendulum). Polymer Testing 2001;20(2):199–204. Available from: https://linkinghub.elsevier.com/retrieve/pii/S0142941800000234 (March 12, 2023).

[85] Dhakar RC. From formulation variables to drug entrapment efficiency of microspheres: a technical review. J Drug Deliv Ther 2012;2(6). Available from: http://jddtonline.info/index.php/jddt/article/view/160 (March 12, 2023).

[86] Rehman Q, Akash MSH, Rasool MF, Rehman K. Role of kinetic models in drug stability. In: Akash MSH, Rehman K, editors. Drug stability and chemical kinetics. Singapore: Springer Singapore; 2020. p. 155–65. Available from: http://link.springer.com/, 10.1007/978-981-15-6426-0_11 (March 12, 2023).

[87] Sharma A, Madhunapantula SRV, Robertson GP. Toxicological considerations when creating nanoparticle-based drugs and drug delivery systems. Expert Opinion Drug Metabolism Toxicol 2012;8(1):47–69. Available from: https://doi.org/10.1517/17425255.2012.637916, http://www.tandfonline.com/doi/full/ (March 12, 2023).

[88] Tacar O, Sriamornsak P, Dass CR. Doxorubicin: an update on anticancer molecular action, toxicity and novel drug delivery systems. J Pharm Pharmacol 2012;65(2):157–70. Available from: https://academic.oup.com/jpp/article/65/2/157-170/6132943 (March 12, 2023).

[89] Gaspar R. Regulatory issues surrounding nanomedicines: setting the scene for the next generation of nanopharmaceuticals. Nanomedicine 2007;2(2):143–7. Available from: https://doi.org/10.2217/17435889.2.2.143, https://www.futuremedicine.com/ (March 12, 2023).

CHAPTER

13

Assessment of nanotoxicology through in vitro techniques and image-based assays

Fernanda Garcia-Fossa[1,*], *Tuanny Leite Almeida*[1,*], *Rafaella Mascarelli Pereira*[1], *Thaís Moraes-Lacerda*[1], *Mariana Rodrigues Da Silva*[1], *Laura de Oliveira-Nascimento*[2] *and Marcelo Bispo de Jesus*[1]

[1]**Department of Biochemistry and Tissue Biology, Institute of Biology, University of Campinas (UNICAMP), Campinas, SP, Brazil** [2]**Faculty of Pharmaceutical Sciences, University of Campinas (UNICAMP), Campinas, SP, Brazil**

13.1 Introduction

Capable of manipulating matter at the nanometer scale, nanotechnology offers a wide range of applications with the potential to revolutionize many fields, including medicine. The application of nanotechnology in the medical field, called nanomedicine, has attracted the attention of scientists over the last few decades, making it possible to monitor, repair, control, and even build biological systems at the molecular level [1,2]. Nanomedicine is an interdisciplinary field that includes biology, chemistry, physics, medicine, materials science, and biomedical engineering. It has proven to be a fertile research field, in which applications have increased in recent years [3,4]. One of the main reasons for the development of this field is the fact that nanomedicine offers therapeutic and diagnostic approaches for diseases that cannot be reached with traditional strategies [2,5–8].

Global analysis shows that the current landscape of nanomedicine is promising and has made significant strides in recent years. More than 280 products containing nanomaterials

* These authors contributed equally to this work.

DOI: https://doi.org/10.1016/B978-0-323-91924-1.00003-4

have been approved by FDA, mostly for medical applications, of which about 100 are already on the market [4,9]. As a result, this market size is reaching significant numbers, estimated at US$53 billion in 2009, which grew to approximately US$134 billion in 2017 and forecasted to reach about US$334 billion by 2025 [3,9]. While the market share remains mostly with therapeutics for the treatment of cancer, which account for about 50% of these sales, there has already been significant growth in other areas in recent years. Emerging segments include chronic respiratory disease, antiinflammatory drug delivery, cardiology, vascular disease, neurology, antiinfectives, diabetes, and regenerative medicine [3,9]. In addition, the patent expiry dates for the first generations of nanotherapeutics are approaching fast, which together with the commercialization of a growing number of new devices, promise to flood the market with even more nanoproducts.

Despite all this progress, leaving laboratories and reaching hospitals is one of the most significant barriers to nanomedicine. However, the main advantage of nanomedicine lies precisely in reducing the toxicity of chemotherapy [10–12] and not in a significant improvement in therapeutic efficacy, as initially conceived. Moreover, two nanoparticles containing magnetic resonance contrast agents (Feruglose and Resovist) have recently been withdrawn from the market because of safety concerns. Therefore, in addition to the challenges and uncertainties, the development of nanotherapeutics requires more efficient methods for assessing toxicity and models that more closely resemble the in vivo environment [13]. Improving toxicological questions is undoubtedly one of the building blocks for establishing nanomedicine and the solution to urgent clinical needs.

This chapter provides an overview of the development of nanotoxicology from its conception to the present day, focusing on silver nanoparticles (AgNPs) and nanoplastics regarding their widespread use and presence in our daily lives. Furthermore, we place the in vitro approaches as a promising tool in developing nanotechnology and nanomedicine. We also critically discuss the techniques and strategies currently used in the field to promote the rationale assessment of nanotoxicity. Particular attention is paid to image-based approaches to assess nanotoxicity. This approach has a significant potential to contribute to the urgent needs in this field (i.e., to evaluate subtle changes caused by low concentrations of nanomaterials). Finally, we conclude with a section on current regulatory challenges.

13.2 Nanotoxicology

Advances in nanotechnology led to the development of risk assessment strategies and toxicity evaluation of effects caused by nanomaterials, an area that has come to be known as *nanotoxicology*. Several events led to the establishment of nanotoxicology in the mid-2000s. In 2004, the National Toxicology Program, the National Institutes of Environmental Health, and the National Institutes of Health created a multidisciplinary research program called "Environmental Protection" to study the effects of nanoparticles on human health and the environment. In the same year, three studies evaluating the impact of carbon nanotubes on rodent lungs prompted great interest in the toxicology community [14]. These studies showed that single-walled or multiwalled carbon nanotubes caused significant acute pulmonary inflammatory effects that were transient in rats [15] but persistent in mice [14]. Around the same time, a study investigating the effects of carbon fullerenes reported lipid peroxidation in the brain and gills of fish, which raised concerns about nanomaterials in the field of ecotoxicology [16].

The term nanotoxicology was first used in a 2004 editorial by Donaldson et al. [17]. In 2005, Oberdörster and colleagues published a seminal review article entitled "Nanotoxicology: an Emerging Discipline Evolved from Studies on Ultrafine Particles," which is cited more than 9000 times [18]. In 2007, the Society of Toxicology published a special issue called nanotoxicology, and the journal of the same name was founded. These events mark the beginning of nanotoxicology [17,19]. After that, a lot of attention has been paid to this topic, and since then, several other reviews have been published [19–22] in addition to several books dedicated exclusively to this topic [23–26]. Although studies were conducted in this field before it was formally established, constant efforts have been made to develop new strategies or to improve techniques previously developed for the study of small molecules, to better assess the toxicology and safety assessment of nanomaterials [27–31].

Nanomaterials have emerged as a promising tool for solving many of our daily problems, and today there are approximately 9000 products containing nanomaterials, ranging from household products to medical applications [32]. The widespread use of nanomaterials in commercial products has undoubtedly increased their production, consumption, and disposal: 1.5 million tons of nanomaterial waste are generated worldwide every year [33]. In addition, products containing nanomaterials, such as personal care products, coatings, paints, and pigments, are the most responsible for soil, water, and air contamination. Therefore, there is a growing need to assess the environmental and potential adverse health effects of these nanomaterials [34,35].

Two sources contribute significantly to the dissemination of nanomaterials in the environment: intentionally manufactured nanomaterials and unintentionally produced nanomaterials, the latter resulting from environmental degradation of bulk materials. Among the intentionally produced nanomaterials, many types have been described, which can be grouped into three categories: carbon-based nanomaterials, organic-based nanomaterials, and inorganic-based nanomaterials. One of the most commercialized inorganic-based nanomaterials, AgNPs, is estimated to be present in 50% of products containing nanomaterials [36]. AgNPs have antimicrobial, antifungal, antiseptic, and deodorant properties, explaining the large number of products being developed in the industry. According to the Nanotechnology Products Database, 935 silver-containing nanoproducts were registered in 2020 [37]. Therefore, the amount of silver in the environment tends to increase. It is estimated that global production of AgNP was 530 tons in 2018, and the overall trend indicates an increase in production [36]. Consequently, the effects of AgNP and its interactions with biological systems remain a great deal of debate.

Among the unintended nanomaterials, micro- and nanoplastics have received much attention due to the widespread production and use of plastics worldwide, which has led to global contamination in recent decades [38]. This contamination has recently come to society's attention due to the ubiquity of plastic waste in surface, ground, and drinking water [39,40]. For instance, the increasing production and ubiquity of plastic waste may have increased the toxic effects of microplastic particles in recent years, particularly microplastic (<5 mm) and nanoplastic (<0.1 m) [41]. This situation is even more precarious due to the proliferation of products containing nanoplastics (e.g., paints, adhesives, and drug delivery systems) summed to the environmental degradation that can lead to the production of nanoplastics and increased human exposure. Among the nanoplastics, polystyrene derivatives are among the most commonly found in drinking water. Some evidence points to the greater ability of these particles to promote the spread of nonpolar and weakly polar organic pollutants in the environment [42]. Consequently, due to their small size, they can migrate into the human body and reach many organs and systems [41,43,44].

Although environmental contamination from nanomaterials is increasing, it is still significantly lower than the concentration ranges used in most studies to assess cytotoxicity [45]. The half-maximal inhibitory concentrations (IC_{50}) used in cytotoxicity studies of nanomaterials are approximately 1000-fold higher than values reported in the environment. For example, the IC_{50} for human keratinocyte line HaCaT cells exposed to different sizes of AgNPs is $\sim 1\ \mu g/mL$ [46], while the predicted concentration range in the effluent is $0.05-0.2\ \mu g/L$ (data from San Francisco Bay Area) [47]. Even accounting for concerns about the trophic transfer, if plants and animals could transfer nanoparticles through food chains (e.g., zucchini to cricket [48] and lettuce to cricket to beetles [49]), the potential human exposure would still be closer to environmental concentrations. However, it should be noted that IC_{50} is often given for 24-hour exposure, which may not compare to lifetime human exposure to lower concentrations [45].

Many studies have estimated the concentration of nanomaterials in the environment [33,47,50,51]. Taken together, these studies indicate worldwide contamination present at low levels ($\sim\mu g/L$ in effluents and $\sim mg/kg$ in biosolids). Therefore, there has been considerable debate regarding the conditions used in the toxicity evaluation of nanomaterials. Many authors argue that these materials need to be evaluated under more relevant exposure conditions (e.g., physical state, environmental transformation, and low concentrations). Therefore, experimental conditions should be kept as close to ambient conditions as possible to maximize translation efficiency. However, the current methods used to assess nanotoxicity are not optimum, posing a challenge once mild alterations are expected at more realistic concentrations, rather than cell death induced by higher concentrations [52]. In recent years, the cytotoxic effects of nanomaterials under these conditions have seen significant advances. Nevertheless, the overall understanding of the cytotoxic effects is not yet accomplished [53].

In addition to the limitations in assessing subtle cellular changes, the variety of cellular responses introduces another layer of complexity. Most current methods often overlook the heterogeneous cellular response, since they focus on metabolic viability and live-dead responses (e.g., 3-(4,5-dimethylthiazol-2-yl)-2,5-diphenyltetrazolium bromide [MTT] assay, neutral red, lactate dehydrogenase release, and calcein/propidium iodide live-dead assay). These techniques neglect smaller subpopulations of cells [54,55], even though these changes are essential to fully understand the mechanisms of nanoparticle-cell interactions. Conversely, some studies attempted to examine the single-cell response to nanoparticles. For example, mass cytometry was used to identify distinct subpopulations of T lymphocyte cells exposed to increasing concentrations of AgNP [56]. Most omics approaches combined with bioinformatics can identify cellular changes caused by nanomaterials at the single-cell level [57]. For example, macrophages exposed to low doses of iron oxide nanoparticles suffered significant transcriptional reprogramming [58]. As mentioned above, the variety and subtlety of cellular responses characterize their multiparametric nature and require a methodology capable of measuring and quantifying these alterations.

13.2.1 In vitro toxicity assessment

In the last decade, non-animal methods have received increasing industry and market attention for assessing toxicity because of the increasing exposure to chemicals and nanomaterials in our daily lives. Therefore, new regulatory risk assessments are required [59], making the new approach methodology (NAM) a promising way to estimate potential risks [60]. A particular advantage of NAM is that it avoids the use of intact animals and uses strategies that involve any technology, procedure, approach, or combination of them, including in vitro assays, to provide information on the toxicological profile of compounds. In this regard, government efforts have been made to regulate animal testing, such as the 7th Amendment of the European Union Cosmetics Directive that bans animals in cosmetic testing [61]; the European Registration, Evaluation, Authorization, and Restriction Regulation for Chemicals, which only allows animal testing in certain circumstances [62]; and the 3-R principle, which includes replacing, reducing, and refining in the research ethics [63]. Therefore, institutions worldwide have become a reference for the regulation of in vitro tests, such as the Centers for the Validation of Alternative Methods (CVAM), established in Europe (ECVAM), Japan (JCVAM), the USA (ICCVAM), Brazil (BraCVAM), and the Organization for Economic Cooperation and Development (OECD). They provide open access guidelines for in vitro and in vivo toxicological testing.

These institutions have also promoted integrated approaches to determine the biological and toxicological relevance of new assays. Two of the more critical approaches are integrated approaches to testing and assessment (IATA) and adverse outcome pathways (AOP). IATA will guide future efforts based on scientific knowledge gaps once this approach gathers information from various sources to identify the toxicological profile of compounds [60]. AOP begins with a molecular event, the trigger (toxicity), which initiates a series of key events linked by causally plausible key event relationships, ultimately leading to an undesirable outcome [64]. The combination of IATA and AOP can guide the scientific community to ensure a complete toxicity profile of a compound that considers the 3Rs principles and other regulatory requirements that concern ethical issues of in vivo testing.

Aside from ethical concerns related to animal testing, the clinical gap between different species is an issue that can be avoided with in vitro testing, considering that some animal testing sometimes shows poor human correlation. For instance, the low correlation between rat and human skin [65] and the differences between human and rodent xenobiotic metabolism led to several late-stage and post-marketing drug withdrawals. Finally, with regard to nanomaterials, some early studies have shown that dogs are susceptible to polysorbate surfactants. These examples highlight the differences within the biological systems and reproductive cycles of different mammals or other laboratory animals phylogenetically distant from humans [66]. These interspecific differences limit the predictive ability of in vivo tests to infer the effects of foreign substances on the human physiological system [65–68]. Additionally, in vivo tests can be difficult to replicate because they are labor-intensive, costly, and time-consuming due to the inherent complexity of each organism.

Creating a new toxicity profile has become a necessity, as more chemicals have been introduced into the market. The scenario is somewhat complex for nanomaterials due to the physical and chemical complexity, for example, multiple sizes, surface functionalization, and composition, resulting in an arduous effort and significant cost to access the in vivo toxicological profile of nanomaterials [59]. For example, a single nanomaterial can be fabricated in various sizes with different surface properties and shapes, which can confer unique properties that can negatively or positively impact biological systems [59]. The heterogeneity of nanomaterials complicates their testing on a case-by-case basis, traditionally (in vivo) assessing the toxicity of a wide variety of existing nanomaterials. However, many safety assessments and a large number of animals would be required [69], making risk assessments prohibitive in terms of cost and time, and the 3Rs would not be respected [70].

Non-animal approaches seem to better fill this need, particularly in vitro methods, as they offer an alternative to using animals. They are being developed for various purposes, such as cytotoxicity, proliferation, genotoxicity, and altering gene expression [30,60,65]. In vitro assays as predictive screens to assess nanoparticle toxicity are simpler, faster, and cheaper than in vivo assays [59,68–70]. Furthermore, the in vitro approach commits to faithfully reproducing the function and organization of the specific tissue or biological system, and the selection of the appropriate in vitro cell model depends on the compound of interest and how it compares to the in vivo exposure [71].

Therefore, in vitro methods have emerged as a promising tool to circumvent these limitations for the toxicological assessment of nanomaterials. The use of cells, tissues, and organoids of human origin allows for more relevant information on nanotoxicological outcomes. Furthermore, in vitro methods provide a comprehensive study of nanocell interactions and cell-specific responses, generating a mechanistic understanding of cellular events that cannot be obtained from animal experiments [59,68,69], which may lead to a better mechanistic understanding of nanoparticle-induced toxicity. Strategic combinations of in vitro test methods in an IATA have great potential to generate results that can identify AOP elements in detail. When applied to nanomaterials, this can provide a broad view of the potential adverse health effects. Therefore, in vitro assays can be controlled and generate more reproducible data [45]; additionally, they are simpler than in vivo tests, avoid the use of animals, are sensitive and time-efficient, and, from a high-throughput screening perspective [71], can be used to generate robust toxicological data. For example, multiparametric approaches such as High-Content Screening have demonstrated high sensitivity and specificity, significantly higher than traditional in vitro assays and comparable to in vivo assays [72]. Therefore, advances in in vitro assays show that they can be a valuable tool for pivotal preclinical studies.

13.2.2 Assessing the nanotoxicity in vitro

In vitro assays can be used to determine the nanotoxicity and its underlying molecular mechanisms. As previously discussed, nanomaterials can have more subtle effects such as disturbing cell signaling, altering biological processes (e.g., cell proliferation and migration), or even leading to more late-stage toxic effects (e.g., cell death). Next, some techniques are discussed in more detail to highlight some key issues. Thus, the major challenges are presented, as well as recommendations to reduce the pitfalls and help to design the toxicity evaluation.

13.2.3 Cytotoxicity

Classical assays estimate cell viability through dye-exclusion assays, for example, propidium iodide, allowing for the evaluation of plasmatic membrane integrity and enzymatic activity. Standard Guidelines often comprehend some of these techniques for cellular state evaluation, such as OECD Guideline 432 that includes neutral red assay and OECD Guideline 491 that includes short time exposure test, which uses MTT assay.

The MTT assay is a colorimetric, quantitative, indirect method for assessing cell viability that can also be used to estimate proliferation in mammalian cells. The assay is based on the reduction of the original yellow tetrazolium bromide salt (MTT) to the water-insoluble violet formazan salt. When solubilized, formazan salt can be quantified by optical density by measuring its absorbance at a wavelength of 570 nm [73]. Salt reduction mainly occurs within the mitochondria and could represent this organelle activity and thus the cellular viability state. However, tetrazolium salt can also be reduced on the endoplasmic reticulum, cytoplasm, and cell membrane [74]. It is well known that variations in conditions such as glucose levels in the culture medium, incubation period, and different cell lineages can significantly affect MTT test results and should be carefully controlled [75]. Special care should be taken in nanotoxicity applications; many nanoparticles are said to interfere with the MTT assay and lead to unreliable results, including liposomes, solid lipid nanoparticles, silica nanoparticles, and others [76,77]. Therefore, appropriate controls (e.g., placebo formulations and bare nanoparticles) should guarantee that nanoparticles do not scatter light or directly reduce MTT. In addition, to avoid other potential artifacts, we recommend using supplemental assays with orthogonal display (e.g., fluorescence microscopy images). When performed under the appropriate conditions, viability tests can be useful to determine the initial parameters for studying the nanotoxicity (e.g., dose- and time-dependent cellular injury responses).

13.2.4 Cell migration

Cellular migration is part of an organism's homeostasis being essential in many biological processes such as organism development, tissue regeneration, and the development of diseases like cancer. For example, in adult humans, wound healing is a cascade of events involving chemotaxis, cell division, neovascularization, and deposition of a new extracellular matrix [78]. Although essential in physiological situations, migration is an undesirable process in tumor progression, as it increases the motility of these cells, increasing the likelihood of metastasis.

The cell migration assay (also known as the wound healing assay or scratch assay) is performed by making a scratch in the center of the well and filling the subsequent area with cell migration. Researchers report that nanoparticles inhibit tumor cell migration and increase migration in tissue regeneration. For example, zinc nanoparticles reduced the migration of retinal tumor cells in a concentration-dependent manner, or graphene nanoparticles inhibited the migration of glioblastoma cells by reducing adhesion molecules [79,80]. Similarly, biogenic AgNPs could inhibit migration and reduce colony formation of human bladder carcinoma cell lines 5637 [81]. Increased migration was reported for chitosan-copper nanoparticles in corneal cell regeneration [82], and silver-tannin nanoparticles increased keratinocyte migration [83]. Such studies are essential for the discovery of new therapies but also offer an opportunity to explore a new and relatively unexplored area of the adverse effects of nanoparticles on cell migration. However, as described for MTT, many articles were published without reporting the effects of empty nanoparticles.

13.2.5 Cell proliferation

Cell proliferation is a complex and controlled cellular process defined as an increase in cell number resulting from a division of mother cells giving rise to a population of daughter cells [84,85]. Cell proliferation leads to the production of new cells to replace dead cells by activating a cell cycle that ensures tissue maintenance, repair, and development [84,86]. Proliferation is a key process used as a parameter in cytotoxicity studies and anticancer drug screening [87]. However, in cancer cells, the signals regulating proliferation and survival pathways are dysregulated by genetic mutations; these mutations cause cells to acquire increased cell proliferation and suppress the ability for cell death, characterizing neoplastic progression [86]. For this reason, the use of anticancer drugs tends to decrease the ability of cancer cells to reproduce and survive [84,88]. Cytotoxicity studies measure proliferative ability to understand whether the drug, compound, or nanoparticle can increase, decrease, or inhibit proliferation [89–92].

Many assays can be used as initial indicators of cell proliferation such as cell count and viability, for example, trypan blue dye count, 3H-thymidine incorporation, and measurement of dsDNA concentration by fluorescent assays (commercial kits such as CyQUANT, Quant-IT PicoGreen) [90,93]. Proliferation can be indirectly measured by determination of ATP content, for example, CellTiter-Glo, ATP lite based on the luciferin/luciferase generation [94], or measurement of a biochemical marker to assess the metabolic activity of the cell, for example, MTT, MTS, WTS, and Alamar Blue/Resazurin assays [90,95]. Cell proliferation can be properly monitored by markers that undoubtedly report the rise of new cells such as Ki67 antibody, 5-Bromo-2'-Deoxyuridine (BrdU), or 50-ethynyl-20-deoxyuridine (EdU). The Ki67 antibody, present during the cell cycle, reports cell proliferation by detecting Ki67 protein, noticeably increasing during the S-phase of the cell cycle. BrdU is a synthetic thymidine analog that can be incorporated into the DNA of actively dividing cells during the cell cycle. EdU is also a synthetic thymidine analog that incorporates nascent DNA and measured by fluorescence after azide binding to DNA conjugated with a fluorophore [96]. These methods of studying cell proliferation are used to identify drugs and nanoparticles that interfere with the cell cycle, and their use has been described for different cell types [89,91,92].

13.2.6 Cell death

The process of cell death is involved in maintaining homeostasis in organisms [97,98] and can be divided into two broad groups: regulated cell death (RCD) and accidental cell death (ACD). The ACD type occurs when cells are subjected to physical, chemical, or mechanical stress and lack signaling or regulatory involvement [99]. In contrast, RCD (such as apoptosis, necroptosis, ferroptosis, pyroptosis, entotic cell death, netotic cell death, parthanatos, lysosome-dependent cell death, autophagy-dependent cell death, alkaliptosis, and oxeiptosis) involves a well-regulated cascade of signaling molecules [97,99–102]. Cell death can be a hallmark of clinical conditions such as cancer and autoimmune and neurodegenerative diseases [103]; it can also indicate the toxic potential of compounds and nanocompounds [104–110]. Some examples of the application of cell death assays are the assessment of the cytotoxic potential of nanomaterials to track potential exposure risks [104–110] or identify new antitumor effects of nanomaterials for application in cancer therapies [111,112].

In this regard, nanoparticles have been reported to induce cell death through different mechanisms such as apoptosis, necroptosis, ferroptosis, and autophagy. However, there are still concerns regarding the cytotoxic effects and adverse outcomes that the application of nanoparticles to fight cancer may promote [113]. For this reason, the properties and in vitro toxicity of therapeutical nanomaterials still need to be explored [45]; therefore, many mechanistic assays can be employed, such as fluorescent labeled assays: TUNEL assay, comet assay, caspase activity assay, and annexin V/propidium iodide assay. Also, activity determination of specific proteins associated with cell death can be employed by Western blotting or immunoblotting [114–116]. As discussed above, nanomaterials have been reported to interfere with some assay components, such as the comet assay and the determination of cytokines, chemokines, and growth factors. The cytotoxic assays described in this section are summarized in Fig. 13.1.

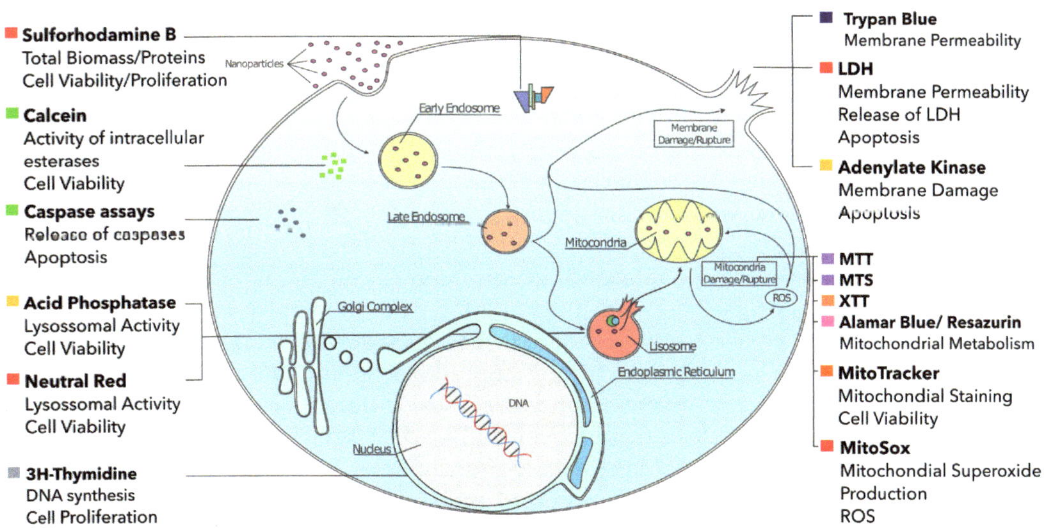

FIGURE 13.1 **In vitro cytotoxic assays for assessing nanotoxicity.** Schematic representation of the uptake of nanoparticles by the cell via endocytosis and some intracellular nanotoxic effects caused by them. Each colored square (outside the cell) indicates a different cytotoxic assay that describes the target structures and associated cellular state.

13.2.7 Considerations for better assay quality outcomes

In vitro assays are the ideal entry point for nanotoxicity assessment because they can be rapid, flexible, and inexpensive and reduce the use of animals and the steps in the safety assessment pathway [117]. However, different, even conflicting, in vitro toxicity results for very similar nanoparticles have been reported in the literature. In addition, the wide range of elements surrounding the design and layout of these methods makes it more difficult to mimic settings across studies and consequently to compare results. Therefore, a critical overview of the assay and its conditions, such as nanomaterial properties, biological models, controls, measurements, and analyzes, is essential to obtain more accurate information that supports better decisions regarding the risks of nanomaterials to organisms and the environment [118–120].

Tissues and cells are specialized, having exclusive biological processes that lead to cell-dependent responses to stimuli. Choosing a relevant model to test the hypothesis increases the likelihood of a well-done translation of knowledge from in vitro to in vivo, primarily when human cells are evaluated to predict human toxicity. Many factors must be taken into consideration while designing the in vitro assays: available systems include cancer, healthy lineages, and primary cells; co-cultures; 2D versus 3D cultures; spheroids, organoids, or even the most complicated induced pluripotent stem cells. A cost-benefit analysis must be performed regarding the purpose of the assay and the significance of the result to determine which model falls between informative and costly, that is, time, money, and effort [121]. Handling, maintenance, and storage practices are also very influential factors and can directly affect viability test results: cell count, seeding density, rinsing, the maximum of cells passage number, and confluence status at treatment; therefore culture media conditions must be carefully assessed, registered, and reported [117,120]. In addition, factors such as cell culture function, genotype, and phenotype, as well as possible contamination with external agents (such as mycoplasma) or other cells (cross-contamination), must be monitored [121,122].

Minimizing interferences in assay results is possible by evaluating nanomaterial properties such as size, polydispersion, and colloidal stability of nanoparticles in different solutions; observation of reagent conditions as pH values in culture media; and identification of any interaction between the material and the reagents or containers used [118]. For example, size and shape can affect nanoparticle uptake and cellular redox metabolism, leading to an over- or underestimation of viability measured by tetrazolium salt-based assay methods, emphasizing the relevance of interference control in verifying whether the assay is functioning as properly documented [120]. Furthermore, other controls and experimental designs must be carefully considered once they severely impact the results. For instance, since cells are not exposed to any conditions other than their regular maintenance, negative controls are essential and are most commonly conceived with assay design. However, cytotoxic effects can be overestimated without positive controls, so a stable, easily assayed positive control is critical to experimental design [123]. Finally, the plate layout for cellular assays can also be optimized to include pipetting, seeding density, and operational controls, making possible not only comparisons of results generated in the same laboratory but also between different study groups [117,124].

After the optimization of controls, determining nanoparticles concentration of use is the next higher influencing factor on cell-based assays. First, the effective bulk concentration of nanoparticles is a complex metric to accurately determine, taking into account internalization and adsorption to cells. Therefore, it would be more appropriate to use the exposure dose or the total number of particles [118,119]. Moreover, nanoparticles are often tested in in vitro assays at high concentrations compared to what reaches cells in an in vivo situation, thus drawing unrealistic toxicity scenarios and precluding the translations of these results between biological models [118]. These high doses also trigger the appearance of artifacts: high rates of particle internalization led to intense mitochondrial activity and consequent stress, generating reactive oxidative stress species that can even induce autophagy in exposed cells [125]. Therefore, failure to adjust the concentration factor for the study can directly lead to less realistic toxicity assessments.

Avoiding different cytotoxicity profiles on the same nanomaterial is done by standardizing in vitro assays, including careful documentation steps and an orthogonal assessment approach. OECD has published a guideline for reporting in vitro toxicity results (GD122), targeting nonstandardized assays [126]. Other templates such as ToxTemp proposed catalog five main test elements, purpose, system, exposure scheme, endpoint, and predictive model, which provide basic information to appropriately classify the reported result [127]. Also, using more than one methodology with different endpoints (metabolic status, ATP consumption, and reactive oxygen species generation) improves the robustness of the results, preventing method-related bias, and allows for a more holistic view of understanding the mechanisms of toxicity associated with chronological information [118,120,128]. Some suggestions for developing more robust assays are listed: use of reliable positive and negative controls; confirmation of cell death and mechanistic details using orthogonal assays; consideration of the therapeutic conditions (e.g., target tissues, presence or absence of a protein corona, and route of administration); and use of more than two cell lines to confirm and discuss [45]. However, it must be considered that in the development of nanoparticles for therapeutic purposes, the insufficient understanding of the toxicological and possible side effects can lead to undesirable clinical results and further impede the implementation of promising nanotechnologies.

13.3 Image-based approaches for assessing nanotoxicity

Cellular imaging used to be known as a descriptive and qualitative science incapable of performing high-throughput experiments. However, this scenario changed in the mid-1990s with the advance of three areas: automated fluorescence microscopy, automated image analysis algorithms, and machine learning methods for processing and recognizing subcellular patterns [129,130]. These advances promoted high-throughput and high-resolution analysis and paved the way for multiple types of scientific studies, such as kinetic studies, target-based drug discovery studies, drug screening studies, safety assessment in drug discovery, mode of action studies, and predictive toxicology. The image-based approach applied to cellular imaging consists of acquiring images, labeling subcellular structures and organelles, and extracting multiparametric data from individualized cells to visualize the data at the cell or well population level [131,132].

Nowadays, the image-based platform is considered a robust approach and plays an important role in pharmaceutical discovery and industry, mainly in drug discovery studies

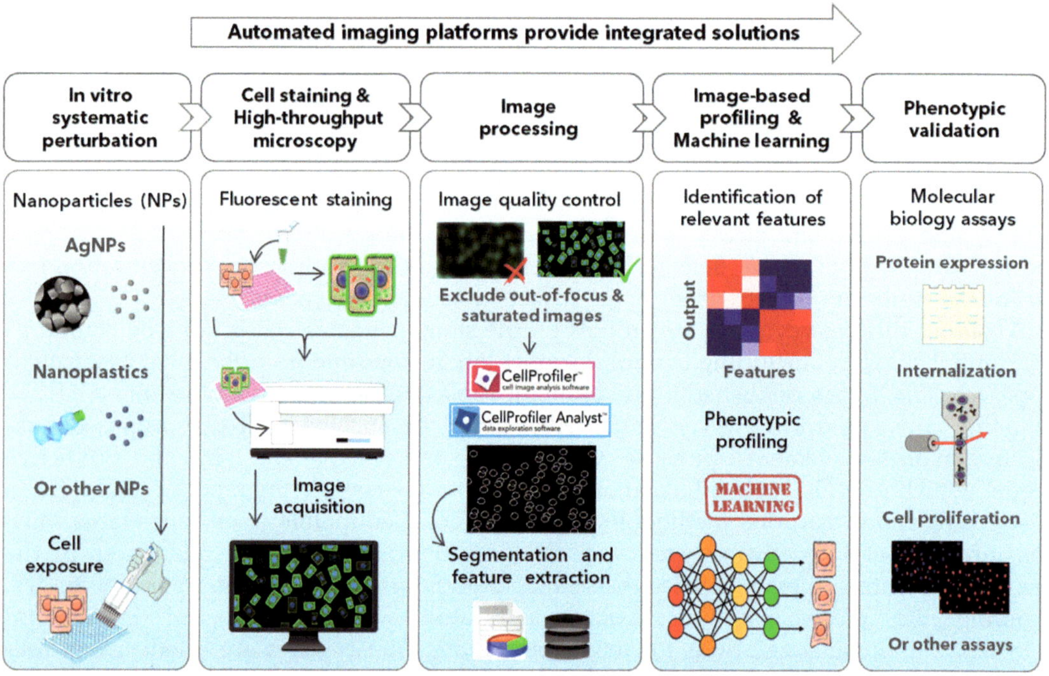

FIGURE 13.2 The main components of the automated high-content screening and analysis (HCS/A) to study the interactions between nanoparticles and cells. The essential elements of these HCS/A systems are cellular exposure to nanoparticles (systematic in vitro perturbation), cell staining and image acquisition, image processing, data analysis (image-based profiling and machine learning), and phenotypic profile validation for the determination of nanoparticle-triggered cytotoxic effect profiles in vitro. HCS/A assay development involves optimizing cell exposure, image acquisition methods, and image analysis algorithms.

and early safety evaluation [131,133]. In this context, high-content screening (HCS) and high-content analysis (HCA) became mainstream technologies, as shown in Fig. 13.2 [134,135]. During drug development, these approaches can help identify hits and play a critical role in compound prioritization and optimization. The HCA/HCS pipeline typically consists of treating cells with the agent of interest (e.g., siRNA, drugs, toxins, and nanomaterials) and autonomously acquires a large set of images of cells labeled with different probes (e.g., fluorophores, fluorescent antibodies, or gene reporters). These approaches have been used to label biological processes, organelles, proteins, molecules, or even use genetically engineered cells expressing fluorescent proteins (FPs) [132,136]. Typically, multiple morphological (e.g., cell shape, membranes, nucleus, and mitochondria) or functional (e.g., cell signaling, gene expression, and metabolism) parameters of cells are captured, but cell systems, tissues, small organisms, or even whole organisms can also be imaged. Image analysis algorithms can extract multiparametric data from cellular properties to assess cell physiology by quantifying multiple phenotypes or functional parameters [133,137]. To be analyzed, the multiparametric data of individual cells require approaches from bioinformatics, computer vision, systems biology, and machine learning. These analyses serve as a basis for identifying subpopulations;

uncovering patterns, trends, and associations; identifying phenotypes; and pattern recognition for data-mining, for example, the classification of compounds according to their pharmacological or toxicological mode of action. This approach can also be used for screening assays, aiming to assess many interferents in a biological context to identify hits for future mechanistic assays [132,138–140].

In toxicology, the HCS and HCA approaches can be used in in vitro tests for toxicity screening of compounds, drugs, and nanomaterials [141,142]. More specifically, in the toxicology field, genotoxicity and hepatotoxicity are parameters that we can measure and evaluate using robust assays such as the Ames test, mouse lymphoma assay, micronucleus assay, comet assay, and chromosomal aberration assay to identify possible DNA damage [132,142]. The use of dyes, probes, and immunofluorescence can measure mitochondrial function and membrane potential, calcium homeostasis, apoptotic activation, and oxidative stress to identify potential hepatotoxicity [132,140]. Furthermore, these approaches could be used to elucidate the mechanism of action and possible adverse health effects of nanoparticles, drugs, and compounds, providing detailed information at the cellular level as spatial distribution and interaction data permeating a biological system environment [132,141].

13.3.1 Phenotypic profiling

Many approaches can generate single-cell multiparametric data, such as deep sequencing, proteomics, and cell imaging. All information collected about the cells (morphological, biochemical, and structural) can describe their phenotype. Image-based phenotypic profiling uses the information at the cellular and subcellular levels to assess cell health and homeostasis. This multivariate information is extracted from cell images using morphological, intensity, and texture measurements, which can be done in the presence or absence of perturbing agents (e.g., siRNA, toxins, and nanoparticles). Phenotypic profiling has been used to diagnose complex cell phenotypes [143], contribute to drug repurposing while predicting the biological activity of compounds [144], and accelerate discoveries that usually rely only on the genetic profile. Similarly, phenotypic analysis can characterize the differences between healthy cells and nanoparticle-treated cells. In addition, different profiles can be used to gain insight into the mechanisms of action of nanoparticles [54,141,145,146]. For example, machine learning algorithms can be used to classify or cluster nanoparticle-treated cells with different known injuries using the specific phenotype they induce [138,147]. Although phenotypic profiling has become an essential framework in biology, pharmacology, and toxicology, this approach to nanotoxicity remains largely unexplored, particularly to unveil mechanistic details of nanotoxicity under relevant conditions.

13.3.2 Use of fluorescent dyes for nanotoxicology assessment

Multichannel fluorescence microscopy is at the heart of image-based phenotypic profiling and acts as a powerful tool to assess single-cell and spatiotemporal mechanisms of nanotoxicity [141,148,149]. Cell fluorescent labeling follows three strategies: the use of fluorophores, also called fluorescent dyes or probes; fluorescent antibodies; and genetically encoded FPs. Some illustrative examples of each strategy are shown in Table 13.1. Fluorophores target

TABLE 13.1 Fluorophores, antibodies, and fluorescent proteins applied in high-content screening (HCS) and high-content analysis (HCA).

Fluorophores	Applications	λexcitation	λemission	References
Hoechst33258	Labels cellular nuclei, cell count	356	465	[150]
Hoechst33342	Labels cellular nuclei, cell count and *cell painting*	361	486	[151]
Calcein AM	Labels live cells/cell viability	495	515	[150]
Propidium Iodide	Labels nuclei of dead cells/cell viability	536	617	[152]
Sytox Orange	Labels nuclei of dead cells	547	570	[153]
DRAQ5	Labels nuclei and lipids	655	730	[154]
SYT0 14	Nucleoli and cytoplasmic RNA	*517(DNA)*	*549(DNA)*	[151]
		521(RNA)	*547(RNA)*	
Acridine Orange	Labels DNA/RNA/acid vesicles	*468(DNA, RNA, acidic vesicles)*	*560 (DNA, RNA)*	[155]
			660 (acidic vesicles)	
Lysotracker Green, Blue, Yellow, Red and Deep Red	Lysosomal location	504/373/465/577/647	511/422/535/590/668	[156]
Concanavalin A + AlexaFluor488	Labels endoplasmic reticulum and *cell painting*	495	519	[151]
Phalloidin + Alexa Fluor568	F-actin cytoskeleton, Golgi, plasma membrane and *cell painting*	578	600	[151]
Fluo-4 AM	Reports intracellular calcium	494	516	[154]
Mitotracker Green, Orange and Deep Red	Reports mass/morphology; mitochondrial location and *cell painting*	*490/551/644*	*516/576/665*	[151]
JC-1 Red and Green	Reports changes in MMP (Δψ)	*585/514*	*590/525*	[157]
Tetramethylrhodamine methyl ester (TMRM)	Reports changes in MMP (Δψ)	549	576	[150]
TOTO-3	Reports plasma membrane integrity	642	660	[154]
YOYO-1	Reports plasma membrane integrity	491	509	[154]
BODIPY665/676	Reports lipid peroxidation	665	676	[154]
BODIPY493/503	Labels membrane lipids	493	503	[152]
BODIPY558/568 C12	Labels membrane lipids	558	568	[154]
CellROX Green	Reports levels of ROS	485	520	[158]
CM-H2DCFDA	Reports levels of ROS	495	527	[152]

(Continued)

TABLE 13.1 (Continued)

Fluorophores	Applications	λexcitation	λemission	References
MitoSOX Red	Reports mitochondrial superoxide production	510	580	[154]
ThiolTracker Violet	Reports reduced glutathione levels	405	526	[159]
Antibodies				
Anti-casp3 + AlexaFluor488	Reports apoptosis	490	525	[146]
Anti-SLC6A19 + AlexaFluor488	Reports cellular amino acid transport	495	519	[160]
Anti-E-chaderin + AlexaFluor647	Reports cellular adherence	652	668	[160]
Anti-p53 + PE	Report tumor formation	565	574	[161]
AntiZO-1 + AlexaFluor594	Reports cellular junction	590	617	[160]
Genetically encoded fluorescent proteins (FPs)				
G-protein + Green GP (GFP)	Reports ligand-dependent homologous desensitization and internalization	483	500	[162]
Clathrin + GFP	Reports acid vesicles formation	483	500	[163]
NADH-NAD$^+$ + GFP	Reports cellular redox state	483	500	[164]
MitoTimer + GFP	Reports protein maturation	483	500	[165]
	Mitochondria turnover			
MitoTimer + Red fluorescent protein (RFP)	Reports protein maturation	558	583	[166]
	Mitochondria turnover			
MitoSypHer + Yellow fluorescent protein	Reports pH	430	480	[166]
	Mitochondrial matrix			
mtKeima + RFP	Mitophagy	561	620	[166]
Histone + GFP	Reports chromosomal condensation state	483	500	[167]

different cellular environments based on chemical properties such as lipophilicity, net charge, or pH. For example, cationic lipophilic dyes can target mitochondria; one of the most commonly used is tetramethylrhodamine methyl ester (TMRM), which reports changes in mitochondrial membrane potential (MMP, $\Delta\psi$). In addition, they can be nonfluorescent enzyme substrates that become fluorescent upon enzymatic activity. For example, the DEVD peptide (Asp-Glu-Val-Asp), a substrate of Caspase-3 or 7, is one of the most commonly used substrates linked to a fluorophore (e.g., rhodamine 110) to report apoptosis induction recorded in live-cell imaging. Fluorescent antibodies rely on antibody epitope-specific recognition of the protein of interest. Primary fluorescent antibodies or nanobodies can be used, or nonfluorescent primary antibodies subsequently labeled with secondary fluorescent antibodies. For example, antibodies against Lysosomal-associated membrane protein 1 (LAMP-1) can be used for colocalization studies of nanomaterials in the endosome-lysosome pathway. Alternatively, cells expressing FPs can be used to report cell structures, biological processes, or even recently evolved proteins to report sensors capable of reporting cellular physiological changes. FPs are particularly useful for live cell imaging and tracking biological phenomena on time. Table 13.1 organizes the three strategies to design setups for phenotypic profiling. Multiplexing of these different strategies relies on determining which cellular structures or processes to label and depends on selecting compatible spectral properties. It means minimizing crosstalk, unintentionally exciting one dye when another is excited, and bleed-through, detecting the emission of an unintentional dye in the channel of another dye. Many publications have focused on developing guidelines to increase rigor and reproducibility in fluorescence microscopy.

A promising approach to analyze nanotoxicity is based on the *Cell Painting assay* [151]. This generalized method stains subcellular structures with fluorescent dyes to determine a wide range of phenotypic effects. After concentration optimization, phenotypic cytotoxic signatures can be generated using known compounds and then compared to the cells incubated with nanoparticles. Furthermore, the single-cell analysis makes this approach an unbiased tool that allows for evaluating a broad spectrum of cytotoxic phenotypic effects in subpopulations neglected by most conventional techniques. In Cell Painting, fluorescent dyes stain subcellular components, the nuclei, the endoplasmic reticulum, the F-actin cytoskeleton, and the mitochondria. Dozens of metrics extracted from each stain image are combined to create a profile. Assessing the phenotypic profile using staining unrelated to any specific outcome provides an unbiased understanding of the underlying mechanisms, which can be interpreted using tools such as Morpheus and Jupyter Notebooks [168]. This allows us to gain a more comprehensive understanding of the cytotoxic effects of nanoparticles [151].

13.3.3 Automated microscopy

Depending on the nanotoxicological question, many parameters have to be selected for the image acquisition: the type of microscopy chosen, the number of channels and times, several viewpoints, and the objective magnification. Therefore, automated microscopes become indispensable to enable the acquisition of large image-based datasets of treated cells stained for many organelles and structures [130,169]. For example, in the subsequent single-cell analysis, one must never forget to acquire a channel for segmenting the objects; typically the first step consists of segmenting the cell and/or the nuclei from the background. The objective magnification must be chosen depending on the analyzed structure. Analysis of subcellular compartments may require higher objectives, 20× or 40×, while lower objectives (10× or 4×) may be required for whole population analysis based on cell count events. One challenge is determining how many images to take. Although the general rule is that the more data the better, the bottleneck associated with storage capacity can be easily reached. Adequate performance of supervised learning to learn a new category may require as little as 50–100 cells, but much more data may be required for other approaches [130]. All of these points need to be considered when conducting a high content analysis. These large datasets require automated image analysis performed by software capable of extracting as much information as possible from the imaged cells [170,171].

13.3.4 Machine learning models for nanotoxicology analysis

Automated microscopy produces images at speeds and complexity beyond the human ability to analyze them, making it impossible to handle, process, or even detect subtle changes caused by nanomaterials. In this context, computational analysis is imperative to improve the efficiency and reproducibility of bioimage research, which is heavily based on statistical learning tools. In short, supervised machine learning algorithms learn the results from the provided data (training set) and use the learned rules to predict the results from unseen data (test set). The training set is used to learn a function from the data, which can be applied to the training set and the test set (which the learner has not seen before). The main goal is that the learning algorithm generalizes well without losing performance [172]; for this purpose, these algorithms can be scored on the accuracy using many strategies such as the confusion matrix [173]. When working with categorical data, the result of the algorithm splits the data into classes, while continuous data has the result as a regression function. Many algorithms are available, and some are discussed in this chapter to illustrate their applications [173].

Many algorithms support supervised machine learning analysis on continuous or categorical data. For example, logistic regression, rather than a continuous value, predicts whether something is true or false by looking at an S curve in the data. Meanwhile, a decision tree recursively splits the data into smaller subsets by grouping more similar data based on the characteristics provided and setting thresholds [174]. Supervised learning can be used in nanotoxicology to predict trends and analyze complex data. Mathematical models make it possible to use the already existing data on the known physiology (organs and tissues) at the organism level and to combine information from the studied nanoparticles to simulate drug/nanoparticle concentration profiles, which are defined as physiologically based pharmacokinetics/pharmacodynamics [175]. Regression models and random forest can also be used to distinguish between classes, for example, when designing a new formulation [176]. Therefore, we see the potential to integrate these common types of data collected in toxicology (e.g., dose-response curves) with image data from cells in vitro to have a robust model to predict nanotoxicological patterns.

Unsupervised learning approaches recognize patterns from unlabeled data, such as principal component analysis (PCA). They are often used to reduce the dimensionality of the dataset while maintaining the variability of the data [177]. For example, the PCA algorithm identified four nanoparticles that reduce acute toxicity profiles (zinc oxide, polystyrene latex amine, nanotubes, and nickel oxide) by measuring cell viability, apoptosis, necrosis, and other characteristics of cells treated with different nanoparticles [79]. Another promising approach is deep learning (DL), a family of machine learning based on neural networks (NN), an algorithm trained to tune many parameters to predict the relationship between the input data and the output (labels). Each layer of a neural network consists of neurons that process data nonlinearly. Each layer transforms the data to become more complex and abstract, turning the relationships between input and output nonlinear [178]. Much of the potential of DL remains unexplored in nanotoxicology.

13.3.5 Software available for image processing

Processing all the images acquired with high-content screening can be tedious, and many software have been developed and improved for this purpose over the last decades [179,180]. The most popular example is ImageJ, more specifically Fiji, which focuses on bioimage analysis and allows for general image processing and macroprogramming to automate tasks [181]. Other versatile and powerful tools are CellProfiler and CellProfiler Analyst software, which are capable of performing a typical image analysis workflow and using the same pipeline for many images. CellProfiler is an open-source software introduced in 2005 that segment, extract information, and analyzes images with built-in modules [182,183]. These modules can perform many tasks like cell segmentation, feature extraction, image quality control, and illumination correction, even allowing for integration of CellProfiler with software like ImageJ or Cellpose [170]. When using CellProfiler, researchers must determine which features are important to answer the biological question. Created as image data exploration using machine learning tools, CellProfiler Analyst helps users filter and choose relevant features from the data [184]. In addition, CellProfiler Analyst provides the tools to train machine learning models and visualize data with histograms and scatterplots. Furthermore, a quality control pipeline is performed by CellProfiler and CellProfiler Analyst [185], which excludes blurred and saturated images from the analysis.

Image processing using CellProfiler and CellProfiler Analyst translates morphological features (i.e., phenotypes) into more compact datasets containing hundreds to thousands of morphological features. This approach improves the chances of finding new mechanisms and unexpected phenotypes of nanoparticle-treated cells that are particularly powerful for subtle changes missed by conventional techniques. Many assays could be evaluated with this technique, for example, when cells are treated with nanomaterials and images are taken for cell viability, oxidative stress, DNA damage, and more [186]. Alternatively, different assays can generate an excessive number of images, which benefits from automated image analysis. For example, cell migration is often assessed by a scratch assay, also called a wound-healing assay, and many images are taken to track the closure of the cell migration area. Some software alternatives are available that perform this measurement, such as ImageJ/Fiji [181]; however, this analysis must be performed manually, frame by frame. A friendly alternative was developed and implemented in the Python programming language, PyScratch, which is open-source software that analyzes migration images in an automated way, eliminating user influence at the time of analysis and allowing quantitative and reproducible analysis of data [155].

13.4 Regulations

As pointed out before, nanomaterials differ in composition, shape, and size range, resulting in various properties that are enabled or enhanced by their dimensions. This fact poses hurdles to standardizing tests and regulations. However, the number of products containing nanosized parts is increasing and requires proper regulatory evaluation. For example, the FDA has reported new nanoscale-related applications since 1970, but half of each from the last 10 years (to 2019). Applications included new cosmetics, human and veterinary medicinal products, and specific claims for nanomaterials ranging from antimicrobial activity to cell proliferation and tissue integration (dental implants) [187].

Several forums and health agencies worldwide screened scientific evidence concerning physiological and environmental effects, particularly of nanosized products. The FDA did not release specific legislation but offers five guidelines to industry, each for a type of product: cosmetics, food ingredients, food contact products, food for animals, liposomal drugs, and drug-containing nanomaterials [188–192] The sixth one states what they consider a nanotechnology-containing product, if it contains material with one dimension at the nanoscale range (1–100 nm) or if it contains submicron dimensions (down to 1 micron) if they are designed to have specific characteristics related to their size [193]. This definition is broader than most standard documents, which only consider the nanoscale. The FDA cooperates with the American Society for testing and materials (ASTM) to provide standard definitions and techniques for US regulatory processes and other countries. When it comes to the drug regulatory field, the FDA is in conjunction with the United States Pharmacopeia (USP); they just released a new chapter focusing on products containing nanomaterials [194]. The document will reflect the legislation of several other countries, as USP is recognized worldwide when it comes to analytical methods for drug testing.

Governments of many countries constantly rely on the guides of the International Organization for Standardization (ISO standards) to assess quality and safety parameters. The ISO Nanotechnology Committee was responsible for publishing 98 standards, and 28 standards are under development (by 2022). They approach definitions, physicochemical characterization, toxicity assessments, detection assays, and considerations for specific materials such as carbon nanotubes and gold nanoparticles. Another relevant institution for standards is the Organization for Economic Cooperation and Development (OECD). Their guidelines are intended to support regulatory testing for any chemical or nanomaterial and often refer to ISO or other standards to avoid and complement ISO or other standards. OECD Testing Guidelines for Chemicals (including nanomaterials) are accepted in all OECD member countries and adherents. This practice reduces duplication of testing, use of animals, and trade barriers when testing is within guidelines. In addition to the cytotoxicity and toxicology protocols cited above, they also address physicochemical and environmental aspects.

Allan and colleagues have thoroughly reviewed international legislation and regulation of nanomaterials and nanoplastics, revealing the diverse landscape discussed at the 2019 Global Summit on Regulatory Sciences. As challenges, stakeholders (scientists, industry, and government agencies) highlighted the development of sufficient reference standards for nanomaterials, the replacement of quality tests with high costs/time/skills, the robustness of interlaboratory assessments, and the global harmonization of definitions and practices. For nanoplastics, in particular, there are few standards affecting toxicity protocols, and regulatory tools to control unintended releases throughout the life cycle of products are lacking [195]. However, it is noteworthy that several guidelines, harmonizations, and reference standards are in preparation so that the regulatory picture is in a constant flow of improvement.

13.5 Conclusions

In recent decades, the trend toward nanotoxicity has led to a deeper understanding of the toxic effects of intentionally and unintentionally produced nanomaterials. Advancing nanotoxicity requires the development of methods capable of handling a variety of nanomaterials and subtle and heterogeneous cellular responses. In this scenario, a multiparametric approach is an appropriate alternative for understanding this cellular phenomenon. Among the many options, the HCA appears as a cost-effective, fast, and powerful tool. Furthermore, they are becoming increasingly powerful with advances in machine learning and deep learning techniques. HCS/HCA can perform phenotypic profiling to understand functional heterogeneity in many toxicologically relevant in vitro models, with a great capacity to translate these results into more clinically relevant in vivo studies. However, regulatory agencies worldwide face a testing backlog due to the limitations of in vivo testing, particularly because it is too slow and expensive. Therefore, the further development of in vitro methods for nanosafety assessment will be crucial to ensure safety and accelerate the introduction of nanotechnology into the market.

References

[1] Suk R, Montealegre JR, Nemutlu GS, Nyitray AG, Schmeler KM, Sonawane K, et al. Public knowledge of human papillomavirus and receipt of vaccination recommendations. JAMA Pediatrics 2019;173(11):1099–101. Available from: https://doi.org/10.1001/jamapediatrics.2019.3105.

[2] El-Ansary A, Al-Daihan S, Al-Dbass A, Al-Ayadhi L. Measurement of selected ions related to oxidative stress and energy metabolism in Saudi autistic children. Clin Biochem 2010;43(1–2):63–70. Available from: https://doi.org/10.1016/j.clinbiochem.2009.09.008.

[3] Bosetti R, Jones SL. Cost-effectiveness of nanomedicine: estimating the real size of nano-costs. Nanomedicine 2019;14(11):1367–70. Available from: https://doi.org/10.2217/nnm-2019-0130.

[4] Kad A, Pundir A, Arya SK, Bhardwaj N, Khatri M. An elucidative review to analytically sieve the viability of nanomedicine market. J Pharm Innov 2020;. Available from: https://doi.org/10.1007/s12247-020-09495-5.

[5] Rajendran L, Veilumuthu R, Ramachandran. A study on the effectiveness of virtual lab in E-learning. Int J Computer Sci Eng 2010;2.

[6] Yan Y, Such GK, Johnston APR, Best JP, Caruso F. Engineering particles for therapeutic delivery: prospects and challenges. ACS Nano 2012;6(5):3663–9. Available from: https://doi.org/10.1021/nn3016162.

[7] Cabral H, Nishiyama N, Kataoka K. Supramolecular nanodevices: from design validation to theranostic nanomedicine. Acc Chem Res 2011;44(10):999–1008. Available from: https://doi.org/10.1021/ar200094a.

[8] Farjadian F, Moghoofei M, Mirkiani S, Ghasemi A, Rabiee N, Hadifar S, et al. Bacterial components as naturally inspired nano-carriers for drug/gene delivery and immunization: set the bugs to work? Biotechnol Adv 2018;36:968–85. Available from: https://doi.org/10.1016/j.biotechadv.2018.02.016.

[9] Gadekar V, Borade Y, Kannaujia S, Rajpoot K, Anup N, Tambe V, et al. Nanomedicines accessible in the market for clinical interventions. J Control Rel 2021;330:372–97. Available from: https://doi.org/10.1016/j.jconrel.2020.12.034.

[10] Maranhão RC, Vital CG, Tavoni TM, Graziani SR. Clinical experience with drug delivery systems as tools to decrease the toxicity of anticancer chemotherapeutic agents. Expert Opin Drug Delivery 2017;14(10):1217–26. Available from: https://doi.org/10.1080/17425247.2017.1276560.

[11] Caster JM, Patel AN, Zhang T, Wang A. Investigational nanomedicines in 2016: a review of nanotherapeutics currently undergoing clinical trials. Wiley Interdiscip Rev Nanomed Nanobiotechnol 2017;9(1). Available from: https://doi.org/10.1002/wnan.1416.

[12] Hare JI, Lammers T, Ashford MB, Puri S, Storm G, Barry ST. Challenges and strategies in anti-cancer nanomedicine development: an industry perspective. Adv Drug Deliv Rev 2017;108:25–38. Available from: https://doi.org/10.1016/j.addr.2016.04.025.
[13] Satalkar P, Elger BS, Hunziker P, Shaw D. Challenges of clinical translation in nanomedicine: a qualitative study. Nanomed Nanotechnol Biol Med 2016;12(4):893–900. Available from: https://doi.org/10.1016/j.nano.2015.12.376.
[14] Shvedova AA, Kisin ER, Mercer R, Murray AR, Johnson VJ, Potapovich AI, et al. Unusual inflammatory and fibrogenic pulmonary responses to single-walled carbon nanotubes in mice. Am J Physiol—Lung Cell Mol Physiol 2005;289(5):L698–708. Available from: https://doi.org/10.1152/ajplung.00084.2005.
[15] Warheit DB, Laurence BR, Reed KL, Roach DH, Reynolds GAM, Webb TR. Comparative pulmonary toxicity assessment of single-wall carbon nanotubes in rats. Toxicol Sci 2004;77(1):117–25. Available from: https://doi.org/10.1093/toxsci/kfg228.
[16] Oberdörster E. Manufactured nanomaterials (fullerenes, C 60) induce oxidative stress in the brain of juvenile largemouth bass. Environ Health Perspect 2004;112(10):1058–62. Available from: https://doi.org/10.1289/ehp.7021.
[17] Donaldson K, Stone V, Tran CL, Kreyling W, Borm PJA. Nanotoxicology. Occup Environ Med 2004;61(9):727–8. Available from: https://doi.org/10.1136/oem.2004.013243.
[18] Oberdörster G, Oberdörster E, Oberdörster J. Nanotoxicology: an emerging discipline evolving from studies of ultrafine particles. Environ Health Perspect 2005;113(7):823–39. Available from: https://doi.org/10.1289/ehp.7339.
[19] Singh AV, Laux P, Luch A, Sudrik C, Wiehr S, Wild AM, et al. Review of emerging concepts in nanotoxicology: opportunities and challenges for safer nanomaterial design. Toxicol Mech Methods 2019;29(5):378–87. Available from: https://doi.org/10.1080/15376516.2019.1566425.
[20] Santamaria A. Historical overview of nanotechnology and nanotoxicology. Methods Mol Biol 2012;926:1–12. Available from: https://doi.org/10.1007/978-1-62703-2-1_1.
[21] Buzea C, Pacheco II, Robbie K. Nanomaterials and nanoparticles: sources and toxicity. Biointerphases 2007;2(4):MR17–71. Available from: https://doi.org/10.1116/1.2815690.
[22] Ai J, Biazar E, Jafarpour M, Montazeri M, Majdi A, Aminifard S, et al. Nanotoxicology and nanoparticle safety in biomedical designs. Int J Nanomed 2011;6:1117–27. Available from: https://doi.org/10.2147/IJN.S16603.
[23] Kumar V, Dasgupta N, Ranjan S. Nanotoxicology: toxicity evaluation, risk assessment and management. 1st ed. CRC Press; 2018.
[24] Sahu SC, Casciano DA. Handbook of nanotoxicology, nanomedicine and stem cell use in toxicology. Handbook of nanotoxicology, nanomedicine and stem cell use in toxicology. Wiley Blackwell.; 2014. p. 1–417. Available from: https://doi.org/10.1002/9781118856017.
[25] Durán N, Guterres SS, Alves OL, editors. Nanotoxicology: materials, methodologies, and assessments, nanomedicine and nanotoxicology. New York: Springer; 2014. Available from: https://doi.org/10.1007/978-1-4614-8993-1.
[26] Gatti AM, Montanari S. Case studies in nanotoxicology and particle toxicology. Case studies in nanotoxicology and particle toxicology. Elsevier Inc.; 2015. p. 1–260. Available from: https://www.sciencedirect.com/book/9780128012154/case-studies-in-nanotoxicology-and-particle-toxicology.
[27] Lai DY. Toward toxicity testing of nanomaterials in the 21st century: a paradigm for moving forward. WIREs Nanomed Nanobiotechnol 2012;4(1):1–15. Available from: https://doi.org/10.1002/wnan.162.
[28] Love SA, Maurer-Jones MA, Thompson JW, Lin YS, Haynes CL. Assessing nanoparticle toxicity. Annu Rev Anal Chem 2012;5:181–205. Available from: https://doi.org/10.1146/annurev-anchem-062011-143134.
[29] Marquis BJ, Love SA, Braun KL, Haynes CL. Analytical methods to assess nanoparticle toxicity. Analyst 2009;134(3):425–39. Available from: https://doi.org/10.1039/b818082b.
[30] Hillegass JM, Shukla A, Lathrop SA, MacPherson MB, Fukagawa NK, Mossman BT. Assessing nanotoxicity in cells in vitro. Wiley Interdiscip Rev Nanomed Nanobiotechnol 2010;2(3):219–31. Available from: https://doi.org/10.1002/wnan.54.
[31] Hussain SM, Warheit DB, Ng SP, Comfort KK, Grabinski CM, Braydich-Stolle LK. At the crossroads of nanotoxicology in vitro: past achievements and current challenges. Toxicol Sci 2015;147(1):5–16. Available from: https://doi.org/10.1093/toxsci/kfv106.

[32] Lazareva A, Keller AA. Estimating potential life cycle releases of engineered nanomaterials from wastewater treatment plants ACS Sustain Chem Eng 2014;2(7):1656–65 American Chemical Society. Available from: https://doi.org/10.1021/sc500121w.

[33] Younis SA, El-Fawal EM, Serp P. Nano-wastes and the environment: potential challenges and opportunities of nano-waste management paradigm for greener nanotechnologies. In: Hussain CM, editor. Handbook of environmental materials management. Cham: Springer International Publishing; 2019. p. 2063–134. Available from: https://doi.org/10.1007/978-3-319-73645-7_53.

[34] Cervantes-Avilés P, Huang Y, Keller AA. Incidence and persistence of silver nanoparticles throughout the wastewater treatment process. Water Res 2019;156:188–98. Available from: https://doi.org/10.1016/j.watres.2019.03.031.

[35] Giese B, Klaessig F, Park B, Kaegi R, Steinfeldt M, Wigger H, et al. Risks, release and concentrations of engineered nanomaterial in the environment. Sci Rep 2018;8(1). Available from: https://doi.org/10.1038/s41598-018-19275-4.

[36] Temizel-Sekeryan S, Hicks AL. Global environmental impacts of silver nanoparticle production methods supported by life cycle assessment. Resources, Conserv Recycling 2020;156:104676. Available from: https://doi.org/10.1016/j.resconrec.2019.104676.

[37] StatNano. Nanotechnology products database | NPD [WWW Document]. https://product.statnano.com; 2020 [accessed 10.29.21].

[38] Peng L, Fu D, Qi H, Lan CQ, Yu H, Ge C. Micro- and nano-plastics in marine environment: source, distribution and threats—a review. Sci Total Environ 2020;698:134254. Available from: https://doi.org/10.1016/j.scitotenv.2019.134254.

[39] Uurasjärvi E, Hartikainen S, Setälä O, Lehtiniemi M, Koistinen A. Microplastic concentrations, size distribution, and polymer types in the surface waters of a northern European lake. Water Environ Res 2020;92(1):149–56. Available from: https://doi.org/10.1002/wer.1229.

[40] Winton DJ, Anderson LG, Rocliffe S, Loiselle S. Macroplastic pollution in freshwater environments: focusing public and policy action. Sci Total Environ 2020;704. Available from: https://doi.org/10.1016/j.scitotenv.2019.135242.

[41] Koelmans AA, Bakir A, Burton GA, Janssen CR. Microplastic as a vector for chemicals in the aquatic environment: critical review and model-supported reinterpretation of empirical studies. Environ Sci Technol 2016;50(7):3315–26. Available from: https://doi.org/10.1021/acs.est.5b06069.

[42] Liu J, Ma Y, Zhu D, Xia T, Qi Y, Yao Y, et al. Polystyrene nanoplastics-enhanced contaminant transport: role of irreversible adsorption in glassy polymeric domain. Environ Sci Technol 2018;52(5):2677–85. Available from: https://doi.org/10.1021/acs.est.7b05211.

[43] Bouwmeester H, Hollman PCH, Peters RJB. Potential health impact of environmentally released micro- and nanoplastics in the human food production chain: experiences from nanotoxicology. Environ Sci Technol 2015;49(15):8932–47. Available from: https://doi.org/10.1021/acs.est.5b01090.

[44] Wright SL, Kelly FJ. Plastic and human health: a micro issue? Environ Sci Technol 2017;51(12):6634–47. Available from: https://doi.org/10.1021/acs.est.7b00423.

[45] Drasler B, Sayre P, Steinhäuser KG, Petri-Fink A, Rothen-Rutishauser B. In vitro approaches to assess the hazard of nanomaterials. NanoImpact 2017;8:99–116. Available from: https://doi.org/10.1016/j.impact.2017.08.002.

[46] Perde-Schrepler M, Florea A, Brie I, Virag P, Fischer-Fodor E, Vâlcan A, et al. Size-dependent cytotoxicity and genotoxicity of silver nanoparticles in cochlear cells in vitro. J Nanomater 2019;2019:1–12. Available from: https://doi.org/10.1155/2019/6090259.

[47] Keller AA, Lazareva A. Predicted releases of engineered nanomaterials: from global to regional to local. Environ Sci Technol Lett 2013;1(1):65–70. Available from: https://doi.org/10.1021/ez400106t.

[48] Hawthorne J, De La Torre Roche R, Xing B, Newman LA, Ma X, Majumdar S, et al. Particle-size dependent accumulation and trophic transfer of cerium oxide through a terrestrial food chain. Environ Sci Technol 2014;48(22):13102–9. Available from: https://doi.org/10.1021/es503792f.

[49] De La Torre Roche R, Servin A, Hawthorne J, Xing B, Newman LA, Ma X, et al. Terrestrial trophic transfer of bulk and nanoparticle La_2O_3 does not depend on particle size. Environ Sci Technol 2015;49(19):11866–74. Available from: https://doi.org/10.1021/acs.est.5b02583.

[50] Keller AA, McFerran S, Lazareva A, Suh S. Global life cycle releases of engineered nanomaterials. J Nanopart Res 2013;15(6). Available from: https://doi.org/10.1007/s11051-013-1692-4.
[51] Keller AA, Wang H, Zhou D, Lenihan HS, Cherr G, Cardinale BJ, et al. Stability and aggregation of metal oxide nanoparticles in natural aqueous matrices. Environ Sci Technol 2010;44(6):1962–7. Available from: https://doi.org/10.1021/es902987d.
[52] Falagan-Lotsch P, Grzincic EM, Murphy CJ. One low-dose exposure of gold nanoparticles induces long-term changes in human cells. Proc Natl Acad Sci U S A 2016;113(47):13318–23. Available from: https://doi.org/10.1073/pnas.1616400113.
[53] Grün AL, Emmerling C. Long-term effects of environmentally relevant concentrations of silver nanoparticles on major soil bacterial phyla of a loamy soil. Environ Sci Eur 2018;30(1). Available from: https://doi.org/10.1186/s12302-018-0160-2.
[54] Murschhauser A, Röttgermann PJF, Woschée D, Ober MF, Yan Y, Dawson KA, et al. A high-throughput microscopy method for single-cell analysis of event-time correlations in nanoparticle-induced cell death. Commun Biol 2019;2(1). Available from: https://doi.org/10.1038/s42003-019-0282-0.
[55] Altschuler SJ, Wu LF. Cellular heterogeneity: do differences make a difference? Cell 2010;141(4):559–63. Available from: https://doi.org/10.1016/j.cell.2010.04.033.
[56] Ivask A, Mitchell AJ, Hope CM, Barry SC, Lombi E, Voelcker NH. Single Cell Level quantification of nanoparticle-cell interactions using mass cytometry. Anal Chem 2017;89(16):8228–32. Available from: https://doi.org/10.1021/acs.analchem.7b01006.
[57] Costa PM, Fadeel B. Emerging systems biology approaches in nanotoxicology: towards a mechanism-based understanding of nanomaterial hazard and risk. Toxicol Appl Pharmacol 2016;299:101–11. Available from: https://doi.org/10.1016/j.taap.2015.12.014.
[58] Kodali V, Littke MH, Tilton SC, Teeguarden JG, Shi L, Frevert CW, et al. Dysregulation of macrophage activation profiles by engineered nanoparticles. ACS Nano 2013;7(8):6997–7010. Available from: https://doi.org/10.1021/nn402145t.
[59] Halappanavar S, Nymark P, Krug HF, Clift MJD, Rothen-Rutishauser B, Vogel U. Non-animal strategies for toxicity assessment of nanoscale materials: role of adverse outcome pathways in the selection of endpoints. Small 2021;17(15). Available from: https://doi.org/10.1002/smll.202007628.
[60] Madden JC, Enoch SJ, Paini A, Cronin MTD. A review of in silico tools as alternatives to animal testing: principles, resources and applications. Altern Lab Animals: ATLA 2020;48(4):146–72. Available from: https://doi.org/10.1177/0261192920965977.
[61] European Parliament & European Council. Directive 2003/15/EC of the European Parliament and of the Council of 27 February 2003. https://eur-lex.europa.eu/legal-content/EN/TXT/?uri = celex%3A32003L0015; 2003.
[62] European Parliament & European Council. Regulation (EC) No 1907/2006 of the European Parliament and of the Council of 18 December 2006. https://eur-lex.europa.eu/legal-content/EN/TXT/?uri = CELEX%3A02006R1907-20140410; 2006.
[63] European Parliament & European Council. Directive 2010/63/EU of the European Parliament and of the Council of 22 September 2010 on the protection of animals used for scientific purposes. https://eur-lex.europa.eu/legal-content/EN/TXT/?uri = celex%3A32010L0063; 2010.
[64] Draskau MK, Spiller CM, Boberg J, Bowles J, Svingen T. Developmental biology meets toxicology: contributing reproductive mechanisms to build adverse outcome pathways. Mol Hum Reprod 2020;26(2):111–16. Available from: https://doi.org/10.1093/molehr/gaaa001.
[65] Dellambra E, Odorisio T, D'Arcangelo D, Failla CM, Facchiano A. Non-animal models in dermatological research. Altex 2019;36(2):177–202. Available from: https://doi.org/10.14573/altex.1808022.
[66] Clift MJD, Jenkins GJS, Doak SH. An alternative perspective towards reducing the risk of engineered nanomaterials to human health. Small 2020;16(36). Available from: https://doi.org/10.1002/smll.202002002.
[67] Clark M, Steger-Hartmann T. A big data approach to the concordance of the toxicity of pharmaceuticals in animals and humans. Regul Toxicol Pharmacol 2018;96:94–105. Available from: https://doi.org/10.1016/j.yrtph.2018.04.018.
[68] Fritsche E, Haarmann-Stemmann T, Kapr J, Galanjuk S, Hartmann J, Mertens PR, et al. Stem cells for next level toxicity testing in the 21st century. Small 2021;17(15). Available from: https://doi.org/10.1002/smll.202006252.

[69] Chen RJ, Chen YY, Liao MY, Lee YH, Chen ZY, Yan SJ, et al. The current understanding of autophagy in nanomaterial toxicity and its implementation in safety assessment-related alternative testing strategies. Int J Mol Sci 2020;21(7). Available from: https://doi.org/10.3390/ijms21072387.

[70] Basei G, Hristozov D, Lamon L, Zabeo A, Jeliazkova N, Tsiliki G, et al. Making use of available and emerging data to predict the hazards of engineered nanomaterials by means of in silico tools: a critical review. NanoImpact 2019;13:76–99. Available from: https://doi.org/10.1016/j.impact.2019.01.003.

[71] Fizesan I, Cambier S, Moschini E, Chary A, Pop A, Kiss B, et al. In vitro cellular models, a resourceful tool in respiratory toxicology. Farmacia 2018;66(4):573–80. Available from: https://doi.org/10.31925/farmacia.2018.4.2.

[72] Olson H, Betton G, Robinson D, Thomas K, Monro A, Kolaja G, et al. Concordance of the toxicity of pharmaceuticals in humans and in animals. Regul Toxicol Pharmacol 2000;32(1):56–67. Available from: https://doi.org/10.1006/rtph.2000.1399.

[73] Mosmann T. Rapid colorimetric assay for cellular growth and survival: application to proliferation and cytotoxicity assays. J Immunol Methods 1983;65(1–2):55–63. Available from: https://doi.org/10.1016/0022-1759(83)90303-4.

[74] Bernas T, Dobrucki J. Mitochondrial and nonmitochondrial reduction of MTT: interaction of MTT with TMRE, JC-1, and NAO mitochondrial fluorescent probes. Cytometry 2002;47(4):236–42. Available from: https://doi.org/10.1002/cyto.10080.

[75] Vistica DT, Monks A, Pittman A, Boyd MR. Tetrazolium-based assays for cellular viability: a critical examination of selected parameters affecting formazan production. Cancer Res 1991;51(10):2515–20.

[76] Angius F, Floris A. Liposomes and MTT cell viability assay: an incompatible affair. Toxicol Vitro 2015;29(2):314–19. Available from: https://doi.org/10.1016/j.tiv.2014.11.009.

[77] Guilherme VA, Ribeiro LNM, Tofoli GR, Franz-Montan M, de Paula E, de Jesus MB. Current challenges and future of lipid nanoparticles formulations for topical drug application to oral mucosa, skin, and eye. Curr Pharm Des 2017;23(43):6659–75. Available from: https://doi.org/10.2174/1381612823666171122103849.

[78] Kaplani K, Koutsi S, Armenis V, Skondra FG, Karantzelis N, Champeris Tsaniras S, et al. Wound healing related agents: ongoing research and perspectives. Adv Drug Deliv Rev 2018;129:242–53. Available from: https://doi.org/10.1016/j.addr.2018.02.007.

[79] Wang XZ, Yang Y, Li R, Mcguinnes C, Adamson J, Megson IL, et al. Principal component and causal analysis of structural and acute in vitro toxicity data for nanoparticles. Nanotoxicology 2014;8(5):465–76. Available from: https://doi.org/10.3109/17435390.2013.796534.

[80] Wierzbicki M, Jaworski S, Kutwin M, Grodzik M, Strojny B, Kurantowicz N, et al. Diamond, graphite, and graphene oxide nanoparticles decrease migration and invasiveness in glioblastoma cell lines by impairing extracellular adhesion. Int J Nanomed 2017;12:7241–54. Available from: https://doi.org/10.2147/IJN.S146193.

[81] Ferreira LAB, Garcia-Fossa F, Radaic A, Durán N, Fávaro WJ, de Jesus MB. Biogenic silver nanoparticles: in vitro and in vivo antitumor activity in bladder cancer. Eur J Pharm Biopharm 2020;151:162–70. Available from: https://doi.org/10.1016/j.ejpb.2020.04.012.

[82] Tellios V, Liu H, Tellios N, Li X, Hutnik CML. Administration of nitric oxide through a novel copper- chitosan delivery system in human corneal and limbal epithelial cell injury. Investig Ophthalmol Vis Sci 2018;59(2):967–77. Available from: https://doi.org/10.1167/iovs.17-23044.

[83] Orlowski P, Zmigrodzka M, Tomaszewska E, Ranoszek-Soliwoda K, Czupryn M, Antos-Bielska M, et al. Tannic acid-modified silver nanoparticles for wound healing: the importance of size. Int J Nanomed 2018;13:991–1007. Available from: https://doi.org/10.2147/IJN.S154797.

[84] Yang N, Ray SD, Krafts K. Cell proliferation. In: Wexler P, editor. Encyclopedia of toxicology. 3rd ed. Oxford: Academic Press; 2014. p. 761–5. Available from: https://doi.org/10.1016/B978-0-12-386454-3.00274-8.

[85] Gratzner HG. Monoclonal antibody to 5-bromo- and 5-iododeoxyuridine: a new reagent for detection of DNA replication. Science 1982;218(4571):474–5. Available from: https://doi.org/10.1126/science.7123245.

[86] Evan GI, Vousden KH. Proliferation, cell cycle and apoptosis in cancer. Nature 2001;411(6835):342–8. Available from: https://doi.org/10.1038/35077213.

[87] Towne DL, Nicholl EE, Comess KM, Galasinski SC, Hajduk PJ, Abraham VC. Development of a high-content screening assay panel to accelerate mechanism of action studies for oncology research. J Biomol Screen 2012;17(8):1005–17. Available from: https://doi.org/10.1177/1087057112450050.

[88] Chan GKY, Kleinheinz TL, Peterson D, Moffat JG. A simple high-content cell cycle assay reveals frequent discrepancies between cell number and ATP and MTS proliferation assays. PLoS One 2013;8(5). Available from: https://doi.org/10.1371/journal.pone.0063583.

[89] Özkan İ, Koçak P, Yıldırım M, Ünsal N, Yılmaz H, Telci D, et al. Garlic (Allium sativum)-derived SEVs inhibit cancer cell proliferation and induce caspase mediated apoptosis. Sci Rep 2021;11(1). Available from: https://doi.org/10.1038/s41598-021-93876-4.

[90] Präbst K, Engelhardt H, Ringgeler S, Hübner H. Basic colorimetric proliferation assays: MTT, WST, and resazurin. Methods in molecular biology, 1601. Humana Press Inc.; 2017. p. 1–17. Available from: https://doi.org/10.1007/978-1-4939-6960-9_1.

[91] Ryoo SR, Kim YK, Kim MH, Min DH. Behaviors of NIH-3T3 fibroblasts on graphene/carbon nanotubes: proliferation, focal adhesion, and gene transfection studies. ACS Nano 2010;4(11):6587–98. Available from: https://doi.org/10.1021/nn1018279.

[92] Javed Z, Khan K, Herrera-Bravo J, Naeem S, Iqbal MJ, Sadia H, et al. Genistein as a regulator of signaling pathways and microRNAs in different types of cancers. Cancer Cell Int 2021;21(1). Available from: https://doi.org/10.1186/s12935-021-02091-8.

[93] Jones LJ, Gray M, Yue ST, Haugland RP, Singer VL. Sensitive determination of cell number using the CyQUANT® cell proliferation assay. J Immunol Methods 2001;254(1–2):85–98. Available from: https://doi.org/10.1016/S0022-1759(01)00404-5.

[94] Hannah R, Beck M, Moravec R, Riss T. CellTiter-GloTM luminescent cell viability assay: a sensitive and rapid method for determining cell viability. Promega Cell Notes 2001;2.

[95] Quent VMC, Loessner D, Friis T, Reichert JC, Hutmacher DW. Discrepancies between metabolic activity and DNA content as tool to assess cell proliferation in cancer research. J Cell Mol Med 2010;14(4):1003–13. Available from: https://doi.org/10.1111/j.1582-4934.2010.01013.x.

[96] Mandavilli BS, Yan M, Clarke S. Cell-based high content analysis of cell proliferation and apoptosis. In: Johnston PA, Trask OJ, editors. High content screening: a powerful approach to systems cell biology and phenotypic drug discovery, methods in molecular biology. New York: Springer; 2018. p. 47–57. Available from: https://doi.org/10.1007/978-1-4939-7357-6_4.

[97] Bedoui S, Herold MJ, Strasser A. Emerging connectivity of programmed cell death pathways and its physiological implications. Nat Rev Mol Cell Biol 2020;21(11):678–95. Available from: https://doi.org/10.1038/s41580-020-0270-8.

[98] Yan G, Elbadawi M, Efferth T. Multiple cell death modalities and their key features (Review. World Acad Sci J 2020;2(2):39–48. Available from: https://doi.org/10.3892/wasj.2020.40.

[99] Tang D, Kang R, Berghe TV, Vandenabeele P, Kroemer G. The molecular machinery of regulated cell death. Cell Res 2019;29(5):347–64. Available from: https://doi.org/10.1038/s41422-019-0164-5.

[100] Chen Y, Hua Y, Li X, Arslan IM, Zhang W, Meng G. Distinct types of cell death and the implication in diabetic cardiomyopathy. Front Pharmacol 2020;11. Available from: https://doi.org/10.3389/fphar.2020.00042.

[101] Tonnus W, Belavgeni A, Beuschlein F, Eisenhofer G, Fassnacht M, Kroiss M, et al. The role of regulated necrosis in endocrine diseases. Nat Rev Endocrinol 2021;17(8):497–510. Available from: https://doi.org/10.1038/s41574-021-00499-w.

[102] Galluzzi L, Aaronson SA, Abrams J, Alnemri ES, Andrews DW, Baehrecke EH, et al. Guidelines for the use and interpretation of assays for monitoring cell death in higher eukaryotes. Cell Death Differ 2009;16 (8):1093–107. Available from: https://doi.org/10.1038/cdd.2009.44.

[103] Smith BA, Smith BD. Biomarkers and molecular probes for cell death imaging and targeted therapeutics. Bioconjugate Chem 2012;23(10):1989–2006. Available from: https://doi.org/10.1021/bc3003309.

[104] Lee YH, Cheng FY, Chiu HW, Tsai JC, Fang CY, Chen CW, et al. Cytotoxicity, oxidative stress, apoptosis and the autophagic effects of silver nanoparticles in mouse embryonic fibroblasts. Biomaterials 2014;35 (16):4706–15. Available from: https://doi.org/10.1016/j.biomaterials.2014.02.021.

[105] Li J, Zhang B, Chang X, Gan J, Li W, Niu S, et al. Silver nanoparticles modulate mitochondrial dynamics and biogenesis in HepG2 cells. Environ Pollut 2020;256:113430. Available from: https://doi.org/10.1016/j.envpol.2019.113430.

[106] Suliman YAO, Ali D, Alarifi S, Harrath AH, Mansour L, Alwasel SH. Evaluation of cytotoxic, oxidative stress, proinflammatory and genotoxic effect of silver nanoparticles in human lung epithelial cells. Environ Toxicol 2015;30(2):149–60. Available from: https://doi.org/10.1002/tox.21880.

[107] Sun C, Yin N, Wen R, Liu W, Jia Y, Hu L, et al. Silver nanoparticles induced neurotoxicity through oxidative stress in rat cerebral astrocytes is distinct from the effects of silver ions. NeuroToxicol 2016;52:210–21. Available from: https://doi.org/10.1016/j.neuro.2015.09.007.

[108] Tomankova K, Horakova J, Harvanova M, Malina L, Soukupova J, Hradilova S, et al. Cytotoxicity, cell uptake and microscopic analysis of titanium dioxide and silver nanoparticles in vitro. Food Chem Toxicol 2015;82:106–15. Available from: https://doi.org/10.1016/j.fct.2015.03.027.

[109] Xue Y, Zhang T, Zhang B, Gong F, Huang Y, Tang M. Cytotoxicity and apoptosis induced by silver nanoparticles in human liver HepG2 cells in different dispersion media. J Appl Toxicol 2016;36(3):352–60. Available from: https://doi.org/10.1002/jat.3199.

[110] Cheung TS, Lau PM, Lu H, Ho HP, Lui PPY, Kong SK. Cytotoxic and sublethal effects of silver nanoparticles on tendon-derived stem cells—implications for tendon engineering. Toxicol Res 2015;5(1):318–30. Available from: https://doi.org/10.1039/c5tx00349k.

[111] Dou L, Meng X, Yang H, Dong H. Advances in technology and applications of nanoimmunotherapy for cancer. Biomarker Res 2021;9(1). Available from: https://doi.org/10.1186/s40364-021-00321-9.

[112] Fan T, Ye W, Zhao P, Zhou W, Chen Y, He C, et al. pH-responsive core-shell nanogels induce in situ antigen production for cancer treatment. Chem Eng J 2021;426:130839. Available from: https://doi.org/10.1016/j.cej.2021.130839.

[113] Sepand MR, Ranjbar S, Kempson IM, Akbariani M, Muganda WCA, Müller M, et al. Targeting nonapoptotic cell death in cancer treatment by nanomaterials: recent advances and future outlook. Nanomed Nanotechnol Biol Med 2020;29:102243. Available from: https://doi.org/10.1016/j.nano.2020.102243.

[114] Jurišić V, Bumbaširević V. In vitro assays for cell death determination. Archive Oncol 2008;16(3–4):49–54. Available from: https://doi.org/10.2298/AOO0804049J.

[115] Kabakov AE, Gabai VL. Cell death and survival assays. In: Calderwood SK, Prince TL, editors. Chaperones: methods and protocols, methods in molecular biology. New York: Springer; 2018. p. 107–27. Available from: https://doi.org/10.1007/978-1-4939-7477-1_9.

[116] Kepp O, Galluzzi L, Lipinski M, Yuan J, Kroemer G. Cell death assays for drug discovery. Nat Rev Drug Discov 2011;10(3):221–37. Available from: https://doi.org/10.1038/nrd3373.

[117] Elliott JT, Rösslein M, Song NW, Toman B, Kinsner-Ovaskainen A, Maniratanachote R, et al. Toward achieving harmonization in a nanocytotoxicity assay measurement through an interlaboratory comparison study. Altex 2017;34(2):201–18. Available from: https://doi.org/10.14573/altex.1605021.

[118] Azhdarzadeh M, Saei AA, Sharifi S, Hajipour MJ, Alkilany AM, Sharifzadeh M, et al. Nanotoxicology: advances and pitfalls in research methodology. Nanomedicine 2015;10(18):2931–52. Available from: https://doi.org/10.2217/nnm.15.130.

[119] Soenen SJ, Manshian B, Montenegro JM, Amin F, Meermann B, Thiron T, et al. Cytotoxic effects of gold nanoparticles: a multiparametric study. ACS Nano 2012;6(7):5767–83. Available from: https://doi.org/10.1021/nn301714n.

[120] Domey J, Haslauer L, Grau I, Strobel C, Kettering M, Hilger I. Probing the cytotoxicity of nanoparticles: experimental pitfalls and artifacts. In: Wegener J, editor. Measuring biological impacts of nanomaterials, bioanalytical reviews. Cham: Springer International Publishing; 2014. p. 31–44. Available from: https://doi.org/10.1007/11663_2013_8.

[121] Coecke S, Balls M, Bowe G, Davis J, Gstraunthaler G, Hartung T, et al. Guidance on good cell culture practice: a report of the second ECVAM task force on good cell culture practice. ATLA Altern Lab Anim 2005;33(3):261–87. Available from: https://doi.org/10.1177/026119290503300313.

[122] American Type Culture Collection Standards Development Organization Workgroup ASN-0002. Cell line misidentification: the beginning of the end. Nat Rev Cancer 2010;10(6):441–8. Available from: https://doi.org/10.1038/nrc2852.

[123] Labouta HI, Sarsons C, Kennard J, Gomez-Garcia MJ, Villar K, Lee H, et al. Understanding and improving assays for cytotoxicity of nanoparticles: what really matters? RSC Adv 2018;8(41):23027–39. Available from: https://doi.org/10.1039/C8RA03849J.

[124] Rösslein M, Elliott JT, Salit M, Petersen EJ, Hirsch C, Krug HF, et al. Use of cause-and-effect analysis to design a high-quality nanocytotoxicology assay. Chem Res Toxicol 2015;28(1):21–30. Available from: https://doi.org/10.1021/tx500327y.

[125] Manshian BB, Himmelreich U, Soenen SJ. Standard cellular testing conditions generate an exaggerated nanoparticle cytotoxicity profile. Chem Res Toxicol 2017;30(2):595–603. Available from: https://doi.org/10.1021/acs.chemrestox.6b00340.

[126] OECD. Guidance document on good in vitro method practices (GIVIMP). OECD series on testing and assessment. https://doi.org/10.1787/9789264304796-en; 2018.

[127] Krebs A, Waldmann T, Wilks MF, van Vugt-Lussenburg BMA, van der Burg B, Terron A, et al. Template for the description of cell-based toxicological test methods to allow evaluation and regulatory use of the data. Altex 2019;36(4):682–99. Available from: https://doi.org/10.14573/altex.1909271.

[128] Riebeling C, Piret J-P, Trouiller B, Nelissen I, Saout C, Toussaint O, et al. A guide to nanosafety testing: considerations on cytotoxicity testing in different cell models. NanoImpact 2018;10:1–10. Available from: https://doi.org/10.1016/j.impact.2017.11.004.

[129] Abraham VC, Taylor DL, Haskins JR. High content screening applied to large-scale cell biology. Trends Biotechnol 2004;22(1):15–22. Available from: https://doi.org/10.1016/j.tibtech.2003.10.012.

[130] Shariff A, Kangas J, Coelho LP, Quinn S, Murphy RF. Automated image analysis for high-content screening and analysis. J Biomol Screen 2010;15(7):726–34. Available from: https://doi.org/10.1177/1087057110370894.

[131] Lang P, Yeow K, Nichols A, Scheer A. Cellular imaging in drug discovery. Nat Rev Drug Discov 2006;5(4):343–56. Available from: https://doi.org/10.1038/nrd2008.

[132] Li S, Xia M. Review of high-content screening applications in toxicology. Arch Toxicol 2019;93(12):3387–96. Available from: https://doi.org/10.1007/s00204-019-02593-5.

[133] Persson M, Hornberg JJ. Advances in predictive toxicology for discovery safety through high content screening. Chem Res Toxicol 2016;29(12):1998–2007. Available from: https://doi.org/10.1021/acs.chemrestox.6b00248.

[134] Lin S, Schorpp K, Rothenaigner I, Hadian K. Image-based high-content screening in drug discovery. Drug Discov Today 2020;25(8):1348–61. Available from: https://doi.org/10.1016/j.drudis.2020.06.001.

[135] Bullen A. Microscopic imaging techniques for drug discovery. Nat Rev Drug Discov 2008;7(1):54–67. Available from: https://doi.org/10.1038/nrd2446.

[136] Van Vliet E, Daneshian M, Beilmann M, Davies A, Fava E, Fleck R, et al. Current approaches and future role of high content imaging in safety sciences and drug discovery. Altex 2014;31(4):479–93. Available from: https://doi.org/10.14573/altex.1405271 Elsevier GmbH.

[137] Kan A. Machine learning applications in cell image analysis. Immunol Cell Biol 2017;95(6):525–30. Available from: https://doi.org/10.1038/icb.2017.16.

[138] Boutros M, Heigwer F, Laufer C. Microscopy-based high-content screening. Cell 2015;163(6):1314–25. Available from: https://doi.org/10.1016/j.cell.2015.11.007.

[139] Vasilevich AS, Carlier A, de Boer J, Singh S. How not to drown in data: a guide for biomaterial engineers. Trends Biotechnol 2017;35(8):743–55. Available from: https://doi.org/10.1016/j.tibtech.2017.05.007.

[140] Donato MT, Tolosa L. High-content screening for the detection of drug-induced oxidative stress in liver cells. Antioxidants 2021;10(1):106. Available from: https://doi.org/10.3390/antiox10010106.

[141] Mittal D, Kaul G. 5.13 - Towards nano-risk assessment with high throughput screening and high content analysis: an intelligent testing strategy. In: Andrews DL, Lipson RH, Nann T, editors. Comprehensive nanoscience and nanotechnology. 2nd ed. Oxford: Academic Press; 2019. p. 343–60. Available from: https://doi.org/10.1016/B978-0-12-803581-8.10430-8.

[142] Schoonen WGEJ, Westerink WMA, Van de Water FM, Horbach GJ. High content Screening for in vitro toxicity testing. Eur Pharm Rev 2011;.

[143] Doan M, Vorobjev I, Rees P, Filby A, Wolkenhauer O, Goldfeld AE, et al. Diagnostic potential of imaging flow cytometry. Trends Biotechnol 2018;36(7):649–52. Available from: https://doi.org/10.1016/j.tibtech.2017.12.008.

[144] Simm J, Klambauer G, Arany A, Steijaert M, Wegner JK, Gustin E, et al. Repurposing high-throughput image assays enables biological activity prediction for drug discovery. Cell Chem Biol 2018;25(5):611–18. Available from: https://doi.org/10.1016/j.chembiol.2018.01.015 e3.

[145] Li Y, Wang J, Zhao F, Bai B, Nie G, Nel AE, et al. Nanomaterial libraries and model organisms for rapid high-content analysis of nanosafety. Natl Sci Rev 2018;5(3):365–88. Available from: https://doi.org/10.1093/nsr/nwx120.

[146] Hansjosten I, Rapp J, Reiner L, Vatter R, Fritsch-Decker S, Peravali R, et al. Microscopy-based high-throughput assays enable multi-parametric analysis to assess adverse effects of nanomaterials in various cell lines. Arch Toxicol 2018;92(2):633–49. Available from: https://doi.org/10.1007/s00204-017-2106-7.
[147] Meijering E, Carpenter AE, Peng H, Hamprecht FA, Olivo-Marin JC. Imagining the future of bioimage analysis. Nat Biotechnol 2016;34(12):1250–5. Available from: https://doi.org/10.1038/nbt.3722.
[148] Nel A, Xia T, Meng H, Wang X, Lin S, Ji Z, et al. Nanomaterial toxicity testing in the 21st century: use of a predictive toxicological approach and high-throughput screening. Acc Chem Res 2013;46(3):607–21. Available from: https://doi.org/10.1021/ar300022h.
[149] Brayden DJ, Cryan SA, Dawson KA, O'Brien PJ, Simpson JC. High-content analysis for drug delivery and nanoparticle applications. Drug Discov Today 2015;20(8):942–57. Available from: https://doi.org/10.1016/j.drudis.2015.04.001.
[150] Iannetti EF, Smeitink JAM, Beyrath J, Willems PHGM, Koopman WJH. Multiplexed high-content analysis of mitochondrial morphofunction using live-cell microscopy. Nat Protoc 2016;11:1693–710. Available from: https://doi.org/10.1038/nprot.2016.094.
[151] Bray MA, Singh S, Han H, Davis CT, Borgeson B, Hartland C, et al. Cell painting, a high-content image-based assay for morphological profiling using multiplexed fluorescent dyes. Nat Protoc 2016;11(9):1757–74. Available from: https://doi.org/10.1038/nprot.2016.105.
[152] Donato MT, Tolosa L, Jiménez N, Castell JV, Gómez-Lechón MJ. High-content imaging technology for the evaluation of drug-induced steatosis using a multiparametric cell-based assay. J Biomol Screen 2012;17:394–400. Available from: https://doi.org/10.1177/1087057111427586.
[153] Petitte J, Doherty M, Ladd J, Marin CL, Siles S, Michelou V, et al. Use of high-content analysis and machine learning to characterize complex microbial samples via morphological analysis. PLoS One 2019;14:e0222528. Available from: https://doi.org/10.1371/journal.pone.0222528.
[154] Tolosa L, Gómez-Lechón MJ, Donato MT. High-content screening technology for studying drug-induced hepatotoxicity in cell models. Arch Toxicol 2015;89:1007–22. Available from: https://doi.org/10.1007/s00204-015-1503-z.
[155] Garcia-Fossa F, Gaal V, de Jesus MB. PyScratch: an ease of use tool for analysis of scratch assays. Computer Methods Prog Biomed 2020;193:105476. Available from: https://doi.org/10.1016/j.cmpb.2020.105476.
[156] Anguissola S, Garry D, Salvati A, O'Brien PJ, Dawson KA. High content analysis provides mechanistic insights on the pathways of toxicity induced by amine-modified polystyrene nanoparticles. PLoS One 2014;9:e108025. Available from: https://doi.org/10.1371/journal.pone.0108025.
[157] Antczak C, Wee B, Radu C, Bhinder B, Holland EC, Djaballah H. A high-content assay strategy for the identification and profiling of ABCG2 modulators in live cells. ASSAY Drug Dev Technol 2014;12:28–42. Available from: https://doi.org/10.1089/adt.2013.521.
[158] McBee ME, Chionh YH, Sharaf ML, Ho P, Cai MWL, Dedon PC. Production of superoxide in bacteria is stress- and cell state-dependent: a gating-optimized flow cytometry method that minimizes ROS measurement artifacts with fluorescent dyes. Front Microbiol 2017;8. Available from: https://doi.org/10.3389/fmicb.2017.00459.
[159] Mandavilli BS, Janes MS. Detection of intracellular glutathione using thioltracker violet stain and fluorescence microscopy. Curr Protoc Cytometry 2010;53:9.35.1–9.35.8. Available from: https://doi.org/10.1002/0471142956.cy0935s53.
[160] Abtahi S, Gliksman NR, Heneghan JF, Nilsen SP, Muhlich JL, Copeland J, et al. A simple method for creating a high-content microscope for imaging multiplexed tissue microarrays. Curr Protoc 2021;1:e68. Available from: https://doi.org/10.1002/cpz1.68.
[161] Radtke AJ, Chu CJ, Yaniv Z, Yao L, Marr J, Beuschel RT, et al. IBEX: an iterative immunolabeling and chemical bleaching method for high-content imaging of diverse tissues. Nat Protoc 2022;17:378–401. Available from: https://doi.org/10.1038/s41596-021-00644-9.
[162] Conway, Minor, Xu, Gunnet, DeBiasio, D'Andrea, et al. Quantification of G-protein coupled receptor internatilization using G-protein coupled receptor-green fluorescent protein conjugates with the arrayscantrade mark high-content screening system. J Biomol Screen 1999;4:75–86. Available from: https://doi.org/10.1177/108705719900400207.
[163] Snapp EL. Fluorescent proteins: a cell biologist's user guide. Trends Cell Biol, Spec Issue – Imaging Cell Biol 2009;19:649–55. Available from: https://doi.org/10.1016/j.tcb.2009.08.002.

[164] Hung YP, Albeck JG, Tantama M, Yellen G. (2011). Imaging cytosolic NADH-NAD$^+$ redox state with a genetically encoded fluorescent biosensor. Cell Metabolism. 10.1016/j.cmet.2011.08.012. 14(4):545-54.

[165] Cerqueira FM, Kozer N, Petcherski A, Baranovski BM, Wolf D, Assali EA, et al. MitoTimer-based high-content screen identifies two chemically-related benzothiophene derivatives that enhance basal mitophagy. Biochemical J 2020;477:461–75. Available from: https://doi.org/10.1042/BCJ20190616.

[166] Fernandes A, Hosseini V, Vogel V, Lovchik RD. Engineering solutions for biological studies of flow-exposed endothelial cells on orbital shakers. PLoS One 2022;17:e0262044. Available from: https://doi.org/10.1371/journal.pone.0262044.

[167] Neumann B, Held M, Liebel U, Erfle H, Rogers P, Pepperkok R, et al. High-throughput RNAi screening by time-lapse imaging of live human cells. Nat Methods 2006;3:385–90. Available from: https://doi.org/10.1038/nmeth876.

[168] Garcia-Fossa F, Costa Cruz M, Haghighi M, de Jesus MB, Singh S, Carpenter AE, et al. Interpreting image-based profiles using similarity clustering and single-cell visualization. Current Protocols in Cytometry 2023;3(3):e713. Available from: https://doi.org/10.1002/cpz1.713.

[169] O'Brien PJ, Edvardsson A. Validation of a multiparametric, high-content-screening assay for predictive/investigative cytotoxicity: evidence from technology transfer studies and literature review. Chem Res Toxicol 2017;30(3):804–29. Available from: https://doi.org/10.1021/acs.chemrestox.6b00403.

[170] Stirling DR, Swain-Bowden MJ, Lucas AM, Carpenter AE, Cimini BA, Goodman A. CellProfiler 4: improvements in speed, utility and usability. BMC Bioinforma 2021;22(1). Available from: https://doi.org/10.1186/s12859-021-04344-9.

[171] Grys BT, Lo DS, Sahin N, Kraus OZ, Morris Q, Boone C, et al. Machine learning and computer vision approaches for phenotypic profiling. J Cell Biol 2017;216(1):65–71. Available from: https://doi.org/10.1083/jcb.201610026.

[172] Ljosa V, Carpenter AE. Introduction to the quantitative analysis of two-dimensional fluorescence microscopy images for cell-based screening. PLoS Comput Biol 2009;5(12):e1000603. Available from: https://doi.org/10.1371/journal.pcbi.1000603.

[173] Brand JE, Koch B, Xu J. Machine learning. SAGE research methods foundations. London, United Kingdom: SAGE Publications Ltd; 2020.

[174] Pedregosa F, Varoquaux G, Gramfort A, Michel V, Thirion B, Grisel O, et al. Scikit-learn: machine learning in python. J Mach Learn Res 2011;12:2825–30. Available from: http://jmlr.csail.mit.edu/papers/volume12/pedregosa11a/pedregosa11a.pdf.

[175] Kuepfer L, Niederalt C, Wendl T, Schlender JF, Willmann S, Lippert J, et al. Applied concepts in PBPK modeling: how to build a PBPK/PD model. CPT: Pharmacomet Syst Pharmacology 2016;5(10):516–31. Available from: https://doi.org/10.1002/psp4.12134.

[176] Gao H, Wang W, Dong J, Ye Z, Ouyang D. An integrated computational methodology with data-driven machine learning, molecular modeling and PBPK modeling to accelerate solid dispersion formulation design. Eur J Pharm Biopharm 2021;158:336–46. Available from: https://doi.org/10.1016/j.ejpb.2020.12.001.

[177] Pearson K. LIII. On lines and planes of closest fit to systems of points in space. London, Edinburgh, Dublin Philos Mag J Sci 2010;2(11):559–72. Available from: https://doi.org/10.1080/14786440109462720.

[178] Hallou A, Yevick HG, Dumitrascu B, Uhlmann V. Deep learning for bioimage analysis in developmental biology. Development 2021;148(18). Available from: https://doi.org/10.1242/dev.199616.

[179] Smith K, Piccinini F, Balassa T, Koos K, Danka T, Azizpour H, et al. Phenotypic image analysis software tools for exploring and understanding big image data from cell-based assays. Cell Syst 2018;6(6):636–53. Available from: https://doi.org/10.1016/j.cels.2018.06.001.

[180] Eliceiri KW, Berthold MR, Goldberg IG, Ibáñez L, Manjunath BS, Martone ME, et al. Biological imaging software tools. Nat Methods 2012;9(7):697–710. Available from: https://doi.org/10.1038/nmeth.2084.

[181] Schindelin J, Arganda-Carreras I, Frise E, Kaynig V, Longair M, Pietzsch T, et al. Fiji: an open-source platform for biological-image analysis. Nat Methods 2012;9(7):676–82. Available from: https://doi.org/10.1038/nmeth.2019.

[182] McQuin C, Goodman A, Chernyshev V, Kamentsky L, Cimini BA, Karhohs KW, et al. CellProfiler 3.0: next-generation image processing for biology. PLoS Biol 2018;16(7). Available from: https://doi.org/10.1371/journal.pbio.2005970.

[183] Carpenter AE, Jones TR, Lamprecht MR, Clarke C, Kang IH, Friman O, et al. CellProfiler: image analysis software for identifying and quantifying cell phenotypes. Genome Biol 2006;7(10). Available from: https://doi.org/10.1186/gb-2006-7-10-r100.

[184] Stirling David R, Carpenter AE, Cimini BA, Xu J. CellProfiler analyst 3.0: accessible data exploration and machine learning for image analysis. Bioinformatics 2021;37(21):3992–4. Available from: https://doi.org/10.1093/bioinformatics/btab634.

[185] Bray M-A, Carpenter AE. Quality control for high-throughput imaging experiments using machine learning in cellprofiler. In: Johnston PA, Trask OJ, editors. High content screening: a powerful approach to systems cell biology and phenotypic drug discovery, methods in molecular biology. New York: Springer; 2018. p. 89–112. Available from: https://doi.org/10.1007/978-1-4939-7357-6_7.

[186] Harris G, Palosaari T, Magdolenova Z, Mennecozzi M, Gineste JM, Saavedra L, et al. Iron oxide nanoparticle toxicity testing using high-throughput analysis and high-content imaging. Nanotoxicology 2015;9(1):87–94. Available from: https://doi.org/10.3109/17435390.2013.816797.

[187] U.S. Food and Drug Administration. Nanotechnology—over a decade of progress and innovation: a report by the U.S. Food and Drug Administration [WWW Document]. https://www.fda.gov/media/140395/download; 2020 [accessed 02.05.22].

[188] U.S. Food and Drug Administration. Final guidance for industry: assessing the effects of significant manufacturing process changes, including emerging technologies, on the safety and regulatory status of food ingredients and food contact substances, including food ingredients that are color additives [WWW Document]. U.S. Food and Drug Administration. https://www.fda.gov/regulatory-information/search-fda-guidance-documents/guidance-industry-assessing-effects-significant-manufacturing-process-changes-including-emerging; 2014 [accessed 02.05.22].

[189] U.S. Food and Drug Administration. Final guidance for industry: safety of nanomaterials in cosmetic products [WWW Document]. https://www.fda.gov/regulatory-information/search-fda-guidance-documents/guidance-industry-safety-nanomaterials-cosmetic-products; 2014 [accessed 02.05.22].

[190] U.S. Food and Drug Administration. Final guidance for industry: use of nanomaterials in food for animals [WWW Document]. U.S. Food and Drug Administration. https://www.fda.gov/regulatory-information/search-fda-guidance-documents/cvm-gfi-220-use-nanomaterials-food-animals; 2015 [accessed 02.05.22].

[191] U.S. Food and Drug Administration. Draft guidance for industry: drug products, including biological products, that contain nanomaterials [WWW Document]. https://www.fda.gov/regulatory-information/search-fda-guidance-documents/drug-products-including-biological-products-contain-nanomaterials-guidance-industry; 2017 [accessed 02.05.22].

[192] U.S. Food and Drug Administration. Final guidance for industry: liposome drug products: chemistry, manufacturing, and controls; human pharmacokinetics and bioavailability; and labeling documentation [WWW Document]. https://www.fda.gov/regulatory-information/search-fda-guidance-documents/liposome-drug-products-chemistry-manufacturing-and-controls-human-pharmacokinetics-and; 2018 [accessed 02.05.22].

[193] U.S. Food and Drug Administration. Final guidance for industry: considering whether an FDA-regulated product involves the application of nanotechnology [WWW Document]. https://www.fda.gov/regulatory-information/search-fda-guidance-documents/considering-whether-fda-regulated-product-involves-application-nanotechnology; 2014 [accessed 02.05.22].

[194] United States Pharmacopeia. New proposed chapter drug products containing nanomaterials. https://www.uspnf.com/notices/proposed-gc-1153-drug-products-containing-nanomaterials; 2019.

[195] Allan J, Belz S, Hoeveler A, Hugas M, Okuda H, Patri A, et al. Regulatory landscape of nanotechnology and nanoplastics from a global perspective. Regul Toxicol Pharmacol 2021;122:104885. Available from: https://doi.org/10.1016/j.yrtph.2021.104885.

CHAPTER

14

Gene therapy: advocacies, perspectives, and ethical provocations

Rajeev Taliyan, Rajesh Sukhija, Ameya Kothekar, Ansit Mishra, Priyamvada Nair and Shaifali Gurjar

Neuropsychopharmacology Division, Department of Pharmacy, Birla Institute of Technology and Science-Pilani Campus, Rajasthan, India

14.1 Introduction

Gene therapy is a technique for studying missing or abnormal genes, in which a copy of the gene with normal functioning is introduced. In 1990, the National Institutes of Health (NIH) authorized the first clinical application of gene therapy in a patient suffering from severe combined immunodeficiency (SCID), a condition characterized by a deficiency in the adenosine deaminase (ADA) gene. This event marked a significant milestone in the field and sparked widespread interest in the therapeutic potential of genetic manipulation. Since then, gene therapy has experienced significant growth and development, with many clinical trials and studies being approved, initiated, or completed globally. These trials and studies focus on utilizing gene therapy to implement strategies to correct or alter genetic material within cells to treat or prevent various diseases. This is achieved by replacing, modifying, or enhancing dysfunctional or defective genes with functional counterparts. Additionally, gene therapy techniques may involve the targeted elimination of specific cells by introducing "killer" genes or the targeted suppression of gene expression [1,2]. This successful demonstration of the therapeutic potential of the nucleus has sparked tremendous interest in treating severe and debilitating hereditary disorders due to mutation of the genomic structure. Gene therapy presents several advantages over conventional pharmacological treatments, including reduced susceptibility to molecular progression, mutagenicity, variable pharmacokinetics, and a lower risk of drug resistance following repeated treatments [3]. In a broader perspective, repairing, silencing, or substituting faulty genes with transgenes is an innovative approach to treating, curing, or eventually preventing the disease. The therapy uses specific carriers which encapsulate foreign genes.

Molecular Pharmaceutics and Nano Drug Delivery
DOI: https://doi.org/10.1016/B978-0-323-91924-1.00013-7

These specific carriers are called vectors, the functionality of which depends on various factors such as methodology adopted, chemical composition, and efficiency of a vector with safe and effective transfer of transgenes into target cells; therefore, creating a large number of genes of interest (GOIs) is the need for effective gene therapy for curing or preventing genetic diseases. The commonly used gene therapy technologies are nonviral physiochemical methods and recombinant viral technologies [4].

In more than 30 years, this diversified and ever-increasing science has had tremendous opportunities. Ongoing advances in gene transfer technology and biosafety have been complemented by a multidimensional understanding of gene therapy. It includes the attainability of an efficient gene delivery method incorporating the understanding of its characteristics and drawbacks. Also a detailed study of the characteristics of the target cell population and a comprehensive study of the molecular basis of the target disease are needed.

14.1.1 Uncovering the past to shape the future: the significance of gene origin in gene therapy

The human genome is comprised of a vast number of genes, which are the fundamental units of inheritance and determinants of phenotype. Estimates from the Human Genome Project suggest approximately 20,000 to 25,000 genes, in human genome, are responsible for encoding the millions of proteins a cell requires [5]. DNA is wrapped into chromosomes that reside in the cell nucleus, and a single chromosome may contain hundreds or even thousands of genes, each with its locus and position that is crucial for its function. The regulation of gene function within chromosomes is facilitated by a combination of DNA and chemical components. Chromatin, a complex of DNA and proteins, further compacts chromosomes through the wrapping of DNA strands with histone proteins, resulting in the formation of nucleosomes. The human genome is composed of approximately 3×10^9 nucleosomes. The message in each gene contains a specific code for the amino acids in the gene's protein expression. The relationship between genes and DNA is intertwined, with long chains of purine and pyrimidine monomeric units (adenine, cytosine, guanine, and thymine) linked in a complementary manner to form the double-helix structure of DNA. The tiny fragments of this helix structure consist of a specific sequence of base pairs and are referred to as genes [1]. Although humans have similar genomes, the subtle differences in DNA sequences between individuals result in unique cell-specific machinery. The regulation of gene expression is a complex process determined by factors such as tissue type, age, chemical signals, and various other factors and methods. The genomic sequence and its arrangement within chromosomes play a crucial role in determining gene-determined traits, which are often influenced by multiple genes. Certain traits may arise from hereditary mutations or spontaneous gene changes and can result in genetic disorders [5,6].

Genetic disorders arise from abnormalities in the DNA, including mutations in a single gene, multiple genes, or changes in the chromosomal structure or number. These mutations can result in various conditions, from severe to rare diseases to more familiar, milder conditions. Some genetic disorders manifest at birth, while others may develop later. The incidence and distribution of genetic disorders can vary significantly among populations and ethnic groups. The pressing need for early diagnosis and expedited development of therapeutic options for individuals with genetic diseases necessitates prioritizing resources and efforts from the scientific community. An estimated 350 million people worldwide, including approximately 70 million Indians, are suffering from genetic disorders. India has a high burden of genetic disorders. It is also estimated that approximately 4%–5% of infants are born with genetic disorder in India [7,8]. Some most common genetic disorders include thalassemia, sickle cell anemia, beta-thalassemia, hemophilia, Tay–Sachs disease, Gaucher disease, and phenylketonuria. Gene therapy presents a promising approach for treating these genetic disorders, with demonstrated success in various genetic disorders [9,10].

14.2 Types of gene therapy

Gene therapy is primarily limited to research community, and its use remains experimental. Most trials took place in the United States of America, Europe, and Australia. The technique is comprehensive, with the extensive potential to treat the recessive gene defects (cystic fibrosis [CF], hemophilia, muscular dystrophy, and sickle cell anemia) and acquired genetic diseases (cancer) and viral infections [11]. Gene therapy is further categorized as somatic cell gene therapy (SCGT) and germline gene therapy (GGT) based on the type of cells involved in the process. Gene therapy is also categorized into in-vivo and ex-vivo gene therapy based on the treatment administered.

14.2.1 Somatic cell gene therapy

SCGT refers to an experimental gene therapy technique that includes the treatment of damaged somatic tissues or organs in individuals. However, once transmitted to offspring, most pathogenic gene mutations cause irreversible tissue and organ damage, resulting in disorders such as hypertrophic cardiomyopathy, Huntington's disease (HD), and BRCA-associated malignancies. In these instances, it is doubtful that somatic gene therapy would correct the pathology of the illness unless therapy is undertaken before the disease start [12].

Since somatic cells do not participate in reproduction; they cannot be inherited. SCGT is fraught with ethical concerns, although its success rate is notable. Virus-enabled gene transfer and liposome-enabled gene transfer are utilized extensively in somatic cell gene therapy. Although it is suitable for many types of somatic cells, it is primarily targeted at bone marrow cells; they are the only cells that can divide and proliferate into various types of blood cells throughout life. This is why the success rate of SCGT is higher for blood-borne diseases such as thalassemia, sickle cell anemia, and hemophilia.

Despite a commendable success rate, SCGT is accompanied with certain limitations such as:

- A virus can infect a cell by combining with its host's genome (viral escape).
- Also, the normal gene function is impaired if the GOI does not get inserted at the desired location.
- The likelihood of oncogene and proto-oncogene activation is quite high.

14.2.2 Germline gene therapy

GGT can repair disease-causing mutations to wild-type variations in early embryonic development when there is a less number of mutations in embryonic cells. Additionally, GGT will prevent the transmission of genetic illness in newborns as well as to all future generations [13]. Using viral vectors, reproductive tissue cells or undivided embryos are injected. The transformed cells must be grown in a sterile laboratory setting with extreme caution. Other unmodified viral cells must not infect the changed cell. The transformed germ cells are utilized for in-vitro fertilization and other assisted reproductive technologies. However, injecting a transgene directly into an embryo is recommended.

14.2.3 In-vivo gene therapy

The foreign gene is directly introduced into the target cell during in-vivo gene therapy. The target gene is administered into the body through aerosols or injections. In several situations, the effect of in-vivo gene therapy is limited. The GOI is exclusively administered to the afflicted location and not to other body tissues. CF and Duchenne muscular dystrophy (DMD) serve as prime instances of in-vivo gene therapy.

In CF, the exogenous gene (or transgenic) is administered through the nasal route as an aerosol, but in DMD, the GOI is a dystrophin gene, which is injected into the muscle cell. Nonetheless, some adjacent cells might also get infected with no apparent reason, resulting in negative consequences. In-vivo gene therapy is currently not a viable method for treating hereditary disorders [14].

14.2.4 Ex-vivo gene therapy

In ex-vivo gene therapy, diseased cells are extracted, transformed in a laboratory (outside the body), and reintroduced into the body. It is termed as ex-vivo because none of the gene therapy methods or stages are conducted within the body. The entire procedure is under the supervision of the researcher; consequently, the current approach is safer and allows scientists more control. Although the approach applies to cells with the ability to divide, only a few types of tissues or cells can be modified ex-vivo. As bone marrow cells may reproduce throughout life, they are frequently employed in ex-vivo gene therapy. Blood cells are another type of cells that are frequently used. The purpose of selecting actively dividing cells is that the transgene can spread to neighboring cells more rapidly. Blood cells and bone marrow cells are the only viable options that limit the ex-vivo gene therapy for treating certain blood-related illnesses such as thalassemia, sickle cell anemia, thrombosis, and hemophilia [14].

14.3 Basic methodologies for gene therapy

Gene therapy employs a variety of different techniques that were first established for therapeutic uses on somatic tissues. In addition to the mutant, an endogenous copy (or copies) of the gene, one of the earliest methods includes the insertion of a synthetic copy of a normal gene into a nonspecific site within the genome. Utilizing viral vectors, the transgene is typically transported and incorporated into the target genome. Another long-term approach in treating genetic diseases involves the use of genome editing methods like guided endonucleases such as transcription activator-like effector nucleases (TALENs), zinc finger nucleases (ZFNs), and, more recently, clustered regularly interspaced palindromic repeats (CRISPR)-Cas9 and CPF1. These methods involve effector nucleases that resemble transcription activators (TALENs).

14.3.1 Single nucleotide polymorphisms and gene therapy: improving outcomes for genetic disorders

Single nucleotide polymorphisms (SNPs) are single nucleotide variations in the genomic DNA, which differ between individuals within a population. SNPs have the potential to influence the expression and function of genes utilized in gene therapy. Each nucleotide at a specific location corresponds to an allele of the SNP gene. SNPs can be classified into synonymous (no effect on protein sequence) and nonsynonymous (change in the amino acid sequence, potentially leading to missense or nonsense mutations) [15,16]. SNPs are also categorized according to their regions, which include noncoding and coding regions, with the latter further subdivided into missense and nonsense regions. SNPs comprise a significant portion of genetic variability, accounting for approximately 90% of all variations in the genome [17]. This implies that minor nucleotide sequence variations contribute to genetic diversity generation. SNPs are estimated to occur at a high density throughout the genome, with a potential range of 3–17 million occurrences. It is also estimated that 5% of these SNPs may be located within genes. Thus, SNPs give a biological identifier that occurs at a very high density throughout the genome and can thus be utilized to identify genes involved in human disorders. SNPs may affect the regulation of the gene's promoter region, leading to altered gene expression. They may also affect the coding region of a gene, resulting in changes to the produced protein and potentially its function. SNPs can serve as biomarkers for recessive, autosomal, metabolic disorders, cancer, and viral infections. Understanding the effect of SNPs on gene therapy is crucial to optimize treatment outcomes and to improve patient outcomes [17,18].

14.3.2 CRISPR–Cas9 technique

Using genome editing to induce lesions in previously altered genes with the aim of modifying the gene to control illness is an alternate method. In both animal and human cells, genome-editing methods like RNA-guided CRISPR-Cas9 are particularly effective at causing insertion and deletion (indel) alterations at specific loci [19]. The CRISPR-Cas9 complex is derived from bacterial and archaeal adaptive immune systems, in which brief nucleotide sequences (spacers) from invasive pathogens like phages are incorporated into the host genome. From there, they can be used to recognize similar "foreign genetic elements," and when the spacers are combined with the effector protein, the Cas9 endonuclease, the invasive DNA is removed [20]. A new age of genetic engineering began with the discovery that the *Staphylococcus pyogenes* CRISPR-Cas9 system could be altered to specifically cause double-stranded DNA breaks in mammalian cells [21].

In a few instances, the production of new mutations in somatic cells has been proposed for therapeutic uses. Mice models are used to investigate ways to change genes causing DMD. The mouse DMD phenotype is caused by a nonsense mutation in exon 23 of the dystrophin (DMD) gene. Excision of exon 23 restored the synthesis of a shorter form of the dystrophin protein and improved skeletal muscle strength to varying degrees [22].

Another illustration is the C–C chemokine receptor type 5 (CCR5) gene, which encodes a human cell surface protein linked to HIV-1 entry. It is believed that a naturally occurring 32-base-pair (bp) deletion in this gene in some human populations confers homozygous carrier resistance to particular HIV-1 strains as well as a few other immunological or health-related consequences [23,24]. Therefore, it has been postulated that introducing comparable mutations in HIV-positive individuals might be therapeutic.

14.4 Current status and recent trends in gene therapy

Gene variations that are passed down from parent to child through the process of hereditary mutations can lead to familial disorders. To attenuate the spread of potentially harmful mutations, novel gene therapy techniques are now being investigated. Following decades of research and development, the area of gene and cell therapy has had a resurgence during the past 5 years, with the first medicines being licensed for use. These cutting-edge medicines are utilized to treat a variety of therapeutic reasons and tissue targets, including cancer, hereditary blindness, and neuromuscular diseases. These authorized medicines have a profound effect on the patients who receive them, but they also have an even greater influence on the field as a whole since they set the stage for the development of treatments for a wide range of additional disorders.

14.4.1 Mitochondrial replacement therapy

Mutations in mitochondrial DNA (mtDNA) inherited from the mother cause a wide variety of irreversible diseases in children and adults. Those afflicted typically pass away at a young age following an excruciating course of the disease. The mitochondrial genome resists direct DNA alterations brought on by gene-editing methods like CRISPR because it lacks native mtDNA repair and recombination systems. Mitochondrial replacement therapy (MRT) replaces mutant mtDNA in carriers of mutations with donated, mutation-free counterpart mtDNA, enabling women who have mtDNA abnormalities to stop the sickness from passing to their children [25].

The MRT procedure, which was developed in a nonhuman monkey, produced a large number of live births utilizing only donor mtDNA. Preimplantation development of human MRT embryos and controls was comparable, which supports the method's practical applicability [26–29]. A healthy male child with donor mtDNA was delivered to a family in Mexico who had previously undergone MRT for a deadly condition associated with mtDNA mutation. This was the first successful application of MRT in humans, providing optimism for the future of this therapy for people with inherited mtDNA gene abnormalities [30].

Recent studies have shown that animals with defective mtDNA can be precisely targeted and eliminated using ZFNs and TALENs. The results of this proof-of-concept study imply that programmable nucleases may be a viable treatment approach for the decrease of mtDNA mutation burdens in heteroplasmic mtDNA disorders [31,32].

14.4.2 Germline gene therapy for heterozygous mutations

The nuclear genome, in contrast to mtDNA, is associated with potent DNA repair and recombination machinery that has historically been used to construct a variety of gene modifications through experiments. Gene conversion, which does not require an external template, is the unidirectional transfer of genetic material from a donor sequence to a highly homologous acceptor [33]. Double-strand break (DSB) repair serves as the catalyst for gene conversion, which takes place during meiotic noncrossover recombination and results in the copying of entire homologous sequences to the DSB-containing region.

Recent advancements in genome-editing technology permit the very efficient creation of DNA DSBs at specified loci in animal and human cells. The introduction of DNA-scissors with programmable, site-specific DNA-binding domains, such as RNA-guided CRISPR–Cas9 vectors, has substantially assisted in current advances [34–36].

Environmental stress or DNA replication mistakes can result in DSBs in addition to other types of DNNA damage [37]. Nonhomologous end joining (NHEJ) or homology-directed repair procedures are frequently used to repair DSBs. Recent genome-editing studies have shown that NHEJ is the main form of cellular repair in somatic cells. Minor indel changes are frequently introduced at the DSB region using this error-prone method [38]. Rarely, simultaneous severing of both alleles may cause large deletions or difficult rearrangements, increasing the likelihood that nearby genes or regulatory areas would be affected [39].

Utilization of alternate endogenous sequences situated on homologous chromosomes as a repair template utilizing the gene conversion mechanism is the present focus of gamma-glutamyl transpeptidase research in human embryos.

14.4.3 Gene therapy for neurodegenerative disease

14.4.3.1 *Parkinson's disease*

In clinical studies for Parkinson's disease that have been conducted so far using AAV2-mediated gene therapy, two different treatment approaches have been used. First, there are therapies known as "symptomatic therapy" that aim to treat clinical symptoms rather than altering the course of the disease as a whole. Both aromatic L-amino acid decarboxylase, a rate-limiting enzyme for dopamine synthesis, and glutamic acid decarboxylase, which catalyzes the synthesis of -aminobutyric acid from glutamate, have been employed in gene transfer procedures to treat Parkinson's disease. In-vivo gene transfer of a neurotrophic factor, such as neurturin or glial-derived neurotropic factor, has also been used in neurorestorative therapy. These therapies are centered on the goal of attempting to restore cellular functions that have been disrupted by the disease process [40].

14.4.3.2 *Alzheimer's disease*

Alzheimer's disease (AD) is linked to the loss of cholinergic neurons in the nucleus basalis of Meynert. Cholinesterase inhibitors continue to be the principal therapy choice for AD patients, despite providing only a moderate improvement in overall symptomatology. Patients with mild to severe AD were initially studied in a dose-escalating phase 1 clinical trial for neuronal growth factor gene injection using adeno-associated virus-2 [41,42].

14.4.3.3 *Huntington's disease*

It is an autosomal dominant condition that results in polyglutaminated Huntingtin (mHtt) protein [43] due to an excess of CAG repetitions on chromosome 4 exon 1. Therefore, the buildup of mHtt inside striatal medium spiny neurons and pyramidal cortical neurons is responsible for the pathogenic phenotype seen in HD. A popular experimental technique for treating the underlying pathology involves creating drugs that lower mHtt levels in an effort to prevent sickness onset [44]. Given that it allows for the direct targeting of damaged nuclei in an effort to lower mHtt levels, gene therapy is a promising prospective treatment for HD. Preclinical gene therapy methods for HD have been developed, and their present emphasis is on employing RNA interference to lower pathologic levels of mHtt (RNAi). Furthermore, studies on nonhuman primates demonstrated that normal Htt declines of up to 45% could be tolerable [45,46]. AAV5-miHTT, a transgene encoding an engineered miRNA targeting HTT mRNA, has been developed to deliver a tailored microRNA that targets human huntingtin [47–49].

14.4.4 Elimination of inherited blood disorders using CRISPR/Cas-9

Inherited blood disorders are good candidates for gene therapy because they can correct the hematopoietic system by editing the causal gene in autologous hematopoietic stem cells (HSCs). This is due to the hematological system's ability to be corrected by gene therapy. There are two forms of inherited blood illnesses known as thalassemia and sickle cell anemia. β-thalassemia is caused by a variety of mutations in the β-globin gene, some of which are minor insertions, single-point changes, or deletions. These mutations lead to a loss of or a reduction in the amount of β-globin that is synthesized [50]. A mutation known as Glu- > Val, which occurs in the β-globin subunit of hemoglobin [50,51], is the root cause of sickle cell disease. This mutation results in aberrant hemoglobin S. Any ailment that is brought on by -globin may be treated by re-expression of the paralogous globin genes. Both CRISPR Therapeutics and Allife Medical Science and Technology Co., Ltd launched clinical studies in 2018 and 2019, respectively, with the goal of healing patients with severe sickle cell disease and thalassemia through the transfusion of CRIPSR/Cas9 altered CD34 + human HSCs (CTX001).

To date, there have been three of these clinical trials conducted, which have been summarized below (Table 14.1).

TABLE 14.1 Clinical trials of gene therapy for β-thalassemia and sickle cell anemia.

Disease	Study title	Strategy	Study phases	Patients parameters	Company
β-Thalassemia Dependent transfusion	Evaluation of CTX001; efficacy and safety in patients with transfusion-dependent -thalassemia	CTX001	Phase 1 Phase 2	45 Patients (>18 years and <35 years age)	Vertex Pharmaceuticals Incorporated and CRISPR Therapeutics
Sickle cell disease	Assessment of CTX001; efficacy and safety in patients with severe sickle cell disease	CTX001	Phase 1 Phase 3	45 Patients (>18 years and <35 years age)	Vertex Pharmaceuticals Incorporated and CRISPR Therapeutics
β-Thalassemia	Subjects with thalassemia mutations whose genes were corrected using the HBB intergenic region	HBB HSC-01	Early phase 1	12 patients, ≥2 and ≤60 years of age	Allife Medical Science & Technology Co., Ltd

14.5 Delivery systems in gene therapy

The efficient incorporation of genetic material (such as a transgene or nuclease) into the cell's nucleus is essential for gene therapy to be effective. A "vector" is a device that transmits genetic material. All the above-mentioned gene therapy types would fail if the vector was not chosen appropriately. The target cells and their characteristics, the length of expression, and the quantity of genetic material to be inserted into the vector all influence the selection of the best vector and delivery method. Viral, nonviral, and engineered vectors are the three general categories of current gene therapy delivery systems.

14.5.1 Viral vectors

Gene therapies come in two flavors: in-vivo and ex-vivo, as was previously mentioned. The majority of in-vivo gene therapies employ vectors to facilitate the gene therapies' uptake by the target cells. A class of viral-based medications called as virotherapy [52] includes viral therapy, which has been used for a very long period. The primary benefit of utilizing a virus as a vector for gene delivery is that it can efficiently transport gene components into host cells while naturally infecting cells. There are a number of promising techniques to cure genetic problems that are spread by viruses, thanks to the nearly 40 years of virus research. Even more effective treatment options are available for some human disorders. A viral vector typically consists of three components: the protein envelope and/or capsid, which contain the genetic payload and define the vector's tissue and antigen recognition; the transgene of interest, which, when expressed in cells, has the desired effect; and the "regulatory cassette," which is a collection of enhancers, promoters, and auxiliary elements that regulate the transgene's stable or transient somatic expression.

The numerous viral vectors utilized in gene therapy are depicted in Fig. 14.1. The DNA of the host cell is fused with a portion of the genetic material used by viral vectors that

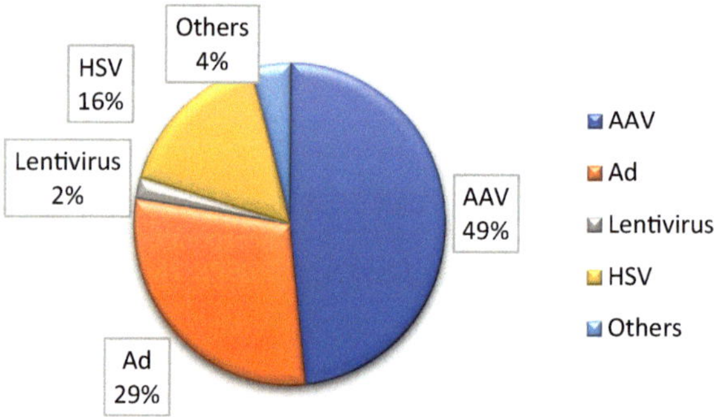

FIGURE 14.1 Commonly used viral vectors in gene therapy.

integrate, such as lentivirus (LV) and gamma retrovirus vectors. Nonintegrating viral vectors, such as AAV and adenovirus (Ad) vectors, maintain their episomal structure in the cell cytoplasm. The key advantage is that insertional mutagenesis poses less danger of genotoxicity.

Ad, AAV, LV, and herpes simplex virus (HSV) are examples of viral vectors that have shown the capacity to deliver gene therapies effectively and safely (Fig. 14.1). Vesicular stomatitis virus, Sendai virus, modified vaccinia virus Ankara, arenavirus, and measles virus are some more viral models that are less frequently used [53]. Ad, AAV, and LV vectors will now be briefly discussed among other viral delivery systems.

14.5.1.1 Adenovirus

One of the viral vectors that is most frequently employed in gene therapy is the Ad. It is a DNA virus with an icosahedral viral particle enclosing its 34–43 kb genome. Ad vectors have a number of beneficial qualities, including the following: (1) the capacity to deliver multiple genome copies into one host cell, resulting in high levels of gene expression; (2) transient gene expression because of episomal DNA that does not get integrated into the host genome; (3) the capacity to transduce both dividing and nondividing cells; and (4) high immunogenicity [54]. Ads are widely used as vectors in gene therapy because of these distinctive qualities. Advertisements have also been used to promote immunizations that prevent cancer. The overall approach for immunizing against tumor cells involves promoting the development of tumor-associated antigens and/or oncolytic mechanisms that enhance anticancer immune responses by Ad-mediated gene delivery. The p53 tumor repressor pathway is known to fail in a number of different tumor types. Ad vectors have been created to encourage the expression of the tumor suppressor gene (p53), which results in cell-cycle arrest and apoptosis. Additionally, immune-regulating genes can be added to Ad vectors to improve the patient's antitumor immune responses. Malignant pleural mesothelioma can be safely treated with intrapleural injections of IFN-2b or Ad-delivered interferon (IFN). Due to the high prevalence of preexisting immunity to major human Ad serotypes, particularly human, immunogenicity and cellular toxicity continue to be significant obstacles to Ad gene therapy (Had5). It has been demonstrated that Had5 vectors are significantly less able to transduce target cells when there are anti-Had5 antibodies present in the blood [55]. Many different nonhuman Ad vectors were created from bovine (Bad), chimpanzee

(ChAd), ovine (Oad), porcine (Pad), and chicken to lessen cross-reactive immunity (Fad). They are the most frequently used [56] because Nabs against chimp-derived Ad vectors are significantly lower in human blood circulation.

14.5.1.2 Adeno-associated viruses

Certain viruses require other viruses for the completion of their own life cycle. These are termed as dependo-parvovirus. The 4.7 kb DNA genome of the nonpathogenic parvovirus AAV is housed in an icosahedral, nonenveloped capsid. The critical genes required for AAV's genome expression and replication are missing. In 1995, a patient with CF received the CF transmembrane regulator (CFTR) gene packed with an AAV2 capsid, marking the first time an AAV vector was used on a human (rAAV2-CFTR). The capacity of vectors based on the wild-type genome, which is around 4.7 kb in size, is irrevocably constrained to 5 kb. Another crucial component of vector design is the regulatory cassettes, which are the promotors utilized in AAV vectors to stimulate transgene expression. Over 100 variations and 11 natural serotypes exist for AAV. The central nervous system (CNS) organs are preferred by some variants, such as AAV9, but the pancreas can be successfully transduced by AAV8. AAV vectors can transduce both diving and nondividing cells; they can permit long-term, stable gene expression, and they have low immunogenicity. These are the three key advantages of AAV vectors. They do not additionally incorporate DNA into the genome of the host.

The first AAV-based gene therapy in the world, Glybera (alipogene tiparvovec), received regulatory approval for commercialization from the European Medicines Agency in 2012. The U.S. Food and Drug Administration (FDA) approved Luxturna, an AAV2-based vector, for the delivery of the retinoid isomerohydrolase RPE65,213 (2017). Leber's congenital amaurosis is a disorder that causes gradual blindness. Since then, more than 200 AAV-based clinical trials have been carried out globally. Muscular dystrophy and the deadly disease hemophilia, a group of significant blood clotting disorders, have long been the subject of research and development. SRP-9001 stands out among the numerous therapy options for muscular dystrophy because it is an AAVrh.74 capsid-based vector that carries a shrunken form of dystrophin. The first AAV-based hemophilia treatments for hemophilia B exhibited no toxicity and sustained transgene presence for years after delivery. These treatments were meant to target muscle tissues as habitats for expressing factor IX (F.IX). Five pharmaceutical companies are pursuing at least 12 clinical trials that are currently in progress. Many of them are highly promising and in phase II or phase 3. These include medicines like Valrox (valoctocogene roxaparvovec, also known as BMN 270), as well as a number of others, like the gene therapy SPK-8011 for hemophilia A. For AAV-mediated gene therapy, innate immunity, which can obstruct transgene expression, is a challenge. Unmethylated CpG dinucleotides cause the activation of MyD88 and the Toll-like receptor 9 (TLR9). One method to reduce immune system activation is to introduce binding sites for microRNAs (miRNAs), such as miR142, which are extensively expressed in various cell types, to the cell's own RNA interference machinery to limit production in antigen-presenting cells [57,58]. The effectiveness and long-term safety profiles of AAV vectors have come under scrutiny, despite the fact that they have historically been thought to be quite safe [59]. New evidence suggests integration of the AAV vector genomes carrying CRISPR components into the genome of host cells at the point of DSBs. Despite the overall positive safety record for AAV therapies in people, it is undoubtedly required to conduct more study into the long- and short-term safety of AAV vectors.

14.5.1.3 Lentiviruses

The first virus used in clinical studies to examine in-vivo gene therapy was a retrovirus. A retrovirus is an encapsulated, spherical virus with RNA as its genetic makeup. A subfamily of the Retroviridae family is the LVs. The first generation of LV vectors was created using the human immunodeficiency viral 1, or HIV. CNS organs transduced in-vivo demonstrated the effectiveness of these vectors [60]. By engaging with specific cell receptors and glycoproteins attached to the outer envelope, lentiviral particles can infect a cell. Lentiviral vectors, as opposed to retrovirus vectors, have a number of advantageous qualities, such as: (1) a capacity of up to 9 kb; (2) the capacity to transduce both dividing and nondividing cells; (3) the capacity to enable long-term gene expression; and (4) a lower risk of insertional mutagenesis and genotoxicity. More current LV vectors are created from nonhuman LVs because they cannot infect humans [61]. Lentiviral vectors are favored in many advanced (phase III) clinical trials for CAR-T cell therapies. The first FDA-approved treatment for B-cell in children is CAR-T therapy, sold under the trade name Kymriah. It expresses a CAR that attaches to CD19 and transforms autologous T cells using lentiviral vectors carrying a transgene. LVs were utilized to treat a variety of ailments, including metabolic abnormalities, cancer, immune system issues, and unusual birth defects, in more than a dozen completed clinical trials. These include autologous A-T87Q-globin LV CD34 + cells for the treatment of beta-thalassemia and sickle cell anemia (anemia III), as well as autologous ABCD1 LV CD34 + cells for the treatment of cerebral adrenoleukodystrophy. Primary immunodeficiency ADA-SCID is uncommon and frequently deadly. It results from a deficiency in the enzyme ADA. Following a nonrandomized clinical experiment that demonstrated that enzyme replacement therapy increased patient survival for more than 2 years without any complications, OTL-101, a lentiviral vector, was included to a phase III clinical investigation to treat ADA-SCID. It has been demonstrated that lentiviral vectors can lead to biological transcripts being spliced improperly. It has been demonstrated that even self-inactivating lentiviral vectors with strong promoter and enhancer regions can activate adjacent genes. To offset the influence of enhancers acting in trans, insulator sequences can be added to lessen these effects. In order to support a greater spectrum of gene therapies in the future, lentiviral vectors are being enhanced and developed. Lentiviral vectors with integrase deficiencies have been created as a means of delivering vaccinations against the flu and malaria antigens. Lentiviral vectors will be used to treat human diseases more widely as a result of this effort.

14.5.2 Nonviral vectors

Utilizing viral vectors has several disadvantages, including its immunogenicity, cytotoxicity, and insertional mutagenesis, or the ectopic integration of viral DNA into chromosomes. This may result in the expression of oncogenes being expressed and activated or tumor-suppressor gene expression being inhibited, which would cause the cells to become malignant. Human investigations have also demonstrated the possibility of an immunological reaction. The nonviral vectors are inexpensive and simple to produce, nonimmunogenic, tissue-specific, and nontoxic. Transposons, liposomes, naked DNA, nucleofection, and other nonviral vector-mediated techniques are employed for gene therapy (Fig. 14.2). Low transfection effectiveness, which is brought on by nonspecific vector uptake by epithelial barriers and extracellular matrix as well as poor transport into therapeutic target cells, limits their clinical utility, nevertheless. Nonviral vectors use physical and chemical approaches as discussed below.

14.5.2.1 *Physical approach*

Physical approaches include the direct breaking of (target) cell membranes to transfer bare plasmids. Microinjection, particle bombardment, and electroporation were among the first methods used to deliver recombinant DNA to cellular targets. Some other advanced methods include sonoporation, laser irradiation, and magnetofection (Table 14.2).

14.5.2.2 *Chemical approaches*

Chemical approaches use lipids, peptides, or polymers in the form of nanocarriers and liposomes to improve plasmid uptake by targeted cells carriers.

14.5.2.2.1 Liposomes

The creation of liposomes, which are spherical vesicles made of one or more phospholipid bilayers, which are the same lipids found in biological membranes, is a method that enhances therapeutic gene transfer into cells. Furthermore, liposomes show reduced immunogenicity and toxicity due to the alteration of composition, size, and charge. Cationic, anionic, neutral, or a combination of these lipids can be used to create liposomes. The lipid used to make liposomes has the potential to change how nanoformulations are administered into the body (Fig. 14.2).

DNA and other molecules are regularly transported via liposomes for medicinal purposes. Cationic, anionic, neutral, or a combination of these lipids can create lipoplexes. The target cell's plasma membrane and the liposome shell converge, enabling transgene entry.

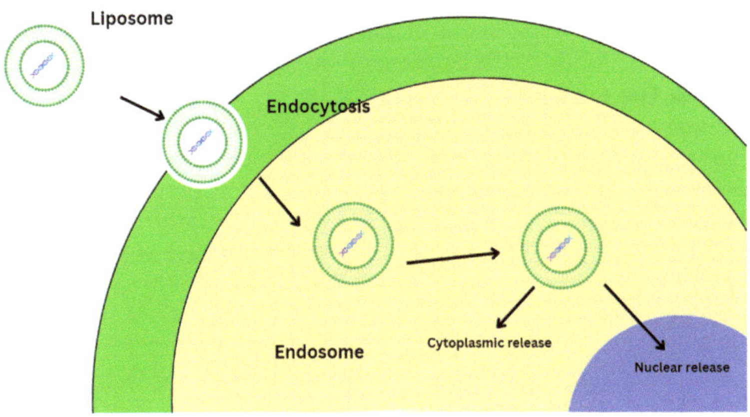

FIGURE 14.2 Process of liposomal uptake by target cells.

TABLE 14.2 Different physical approaches of gene insertion in target cells.

Method	Mechanism
Microinjection	The most direct method, microinjection, is being used for many different things. Very tiny glass needles (usually with an outer diameter of less than 0.2 m) are used to inject DNA or other materials into the cell for later integration and/or expression. The approach's directness enables delivery in almost every cell treated, unlike many other approaches [62].
Particle bombardment/ Biolistic	The method of particle bombardment, commonly referred to as biolistic, is frequently used to genetically alter plants and other organisms. Target cells or tissues are shot at with metal particles coated with DNA using a biolistic device or gene gun [63].
Electroporation	The applied electric field is greater than the capacitance of the membrane. As a result, oppositely polarized charges align on both sides of the cell membrane, creating a potential difference at a particular location on the cell surface. A pore forms as a result of membrane rupturing, allowing the molecule to pass [64].
Sonoporation	A noninvasive method called sonoporation uses an ultrasonic pulse to momentarily permeate the cell membrane, allowing DNA to be taken up by the cells. Interest-related genetic material is integrated into a microbubble and given to the body's circulatory system. Following that, external ultrasound application takes place [65].
Photoporation	In the photoporation technique, the cell membrane pores caused by the laser allow for the introduction of a transgene. The frequency of the laser light and the focal length are key factors in the success of the gene delivery [66].
Hydroporation	A significant volume of DNA solution is directly injected under hydrodynamic pressure. The DNA enters the host cell through a channel that is opened by the pressure. In hepatic cells, the method is widely employed for gene transfer [67].
Magnetofection	Particles with magnetic charges mated with the plasmid. In the presence of a greater magnetic field, the transgene is inserted into the cell or cell line. Ex-vivo applications are more suited for magnetoreception [68].

Lipids have been used to carry genes for a very long time. A majority of lipids have positively charged headgroups that bind electrostatically with nucleic acid anionic phosphate groups to form lipoplexes, which are cationic liposomes coupled to negatively charged plasmids [69]. N-[1-(2,3-dioleyloxy) propyl] is a group of cationic lipids, N-[1-(2,3-dioleoyloxy) propyl]-N,N,N-trimethylammonium chloride, dioctadecanoyl spermines, and -N,N,N-trimethylammonium methyl sulfate. The formation of a lipoplex begins with the electrostatic connection, which causes a fleeting contact. Functionalizing liposomes can increase gene trafficking into tumor cells, leading to increased antitumoral activity when compared to unmodified liposomes, according to in-vitro and in-vivo experiments using a variety of targeting ligands. To the best of our knowledge, however, only a few number of clinical trials utilizing liposomes filled with nucleic acids for the treatment of cancer have been carried out [70].

14.5.2.2.2 Peptides

Eptides are new drug/gene delivery systems since they have short amino acid chains (50 amino acids or less). They have alterable amino acid chains, are biocompatible and biodegradable, and can penetrate barriers more quickly. They can also target gene cargo more quickly. Compared to proteins, peptides are easier to manufacture (in bacterial or mammalian cells, or through solid phase peptide synthesis), have a longer shelf life, and are more stable when handled at room temperature. Studies on peptides, also referred to as cell penetrating peptides, have focused on their effects on integrin receptors (such as v3, v5, and 51), growth factor receptors (such as EGFR, PDGFR, and VEGFR), and G-protein coupled receptors (e.g., octreotide, exenatide, leuprolide, and abarelix). Through clathrin-dependent endocytosis, caveolae-mediated endocytosis, and micropinocytosis, these CPPs are endocytosed in the cells [71]. Mutations in the mitochondrial genome have been associated with a number of disorders, including cancer, diabetes, Parkinson's disease, and, more recently, viral and autoimmune diseases [72]. Negatively charged DNA is shielded by carrier molecules such amphiphilic and cationic peptides for effective mitochondrial transport due to the hydrophobicity and negative charge of mitochondrial membranes. There is a possibility of interference with the many activities with peptide-based delivery techniques. Significant research is being done on a number of levels to create peptide systems that are purely stimuli-responsive and have adequate physicochemical properties for delivering nucleic acids. The development of innovative materials and a full understanding of the mechanisms by which peptide-based delivery systems bypass membrane barriers portend well for the future of peptide-based delivery systems in gene therapy [73].

14.5.2.2.3 Polymers

Another type of gene carrier is cationic polymers, which can be created artificially or naturally. These polymers interact with DNA to form polyplexes, which are nanoscale complexes. In general, polyplexes are more stable than lipoplexes. The most widely used cationic polymer for gene transport during the past 20 years has been polyethyleneimine (PEI). The degree of free amine content, MW, polymer-to-DNA ratios, and the fluid used to create the polyplexes are crucial factors for in-vivo transfection. However, high molecular weight PEI has been linked to cytotoxicity that causes apoptosis (disruption of the mitochondrial membrane) and necrotic cell death after internalization (Wightman et al., 2001). In addition to PEI and more contemporary polyamines of various topologies, synthetic or natural polypeptides and their derivatives have been researched as gene delivery vehicles. Amino esters or polyamino acid derivatives with high DNA condensing properties include poly (l-lysine), polyornithine, polyarginine, histones, and poly (l-lysine) (PLL). Dendrimers, chitosan, synthetic amino derivatives of dextran, and cationic acrylic polymers are other polymers with high gene transfer activity.

14.5.2.2.4 Inorganic nanoparticles

The phosphate backbone of molecules like DNA and small interfering RNA (siRNA) causes them to have a negative charge. As a result, positively charged surface groups on nanostructures can noncovalently connect to DNA or RNA by electrostatic attractions, as has been exploited extensively in a number of nanodelivery systems (Fig. 14.3).

Numerous inorganic nanoparticles are frequently produced using metals (such as iron, gold, and silver), inorganic salts, or ceramics (e.g., phosphate or carbonate salts of calcium, magnesium, or silicon). Cells readily absorb gold nanoparticles, which typically have diameters between 10 and 20 nm. Thiols and oligonucleotides are capable of functionalizing

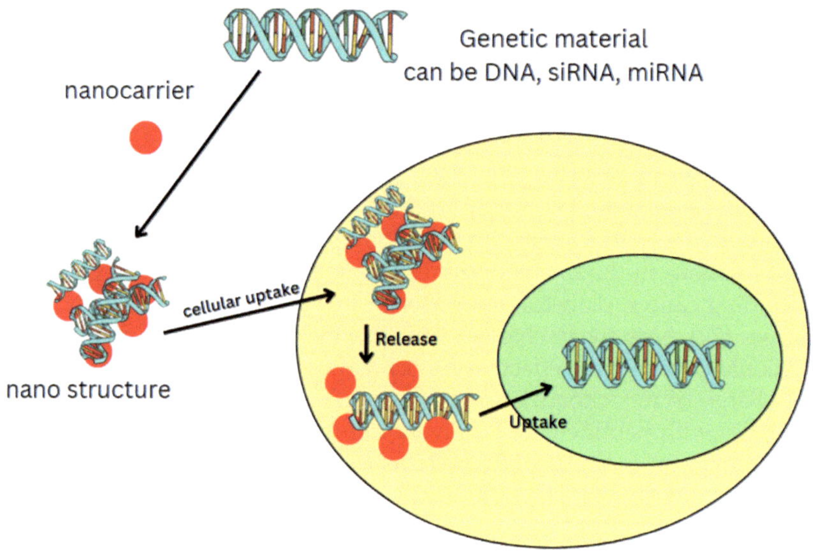

FIGURE 14.3 Schematic representation of nanoparticals as a DNA carrier and their process of gene transfer.

the surface of gold and are simple to covalently connect. This techniques have the substantial drawback of requiring multistep surface functionalization, followed by conjugation with cationic moieties throughout the synthesis process. This reduces the effectiveness of these gene carriers by producing a heterogeneous mixture of polyelectrolyte complexes. Gold nanoparticles functionalized with single-stranded DNA were created by Mirkin et al., and they have shown exceptional gene transport efficiency. These nanoparticles performed better in terms of repression of gene expression, binding affinity for target DNA, immunity to nuclease, and cell toxicity than antisense DNA delivered by Lipofectamine or Cytofectin [74]. Since their discovery in 1991, carbon nanotubes (CNTs) have been the subject of intense research for potential biomedical applications. CNTs are rolled-up graphene layers that are arranged into one-dimensional tubes with lengths ranging from hundreds of nanometers to tens of microns. Surface functionalization of single-walled CNTs with cationic glycopolymers was seen when they were used as an in-vitro gene transfer method. Because of their luminosity, QDs are being employed for in-vivo cancer targeting and diagnostics, fluorescent probes for living cells, and other applications that are attracting attention. One of the most effective methods for delivering genes is using them as siRNA carriers. The QDs are designed to generate a strong and consistent fluorescent signal for intracellular siRNA imaging. Amphiphilic PEI derivatives (amPEIs) were created for the encapsulation of QDs [75]. Inorganic nanoparticles are now being researched for effective gene delivery, and numerous experts are anticipated to present examples of their development. The following areas need to be created and worked on: (1) creation of novel nanomaterials for efficient gene delivery; (2) analysis of critical structure–property relationships on cytotoxicity and transfection productivity; (3) longevity studies; and (4) in-vivo experimental research. The synthesis of nanoparticles using soft materials, like as hydrogels, has the potential to advance gene delivery [76].

14.6 Ethical concerns of gene therapy

Gene therapy involves editing and modifying the natural design of DNA, which poses some concerns. There is a certain group of thinkers, which might approve and encourage using science and technology to alter and "handpick" desirable traits, or genes, in our DNA; other thinker's might oppose this unorthodox method of curing diseases. Others will argue that letting the disease run its course is the best option as it does not retaliate against various aspects such as religious beliefs and practices and side effects of the treatment. This conflict of interest gives rise to several ethical concerns. These ethical concerns are one of the several hurdles that must be overcome to make advancements in medicine.

Patients receiving SCGT for conditions like CF or DMD have therapeutic genes added to their somatic cells [77]. Lymphocytes were taken from the patient's body and grown in culture in the first clinical gene therapy carried out by W. French Anderson and his colleagues at the NIH on a 4-year-old girl with SCID brought on by the absence of the gene for ADA enzyme [78]. Then, using a retroviral vector LNL6, a functional cDNA was introduced into these lymphocytes and returned to the patient's body [14]. Nevertheless, since these lymphocytes are not immortal, they will have to be periodically replaced by new genetically modified lymphocytes [79]. A solution is adding the gene for ADA to the cells at embryonic stages. Contrary to SCGT, human GGT, also known as HGLGT or human germline genome modification, modifies the DNA of human germ cells rather than somatic cells in order to avoid the development of a certain hereditary disease in future generations [80]. This method carries risks of its own. This genetic modification is essentially an alteration in the gene that may result in unforeseen adverse effects, with or without the originally intended therapeutic changes. A majority of scientists support gene therapy using somatic cells; however, it is still debatable whether or not to change embryonic stem cells, which are formed from an embryo, and embryonic germ cells, which are derived from fetal primordial germ cells [81].

A few Chinese researchers took it a step further; they used embryonic cells and modified the DNA using CRISPR-Cas9 technology. Another group of Chinese researchers, to introduce HIV resistance by incorporating the CCR5 gene, successfully modified only 4 out of the 26 embryos. This was not a good ratio considering an embryo is a potential life and demanded immediate measures and improvement of the technique. The attention brought by these publications led to several countries approving experimentation on embryonic cells. While Japan and the United Kingdom were on board, the American research groups remained orthodox. They held off testing on embryonic cells in the hopes of coming across some other way [77].

The origin, technique of development, and usage of embryonic stem cells or embryonic germ cells raise ethical and moral concerns about this approach. What extremities are we willing to meet in the name of science? The control and usage of information gained from genetic testing pose another ethical concern for us. How much and what kind of information should be allowed to the public, employees, insurers, and patients need to be discussed, and rules must be set for the same. Maintenance of the privacy of the patient's results can turn out to be challenging, as employers and medical or life insurers have a stake in knowing the medical profiles of their employees and clients, respectively. This is because employers might want to know which of their workers are at high risk of genetic disorders that may affect their performance at work or whether the workplace could cause the onset of any disease. Employers often must provide insurance that will cover for medical expenses of the employees in case they become aware of any genetic predisposition toward diseases requiring expensive medical treatments. In that case, the chances of these employees getting hired will become less, or they will be denied such medical insurance. Hence, this will affect the person's chances of getting employed or receiving medical benefits, despite being efficient and skilled in his field [82]. There are several risks of invoking psychological harm upon revealing the genetic information, as they might indicate the progeny or a family member carrying a diseased gene.

Now, since a disease occurring is not guaranteed by having faulty genes and is dependent on many other factors, it is ultimately the parent's decision whether they want to continue with the pregnancy or to abort the child. Moreover, if they decide to carry the baby, and the baby develops the predicted disease, the psychological burden on the parents holds them responsible for the unfortunate outcomes. Furthermore, if they decide to abort the child before it is born, the guilt and pain of losing a child will weigh them down [82].

One of the main reasons for such strong objections toward a new method that aims at curing many diseases by targeting the root cause at the genetic level is the lack of thorough and complete understanding of what gene therapy is and what it offers. Some base their opinions on whatever information they have on their hand or have heard from some source or their beliefs and rule it out as a practical treatment course. This reason can be found to be evident in all scientific endeavors, for example, anti-vaxxers, who oppose the use of vaccines and promote and believe in baseless rumors, despite being given solid evidence of how important it is to get vaccinated.

In cases such as these, eugenics and uncertainty of safety and outcomes outweigh the purpose of the treatment. Unless and until we find concrete proof of benefits dominating the side effects, subjecting these therapies to human trials cannot be approved, since, in science, to find a solution to an inevitable conundrum, there are always different trains of thought. Everyone might not agree with each other, but issues related to ethics in medicine deal with so much more than just diseases and their prevention and cure, but also human sentiments and psychology, economic feasibility, and equal availability for the common folk.

14.7 Challenges to gene therapy

In simplest terms, gene therapy is the direct or indirect editing, deletion, or insertion of genes into the DNA. These genes cannot be introduced into the host cells; if they could, their efficacy would be far too low to be considered therapeutic. Instead, it is intended to successfully transfer the desired gene into the patient's body by delivering these genes via a genetically engineered carrier, or vector. Consequently, nonviral or viral vector delivery techniques can be used for gene therapy. Aside from the delivery of these vectors, which is difficult, this therapy also depends on careful vector selection and avoiding vector distribution to nontarget tissues.

These vectors can trigger the body's natural defense system, the immune system. These response might get detected by the body's cells and set off an immune response against them—both T-cell mediated and humoral immune response to the proteins from the viral vectors or transgene products—as they are viewed as foreign bodies by the host's body, and the immune system will try to get rid of them [83]. This would result in altered or ineffective therapeutic gene expression and may even cause side effects.

A vital incident highlighting this issue occurred in 1999 when an 18-year-old named Jesse Gelsinger was treated for ornithine trans carboxylase (OTC) deficiency. OTC is a liver enzyme involved in the urea cycle and is responsible for the breakdown and removal of nitrogen in the body. Its deficiency will lead to the excretion of excess nitrogen in the form of ammonia in the blood. In this case, Gelsinger's immune system reacted to the Ad vectors administered, and the boy died a few days later due to multiorgan failure [84]. In viral vectors, the infectious genetic material is replaced with the therapeutic genes, whereas in nonviral vectors, circular DNA (plasmids) with therapeutic genes incorporated is used. The latter method produces less severe side effects and degeneration of the modified DNA.

In protein replacement gene therapy, antibodies that neutralize the therapeutic genes are produced for patients in whom an essential protein is deficient or absent. One other challenge that arises using viral vectors is nonspecificity. Since viruses can affect more than one type of cell due to a lack of specificity, they may infect cells other than the targeted ones. This may result in a new disease while curing the intended one [83].

As we know, the infectious part of the virus is the genetic material, either the RNA or the DNA. Sometimes, it may so happen that the altered viral vectors introduced into the body regain their ability to cause diseases (as recombinant viruses can produce infectious parental viruses if the therapeutic gene is somehow removed). If the new genes get inserted at the wrong position in the DNA or if the DNA is incorrectly altered, it may lead to uncontrolled growth and multiplication of cells, causing cancer. Tumor suppressor genes and oncogenes control cancer—a decrease in the tumor suppressor genes and an increase in the expression of oncogenes will result in cancer. This possible insertional mutagenesis or induced oncogenicity can be seen as a significant threat. An attempt was made at treating Wiskott–Aldrich syndrome, a disease caused due to mutation in the WAS gene responsible for the production of WAS proteins or WASp, which signals cells to adhere to other cells and tissues and form clots [85]. The treatment used a γ-retrovirus, and the result was seven in nine patients had developed leukemia [86]. There are challenges about the cost-efficiency of the treatment as well. Gene therapy involves incorporating several methods and technologies, as discussed in the previous section, such as electroporation, sonoporation, microinjection, magnetofection, and photoporation, whose equipment and inventory may prove to be costly for trials and testing [3]. The International Summit on Human Gene Editing, held in DC, raised issues like inaccurate or incomplete gene edition, difficulty in predicting adverse effects, inability to reverse the treatment, implications of passing on to future generations, and ethical considerations of intended manipulation of the DNA and, hence, also the human evolution.

The organizing committee of the international summit concluded the following:

1. Basic and intensive preclinical research, keeping in mind the biology of the embryos and germline cells, technologies for gene editing, sequence, benefits, and potential threats and risks.

2. It would be dangerous to advance germline cell gene therapy until all safety and efficacy concerns have been addressed and there is widespread social consensus regarding the necessity of this treatment.
3. Ultimately, each country is free to regulate activities under its jurisdiction, and the international community must aim to establish standard norms and prevent improper or unacceptable activities [87].

14.8 A summary of progress and prospects of gene therapy

It has been a desire in the medicine field to be able to alter precise locations in the human genome ever since it was discovered that genes are the fundamental unit of inheritance. In 1990, the NIH approved the first case of gene therapy for SCID, bringing attention to the potential future use of genes for therapeutic purposes. Numerous therapies have been accepted, started, or finished since that time. Gene therapy is now possible because of genetics and bioengineering, which have made it possible to employ vectors (or carriers) to transfer extrachromosomal material to target cells. Gene therapy kills cells by introducing killer genes, replaces dysfunctional or damaged genes with good ones, and inhibits gene expression. Additionally, SNPs account for 90% of all variations, demonstrating that genetic diversity is produced daily by changes in the nucleotide sequence. SNPs offer a high-density biological identifier that can be used to locate genes linked to human disease. Familial disorders are caused by many gene variants that are passed down to offspring (known as heritable or germline mutations) and persist in particular human lineages. Innovative strategies for preventing the transmission of dangerous defects from parent to child have become more popular as a result of the prevalence of genetic diseases. SCGT, GGT, in-vivo gene therapy, and ex-vivo gene therapy are now categories for gene therapy procedures based on the cell type involved in the process. During early embryonic development, when the mutation is present in a small number of embryonic cells, GGT has the ability to transform disease-causing mutations into wild-type variants. Somatic gene therapy refers to experimental gene therapy procedures that treat people's damaged somatic tissues or organs. Today, a wide range of diseases, including cancer, cardiovascular, monogenic, neurological, ophthalmic, and metabolic problems, are treated with gene therapy. The use of GGT to repair mtDNA mutations, which if left untreated may result in a wide range of chronic, irreversible disorders in both children and adults, is on the rise. Today, gene therapy is also utilized to repair DNA double strand breaks brought on by stress from the environment or errors in DNA replication during the S phase of the cell cycle. Numerous new prospects for the management and treatment of previously incurable diseases are now available because of recent advancements in gene therapy techniques. Gene delivery techniques are vital for employing gene therapy to cure human genetic illnesses. Gene therapy is only effective if the genetic material is successfully incorporated into the cell's nucleus. The capacity for viruses to stick to their hosts and effectively transfer their genetic material into the host cell is a natural trait. HSV, LV, Ad, and AAV are a few examples of viral vectors that have demonstrated efficacy and safety in delivering drugs. The immunogenicity, cytotoxicity, and insertional mutagenesis—the ectopic integration of viral DNA into chromosomes—of viral vectors are just a few of their downsides. The creation of nonviral systems is the result of these limitations. Physical nonviral systems include plasmids, DNA bombardants, electroporation, hydrodynamic ultrasound, and magnetofection (chemical: cationic lipids, different cationic polymers, and lipid polymers). Nonviral vectors have a far lower immunogenicity and are less likely to result in homologous recombination or insertional mutagenesis after being taken up by the cells. Their clinical usefulness is restricted by low transfection efficiency, which is brought about by nonspecific vector uptake by epithelial barriers and extracellular matrix as well as poor transport into therapeutic target cells. Since gene therapy entails changing the DNA of a patient's inherent genetic makeup, it raises ethical questions in the eyes of some. One of the many challenges that must be solved in order to develop medicine is these ethical issues. As an illustration, HGLGT, which modifies the DNA of human germ cells rather than somatic cells to prevent the disease in future generations, is not without danger. Eugenics and the uncertainty of safety and results trump the treatment's original intended goal in situations like these. Human trials for these medicines cannot be permitted until there is clear evidence that the benefits outweigh the side effects. Issues related to medical ethics deal with much more than just diseases and their prevention and treatment because there are often divergent schools of thought in science about a particular conundrum and people may not agree with one another. Instead, they also take into account human sentiments, economic viability, and equal accessibility for the general public. The goal of this chapter is to discuss the ethical concerns associated with genome editing, while highlighting the many types of gene therapies and vectors use.

References

[1] Susman M. Genes: definition and structure. eLS. Wiley; 2001.

[2] Wu H, Chaudhary AK, Mahato RI. Gene therapy. Pharmaceutical biotechnology: fundamentals and applications. Springer International Publishing; 2019. p. 323–55.

[3] Cring MR, Sheffield VC. Gene therapy and gene correction: targets, progress, and challenges for treating human diseases. Gene Ther 2022;3–12 Springer Nature.

[4] Paul A, Collins MG, Lee HY. Gene therapy: the next-generation therapeutics and their delivery approaches for neurological disorders. Front Genome Ed 2022;4.

[5] Vaishnav ED, de Boer CG, Molinet J, Yassour M, Fan L, Adiconis X, et al. The evolution, evolvability and engineering of gene regulatory DNA. Nature. 2022;603(7901):455–63.

[6] Valeur E, Guéret SM, Adihou H, Gopalakrishnan R, Lemurell M, Waldmann H, et al. Neue Modalitäten für schwierige Zielstrukturen in der Wirkstoffentwicklung. Angew Chem 2017;129(35):10428–59.

[7] Barua S., Rege K., Meldrum D., Voelkel-Johnson C., Dai L., Sierks M. Enhancement of polymer-mediated gene expression using chemotherapeutic modulators of intracellular trafficking and cell cycle progression; 2011.

[8] Epidemiology of Genetic Diseases in the India 2022—Google Search [Internet]. [cited 2023 Feb 5]. https://www.google.com/search? q = Epidemiology + of + Genetic + Diseases + in + the + India + 2022&rlz = 1C1ONGR_enIN1022IN1022&oq = Epidemiology + of + Genetic + Diseases + in + the + India + 2022&aqs = chrome.69 i57j33i22i29i30.8034j0j15&sourceid = chrome&ie = UTF-8.

[9] Angural A, Spolia A, Mahajan A, Verma V, Sharma A, Kumar P, et al. Review: understanding rare genetic diseases in low resource regions like Jammu and Kashmir – India. Front Genet 2020;11.

[10] Sivasubbu S, Scaria V. Genomics of rare genetic diseases-experiences from India. Hum Genomics 2019;14(1):52.

[11] Misra S. Human gene therapy: a brief overview of the genetic revolution. J Assoc Phys India 2013;61 (2):127–33.

[12] Rossidis AC, Stratigis JD, Chadwick AC, Hartman HA, Ahn NJ, Li H, et al. In utero CRISPR-mediated therapeutic editing of metabolic genes. Nat Med 2018;24(10):1513–18.

[13] Wolf DP, Mitalipov PA, Mitalipov SM. Principles of and strategies for germline gene therapy. Nature Medicine 2019; Nature Publishing Group.

[14] Gonçalves GAR, Paiva R, de MA. Gene therapy: advances, challenges and perspectives. Einstein (Sao Paulo, Braz) 2017;369–75.

[15] Kaur S, Ali A, Ahmad U, Siahbalaei Y, Pandey AK, Singh B. Role of single nucleotide polymorphisms (SNPs) in common migraine. Egypt J Neurol Psychiatr Neurosurg 2019;55(1).
[16] Vallejos-Vidal E, Reyes-Cerpa S, Rivas-Pardo JA, Maisey K, Yáñez JM, Valenzuela H, et al. Single-nucleotide polymorphisms (SNP) mining and their effect on the tridimensional protein structure prediction in a set of immunity-related expressed sequence tags (EST) in Atlantic Salmon (Salmo salar). Front Genet 2020;10.
[17] Martínez T, Wright N, López-Fraga M, Jiménez AI, Pañeda C. Silencing human genetic diseases with oligonucleotide-based therapies. Hum Genet 2013;132(5):481–93.
[18] Varela MA, Curtis HJ, Douglas AGL, Hammond SM, O'Loughlin AJ, Sobrido MJ, et al. Transfer of genetic therapy across human populations: molecular targets for increasing patient coverage in repeat expansion diseases. Eur J Hum Genet 2016;24(2) [Internet]. 2015 May 20 [cited 2023 Feb 5];24(2):271–6. https://www.nature.com/articles/ejhg201594.
[19] Genovese P, Schiroli G, Escobar G, di Tomaso T, Firrito C, Calabria A, et al. Targeted genome editing in human repopulating haematopoietic stem cells. Nature. 2014;510(7504):235–40.
[20] Horvath P., Barrangou R. CRISPR/Cas, the immune system of bacteria and archaea [Internet]. Available from: http://science.sciencemag.org/.
[21] Kim S, Broströmer E, Xing D, Jin J, Chong S, Ge H, et al. Probing allostery through DNA. Science (1979) 2013;339(6121):816–19.
[22] Tabebordbar M, Zhu K, Cheng JKW, Chew WL, Widrick JJ, Yan WX, et al. In vivo gene editing in dystrophic mouse muscle and muscle stem cells. Science (1979) 2016;351(6271):407–11.
[23] Liu R, Paxton WA, Choe S, Macdonald ME, Stuhlmann H. Homozygous defect in HIV-1 coreceptor accounts for resistance of some multiply-exposed individuals to HIV-1 infection. Cell 1996;.
[24] Haworth KG, Peterson CW, Kiem HP. CCR5-edited gene therapies for HIV cure: closing the door to viral entry. Cytotherapy 2017;19:1325–38 Elsevier B.V.
[25] Wolf DP, Mitalipov N, Mitalipov S. Mitochondrial replacement therapy in reproductive medicine. Trends Mol Med 2015;21:68–76 Elsevier Ltd.
[26] Tachibana M, Amato P, Sparman M, Woodward J, Sanchis DM, Ma H, et al. Towards germline gene therapy of inherited mitochondrial diseases. Nature 2013;493(7434):627–31.
[27] Lee HS, Ma H, Juanes RC, Tachibana M, Sparman M, Woodward J, et al. Rapid mitochondrial DNA segregation in primate preimplantation embryos precedes somatic and germline bottleneck. Cell Rep 2012;1(5):506–15.
[28] Kang E, Wu J, Gutierrez NM, Koski A, Tippner-Hedges R, Agaronyan K, et al. Mitochondrial replacement in human oocytes carrying pathogenic mitochondrial DNA mutations. Nature 2016;540(7632):270–5.
[29] Paull D, Emmanuele V, Weiss KA, Treff N, Stewart L, Hua H, et al. Nuclear genome transfer in human oocytes eliminates mitochondrial DNA variants. Nature 2013;493(7434):632–7.
[30] Alikani M, Fauser BCJ, García-Valesco JA, Simpson JL, Johnson MH. First birth following spindle transfer for mitochondrial replacement therapy: hope and trepidation. Reproductive BioMedicine Online 2017;333–6 Elsevier Ltd.
[31] Gammage PA, Viscomi C, Simard ML, Costa ASH, Gaude E, Powell CA, et al. Genome editing in mitochondria corrects a pathogenic mtDNA mutation in vivo. Nat Med 2018;24(11):1691–5.
[32] Bacman SR, Kauppila JHK, Pereira CV, Nissanka N, Miranda M, Pinto M, et al. MitoTALEN reduces mutant mtDNA load and restores tRNAAla levels in a mouse model of heteroplasmic mtDNA mutation. Nat Med 2018;24(11):1696–700.
[33] Kosicki M, Tomberg K, Bradley A. Repair of double-strand breaks induced by CRISPR–Cas9 leads to large deletions and complex rearrangements. Nat Biotechnol 2018;36(8):765–71.
[34] Yusa K, Rashid ST, Strick-Marchand H, Varela I, Liu PQ, Paschon DE, et al. Targeted gene correction of alpha 1-antitrypsin deficiency in induced pluripotent stem cells. Nature 2011;478(7369):391–4.
[35] α1-antitrypsin deficiency in induced pluripotent stem cells. Nature 2011;478(7369):391–4.
[36] Suzuki K, Yu C, Qu J, Li M, Yao X, Yuan T, et al. Targeted gene correction minimally impacts whole-genome mutational load in human-disease-specific induced pluripotent stem cell clones. Cell Stem Cell 2014;15(1):31–6.
[37] Schwank G, Koo BK, Sasselli V, Dekkers JF, Heo I, Demircan T, et al. Functional repair of CFTR by CRISPR/Cas9 in intestinal stem cell organoids of cystic fibrosis patients. Cell Stem Cell 2013;13(6):653–8.
[38] Kowalczykowski SC. An overview of the molecular mechanismsof recombinational DNA repair. Cold spring harbor perspectives in biology, 7. Cold Spring Harbor Laboratory Press;; 2015.

[39] Spies M, Fishel R. Mismatch repair during homologous and homeologous recombination. Cold Spring Harb Perspect Biol 2015;7(3).

[40] Chen JM, Cooper DN, Chuzhanova N, Férec C, Patrinos GP. Gene conversion: mechanisms, evolution and human disease. Nat Rev Genet 2007;762–75.

[41] O'Connor DM, Boulis NM. Gene therapy for neurodegenerative diseases. Trends in molecular medicine 2015;504–12 Elsevier Ltd.

[42] Sudhakar V, Richardson RM. Gene therapy for neurodegenerative diseases Springer New York LLC Neurotherapeutics, 16. 2019. p. 166–75.

[43] Rafii MS, Tuszynski MH, Thomas RG, Barba D, Brewer JB, Rissman RA, et al. Adeno-associated viral vector (serotype 2)-nerve growth factor for patients with Alzheimer disease a randomized clinical trial. JAMA Neurol 2018;75(7):834–41.

[44] MacDonald ME ACDM. A novel gene containing a trinucleotide repeat that is expanded and unstable on Huntington's disease chromosomes. The Huntington's disease collaborative research group. Cell. 1993;72(6):971–83.

[45] Yamamoto A, Lucas JJ, Hen R. Reversal of neuropathology and motor dysfunction in a conditional model of Huntington's disease. Cell 2000.

[46] McBride JL, Pitzer MR, Boudreau RL, Dufour B, Hobbs T, Ojeda SR, et al. Preclinical safety of RNAi- mediated HTT suppression in the rhesus macaque as a potential therapy for Huntington's disease. Mol Ther 2011;19(12):2152–62.

[47] Grondin R, Kaytor MD, Ai Y, Nelson PT, Thakker DR, Heisel J, et al. Six-month partial suppression of Huntingtin is well tolerated in the adult rhesus striatum. Brain 2012;135(4):1197–209.

[48] Miniarikova J, Zanella I, Huseinovic A, van der Zon T, Hanemaaijer E, Martier R, et al. Design, characterization, and lead selection of therapeutic miRNAs targeting Huntingtin for development of gene therapy for Huntington's disease. Mol Ther Nucleic Acids 2016;5:e297.

[49] Miniarikova J, Zimmer V, Martier R, Brouwers CC, Pythoud C, Richetin K, et al. AAV5-miHTT gene therapy demonstrates suppression of mutant huntingtin aggregation and neuronal dysfunction in a rat model of Huntington's disease. Gene Ther 2017;24(10):630–9.

[50] Thein SL. The molecular basis of β-thalassemia. Cold Spring Harb Perspect Med 2013;3(5).

[51] Reticulocytes T., David Heywood J., Karon M., Weissman S. Amino acids: incorporation into α-and β- chains of hemoglobin by normal and. Source: Science, New Series, vol. 146; 1964.

[52] Telen MJ, Malik P, Vercellotti GM. Therapeutic strategies for sickle cell disease: towards a multi-agent approach. Nat Rev Drug Discov 2019;139–58 Nature Publishing Group.

[53] Finer M, Glorioso J. A brief account of viral vectors and their promise for gene therapy. Gene Ther 2017;1–2 Nature Publishing Group.

[54] Felt SA, Grdzelishvili VZ. Ecent advances in vesicular stomatitis virus-based oncolytic virotherapy: a 5-year update. J Gen Virol 2017;2895–911 Microbiology Society.

[55] Lasaro MO, Ertl HCJ. New insights on adenovirus as vaccine vectors. Mol Ther 2009;1333–9 Nature Publishing Group.

[56] Zak DE, Andersen-Nissen E, Peterson ER, Sato A, Hamilton MK, Borgerding J, et al. Merck Ad5/HIV induces broad innate immune activation that predicts CD8 + T-cell responses but is attenuated by preexisting Ad5 immunity. Proc Natl Acad Sci U S A 2012;109(50):E3503–12.

[57] Quinn KM, da Costa A, Yamamoto A, Berry D, Lindsay RWB, Darrah PA, et al. Comparative analysis of the magnitude, quality, phenotype, and protective capacity of simian immunodeficiency virus gag-specific CD8 + T cells following human-, simian-, and chimpanzee-derived recombinant adenoviral vector immunization. J Immunol 2013;190(6):2720–35.

[58] Brown BD, Venneri MA, Zingale A, Sergi LS, Naldini L. Endogenous microRNA regulation suppresses transgene expression in hematopoietic lineages and enables stable gene transfer. Nat Med 2006;12(5):585–91.

[59] Majowicz A, Maczuga P, Kwikkers KL, van der Marel S, van Logtenstein R, Petry H, et al. Mir-142-3p target sequences reduce transgene-directed immunogenicity following intramuscular adeno-associated virus 1 vector-mediated gene delivery. J Gene Med 2013;15(6–7):219–32.

[60] Hanlon KS, Kleinstiver BP, Garcia SP, Zaborowski MP, Volak A, Spirig SE, et al. High levels of AAV vector integration into CRISPR-induced DNA breaks. Nat Commun 2019;10(1).

[61] Naldini L., Blomer U., Gallay P., Ory D., Mulligan R., Gage F.H., et al. In vivo gene delivery and stable transduction of nondividing cells by a lentiviral vector [Internet]. http://www.sciencemag.org.

[62] Cavalieri V, Baiamonte E. Iacono M lo. Non-primate lentiviral vectors and their applications in gene therapy for ocular disorders. Viruses 2018; MDPI AG.
[63] Herweijer H, Wolff JA. Progress and prospects: naked DNA gene transfer and therapy. Gene Ther 2003;453–8.
[64] Al-Dosari MS, Gao X. Nonviral gene delivery: principle, limitations, and recent progress. AAPS J 2009;671–81.
[65] Geboers B, Scheffer HJ, Graybill PM, Ruarus AH, Nieuwenhuizen S, Puijk RS, et al. High-voltage electrical pulses in oncology: irreversible electroporation, electrochemotherapy, gene electrotransfer, electrofusion, and electroimmunotherapy. Radiology 2020;254–72 Radiological Society of North America Inc.
[66] Sitta J, Howard CM. Applications of ultrasound-mediated drug delivery and gene therapy. Int J Mol Sci 2021; MDPI.
[67] Li SD, Huang L. Non-viral is superior to viral gene delivery. J Contr Rel 2007;181–3.
[68] Herweijer H, Wolff JA. Gene therapy progress and prospects: hydrodynamic gene delivery. Gene Ther 2007;99–107.
[69] Luiz MT, Dutra JAP, Tofani LB, de Araújo JTC, di Filippo LD, Marchetti JM, et al. Targeted Liposomes: a nonviral gene delivery system for cancer therapy. Pharmaceutics 2022; MDPI.
[70] Buck J, Grossen P, Cullis PR, Huwyler J, Witzigmann D. Lipid-Based DNA therapeutics-hallmarks of non-viral gene delivery [Internet]. 2019. http://www.lib.ed.ac.uk.
[71] Jones CH, Chen CK, Ravikrishnan A, Rane S, Pfeifer BA. Overcoming nonviral gene delivery barriers: perspective and future. Mol Pharm 2013;4082–98.
[72] Thapa RK, Sullivan MO. Gene delivery by peptide-assisted transport. Current opinion in biomedical engineering 2018;71–82 Elsevier B.V.
[73] Nicolson G.L. Mitochondrial dysfunction and chronic disease: treatment with natural supplements.
[74] Integrative Medicine. 2014;13.
[75] Tarvirdipour S, Skowicki M, Schoenenberger CA, Palivan CG. Peptide-assisted nucleic acid delivery systems on the rise. Int J Mol Sci 2021; MDPI.
[76] Hurst SJ, Lytton-Jean AKR, Mirkin CA, Maximizing DNA. Loading on a range of gold nanoparticle sizes. Anal Chem 2006;78(24):8313–18.
[77] Yang W., Guo W., Zhang T., Yang W., Su L., Fang L., et al. Synthesis of aqueous AgInS/ZnS@PEI as self-indicating nonviral vector for plasmid DNA self-tracking delivery corresponding authors ABSTRACTI I I I [Internet]. http://www.rsc.org/materialsB.
[78] Kai D, Liow SS, Loh XJ. Biodegradable polymers for electrospinning: towards biomedical applications. Mater Sci Eng C 2015;45:659–70.
[79] Scheller EL, Krebsbach PH. Gene therapy: design and prospects for craniofacial regeneration. J Dental Res 2009;585–96.
[80] Miller AD. Retroviral vectors: from cancer viruses to therapeutic tools. Human Gene Therapy 2014;989–94 Mary Ann Liebert Inc.
[81] Resnik DB, Langer PJ. Human germline gene therapy reconsidered Mary Ann Liebert, Inc Human gene therapy, 12. 2001.
[82] Julia. Published by nuffield council on bioethics 28 bedford square London WC1B 3EG [Internet]. 2000. http://www.nuffieldfoundation.org/bioethics.
[83] Penticuff J. Ethical issues in genetic therapy.
[84] Zhou HS, Liu DP, Liang CC. Challenges and strategies: the immune responses in gene therapy. Med Res Rev 2004;748–61.
[85] Wirth T, Parker N, Ylä-Herttuala S. History of gene therapy. Gene 2013;525(2):162–9.
[86] Institute of Allergy N, Diseases I. Wiskott-Aldrich syndrome.
[87] Du X, Wang J, Zhou Q, Zhang L, Wang S, Zhang Z, et al. Advanced physical techniques for gene delivery based on membrane perforation. Drug Deliv 2018;25(1):1516–25.

Index

Note: Page numbers followed by "*f*" and "*t*" refer to figures and tables, respectively.

B

D

H

J

K

L

M

Q

R

U

V